D1244035

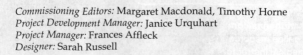

Commissioning Editors: Margaret Macdonald, Timothy Horne
Project Development Manager: Janice Urquhart
Project Manager: Frances Affleck
Designer: Sarah Russell

Essentials of
Pathology

SAUNDERS
An imprint of Elsevier Science Limited

The right of Neville Woolf, Andrew Wotherspoon and
Martin Young to be identified as authors of this work has been
asserted by them in accordance with the Copyright,
Designs and Patents Act 1988

First published 2002

ISBN 07020 23949

British Library Cataloguing in Publication Data
A catalogue record for this book is available from the British
Library

Library of Congress Cataloging in Publication Data
A catalog record for this book is available from the Library of
Congress

Note
Medical knowledge is constantly changing. As new
information becomes available, changes in treatment,
procedures, equipment and the use of drugs become necessary.
The authors and the publishers have taken care to ensure that
the information given in this text is accurate and up to date.
However, readers are strongly advised to confirm that the
information, especially with regard to drug usage, complies
with the latest legislation and standards of practice.

Printed in China

The
publisher's
policy is to use
**paper manufactured
from sustainable forests**

Essentials of
Pathology

Neville Woolf
PhD FRCPath FRCS
Faculty Tutor in Clinical Sciences,
Royal Free and University College Medical School
of University College London,
London, UK

Andrew Wotherspoon
MB BCh
Consultant Histopathologist,
Department of Histopathology,
Royal Marsden Hospital, London

Martin Young
BSc MRCOG MRCPath
Consultant Histo/Cytopathologist,
Department of Cellular Pathology,
St George's Healthcare NHS Trust, London

SAUNDERS

Edinburgh • London • New York • Philadelphia • St Louis •
Sydney • Toronto • 2002

Preface

....

The study of pathology underlies the ability to understand, diagnose and treat in all aspects of clinical medicine. However the amount of information is ever increasing, with more detailed appreciation of the underlying sub-cellular mechanisms and genetic abnormalities associated with various disease entities. Although it is impossible for each health care professional to have a complete and detailed understanding of all pathology, it is essential that they all have a working understanding of general pathological mechanisms and a superficial knowledge of the pathology of the commoner diseases within each organ.

This is a compact book which presents essential facts in a way that we hope is easy to digest. It is based on the more detailed *Pathology: Basic and Systemic* by Neville Woolf. While it contains the most important facts from that book, the text is shortened for quick reference and revision.

The format and size make this a valuable, portable reference which allows pathological features to be interpreted within the more modern, integrated curriculum. In this setting, pathology is learned in the context of clinical medicine rather than as the isolated and rather tedious basic scientific subject that some members of the health professions have considered this subject in the past.

A. Wotherspoon
London

Contents

BASIC PATHOLOGY   1

1 The nature of pathology   *3*

2 Cell injury and its manifestations   *10*

3 Cell and tissue death   *22*

4 Acute inflammation I: Introduction   *26*

5 Acute inflammation II: Cellular events   *30*

6 Factors that modify the inflammatory reaction   *43*

7 The natural history of acute inflammation I:
Healing   *49*

8 The natural history of acute inflammation II:
Wound healing   *53*

9 The natural history of acute inflammation III:
Chronicity   *62*

10 The immune system   *67*

11 Disorders related to the immune system   *84*

12 Autoimmune disease   *94*

13 Transplantation and the major histocompatibility
complex   *99*

14 Granulomatous inflammation   *108*

15 Some specific granulomatous disorders   *112*

16 Amyloid and the amyloidoses   *123*

17 General pathology of viral infection   *129*

18 Disorders of blood flow: a basis   *141*

19 Ischaemia and infarction   *151*

20 Abnormal accumulations of fluid and disturbances of blood distribution *154*

21 Pigmentation and heterotropic calcification *159*

22 Neoplasia: disorders of cell proliferation and differentiation *164*

23 Non-neoplastic disturbances in cell growth and proliferation *167*

24 Cell proliferation and differentiation in relation to neoplasia *171*

25 Relationship of neoplastic cells with their environment: tumour spread *175*

26 Effects of neoplasms on the host *184*

27 Effect of the host on neoplasms *190*

28 Oncogenesis and the molecular biology of cancer *193*

29 Oncogenesis *203*

30 Genetic disorders *214*

31 Single gene defects *221*

SYSTEMIC PATHOLOGY *229*

32 The cardiovascular system *231*

33 The respiratory system *282*

34 The gastrointestinal system *330*

35 The liver, biliary system and exocrine pancreas *410*

36 The kidney *466*

37 The lower urinary tract *514*

38 The male reproductive system *523*

39 The female reproductive system *551*

40 The endocrine system *613*

41 The haemopoietic system *649*

42 The lymphoreticular system *704*

43 The skin *750*

44 The skeletal system *801*

45 The nervous system *863*

46 Special senses *939*

Index *955*

Basic pathology

The nature of pathology

··

SURGICAL PATHOLOGY, CYTOLOGY AND MORBID ANATOMY

General pathology is the study of the functional and structural changes that occur in cells and tissues as a result of direct damage by or reaction to a wide variety of events. Generally this involves assessment of:

- the cause of the disease (**aetiology**)
- the mechanism by which this causative agent induces changes in the cell/tissue (**pathogenesis**)
- the morphological changes themselves

Study of the pathology of diseases is the synthesis of several different procedures:

- surgical pathology
- cytopathology
- morbid anatomy

using an array of laboratory techniques:

- microscopy (the cornerstone of all diagnostic histopathology)
- histochemistry
- immunohistochemistry
- electron microscopy
- molecular pathology.

Surgical pathology

This is the study of tissue taken from live patients for the purposes of establishing a diagnosis. Examination of the biopsy/excision material gives

- tissue diagnosis
- prognostic information
- insights into aetiology and pathogenesis.

Paraffin sections

This is the cornerstone of the work of a histopathology lab-oratory. Embedding tissue within paraffin wax gives the tissue a rigidity that will allow thin (3–5 µm) sections to be cut. These can then be stained and examined under a light microscope.

The paraffin block and the cut sections are permanent and may be kept indefinitely. Paraffin sections provide the best material for histological assessment; processing of tissue for paraffin sections takes 24–48 hours from the removal of the tissue from the patient to production of a written report with the diagnosis. Several steps are required.

Fixation This can be achieved by a variety of solutions; one of the most widely used is formalin. Fixation time is dependent on the size of the specimen and generally takes 8–24 hours with smaller biopsies taking the shortest time. Whole organs may require to be opened (if hollow) or sliced to aid penetration of formalin into the tissue. Delay in or inadequate fixation results in tissue autolysis and degenera-tion and gives suboptimal histology which in extreme cases may render the sample unassessable.

Decalcification Tissue specimens containing bone need to be softened by decalcification. The time required for this is determined by the size and hardness of the specimen and by the decalcifying medium used.

Tissue selection This is performed by the pathologist who examines the macroscopic appearance of the tissue sample and selects those pieces required for microscopic examina-tion.

Tissue processing This is performed by an automated machine which takes the tissue through a variety of chemi-cal steps. In many laboratories this process is run overnight.

Paraffin embedding The tissue is placed within a block of paraffin wax.

Section cutting Thin sections are cut by skilled technicians using a microtome that passes the paraffin block over a sharp blade. These sections are then placed on a glass microscope slide.

Section staining   The slide upon which the section has been attached is passed through a series of chemicals and stains to colour the section. In general the routine stain used for the initial assessment of histological slides is performed using a mixture of haematoxylin and eosin (H&E). The haematoxylin stains nuclei blue and the eosin stains the cytoplasm and other material pink.

Frozen sections

Tissue sections for microscopy can be cut rapidly from tissue that is frozen. This technique takes 15–20 minutes and can therefore be used to give a histological assessment of tissue while the patient remains in the operating theatre under anaesthetic.

The morphology of frozen sections is generally inferior to that of paraffin sections and the amount of tissue examined is of necessity limited. Although some centres will perform frozen section assessment of all surgical pathological material the indications for frozen sections are limited to situations where the assessment of the lesion will alter immediate surgical management of the patient, e.g.

- diagnosis of a tumour
- the assessment of tumour spread (including lymph node involvement and metastasis)
- assessment of the adequacy of resection of a tumour.

Histochemistry

Different intra- or extracellular components stain differently with certain histological stains. For instance stains can be used to highlight glycogen, mucins, melanin pigment, iron/haemosiderin, calcium, reticulin fibres, argentaffin granules, amyloid and connective tissue components. These are relatively easy and cheap to perform.

Immunohistochemistry

This utilizes the ability of labelled antibodies to bind to specific antigens in tissue sections. The label can then be visualized by using a chromogen and the background tissue can be stained so the labelled cells can be viewed within the context of the tissue in which they are situated.

Many cell types express specific antigens which allows the specific identification of these cells.

Electron microscopy

This allows the detailed study of intra- and extracellular components of cells and tissues. Different cell types have different ultrastructural appearances to the cell membrane and cellular constituents.

This is useful in distinguishing some tumour types and routinely used for the examination of glomerular structure in renal biopsies.

Molecular pathology

In-situ hybdridization   Uses the ability of labelled single strands of nucleic acids to bind to the complementary strand. It may be applied to DNA or RNA, allowing the identification of particular DNA or RNA nucleic acid sequences (which may be host, bacterial or viral) in tissue sections with preservation of cell morphology for morphological localization of the signal. Radioactive or non-radioactive labelling systems may be used.

Blot techniques   These may be used to look for particular proteins, RNA or DNA following extraction from tissues:

- DNA – Southern blot
- RNA – Northern blot
- protein – Western blot.

Southern blot allows the detection of specific DNA sequences by analysis of DNA fragment sizes following digestion by endocleases (which cut DNA at sites containing specific nucleotide sequences) and gel electrophoresis of the products which separates the fragments by size. The fragments are blotted from the fragile gel on to a more durable membrane and may be hybridized with labelled DNA probes.

Polymerase chain reaction   Allows the identification of small amounts of DNA. DNA segments are amplified in quantity using a DNA polymerase and two primer segments of DNA which border the area of DNA to be amplified. As only the segment of DNA between the primers is amplified consistently in each cycle the product can be electrophoresed and the product band visualized by staining with ethydium bromide.

The reaction uses several cycles in which the reaction mixture is taken to different temperature levels:

- denaturation of double stranded DNA into single strands (94°C for 30–90 s)
- primer annealing to each single strand (55°C for 30–120 s)
- extension of primers using heat stable *taq* polymerase (72°C for 60–180 s).

Each cycle doubles the amount of DNA of the target sequence presence. Usually about 30 cycles are used which will amplify the target DNA about a billionfold.

Cytopathology

This is the morphological examination of whole single cells present in body fluids, smears/scrapes of exfoliated cell or as material aspirated from solid tissue. It is separated into two main groups:

- Gynaecological – assessment of cervical smears most of which are derived from national cervical screening services.
- Non-gynaecological – all other samples. Frequently performed for the assessment of lesions thought to be tumours.

Material is spread over a whole microscope slide (fluids are treated to concentrate the cells e.g. by centrifugation). Smears are stained using dyes that highlight nuclear and cytoplasmic detail usually by the Papanicolaou stain (if the slide has been pre-fixed in alcohol) or the May–Grunwald–Giemsa stain (for air-dried material). Some laboratories use haematoxylin and eosin for cytological preparations.

Cytopathology has the advantage of being very rapid and causing minimal trauma to the patient; disadvantages include lower specificity than histology and difficulty in sub-typing some lesions.

Morbid anatomy

The performance of an autopsy is used to determine the exact cause of death and elucidate the disease processes associated with the individual's death. In the UK and in many other countries there are two types of post-mortem.

Hospital post-mortem

Used to study the disease process in a patient in whom the cause of death is known (i.e. for whom a death certificate can be issued). It requires written consent from relatives or next of kin. Without this the autopsy is illegal. The next of kin may specify extent of examination (e.g. excluding head/brain, limited to thorax, etc.) It should not be carried out even if next of kin consent if it is believed that the deceased had expressed an objection to his body being subjected to an autopsy.

Legal post-mortem

This is initiated by the coroner (in England and Wales) or equivalent. In England and Wales it is the responsibility of the coroner to investigate deaths that are either suspected of being 'unnatural' or are considered to be natural but in which a death certificate cannot be issued.

A death certificate cannot be issued if:

- the cause of death is unnatural (including accidents, violent deaths, neglect)
- the medical practitioner did not attend the deceased in the last illness
- the medical practitioner did not see the deceased within 14 days of death
- the medical practitioner did not see the body after death.

Other cases that should be reported to the coroner include:

- deaths associated with industrial disease
- deaths occuring during medical/surgical procedures (or soon afterwards)
- when a mother dies as a result of a termination of pregnancy
- sudden or unexplained infant deaths (cot deaths)
- suicide
- death while in custody (including prison).

Deaths may be reported to the coroner by lay persons. The coroner is required to determine the identity of the deceased, the cause of death and how, where and when the death occurred. In some cases the coroner will be able to determine these facts following consultation with the medical practitioner in which case an autopsy will be unnecessary. Otherwise an autopsy will be carried out. The autopsy report is for the coroner and disclosure to other individuals requires the coroner's consent.

The coroner will hold an inquest into the death if it is determined to be unnatural. Mostly these are held without juries but enrolling a jury is at the discretion of the coroner.

Cell injury and its manifestations

....

CELL ADAPTATION

Under most circumstances cells attempt to maintain a steady state but will adapt to changing circumstances, e.g. increased functional demand. An increase in demand leads either to an increase in the size of individual cells (**hypertrophy**), an increase in the number of cells (**hyperplasia**), or both. When the demand for a function is reduced there is a decrease in cell size (**atrophy**). If the degree of change is too great to allow adaptation then some loss of normal cell structure and functions may occur correlating with **cell injury**, which may be reversible, or irreversible: **cell death**.

Maintenance of the steady state
This requires:

- preservation of normal DNA templates
- normal enzyme content
- intact membranes and transmembrane proteins
- adequate supply of oxygen and substrates.

....

TYPES OF INJURY

There are many types of injury but the reaction patterns are limited. A given degree of injury will have different effects on different cell types. Common types of injury include:

- hypoxia
- anoxia
- reoxygenation: reperfusion of acutely ischaemic tissue may have an incremental effect, possibly due to generation of oxygen free radicals
- extremes of heat or cold

- chemical agents
- immunological mechanisms (cellular or humoral)
- infectious agents
- irradiation
- nutritional deficiencies.

....

SITES OF INJURY
Nucleus

This may be altered as an inherited abnormality (e.g. alteration in chromosome number or the structure of individual chromosomes) or as an acquired abnormality associated with toxic damage and nutritional deficiencies of folic acid and vitamin B_{12}.

Toxic nuclear damage is seen in the treatment of malignant disease by chemotherapy using different types of agent e.g.:

- alkylating agents (e.g. cyclophosphamide) combine with DNA
- alkaloids (e.g. vincristine) damage the mitotic spindle.

Cell membranes

Some inherited defects of membrane structures have been identified which involve either transport or receptor defects. Acquired membrane injuries are related to complement activation or free radicals.

Complement-related membrane injury

Fixation of complement to cell surface bound antigen/antibody complexes leads to the generation of a membrane attack complex mediated by components 8 and 9 of the complement sequence. It is thought that C8 opens and shuts a transmembrane channel which causes lysis when the channel remains open.

Binding of C9 jams the channel open.

FREE RADICALS AND CELL INJURY

Free radicals are the common effector pathway of a number of different types of cell injury including:

- reperfusion injury following ischaemia
- certain drug-induced haemolytic anaemias
- paraquat poisoning
- carbon tetrachloride poisoning (associated with the generation of Cl_3^- in the smooth endoplasmic reticulum of liver cells leading to peroxidation of membrane phospholipids)
- radiation injury (caused by therapeutic irradiation)
- ageing
- oxygen toxicity
- atherogenesis.

A free radical is an atom or molecule that has a single unpaired electron in its outer orbital. These are very active and not only react with molecules within the cell membrane but often convert these to free radicals as well thus forming a positive amplification system.

Generation of free radicals can result from absorption of radiant energy, reduction of molecular oxygen giving the reactive superoxide anion O_2^-. Superoxide plays an important part in bacterial killing by neutrophil leucocytes and macrophages.

Scavenging mechanisms are present within cells to control free radical generation which is probably a common result of intracellular redox reactions. One important scavenger is **superoxide dismutase**, which results in the catalytic dismutation of the superoxide anion to hydrogen peroxide and water.

Effects of free radicals

These include:

- Peroxidation of unsaturated lipids in the cell membranes: *morphologically*, there is bleb formation on the plasma membrane; *functionally*, there is breakdown of mechanisms regulating calcium inflow and calcium

therefore accumulates as deposits in mitochondria. Peroxidation is inhibited by vitamin E and glutathione peroxidase.
- Protein and DNA damage.
- Reaction with molecules and ionic components in the intracellular water compartments.
- Reaction with components of the extracellular space.

Glycosoaminoglycans of connective tissue ground substance may be degraded by free radicals.

LYSOSOMES AND CELL INJURY

Lysosomes may be involved in disease in three ways.

1. *Storage diseases*. Inherited deficiency of a lysosomal enzyme resulting in accumulation of the normal substrate mainly within phagocytic cells but also in liver parenchymal cells, neurones, fibroblasts and renal tubular epithelial cells.

   Substances including glycogen, complex mucopolysaccharides and sphingolipids may be involved.
2. *Disruption of lysosomes*. This leads to release of intralysosomal enzymes into the cell cytoplasm. It is seen in gout (affecting neutrophils) and silicosis (affecting macrophages).

   Phagocytosis of crystalline material is associated with lysosome fusion and formation of abnormal hydrogen bonds between the particle surface and the lysosomal membrane causing rupture and spillage of enzymes into the cell cytoplasm and surrounding area.
3. *Secretion of enzymes (usually from macrophages)*.

STRESS PROTEINS AND CELL INJURY

When cells of any type are exposed to environmental stress (exemplified in the laboratory by heat) an increase occurs in a group of intracytoplasmic proteins termed the **heat shock proteins (hsp)**.

Other stresses associated with rises in hsp include fever, ischaemia, oxidant injury, infection, cancer and many chemical species (including transition metals, alcohol and various oxidants). These proteins are thought to help the cell withstand the stress and protect it from any further stresses that might occur (pre-conditioning).

Classification of stress proteins

Four main groups exist based on molecular weight and electrophoretic migration.

- **hsp 90**: binds to other proteins and regulates their activity; prevents aggregation and refolding of polypeptides
- **hsp 70**: dissociates some polymers. Binds to extended polypeptides. Has ATPase activity
- **hsp 60**: weak ATPase activity. Binds to partly folded polypeptides and helps correct folding
- **hsp 15–30**: unknown functions.

BACTERIAL TOXINS AND CELL INJURY

Classification of bacterial toxins

Divided into **exotoxins** and **endotoxins**.

Exotoxins

- Proteins secreted by a living organism which are immunogenic and usually heat labile.
- Usually target a precise intracellular process, membrane component or neurotransmitter.
- A toxoid (same compound with unimpaired immunogenicity but without toxic properties) can usually be produced from them.

Endotoxins

- Lipopolysaccharides which form part of the structure of the micro-organism and are not secreted but may be released from dead organisms.
- Weakly immunogenic and usually heat stable, they can target a range of cell types and plasma proteins.
- No toxoid can be produced.

Actions of bacterial toxins

Exotoxins

- some enter the cell by endocytosis and act as an enzyme
- commonest action is **irreversible ADP ribosylation** where ADP ribose is transferred from NAD to an intracellular protein the function of which is inhibited. Examples:

Vibrio cholerae toxin

- Causes profuse watery diarrhoea (up to 11–30 litres of stool per day).
- Effects are due to the toxin rather than the organism which does not invade the tissues, remaining in the gut lumen.
- Consists of two portions: a single A portion and a pentagonal B portion. The **A portion** enters the small gut epithelial cell and irreversibly ribosylates the G protein. This inactivates its GTPase function and the production of cAMP continues unabated. In the villous cell cAMP inhibits entry of water sodium and chloride while in the crypt it promotes the pumping out of water sodium, chloride and bicarbonate into the gut lumen. The **B portion** binds irreversibly to and activates a GM1 ganglioside receptor on the luminal aspect of the small gut intestinal cells. This receptor is functionally coupled to adenylate cyclase via a stimulatory G protein, G_s. The end result of this is production of cAMP in a controlled manner.

Diphtheria toxin

- Only strains of *Corynebacterium diphtheriae* which produce the toxin cause diphtheria.
- Toxigenicity is conferred by a bacterial virus (bacteriophage) with the gene encoding the toxin which is incorporated in the bacterial genome.
- Expression of the *tox* gene is usually controlled by a binding with a repressor protein in the presence of ferrous iron. Fall in iron concentrations results in protein production. In mutant strains, which cannot produce the repressor protein, toxin production proceeds uninfluenced by iron concentrations.

- Toxin spreads in the bloodstream and affects many organs (e.g. heart, kidneys and nervous system) while the organism remains localized to the pharynx.
- Toxin consists of two parts, one of which binds to a cell receptor while the other enters the cell and irreversibly ribosylates and inactivates the elongation factor 2 (EF-2) protein which is vital to translation of messenger RNA. Protein synthesis in the affected cell ceases.

Toxins that damage cell membranes   The toxin may act as lytic enzyme causing disruption to the plasma membrane.
- Alpha toxin of *Clostridium perfringens* acts as a lecithinase and cleaves phospholipids in the plasma membrane.
- Haemolysins of *Staphylococcus aureus*.
- Haemolysins of *Streptococcus pyogenes*.

Toxins and neurotransmission   The toxin may inhibit neurotransmission.
Clostridium botulinum
- Very toxic.
- Toxin found in food contaminated by the clostridium.
- Infection by the organism is not required, ingestion of the toxin sufficing to cause damage.
- Toxin exists in eight antigenic forms not all of which cause botulism in humans. Type A accounts for 60% of cases.
- Toxin is carried in the blood stream to peripheral neuromuscular junctions where it blocks the transmission of acetylcholine by inhibiting its release from nerve terminals resulting in flaccid paralysis of affected muscles.

Clostridium tetani
- Produces a toxin responsible for muscle spasm and contracture called tetanospasmin.
- Organisms enter the body and multiply.
- Organisms release the toxin which enters motor nerves and travels to the anterior horn cells of the spinal cord.
- Toxin blocks transmission of glycine from inhibitory interneurones.

RADIATION INJURY

Biological response to radiation

This depends on the interaction of:

- physical factors e.g. dose, character and time of administration
- chemical factors e.g. substrates for generation of free radicals
- biological factors e.g. point in cell cycle at time of irradiation.

Different organs have different sensitivity to radiation damage:

- **very high** – bone marrow, testis, ovary, growing cartilage, lens and the breast in childhood
- **high** – kidney, liver, lung, heart, growing bone, small and large intestine, thyroid, cornea, pituitary, spinal cord, growing muscle, salivary gland, brain, skin
- **intermediate** – adult bone, adult cartilage, mucosa of mouth, oesophagus, bladder
- **low** – uterus, vagina, pancreas, adrenal.

In most organs irradiation may be associated with the subsequent appearance of tumours.

Radiation effects on specific tissues

Blood vessels

In the acute phase there is dilation and increased permeability of arterioles and capillaries.

Later the endothelial cells undergo necrosis and there may be patchy necrosis of smooth muscle of arterioles. In the later stage small blood vessels may still show subendothelial accumulation of ground substance.

Secondary effects in the tissues include atrophic changes in skin associated with scarring of the sub-epidermal tissue, interstitial scarring of myocardium, ulceration of the gut, renal cortical atrophy, necrosis of white matter in the brain and spinal cord damage.

Skin

In the early stages there is erythema, loss of hair and dryness. Atrophy, blood vessel dilation, hyperkeratosis and homogenization of collagen characterizes delayed injury.

Haemopoietic/lymphoid systems

Large doses are associated with leucopenia and decreased size of lymph nodes and spleen.

Heart

Most commonly there is pericarditis followed by scarring. There may be interstitial fibrosis associated with blood vessel damage (see above).

Lung

Initially there is oedema due to increased permeability of the alveolar capillaries. After there is necrosis and desquamation of type 1 pneumocytes with type 2 cell proliferation. Damaged air spaces show hyaline membranes. Later (after 16 weeks) interstitial scarring causes restrictive lung disease.

Gastrointestinal tract

The oral mucosa shows effects similar to the skin. Salivary glands show scarring and loss of acinar tissue giving a dry mouth. In the rest of the GI tract there is loss of surface epithelium due to decreased stem cell regenerative function. In the long term, there may be strictures, chronic ulcers and fistulae.

Liver

Effects usually appear about three months after irradiation. The principal targets are the venous drainage, terminal hepatic venules and the terminal portions of some sinusoids. The endothelial cells become swollen and in some cases necrotic associated with fibrin deposition in the lumen leading to veno-occlusive disease. The end result is congestion and ultimately necrosis of the central part of the liver lobule.

Urinary tract

In the urinary bladder reduced stem cell regeneration leads to ulceration. Scarring in the deeper portions may be associated with reduced bladder capacity.

In the kidney there is vasodilation, interstitial oedema and glomerular damage leading to proteinuria. Functional recovery is the rule but after a long latent period there may be progressive scarring of glomeruli and tubule loss.

Nervous system

Both brain and spinal cord show necrosis associated with myelin loss thought to be associated with small vessel damage. Severe spinal cord damage may lead to paraplegia.

....

MORPHOLOGICAL EXPRESSIONS OF CELL INJURY

Sub-lethal cell injury

Alterations in cell volume (acute cellular oedema)

Mainly the result of breakdown of sodium and potassium transport systems causing isotonic fluid accumulation in cells leading to swelling of mitochondria (giving a granular appearance to the cytoplasm).

Intracellular oedema is associated with hypoxia but may occur with fever or in association with damage due to toxins and chemical poisons.

The normal cell has high potassium and low sodium compared with extracellular fluid which is maintained by an ATP-dependent transport system (the **sodium pump**). Injury associated with hypoxia and the other agents results in the partial failure of the sodium pump due to decreased production of ATP. Potassium diffuses out of the cell and sodium ions enter the cell. Water enters the cell with the sodium ions leading to increased cell volume.

Hypoxia   causes the following sequence of results:

- Low oxygen tension causes decreased mitochondrial phosphorylation causing a fall in ATP.
- The low ATP stimulates the enzyme **phosphofructokinase** which leads to increased anaerobic glycolysis.

- This leads to accumulation of lactate which lowers intracellular pH (morphologically this causes clumping of nuclear chromatin).
- By this time the decreased ATP will have affected the sodium pump.
- Protein production falls, associated with detachment of polysomes from the membranes of endoplasmic reticulum. At this stage the process is reversible. The cytoskeleton also appears to be affected at this stage and the plasma membrane may show blebs or the appearance of microvilli. If hypoxia continues beyond this point the degree of cell damage may reach a point at which reversal becomes impossible and the cell will die.
- Nuclear chromatin undergoes enzymatic attack. As this proceeds the nucleus becomes digested away (**karyolysis**). At this point there is ionic equilibration and other molecules can move across the cell membrane so that dyes can move into the cells and enzymes leak out. Plasma concentrations of intracellular enzymes can provide a marker of cell death (e.g. death of cardiac muscle is associated with the presence of creatinine kinase and β-hydroxybutyric acid dehydrogenase in plasma; liver cell damage is associated with elevated plasma concentrations of aspartate amino-transferase and alanine amino-transferase).

Accumulation of intracellular triglyceride (fatty change)

Fatty change is present where parenchymal cells (mostly liver, heart and kidney) contain stainable triglyceride.

Macroscopic changes

- Organs which have undergone severe fatty change are pale-yellowish brown and may feel greasy.
- In the kidney there may be yellow streaks in the cortex as fatty change tends to affect the cells of the convoluted tubule.
- The excess fat is largely derived from fat stored in adipose tissue rather than fat already present within the cell.

Fatty change in the liver   In the normal state the liver cell receives fat from two sources:

- non-esterified free fatty acid (FFA) from peripheral adipose tissue stores and released during lipolysis
- from the intestine in the form of chylomicrons. Within the liver cells FFAs are released.

Irrespective of their source FFAs are esterified to form triglyceride. Some are incorporated into phospholipid and others are incorporated into cholesterol esters.

The triglyceride within the liver cell is coupled to a lipid-acceptor protein (apoprotein) and secreted from the liver in the form of very low density lipoprotein (VLDL). Triglyceride will accumulate if there is an increase in the amount of lipid, particularly non-esterified fatty acids (NEFA) delivered to the liver or if the liver cell is unable to carry out the normal metabolism of lipid. High NEFA levels in the presence of normal liver cells is seen in:

- Starvation.
- When there is block to normal carbohydrate metabolism e.g. uncontrolled diabetes mellitus, galactosaemia and some forms of glycogen storage disease.
- Normal NEFA in the presence of injury or abnormality in the liver cells can be seen in association with anoxia associated with congestive cardiac failure, severe protein and calorie undernutrition (known as **kwashiorkor** when seen in children) and **chronic alcoholism**.
- In alcohol-induced fatty change interference with oxidation of fatty acids is likely to be the most important cause of triglyceride accumulation.
- Other chemical and bacterial toxins may cause fatty change including carbon tetrachloride, puromycin, ethionine and phosphorus.

Cell and tissue death 3

CELL DEATH

- Cell death occurs when cells cannot achieve a new steady state following environmental changes.
- It is due to breakdown of energy-dependent organized interactions between DNA, membranes and enzymes. All cellular functions cease.
- It occurs regularly under physiological as well as pathological conditions.
- Disease characteristics are often determined by the type of cell involved and the extent of cell death.

MORPHOLOGICAL CHANGES IN CELL DEATH

These are dependent upon whether enzymic digestion or protein denaturation is the dominant process.
Cytoplasmic changes:

- decrease in basophilia due to RNA and protein loss
- increased eosinophilia due to denaturation of cytoplasmic proteins
- loss of glycogen
- fragmentation and clumping of cytoplasmic contents.

Nuclear changes:

- karyolysis – gradual fading away of basophilic nuclear material
- karyorrhexis – fragmentation of nucleus. Debris phagocytosed by other cells or disappears
- pyknosis – nucleus shrinks becoming intensely basophilic.

Heterolysis

This is digestion by enzymes derived from cells other than the dying cell (e.g. neutrophil polymorph or macrophage). It may be the result of:

- endocytosis – ingestion by phagocytes of portions of dying/dead cells and the segregation of the material into phagosomes
- fusion of phagocyte lysosomes and phagosomes (forming secondary phagosomes) results in digestion of the debris.

APOPTOSIS (PROGRAMMED CELL DEATH)

Normal cell turnover implies balance between cell death and replacement by new cells. Apoptosis plays an opposite role to mitosis in regulation of the size of cellular populations. It is important in normal embryonic development (e.g. separation of digits), and differs from necrosis in that there is:

- no breakdown in supply of cellular energy
- no failure in maintenance of normal cell volume
- no plasma membrane rupture
- no associated inflammatory reaction
- energy dependence
- protein synthesis.

Morphological changes

- separation of affected cell from neighbours
- nuclear chromatin becomes condensed
- cell breaks up into membrane-bound fragments (apoptotic bodies)
- Fragments are either shed (if epithelial lining cells involved) or phagocytosed by other cells.

Mechanisms involved in apoptosis

- expression of proto-oncogene c-myc which render the cell susceptible to apoptosis
- protection from apoptosis is associated with products from genes including bcl-2, the proto-oncogene c-abl, the

LMP-1 gene of the Epstein–Barr virus and the early region gene Elb of adenovirus
- normal (wild type) tumour suppressor gene p53 initiates apoptosis after cell injury (especially double stranded DNA breaks).

....

NECROSIS

Cell death occurring in part of an organ/tissue where continuity with neighbouring viable tissue is preserved.

Coagulative necrosis
- dominant process is the denaturation of intracytoplasmic protein
- dead tissue becomes firm and slightly swollen
- tissue shows general retention of microscopic architectural pattern
- typically occurs in ischaemic injury with the exception of ischaemic injury in the brain.

Caseation necrosis
- occurs characteristically in tuberculosis
- macroscopically the tissue appears cheese-like (caseous)
- tissue appears microscopically structureless.

Liquefaction necrosis
- effect of hydrolytic enzymes is dominant factor
- macroscopically there is accumulation of protein rich semi-fluid material
- not common as a primary event except in ischaemic injury to brain
- seen as secondary event when necrotic tissue is infected by pus-forming organisms.

Traumatic fat necrosis
- mostly seen in female breast
- due to rupture of adipocytes and release of their contents
- macroscopic features: may produce hard lump
- microscopic features: numerous granular macrophages containing phagocytosed lipid; foreign body giant cells are often present.

Enzyme mediated fat necrosis
- often seen in association with acute haemorrhagic pancreatitis
- due to release of proteolytic and lipolytic enzymes.

Gangrene

Necrosis of tissues associated with superadded putrefactive necrosis due to micro-organisms (e.g. clostridial species, streptococci and bacteroides species).

Gas gangrene
- refers to rapidly spreading tissue necrosis due to proteolytic clostridia producing CO_2
- the presence of dead tissue and anaerobic conditions favour the multiplication of these organisms leading to spreading of the infection.

Ischaemic gangrene
- may be seen in the gut or in the lower limb
- in the limb it is associated with atherosclerosis of large or medium-sized arteries or in younger people it may be associated with thrombo-angiitis obliterans. If the limb is oedematous with a thick layer of adipose tissue this will be associated with putrefactive infection (wet gangrene). Where this is not present and when the arterial narrowing has been slowly progressive the most distal extremities become desiccated and black (dry gangrene).

Acute inflammation I: Introduction

....

Acute inflammation occurs when living tissue is injured. It is characterized by phagocytic cells and elements of circulating plasma entering the area; symptoms and signs are related to permeability of arterioles, capillaries and venules. Response is mediated via two pathways.

Microcirculation
- increase in calibre of arterioles, capillaries and venules leading to increased amount and speed of blood flow resulting in **redness** and **heat**
- increase in permeability of blood vessels resulting in escape of larger amounts of water, solutes and high molecular weight proteins such as fibrinogen. Results in swelling **(oedema)**.

Involvement of leucocytes
- adhesion of neutrophils and monocytes to endothelial cells
- migration of leucocytes between the endothelial cells
- attachment to infecting micro-organisms or dead/injured cells
- engulfment of organism/cell or tissue debris
- killing of phagocytosed organism or **digestion** of cell debris
- production of chemical mediators with effects on surrounding tissue.

....

CAUSES OF ACUTE INFLAMMATION
- mechanical trauma: e.g. cutting or crushing
- chemical injury: e.g. acid, alkali, phenol

- ultraviolet or X-radiation
- extremes of heat or cold
- reduction in arterial blood supply sufficient to cause death of under-perfused tissue
- organisms: e.g. bacteria, viruses, parasites, worms, fungi
- inappropriate or excessive operation of immune system.

....

CLINICAL CHARACTERISTICS OF ACUTE INFLAMMATION (CARDINAL SIGNS)

- heat (calor)
- redness (rubor)
- swelling (tumor)
- pain (dolor).

Underlying mechanisms for clinical signs

Redness and heat

- Caused by persistent dilation of small vessels and increased blood flow into affected area.
- Occurs at the level of the arteriole.
- Arteriolar circular smooth muscle usually under the control of autonomic nervous system (particularly sympathetic vasoconstrictor nerves); it also reacts to local chemical mediators.

Swelling

- Caused by local accumulation of excess interstitial fluid containing solutes and proteins from plasma (oedema fluid).
- In the normal state endothelium is permeable to a wide range of molecules through a two-pore system.
- Large pores (diameter 50 nm) equivalent to plasmalemmal vesicles which are concentrated along the luminal and abluminal membranes. Once these have incorporated a large molecule by pinocytosis they bud off from the luminal membrane and travel across the endothelial cell to the abluminal aspect, fuse with the plasma membrane and discharge their contents.

- Small pores (diameter about 9 nm) may correspond to the junctions between adjacent endothelial cells.
- Transport of water and solute across the endothelium shows features of ultrafiltration controlled by opposing physical forces.
- Hydrostatic forces within the microcirculation push fluid into the extravascular tissue.
- Intravascular osmotic pressure exerted by the plasma proteins and the hydrostatic pressure of the extravascular tissues pushes fluid back into the vessels. In the normal state this results in a small net outflow of fluid from the microcirculation which drains via the lymphatic channels. In acute inflammation there is protein leakage which combines with increased intravascular hydrostatic pressure to increase oedema fluid accumulation. In mild injury this protein leakage occurs at the level of small venules measuring 80–100 nm and may be due to endothelial cell contraction.
- A major factor affecting these changes is the severity of the injury.
- On the basis of two characteristics – time between injury and recordable changes and duration of these changes – three patterns can be observed:

Immediate transient response
— follows immediately on mild injury
— alteration in vascular permeability reaches peak within 5 min or so and returns to normal within 15 min
— escape of fluid is confined to small venules
— development of leaky venules extends more widely than immediate site of injury suggesting involvement of a chemical mediator (histamine). Blocked by anti-histamines
— short duration of the change suggests that the increased permeability is due to endothelial cell contraction rather than endothelial cell damage.

Delayed persistent response (e.g. sunburn)
— takes longer to develop – peak effect may occur 4–24 h after injury
— not due to histamine (not blocked by antihistamines)

— when the effect is seen after 4 h the leak of fluid and macromolecules occurs at the level of the capillaries
— if the peak is later then both venules and capillaries are involved
— some of the capillaries contain small aggregates of platelets and broken-up endothelial cells
— in venules interendothelial gaps are found but this is thought to be due to direct damage rather than to histamine.

Immediate persistent response (e.g. bad burns or following severe mechanical trauma)
— affected vessels begin to leak within a few minutes of injury
— peak permeability at 15–60 min
— small vessels of all types leak
— there is severe damage to endothelial cells and pericytes. Sloughing of endothelial cells from basement membrane occurs
— exudation continues until the endothelial cells have been replaced by ingrowth of cells from the adjacent uninjured vessel
— leakage may therefore last for many days.

Pain

• is in part the result of increased tissue turgor
• is more severe if the tissue is denser
• may also be related to the action of chemical mediators released as part of the inflammatory response.

Acute inflammation II: Cellular events

....

CELL POPULATION OF THE INFLAMMATORY EXUDATE

Neutrophil

- major cell in early stages of inflammatory process
- present in relatively large numbers in blood (40–75% of circulating white cells)
- replaced rapidly from precursors in bone marrow
- moves more quickly than other leucocytes.

Morphology

- diameter about 15 μm
- segmented nucleus
- granular cytoplasm
- contain two types of granule:
  1. larger granules contain lysozyme (about one third of contents), lysosomal enzymes, peroxidase and certain cationic proteins.
  2. smaller granules (also lysosomal in nature) contain lysozyme (about two thirds of content), alkaline phosphatase, lactoferrin (an iron-binding protein that inhibits multiplication of bacteria).

Operations in acute inflammation

Adhesion to endothelium and emigration

With changes in blood flow the heavier white cells lie at the periphery of the column of blood cells. Some adhere to the endothelium (**margination**) associated with receptor-ligand binding.

Adhesion molecules on endothelial cells

1. **Selectins**:
- glycoproteins with amino terminal lectin-like domain; epidermal growth factor-like domain; many cysteine-rich tandem repeats (similar to those seen in complement-regulating proteins); transmembrane region; short intracytoplasmic region
- not present on resting endothelial cells
- expressed on endothelial stimulated by chemical signals including bacterial endotoxin; interleukin-1; phorbol esters; thrombin; tumour necrosis factor α. Appears within 30 min of stimulation. Peak concentrations after 2–4 h. Expressed for about 24 h.

There are two endothelial selectins: **E-selectin** (endothelial leucocyte adhesion molecule 1; ELAM-1: associated with the ligand **sialylLewisX** found on white cells (neutrophils; monocytes); **P-selectin** (platelet activation-dependent granule to external membrane protein; PADGEM): also present within α granules of platelets. Present constitutively in rod-shaped granules (**Wiebel–Palade bodies**). Transported to luminal surface following stimulation. Associated with the ligand **lacto-n-fucopentaose III (LNF III)**.

2. **Immunoglobulin gene superfamily**
- glycoproteins
- contain several domains which resemble the structure of immunoglobulin
- three molecules identified:

  — Vascular cell adhesion molecule 1 (VCAM-1)
  — Intercellular cell adhesion molecule 1 (ICAM-1; CD54)
  — Intercellular cell adhesion molecule 2 (ICAM-2)

- ICAMs thought to be most involved.
- ICAMs are constitutively expressed by endothelial cells.
- ICAM-1 is expressed at very low levels. Expression is increased by inflammatory stimulants (e.g. interleukin-1; tumour necrosis factor α). Induction of expression takes 4–6 h. Maximum levels at 24 h when plateau occurs.
- Cellular ligands for immunoglobulin gene superfamily are **integrins**. These mediate adhesion of cells to extracellular matrices (e.g. fibronectin; vitronectin),

fibrillar proteins (e.g. collagen; laminin), endothelial cells. Composed of two subunits: α (11 sub-units so far identified) and β (6 sub-units so far identified). At least 16 different integrins from various combinations (some cell-type specific [e.g. pgIIb/IIIa expressed only on megakaryocytes and platelets – mediates platelet aggregation; LFA-1, MAC-1; p150,95 only expressed on leucocytes and adhere to endothelial ICAMs, known as β_2 integrins, composed of same β chain with different α subunit]).

Emigration

- following margination the neutrophils put out pseudopodia
- pseudopodia enter the gap between adjacent endothelial cells and force it open
- neutrophils move into basement membrane substance
- process takes 2–9 min
- leucocytes from newborn and leukaemic myeloblasts cannot attenuate cytoplasm to squeeze through gaps
- chemo-attractants associated with emigration are C-X-C chemokines of which interleukin-8 (IL-8) is the most important in this context.

Neutrophil movement

- crawl forward by protrusion of pseudopodia which become transiently attached to underlying substrate. Rest of cell pulled forwards
- movement driven by peripheral part of cytoplasm and is derived from actin filaments
- actin filaments are attached to the inner side of the leucocyte plasma membrane on the aspect attached to the underlying substrate
- actin filaments assemble in response to chemotactic signals
- in the resting state non-polymerized actin caused by
  1. a molecule that sequesters monomeric actin molecules (**profilin**)
  2. a molecule that binds to the growing ends of actin filaments preventing addition of monomers to the growing end (**gelsolin**)
- myosin powers the contraction of leucocyte cytoplasm.

This is regulated in the same way as in smooth muscle and platelets – a calcium-calmodulin complex activates a myosin light-chain complex. This phosphorylates the myosin light chain.

Chemotaxis

- directional, purposeful movement of phagocytes towards areas of tissue injury, death or bacterial invasion
- mediated by chemical messengers
- different from **chemokinesis** (chemically induced increase in phagocytic cell activity, has no vectorial component)
- has two components:
  1. signals that attract phagocytes
  2. ability of phagocyte to respond to signal and move towards the source of the signal (reception and transduction).

Signals that attract phagocytes

Chemotactic agents

1. Products of invading micro-organisms – formylated peptides.
2. Endogenous compounds. Examples of these include: activated plasma protein cascades: the complement system (C3a, C5a; C567 complex), Kinin system (kallikrein; bradykinin); intrinsic blood clotting pathway (fibrino-peptides); and fibrinolytic pathway (plasmin).

The complement system

This consists of about 20 different proteins. When activated it yields compounds which coat micro-organisms and function as adhesion molecules for neutrophils and macrophages (**opsonins**). This leads to lysis of bacterial cell membranes via membrane attack complex and influences the vascular and cellular pathways of acute inflammation.

It can be activated in at least two ways:

1. The *classical pathway* through formation of antigen-antibody complexes to which C1q binds.

2. The *alternate pathway* operates via the direct cleavage of C3 with consequent activation of the rest of the sequence. Can be activated by:

- certain lipopolysaccharides derived from Gram-negative bacteria (endotoxins)
- cobra venom
- polysaccharides derived from cell walls of certain yeasts (**zymosan**)
- aggregated immunoglobulins (notably IgA and IgE)
- plasmin (product of the fibrinolyitic cascade).

As well as being important in chemotaxis the complement cascade also influences vascular changes in the acute inflammatory reaction by increasing permeability through the formation of **anaphylatoxins** (C3a; C5a). C5a is 1000 times more active than C3a.

C5a and C3a are mediators of both vascular and cellular components of the inflammatory reaction.

- C567 complex is purely chemotactic
- C3 fragments can induce release of neutrophils from bone marrow reserves
- C5a may induce release of lysosomal enzymes
- The effects of C5a on microvessels are probably due to its effect on mast cells which are stimulated to produce large amounts of leukotriene B_4.

The kinin system

This is able to induce change in tone of vascular smooth muscle. Cascade starts with activation of **Hageman factor (clotting factor XII)** which can be cleaved by:

- glass
- kaolin
- collagen
- basement membrane
- cartilage
- trypsin
- sodium urate crystals
- kallikrein (a later member of the kinin-forming cascade)
- plasmin
- clotting Factor XI
- bacterial endotoxins.

Once the Hageman factor is cleaved it acts on three plasma proenzymes:

1. Clotting Factor XI is activated to initiate the intrinsic clotting cascade.
2. Plasminogen proactivator is activated to plasminogen activator with ultimate formation of plasmin (fibrinolytic enzyme).
3. Pre-kallikrein is cleaved to kallikrein leading to kinin formation.

Kallikrein cleaves kininogen to release **bradykinin** (a powerful hypotensive agent producing vascular dilation and increased vascular permeability).

The clotting system

Activation of Hageman factor in turn activates clotting Factor XI which itself activates Hageman factor in a positive feedback loop.

The fibrinolytic system

The eventual product of this cascade is plasmin which is fibrinolytic and feeds back to activate more Hageman factor. It also digests Hageman factor into particles that tend to activate pre-kallikrein rather than Factor XI.

Stored within cells and released on demand: histamine, 5-hydroxytryptamine, lysosomal components.

Vasoactive compounds

Mast cell granules contain histamine, heparin, 5-hydroxytryptamine and other enzymes.

Histamine, which is formed by decarboxylation of histidine, is found in granules of mast cells and gastric parietal cells.

Mast cells may degranulate following physical injury (e.g. heat, mechanical trauma, irradiation) or action of chemical agents (e.g. immunoglobulins, snake venoms, bee venom, dextrans, chymotrypsin, trypsin, certain surfactants and cationic proteins from lysosomes of neutrophils, C3a, C5a, antigenic challenge to IgE coated cells).

Mast cell degranulation is dependent upon increase in cellular cGMP and inhibition of cAMP.

Histamine and 5-hydroxytryptamine cause vascular dilation and increased vascular permeability

Lysosomal compounds
• cationic proteins
• acid proteases
• neutral proteases.

Newly synthesized in and released from cells on demand – prostaglandins; leukotrienes; platelet activating factor; cytokines (e.g. interleukin-1, tumour necrosis factor α).

Products of arachidonic acid peroxidation
Arachidonic acid can be metabolized in two ways:

Cyclo-oxygenase pathway   results in production of stable prostaglandins (e.g. prostaglandin E_2 – vasodilator and increaser of vascular permeability; thromboxane A_2 – a potent vasoconstrictor and platelet aggregator; prostaglandin I_2 – vasodilator and anti-aggregator).

Lipoxygenase pathway   which can occur in platelets, neutrophils and mast cells and results in the formation of **leukotrienes**.

Platelet activating factor (PAF)
• derived from membrane phospholipid
• activates platelets and has many other actions
• generated after activation of phospholipase A2.

Cytokines
Low molecular weight proteins synthesized and released from cells, active in inflammation and in determining immune responses.

IL-8 and other chemokines
• low molecular weight (8–11kD)
• important in initiating and maintaining inflammatory response.

Classified into two families:

1. α **family**, coded for by genes on chromosome 4. Characterized by amino-acid sequence in which the two

terminal cysteines are separated by some other amino acid. Includes interleukin (IL)-8; β-thrombomodulin; gro-α, β and γ; platelet factor 4. Mostly produced by monocytes but some are produced by T-lymphocytes, endothelial cells and platelets. IL-8 mediates the rapid accumulation of neutrophils in inflamed tissues by inducing the formation of neutrophil-binding integrins on the endothelial cells of microvessels in the injured area. Gro (MIP 2-α or 2-β) also acts as a neutrophil chemo-attractant as well as promoting release of lysosomal enzymes which contribute to the inflammatory response. β-thrombomodulin and platelet factor four which are released from activated platelets stimulate the fibroblasts which take part in the organization of thrombi and haematomas.

2. β **family**, coded for by genes located on chromosome 17. They have cysteine–cysteine amino acid arrangement. They include RANTES (regulated on activation, normal T-cell expressed and secreted); macrophage activating factor (MCAF); MIP 1-α; MIP l-β which are produced by T-lymphocytes and monocytes.

Interleukin-1 (IL-1)

- mainly from monocytes and macrophages but also from endothelial cells and some epithelial cells
- molecular weight 17–18kD
- synthesis stimulated by various microbial products (e.g. bacterial endotoxin) and other cytokines
- potent regulator of local and systemic events.

  — Local: upregulation of adhesion molecule expression on endothelium leading to adhesion of leucocytes and platelets, stimulation of macrophage production of chemokines (e.g. IL-8).
  — Systemic: acts as endogenous pyrogen; induces glucocorticoid synthesis; induces release of prostaglandins, collagenase and acute phase proteins.

- lacks ability to cause necrosis of tumour cells and tissue injury; increase expression of MHC coded proteins; mediate the Shwartzman reaction.

Tumour necrosis factor α *(TNF-α)* This belongs to a family of ligands that bind to receptors on target cells which initiate either signals for cell proliferation or for apoptosis. TNF-α exists almost entirely as a secreted protein but others are transmembrane proteins acting through cell–cell contact.

- binds to two transmembrane receptor proteins (one 55kD, the other 75kD) with different effects:
  - 55kD receptor occupied: apoptosis; tumour cell lysis in vitro
  - 75kD receptor occupied: T-lymphocyte proliferation; skin necrosis; insulin resistance
  - both receptors occupied: bone resorption; haemorrhagic necrosis in tumours; endotoxic shock; fever.
- plays an important part in host defence against infections by Gram-negative bacteria
- upregulates expression of MHC class I proteins and cytotoxic potential of CD8 T lymphocytes (increasing defence against intracellular parasites)
- at high concentrations it is a potent mediator concerned in pathogenesis of endotoxin-related shock.

Reception and transduction of signals

The first site of interaction between chemotactic molecule and cell is likely to be a specific receptor. Signal transduction is followed by release of arachidonic acid from the cell; arachidonic acid release may directly or indirectly induce change in membrane ion permeability (especially calcium). Cyclic nucleotides (the balance between cAMP and cGMP) are important in the control of movement.

cGMP:
- enhances chemotactic movement
- enhances release of active substances from mast cells (e.g. histamine, leukotrienes)
- enhances release of lysosomal enzymes from neutrophils and lymphokines from T lymphocytes
- promotes assembly of microtubules when concentration rises.

cAMP:
- has opposite effects to cGMP.

Phagocytosis

Opsonization

This is the coating of particles with proteins (e.g. immunoglobulin) allowing them to be more readily phagocytosed. Opsonins may be specific antibodies of IgG class (Fc fragment must be intact); or C3b fragment of complement.

Engulfment

This results from fusion of pseudopodia projecting from phagocyte plasma membrane, so that the phagocytosed object is locked into **phagosome**.

Phagosome buds off the plasma membrane and moves into the cytoplasm of the cell. Engulfment is an active, energy-dependent process, inhibited by factors interfering with ATP formation.

Lysosomal fusion and killing

Lysosomal granules move towards a phagosome: apposition and fusion of the membranes of the granule and phagosome occurs. The lysosomal granule disappears.

Metabolic events associated with bacterial killing

Respiratory burst

A burst of oxidative activity resulting in the step-wise reduction of molecular oxygen to hydrogen peroxide. It is associated with a 2–20-fold increase in oxygen consumption by the cell and a considerable increase in glucose metabolism via hexose monophosphate shunt. Reduction of molecular oxygen is catalysed by a non-haem protein oxidase.

The hydrogen donor is either NADH or NADPH. In the reduction process, oxygen gains only one electron and is converted into the **superoxide anion** (an oxygen free radical). When two molecules of superoxide anion react one is oxidized and the other is reduced to form **hydrogen peroxide** and **oxygen**. This reaction is catalysed by **superoxide dismutase**. Superoxide itself has little bactericidal activity. Most bactericidal activity is thought to be due to hydrogen peroxide. This is potentiated when hydrogen peroxide reacts with myeloperoxidase and halide ions.

Detoxification of hydrogen peroxide

Necessary to prevent damage to cell's own membranes. The process is performed by catalase and glutathione peroxidase (which needs glutathione as a substrate which is replenished via a process requiring glucose-6-phosphate dehydrogenase which is therefore important in both the formation and detoxification of hydrogen peroxidase).

Other mechanisms of bacterial killing

- low pH in phagolysosome (pH 3.5–4)
- lysozyme (muramidase)
- lactoferrin
- cationic proteins
- lysosomal hydrolases.

DEFECTS IN NEUTROPHIL FUNCTION

Neutropenia

Occurs in various forms of bone marrow failure. May be caused by:

- drugs (e.g. chloramphenicol; benzene)
- infiltration of marrow by metastatic tumour cells
- bone marrow fibrosis
- other forms of marrow aplasia.

Disorders of migration and chemotaxis

Intrinsic cell defects

- lazy leucocyte syndrome: point of defect unknown
- Job's syndrome: typically affects fair-skinned, red-haired girls. Associated with recurrent 'cold' staphylococcal abscesses.
- diabetes mellitus: impaired locomotion associated with poor diabetic control. Reversed by adding glucose and insulin to leucocytes

- Chediak–Higashi syndrome: congenital (autosomal recessive). Associated with partial albinism; giant lysosomal granules in neutrophils; increased susceptibility to bacterial infections. Neutrophils fail to show directed movement to chemotactic stimuli and show delayed intracellular killing due to reduced rate of phagosome/lysosome fusion
- leucocyte adhesion deficiency syndrome.

Inhibition of locomotion
- can be associated with certain drugs (e.g. corticosteroids; phenylbutazone).

Deficiencies in generation of chemotactic signals
- the most important involve complement system.

Disorders of phagocytosis

Opsonin deficiencies
these include deficiencies of complement or IgG.

Defects in engulfment
- can be associated with certain drugs (e.g. morphine analogues)
- associated with hyperosmolar conditions (e.g. diabetic acidosis).

Disorders of lysosomal fusion
- may be associated with drugs (e.g. corticosteroids; colchicine; certain anti-malarials)
- also seen in Chediak–Higashi syndrome.

Disorders of bacterial killing

Chronic granulomatous disease of childhood
- rare, sometimes X-linked
- characterized by recurrent bacterial infections (including *Staphylococcus aureus*; *Aerobacter aerogenes*; fungi including *Aspergillus* species) involving skin, lung, bones and lymph nodes
- neutrophils respond normally to chemotaxis and show normal phagocytosis

- no associated respiratory burst. No superoxide or hydrogen peroxide formation
- defect due to lack of **cytochrome b-245**.

....

MONONUCLEAR PHAGOCYTES

These are seen in two forms: a circulating **monocyte** which matures or differentiates into a **macrophage** when it migrates into tissues.

A monocyte has a half-life of about 22 hours (three times as long as a neutrophil). Monocytes and macrophages are derived from bone marrow, and the transition from monocyte to macrophage is associated with:

- increased cell size
- more convoluted plasma membrane
- more prominent Golgi and endoplasmic reticulum.

Many pathogenic organisms are phagocytosed by macrophages and a large number are destroyed within the phagosomes.

Some organisms parasitize macrophages and multiply within phagosomes (e.g. *Listeria; Brucella; Salmonella; Mycobacteria; Chlamydia; Rickettsia; Leishmania; Toxoplasma; Trypanosoma; Legionella*). This symbiosis is destroyed by macrophage activation.

Macrophage chemotactic factors include many associated with neutrophil chemotaxis.

Lymphokines (secreted by activated T lymphocytes) trigger a wide range of macrophage functions. This group includes **macrophage chemotactic factor** and a **migration-inhibition factor** (immobilizes macrophages at the site of inflammation and stimulates the secretion of hydrolic enzymes).

Factors that modify the inflammatory reaction

The outcome of an injury is the result of a combination of factors relating to the injurious agent and to the host.

FACTORS RELATED TO THE INJURIOUS AGENT

These include the dose and strength (virulence of micro-organisms) of the agent, the duration of exposure (especially for physical and chemical agents) and the agent's intrinsic nature. The intrinsic nature of the agent may produce a morphological reaction that is quite characteristic.

Suppurative inflammation

Certain organisms (e.g. *Staphylococcus aureus*) elicit inflammatory responses that are characterized by massive emigration of neutrophils which die after phagocytosis of the organism and release large amounts of lysosomal enzymes. This, together with bacteria-derived substances (exotoxins) that also damage tissues, results in an area of liquefaction necrosis containing necrotic debris and dead or dying neutrophils. This forms a thick, opaque yellow-green fluid (**pus**). Organisms that cause this reaction are termed **pyogenic** and the process is called **suppuration**. A localized suppurative lesion is an **abscess**.

Membranous inflammation

Other organisms (e.g. *Corynebacterium diphtheriae*, *Clostridium difficile*) produce exotoxins which kill surface epithelia. Fluid rich in fibrinogen exudes from sub-epithelial blood vessels, is converted to fibrin, becomes densely infiltrated by neutrophils and contains dead epithelial cells. This results in an opaque, grey-white membrane covering the surface.

Predominantly macrophage cellular reactions

Some bacteria (predominantly *Salmonella typhi*) elicit an inflammatory response in vivo that is dominated by macrophages rather than neutrophils.

Haemorrhagic inflammation

Some organisms attack small blood vessels and produce lesions in which bleeding is a prominent feature. This is characteristic of some rickettsial diseases (e.g. typhus), anthrax and some cases of pneumonia caused by influenza virus.

Fibrinoid necrosis

Reactions due to the impaction or formation of antigen-antibody complexes in small vessels or due to irradiation are characterized by the development of a characteristic form of necrosis. In H&E stained sections the vessels or collagen develops a smudgy eosinophilic appearance which can be shown to contain fibrin (**fibrinoid necrosis**).

Extension of the inflammatory reaction

In cases in which the inflammatory reaction is due to infection by a pathogenic micro-organism, whether or not the organism can spread through the tissues is an important modifying factor. It is of prime importance in the natural history of the disease whether the tissue reaction will keep the infection localized or whether spread to the surrounding tissues or to distant sites can occur. Factors that may influence this include:

- The release of **spreading factors** by the organism (such as the hyaluronidase produced by *Streptococcus pyogenes* and *Clostridium perfringens*).
- Lymphatic blockage may assist in localization of the infection. This may be mediated by coagulation of lymph with the formation of fibrin and may be prevented by organisms which produce lytic enzymes.
- Susceptibility of the infecting organism to the normal defensive process of phagocytosis. Some organisms have capsules that make phagocytosis difficult. These capsules may be carbohydrate (as seen in the capsular

polysaccharide of *Pneumococcus*) or protein (such as the protein A in the wall of *Staphylococcus aureus*). *Streptococcus pyogenes* and *Staphylococcus aureus* produce endotoxins that can kill phagocytes.

....

FACTORS RELATED TO THE HOST

These relate mostly to those injuries produced by micro-organisms. The general physiological state of the host is important and if this is impaired a trivial infection may become life threatening. Defects in the phagocyte system render the host more susceptible to infection, as do defects in the B and T cell elements of the immune system. Defects in the B and T cell elements may be seen as part of a congenital syndrome, associated with a disease process (e.g. AIDS or Hodgkin's disease), may be induced by deliberate immunosuppression or as a side effect of another therapy (e.g. cytotoxic therapy for tumours).

....

CLASSIFICATION OF INDIVIDUAL INFLAMMATORY REACTIONS

Inflammatory lesions can be classified in respect to the duration of the reaction, the type of exudate associated with a type of injury and the effect of the anatomical location on the lesion morphology.

Duration If the reaction is fairly short (e.g. days) it is termed acute. A reaction lasting for some weeks is termed sub-acute and longer lasting reactions are termed chronic.

Types of exudate

- *serous exudate* This is characterized by the outpouring of fluid with a low protein content. This is most frequently seen in relation to surfaces that are lined by mesothelium but may also be seen in a blister on the skin.
- *fibrinous exudate* This type of exudate is rather lower in volume than the serous exudate and has a high protein content with large amounts of fibrinogen which is converted to fibrin. This is seen in relation to serosa-

lined cavities and is associated with pain during movement of the underlying viscera. A consequence of two contiguous surfaces being lined by fibrin is a tendency for the surfaces to stick together with formation of permanent bridges of scar tissue.

- *haemorrhagic exudate* This is usually a fibrinous exudate in which there has been some damage to the underlying small blood vessels.
- *purulent exudate* An opaque exudate containing a large number of cells and necrotic debris. This may be seen in combination with fibrinous exudate in relation to serous surfaces such as the peritoneum.
- *catarrhal exudate* Seen mostly when mucous membranes are involved in inflammatory reactions The exude is initially serous but is followed by a profuse discharge of mucus from the glands of the mucosa.
- *membranous and pseudo-membranous exudate*.

The exudate may be protective in a number of ways:

- dilution of the injurious agent
- bacterial killing by antibody and complement contained within the protein compartment of the exudate
- localization of the injurious agent by polymerized fibrin. Fibrin also assists the phagocytosis of non-opsonized organisms (**surface phagocytosis**).

Anatomical location of the inflammatory reaction

Abscess formation

This occurs in the substance of a solid tissue where the causal agent is a pyogenic organism. An abscess is a localized lesion with a necrotic pus-filled centre, but if the process is a spreading one the lesion is termed **cellulitis**.

An abcess has clearly defined zones:

- the centre is made up of partly or completely liquefied dead tissues with dead and dying neutrophils
- this is surrounded by a layer of fibrin and living neutrophils
- at the periphery is a membrane made up of proliferating fibroblasts, new capillaries and young collagen fibres

- the last layer represents the repair process with a layer of fibroblastic proliferation which serves as a barrier to the further spread of the inflammatory process. This layer also serves to prevent the discharge of the abcess contents without which healing cannot occur.

Ulcers
This is a local defect in an epithelial surface produced by the shedding of dead epithelial cells.

Possible harmful effects of inflammation
Oedema
This may have harmful effects if a narrow tube is further obstructed by swollen tissues such as in laryngeal oedema associated with para-influenzal infection. Swelling of the brain (cerebral oedema) within the solid box of the cranium causes increased pressure that is transmitted downwards and backwards through the foramen magnum, causing displacement of the brain and being associated with shearing stresses to the perforating blood vessels; blood supply to important areas may be occluded.

Failure to control mediator release
This is rare but may be seen in a condition known as hereditary angio-neurotic oedema where the patient develops localized areas of oedema. This is thought to be a result of the unrestrained activity of a kinin-like particle released during the course of activation of the C2 component of complement.

Malfunction due to exudates
Exudates may cause mechanical problems such as the loss of functional lung tissue during an episode of lobar pneumonia when the alveolar spaces are filled by exudate.

Phagocyte-mediated tissue damage
This may occur as a result of interruption of phagosome–lysosome fusion (such as is seen in gouty arthritis and silicosis) or through inappropriate triggering of phagocyte secretory or metabolic function.

Release of phagocyte-derived free radicals

Oxygen metabolites released from neutrophils and macrophages may be toxic to red cells, endothelial cells, fibroblasts, platelets and spermatozoa. Damage to the endothelial cells of the pulmonary vascular bed by oxygen-derived free radicals may be important in the production of adult respiratory distress syndrome (ARDS).

Immune complexes

The lodging of antigen-antibody complexes at various locations may cause tissue damage.

Tissue injury may be followed by:

- resolution – complete return to functional and structural normality
- healing by repair – replacement of lost tissue by scar tissue
- chronicity – persistence of the inflammatory process.

Factors determining which of these will follow an inflammatory reaction include:

- the nature of the injury
- the tissue target
- the host response.

RESOLUTION

This indicates **return of the inflamed area to the state existing before the injury occurred** and implies **no significant loss of tissue** (i.e. no necrosis). Central to this is the complete removal of the inflammatory exudate which is largely accomplished by proteolysis and phagocytosis by macrophages.

An example of resolution is provided by **lobar pneumonia**. A severe inflammatory response occurs when the air spaces are invaded by *Streptococcus pneumoniae* organisms. Initially there is an exudate rich in fibrin and poor in cells. The process spreads to adjacent air spaces until an extensive area of lung is involved. Inflammatory cells migrate into the fibrin-rich exudate. Most of the viable organisms are killed by the neutrophils. Many neutrophils also die in the course of this process. At this stage the areas of lung affected are red, fleshy and airless. Microscopy shows dilation of the alveolar capillaries and air spaces filled by exudate but no necrosis of the alveolar septa.

Once the organisms have been cleared macrophages are recruited to the area and become the dominant cellular element. There is lysis of the fibrinous exudate by plasmin derived from plasminogen which is derived from the macrophages.

The macrophages phagocytose much of the cellular and bacterial debris and the material not phagocytosed is broken down by lysosomal enzymes secreted by reverse endocytosis. The lysed exudate drains away via the lymphatics.

Failure to remove all the exudate will result in **organization**.

ORGANIZATION

This occurs if the exudate persists. The residual infiltrate is infiltrated by numerous macrophages followed by migration of fibroblasts and new, small blood vessels similar to that seen in wound healing. Eventually the exudate is replaced by vascularized fibrous tissue in the first instance and eventually by collagen-rich scar tissue.

Organization may lead to highly disadvantageous clinical scenarios such as:

- formation of fibrous adhesions in the peritoneum which may cause bowel obstruction later
- obliteration of the pleural or pericardial spaces (causing constrictive pericarditis).

REGENERATION

Tissue which is lost during injury must be replaced if possible by new living tissue. If this tissue regeneration occurs in an orderly way the tissue elements of the normal organ are replicated (**regeneration**). This depends on the lost cells being replaced by identical cells and the normal architecture of connective tissue and blood vessels either not having been lost or having been replaced.

Regeneration depends on the type of cell lost in the inflammatory response and on the preservation or restoration of a normal stromal framework. If the framework is destroyed the regenerating cells will grow in a disorganized fashion.

There are three main cell types.

Labile cells

These are derived from mitotic division of stem cells and are defined by:

- not themselves being terminally differentiated
- having no fixed limit on their capacity to divide during the lifetime of the animal
- giving rise to daughter cells which can either remain as stem cells or can embark on terminal differentiation.

The stem cell populations exist where there is a need for a replacement mechanism for differentiated cells which cannot themselves divide and which often have a short life.

Labile cells fall into two groups:

1. **Those covering epithelia**. Statified squamous epithelium of the skin, mouth, pharynx, oesophagus, vagina and cervix; transitional epithelium of the urinary tract, gut epithelium; lining epithelium of exocrine gland ducts; endometrial gland epithelium and lining of the Fallopian tubes.
2. **Blood and lymphoid cells**.

Stable cells

These are normally quiescent and have a very low rate of turnover. When these cells are lost replacement is carried out by mitotic division of mature cells. There appears to be no stem cell compartment. Loss is followed by marked upregulation of cell division and the lost cells are rapidly replaced. Such regeneration involves the upregulation of endocrine, paracrine or autocrine mitogenic signals and the possible upregulation of receptor function, signal transduction and expression of DNA-binding proteins. In the liver and the renal tubules one of the most potent factors involved is a multi-functional cytokine hepatic growth factor (HGF; scatter factor) coded for on chromosome 7 and secreted by various cells including fibroblasts, epithelial and endothelial cells, Kupffer cells in the liver sinusoids and lipocytes (Ito cells) in the space of Disse in the liver. HGF production is increased by IL-1 and by a humoral sub-stance, injurin. HGF exerts its effects by binding the gene product of *c-met*.

Stable cells include: liver cells; renal tubular cells; secretory epithelium of endocrine glands, bone cells and fibroblasts.

Permanent cells

These cells never divide in post-natal life and cannot be replaced if lost. Permanent cells include: nerve cells, myocardial cells, the auditory hair cells and the cells of the lens of the eye.

8 The natural history of acute inflammation II: Wound healing

The objectives of wound healing are twofold:

1. Resoration of the integrity of epithelial surfaces if this has been lost.
2. Restoration of tensile strength of the connective tissue.

Whatever the wound the basic mechanisms of healing are the same, with differences in degree rather than kind. Conventionally wound healing is considered to occur in one of two ways. Healing by **primary intention** is when the edges of a cleanly incised wound are in close apposition, and healing by **secondary intention** is when there has been extensive loss of epithelium, a large sub-epithelial tissue defect and wound edges that cannot be brought together by sutures.

....

HEALING OF AN INCISED WOUND

Incision involves division of epidermis, dermal connective tissue, subcutaneous tissue and blood vessels. **Haemorrhage and clot formation** are pivotal events. There is accumulation within the tissue defect of platelets, fibrinogen and fibronectin. Clotting mechanisms are activated, fibrinogen is converted to polymerized fibrin and is stabilized by fibronectin binding. This holds the severed edges together.

Epidermal events

Within a few hours a single layer of epidermal cells migrate to cover the area of epidermal loss. This spreading process is called **epiboly** and depends on the interaction between the keratinocytes and the extracellular matrix glycoprotein fibronectin. Fibronectin provides ligand receptors and the binding of ligand to receptor mediated cell-matrix adhesion. The receptors on the cells that bind to these ligands are called **integrins**.

New epidermal cells, essential for epithelial recovering, are derived from the stem cell compartment which is made up of the basal cells just above the dermo-epidermal junction. From about 12 h after wounding there is a marked increase in mitotic activity of the basal cells about 3–5 cells from the wound edge, and the new epidermal cells grow under the surface of fibrin/fibronectin clot.

Dermal events

Within the first few hours after wounding there is a mild inflammatory reaction with influx of neutrophils in and around the wound (**0–1 day** after wounding) followed by macrophages (**1–2 days** after wounding).

For a successful outcome to the wound healing there should be:

- removal of inflammatory exudate and debris
- restoration of tensile strength, requiring synthesis of collagen and matrix proteins and proliferation of fibroblasts
- ingrowth of new small blood vessels by budding of new endothelial cells and chemo-attraction of these cells into the fibrin/fibronectin gel.

In a surgical incision fibroblasts and myofibroblasts appear in the wound between **2–4 days** after wounding and endothelial cells **one day later**.

Initially the buds of endothelial cells are solid but they soon acquire a lumen. At this stage the new vessels do not have a basement membrane and are extremely leaky. This richly vascularized gel also contains inflammatory cells and collagen-producing fibroblasts and is called **granulation tissue** (as it has a granular appearance when viewed in vivo).

The restoration of tensile strength depends on the production and orientation of collagen. Collagen contains large amounts of the amino acids hydroxyproline and hydroxylycine. Within **24 h** of wounding, protein-bound hydroxyproline appears within the damaged area and within **2–3**

days some fibrillar material can be seen. Within **a few weeks** the amount of collagen in the wounded area is normal although tensile strength is not regained for **some months**.

Collagen consists of three peptide α-chains in a helical pattern which undergo post-translational hydroxylation of of proline and lysine moieties with subsequent glycosylation of the hydroxylysine. Solluble pro-collagen is secreted into the extracellular environment where solubility conferring extra peptides are removed and the molecules are assembled into fibres. Tensile strength is obtained by crosslinkage of the fibres.

....

HEALING OF A WOUND ASSOCIATED WITH A LARGE TISSUE DEFECT

This differs from healing of the incised wound mainly in the quantity of the defect that is present and many of the mechanisms are similar. One feature of the healing process seen in large defects and not seen in healing of the incised wound is **wound contraction**.

Two to three days after formation of a large wound its size decreases in a way that is independent of the rate of covering by new epidermal cells. This occurs at a time when there is little new collagen formation. The currently favoured hypothesis to explain this relates to contraction of **myofibroblasts** which appear at the margins of the wound in the first few days and are connected to collagen via fibronectin.

....

GROWTH FACTORS AND CYTOKINES IN WOUND HEALING

Growth factors

These are peptides that reach specific targets via **endocrine** (secreted at a distance), **paracrine** (secreted in the neighbourhood) or **autocrine** (secreted by the same cell that uses the factor) pathways.

Growth factors can be considered in two groups:

1. Competence factors move a cell out of G_0 and into cell cycle (e.g. platelet derived growth factor; basic fibroblast growth factor).
2. Progression factors have a mitogenic effect only on cells not in G_0 (e.g. insulin-like growth factors 1 and 2 and epidermal growth factor).

Platelet-derived growth factor (PDGF)

PDGF is derived from:

- α-granules of platelets
- endothelial cells
- macrophages
- arterial smooth muscle
- certain tumour cells.

PDGF binds to a receptor which, after ligand-receptor interaction, acts as a tyrosine kinase. It has a number of functions:

- mitogenic effects
- chemotactic to mesenchymal cells (except endothelial cells)
- increases intracellular synthesis of cholesterol, increases binding of low density lipoprotein by increasing the number of LDL receptors on a target cell membrane
- increases prostaglandin secretion
- induces changes in cell shape by reorganization of actin filaments
- induces increased synthesis of RNA and protein
- is a potent vasoconstrictor.

Epidermal growth factor (EGF) and transforming growth factor α (TGFα)

EGF is a 53 amino acid polypetide cleaved from a larger protein. It stimulates mitogenesis in **connective tissue** as well as **epithelial cells**. It is stored in the salivary gland, lacrimal glands and Brunner's glands of the duodenum. Blood-borne EGF is found in platelets (mainly α-granules). EGF accelerates the regeneration of epidermal cells and has a benefit on the dermal component of healing in experimental wounds but there is no evidence that it is produced by any of the cells involved in the healing process (although platelets can store EGF).

Transforming growth factor α shows considerable homology with EGF and is produced by both epidermal cells and macrophages in healing wounds. It binds to the same receptor as EGF, has the same mitogenic effect and may be a direct mediator of wound healing.

Transforming growth factor β (TGFβ)

This is a polypeptide that is produced by almost all cell lines in culture. In the presence of EGF it acts as a mitogen but under certain circumstances may inhibit growth. TGF β is a powerful chemo-attractant for monocytes and its release from the first wave of inflammatory cells in wound healing may recruit further monocytes/macrophages.

Cytokines

This is a group of protein cell regulators that includes lymphokines, monokines, interleukins and interferons. They usually have a low molecular weight and tend to be produced locally in an autocrine or paracrine fashion. Their action is mediated by binding to high affinity receptors. Two cytokines play significant roles in wound healing.

Interleukin-1 (IL-1)

IL-1 is produced by macrophages and activated epithelial cells and has several actions:

* proliferative effect on dermal fibroblasts
* upregulation of collagen synthesis by fibroblasts
* increased collagenase secretion allowing remodelling.

Tumour necrosis factor α (TNF α)

TNF-α is a monocyte/macrophage product responsible for macrophage mediated tumour cell killing and is also responsible for wasting (cachexia) associated with chronic illness. Secretion follows activation of monocytes/macrophages by interaction with fibrin, binding to TGF-β, the action of γ interferon and the action of endotoxin. TNF-α is a potent stimulus for the ingrowth of new blood vessels being responsible both for the chemotaxis of endothelial cells and for the focal breakdown of basement membrane which precedes this.

....

FACTORS THAT INTERFERE WITH WOUND HEALING

These may be divided into systemic and local factors.

Systemic factors

Nutrition

- **Protein**: undernourished patients show evidence of depression of the immune system which may delay healing and deficient protein intake may inhibit collagen formation.
- **Vitamin C**: lack of this inhibits the secretion of collagen by fibroblasts due to a failure of hydroxylation of proline in the endoplasmic reticulum of fibroblasts.
- **Vitamin A**: this is important in morphogenesis, epithelial proliferation and epithelial differentiation. Applied topically to wounds it can accelerate epithelial covering.
- **Zinc**: zinc accerates healing of experimental wounds and zinc deficiency is associated with poor healing (e.g. in patients with burns on prolonged parenteral nutrition feeding).

Steroid hormones

Glucocorticoids have an inhibitory effect on healing and on fibrous tissue production. It is unknown whether this is the result of a diminishing of the immune response or to a more direct affect.

Age

Wounds tend to heal more rapidly in the young, but this might be because of better arterial perfusion in the elderly.

Diabetes

In uncontrolled diabetes there is impairment of the neutrophil response to injury and infection. In addition diabetics may suffer from poor arterial perfusion and sensory neuro-pathy. The first impairs healing while the second makes repeated injury more likely.

Local factors

Foreign body or infection

The presence of a foreign body will increase the intensity and prolong the duration of the inflammatory response. Foreign bodies may include misplaced elements of the patient's own tissues such as necrotic bone, hair or keratin.

Excess mobility

This is of particular relevance to fracture healing but applies to other tissues as well.

Perfusion and venous drainage

Where there is compromise of the arterial perfusion there may be a disproportionate degree of tissue damage and there may be delay or inhibition of healing. Adequate venous drainage is important and impairment of this may play a part in the genesis of chronic ulcers which appear on the legs of elderly patients.

....

REPAIR OF SPECIALIZED TISSUE

Bone

In the early stages this is essentially similar to healing in the skin with the tissue defect in the first instance filled by well-vascularized connective tissue. However, the subsequent stages differ from those in an open wound and there is involvement of specialized cells: **osteoblasts** lay down seams of uncalcified bone (osteoid) and **osteoclasts** resorb bone and are important in remodelling.

Repair of a fracture may be considered in a number of stages.

1. With fracture, tearing of the blood vessels results in haem-orrhage which fills the defect with blood clot and plasma-derived proteins.

2. The injury elicits an inflammatory reaction but with only a mild neutrophil infiltration. The combination of haemorrhage and inflammatory oedema causes loosening of the periosteum and a fusiform swelling at the fracture sight.

3. Some degree of bone necrosis occurs and the morphological evidence of this is apparent after 24–48 h. Initially this is seen as fat necrosis in the marrow and if haemopoietic cells are present they lose their nuclear staining. The necrosis of the bony tissue is dependent on the local blood supply. Some sites are particularly likely to show ischaemic necrosis after fracture: talus, carpal scaphoid and head of the femur.

4. Macrophages invade the site. Granulation tissue is formed (about **day 4**) which replaces the blood clot and extends upwards and downwards in the marrow cavity for a considerable distance. Within the granulation tissue small groups of cartilage cells begin to differentiate from connective tissue stem cells.

5. **Provisional callus** is a cuff of woven bone admixed with islands of cartilage. This unites the severed bone on the external aspect but not across the severed ends. This callus originates from two sources:
   - Periosteum – the inner layer lays down woven bone. Where the periosteum has been raised from the external surface of the bone woven bone fills the gap. The efficiency of formation of this external callus depends on the blood supply around the fracture site.
   - Medullary cavity – fibroblasts and osteoblasts lay down bone matrix some of which is deposited on trabeculae of dead bone while the remainder forms new trabeculae.

6. After the formation of the provisional callus the clot which fills the gap between the bone ends is invaded first by granulation tissue capillaries and then by osteoblasts with eventual ossification. In some instances the fibrous tissue filling is not replaced by bone (non-union).

7. Once union has occurred and the patient is bearing weight the lumpy new bone is gradually resorbed and smoothed out. Excess medullary bone is similarly removed. Woven bone becomes replaced by lamellar bone. Restoration to normal may take up to 1 year.

NERVOUS TISSUES

Central nervous system (CNS)

Most neurones cannot be replaced when they are lost. Necrosis within the CNS elicits a proliferation of glial cells and formation of new glial fibres which together with the ingrowth of capillaries may constitute a barrier to the regeneration of new neuronal fibres.

Peripheral nerves

When an axon is severed the nerve cell shows **chromatolysis** (swelling with disappearance of Nissl granules). The axon swells and the myelin sheath splits and later breaks up. The surrounding Schwann cells proliferate and accumulate some of the lipid derived from the myelin. Neurofibrils start to sprout from the proximal end of the severed axon and invaginate the Schwann cells which act as a template for new fibrils. The neurofibrils push their way through the Schwann cells at a rate of about 1 mm/day and may in the end reach the appropriate end organ. The myelin sheath is reformed by the secretory activity of the Schwann cells and a degree of normal function may be attained. In some instances the neurofibrils do not grow along existing endoneural channels. This results in a haphazard tangle of new nerve fibres embedded in scar tissue (**stump** or **traumatic neuroma**).

The natural history of acute inflammation III: Chronicity

If the inflammatory process lasts for months or years it is termed **chronic**. Chronicity may be defined in terms of:

- duration
- morphological appearance
- the biological processes involved.

CLASSIFICATION

Chronic inflammatory disorders can be considered as members of several major groups.

1. **Following significant acute inflammation** e.g. conditions where there has been a significant phase of acute inflammation (such as peptic ulcer or chronic osteomyelitis) where an inflammatory response continues accompanied by attempts at healing.
2. **Tissue damage caused by non-living agents**. Such irritants can persist within the tissue for a very long time. If such foreign material is cytotoxic the inflammatory response is dominated by macrophages and evidence of repair (e.g. pulmonary silicosis).
3. **Granulomatous inflammation** e.g. conditions where the acute inflammatory response is short-lived and mild but is predestined to become chronic. The lesions are characterized by the accumulation of macrophages and lymphocytes and may be associated with necrosis and scarring. Cell-mediated immunity plays a dominant role.
4. **Antibody-mediated inflammation**. Chronic inflammation dominated by the humoral effector arm of the immune system, such as in immune complex-mediated disorders.

5. **Autoimmune reactions**. Chronic inflammatory disorders associated with plasma auto-antibodies.
6. **Chronic duct obstruction**. Inflammatory disorders due to failure to drain secretions from exocrine glands.

Chronic inflammation as a complication of acute inflammation

This is a failure of the termination of the acute inflammatory reaction, either in resolution or repair, and may result from:

- persistence of the injurious agent
- failure of removal of the exudate
- inadequate arterial perfusion and venous drainage
- failure to maintain adequate drainage of exocrine glands (in the appropriate location).

If any of these are present then a type of pathological process is likely to occur in which there is a mixed morphological picture. This is exemplified by the appearance of a chronic peptic ulcer, in which there is:

- Loss of mucosa, muscularis mucosae and some muscularis propria with debris mixing with fibrin. This is associated with injury sufficient to cause death of the mucosa.
- Immediately beneath this is a zone of typical acute inflammation infiltrated by neutrophils and macrophages which in this case is persistent.
- Beneath this is a zone of granulation tissue with numerous activated macrophages, lymphocytes and plasma cells which reflects attempts at demolition of the exudate and orchestration of vascularization and repair.
- A zone of scar tissue which is vascularized in its superficial part but more deeply consists of dense fibrous tissue. Arteries in this zone show obliteration of their lumen (endarteritis obliterans) and unduly prominent nerve bundles. This zone represents healing by repair, which in this instance is unsuccessful.

The macrophage in chronic inflammation

This plays a dominant role in the natural history of chronic inflammation due to its ability to:

- phagocytose and scavenge micro-organisms and non-living material
- kill many micro-organisms
- synthesize and release tissue-damaging products
- synthesize and release mediators of acute inflammation and fever
- present antigens to both B and T lymphocytes and to initiate immune responses
- become activated by signals from lymphocytes following antigen presentation
- release chemo-attractant mediators involved in repair and angiogenesis
- release growth factors
- regulate its own activities through autocrine loops.

Secretion products are important in the macrophage's functional repertoire. Table 9.1 lists these.

Table 9.1 Macrophage secretion products

Product	Target	Main actions
Prostaglandins and leukotrienes	Smooth muscle, leucocytes	Upregulation of acute inflammation, cause of fever, implicated in pain
Lysosomal cationic proteins	Leucocytes	Chemo-attractant
Oxygen free radicals, hydrogen peroxide, and nitric acid	Proteins, lipids	Microbicidal, implicated in tissue damage
Metalloproteinases	Connective tissue matrix proteins	Connective tissue breakdown
Interleukin 1	T and B lymphocytes, macrophages, osteoclasts, neutrophils, liver cells, endothelium	Induction of proliferation and activation of B and T cells; induction of prostaglandin and cytokine release by macrophages; induction of adhesion molecule expression for leucocytes on endothelium; induction of fever (via prostaglandin release); causation of osteoclast-mediated bone resorption; induction of release of acute phase proteins; upregulation of production of IL-6, GM-CSF and interferon β1
Interleukin 6	T and B cells, thymocytes, liver cells	Stimulation of growth and differentiation of B and T cells and precursors of blood cells; induction of production of acute phase proteins
Interleukin 8	T cells, neutrophils	Chemo-attractant
Interleukin 10	T cells	Down-regulation of mononuclear responses in inflammation, inhibition of interferon γ production; increased TH2 lymphocyte expression

Table 9.1 Macrophage secretion products *(continued)*

Product	Target	Main actions
Granulocyte-monocyte colony stimulating factor (GM-CSF)	Neutrophil and monocyte precursors, macrophages, neutrophils, monocytes	Stimulation of growth of neutrophil and monocyte precursors; activation of mature neutrophils and monocytes
Tumour necrosis factors α and α	T cells, macrophages, fibroblasts, endothelial cells	Activation of phagocytic cells, induces cachexia in cancer, induction of expression of adhesion molecules, induction of production of IL-1, IL-6, TN-α, IFN-γ, GM-CSF and acute phase proteins
Platelet derived growth factor, basic fibroblast growth factor	Fibroblasts, smooth muscle cells	Chemo-attractant; mitogen
Transforming growth factor β	T lymphocytes, fibroblasts, endothelial cells	Inhibition of T cell proliferation; upregulation of connective tissue matrix protein synthesis; promotion of new vessel formation; may inhibit or stimulate connective tissue growth (dependent on local concentration of other growth factors); autocrine effect on its own production by macrophages and on other macrophage derived polypeptides

10   The immune system

COMPONENTS OF THE IMMUNE SYSTEM

Antigens

These are substances capable of inducing a specific response from cellular elements of the immune system, usually protein, polypeptide or polysaccharide.

The chemical sites responsible for recognition by receptors or globulins (antibodies) are small and most antigens have many such sites which are called **epitopes**.

Ability to function as an antigen is determined partly by size. Most have molecular weight in excess of 10 000. Molecular weight of 2500 appears to be the lowest level below which antigens cannot elicit response.

It is possible for certain small molecules which cannot themselves act as antigens to bind to a carrier (usually protein). This complex can elicit an immune response with the antigenic determinant of the small passenger molecule. The small molecules are **haptens**. The antibodies formed in response to the hapten-carrier complex can then react with free hapten.

Most antigens are foreign to the individual and derived from the environment (**exogenous**) but some may be native to the host (**endogenous**).

Endogenous antigens

- Heterologous

    - common to species phylogenetically unrelated
    - may lead to curious cross-reactions important in disease pathogenesis (e.g. suggestion that cross-reactivity of M proteins of some strains of β-haemolytic *Streptococcus pyogenes* with heart muscle leads to acute rheumatic fever).

- Autologous
    - host's own normal constituents
    - usually recognized as self and do not elicit immune response (**tolerance**)
    - tolerance can be broken down allowing anti-self antigen production and resulting in **autoimmune diseases**.

- Homologous
    - also known as iso-antigens
    - distinguish one individual from another (e.g. ABO blood groups system)
    - expression is genetically controlled.

Consequence of encounter between host and antigen

- Antibody formation (humoral response)
    - production of globulins with ability to bind specifically to antigenic determinant
    - produced by plasma cells.

- Clonal proliferation of T lymphocytes (cell mediated immunity)
    - these may directly lyse foreign cells or host cells with antigenic make-up that has been modified (e.g. by viral infection)
    - they release a range of non-antigen specific soluble products (**lymphokines**) which may activate or suppress the function of other cells.

Cellular basis of immune reactions

B Lymphocytes

Functions Production of antibody following terminal differentiation to plasma cell.

T Lymphocytes

Actions Act alone against pathogens which survive and grow intracellularly. They co-operate with B lymphocytes and antigen-presenting cells to upregulate (T helper cells) or down-regulate (T suppressor cells) the immune system.

Mode of action *Cell-to-cell contact* is vital for destruction of abnormal or foreign cells. *Synthesis/secretion of lymphokines* mediates interactions between T and B lymphocytes and between T cells and macrophages.

Functions Important in rejection of allogenic grafts. Appears to be involved in surveillance for altered cells (e.g. tumour cells) and their destruction. Responsible for a variety of inflammatory responses occurring after second and subsequent exposure to certain antigens or haptens (e.g. delayed hypersensitivity reactions).

Table 10.1 lists peptide cytokines secreted by T lymphocytes.

Table 10.1 Peptide cytokines secreted by T lymphocytes

A Interleukins (ILs)

IL-2	• major growth factor for helper and cytotoxic T cells and lymphokine activated killer cells
	• also involved in B cell development
IL-4	• pivotal in development of T_{H2} subset
	• involved in B-cell help
	• causes antibody switching to IgE production
	• growth factor for mast cells
	• stimulates production of VCAM
IL-5	• stimulates growth and differentiation of eosinophils
	• promotes growth and differentiation of B cells
	• acts with other cytokines to induce synthesis of IgA and IgM in mature B cells
IL-6	• causes terminal differentiation of Ig-producing B cells
	• inhibits macrophage production of IL-1 and γ-interferon
	• stimulates liver to produce acute phase proteins (e.g. fibrinogen, serum amyloid A protein, α_2-macroglobulin)
	• promotes formation of osteoclasts
IL-9	• promotes proliferation of T cells
IL-10	• down-regulates production of cytokines (including IL-1, γ-interferon, TNF-α) by macrophages
	• inhibits NO production
	• stimulates B cell proliferation, differentiation and activity
IL-12	• strong stimulator of NK cells
	• growth factor for activated T cells
	• maturation factor for cytotoxic T cells
	• induces formation of γ-interferon thereby enhancing formation of T_{H1} cells
IL-13	• suppresses pro-inflammatory cytokine, chemokine and growth factor production by macrophages

Table 10.1 Peptide cytokines secreted by T lymphocytes (continued)

	• down-regulates NO production • enhances expression of MHC class II proteins • causes immunoglobulin switch to IgE and IgG4 production in B cells
IL-14	• induces proliferation of activated (but not resting) B cells • inhibits immunoglobulin production

B Interferons

γ-Interferon	• antiviral • pivotal for development of T_{H1} cells from T_{H0} cells • inhibits development of T_{H2} cells • the most powerful macrophage activating factor • increases expression of MHC class I and II (enhancing antigen presentation) • causes expression of adhesion molecules on surface of vascular endothelium • causes differentiation of cytotoxic T cells • antagonises several IL-4 actions • promotes synthesis of IgG2 by activated B cells

C Cytotoxins: tumour necrosis factors (TNFs)

TNF-α	*at high concentrations:* • acts systemically • acts as pyrogen • activates clotting system • stimulates production of acute phase proteins by liver • inhibits myocardial contractility by stimulating NO production • over long periods causes cachexia *at low concentrations:* • upregulates inflammatory response • induces expression of adhesion molecules ICAM-1, VCAM- and E-selectin thus promoting leucocyte migration into extravascular compartment • enhances killing of intracellular organisms • activates several leucocyte types leading to macrophage production of cytokines including IL-6, chemokines and more TNF-α
TNF-β	• shares many actions with TNF-α • lyses tumour cells but not normal cells • activates neutrophils • increases adhesion of leucocytes to vascular endothelium and promotes their migration

D Colony stimulating factors (CSFs)

GM-CSF	• stimulates growth of granulocyte and macrophage (GM) colonies • activates macrophages, neutrophils and eosinophils
IL-3	• stimulates growth and differentiation of haemopoietic precursors

Table 10.1 Peptide cytokines secreted by T lymphocytes *(continued)*

E Others

TGF-β
- transforming growth factor β
- family of five closely related proteins
- secreted in inactive form. Must be cleaved before it can bind to receptor.
- has autocrine effect on monocytes/macrophages regulating its own production
- up-regulates production of IL-1, FGF, PDGF and TNF-α
- increases production of connective tissue matrix proteins
- potent angiogenic factor
- has immunosuppressive effect by inhibiting proliferation of T lymphocytes

....

ANTIBODIES

Operations
- agglutination and lysis of bacteria
- opsonization of organisms
- initiation of 'classical' pathway of complement activation
- blocking of entry of micro-organisms from gut, respiratory tract, eyes, urinary tract etc.
- killing of infected cells
- neutralizing bacterial toxins.

Structure
- Y-shaped, 4-chain structure held together by disulphide bonds.
- Two chains have a molecular weight of 22 000 (light chains); the other two have a molecular weight in the range 55 000–72 500 depending on immunoglobulin class (heavy chain).
- Differences in immunoglobulin classes are due to differences in the heavy chains and whether they exist as monomers (IgG, IgD, IgE), dimers (IgA) or pentamers (IgM).
- Two different light chain types exist (kappa and lambda) a pair of which is found in association with the heavy chain in all immunoglobulin classes.
- Monomeric immunoglobulin contains three segments that can be produced by cleaving with the proteolytic

enzyme papain. There are two parts that contain the light chain and its associated portion of heavy chain and have the ability to bind antigen **(Fab – fragment antigen binding)** and a third part **(Fc – fragment crystallizable)** that has important biological functions including complement activation and immune adherence.

Diversity

- Huge numbers of combining sites exist to recognize the vast array of antigenic epitopes.
- Diversity in antibodies is due to the variability of the amino acid sequences in the N terminal antigen combining ends of the heavy and light chains **(variable regions)**.
- This diversity is the result of rearrangement of the genes coding for immunoglobulin synthesis in the early development of each B cell to give a unique genetic code within each cell. This is achieved by the selection of one V region (out of about 70), a J region (from about 5) and in heavy chain genes a D region. Intervening genetic material from unused segments are deleted to give a unique VJ (in light chain genes) or VDJ (in heavy chain genes) sequence in each B cell.

Classes

Immunoglobulin G (IgG)

- makes up about 70–80% of plasma immunoglobulin
- is monomeric
- diffuses rapidly into extravascular compartment and plays important role in toxin neutralization and bacterial opsonization
- two IgG molecules bound closely to an antigen can activate complement but this ability varies with the sub-class of IgG with IgG1 and 3 readily activating complement, IgG2 being less efficient and IgG4 not activating complement at all
- is the only immunoglobulin type that can cross the placenta.

Immunoglobulin A (IgA)

- appears selectively in seromucous secretions, tears, sweat and breast milk

- heavy chains are of high molecular weight compared to IgG
- dimerized by linkage to **J-chain**
- transported across epithelium bound to secretory component
- functions by inhibiting the binding of organisms to mucosal surfaces and therefore
- prevents them from entering cells.

Immunoglobulin M (IgM)
- largest of immunoglobulins (weight 900 000)
- consists of a pentamer of molecules joined by J-chains
- first type of immunoglobulin formed after initial antigen contact
- synthesis falls as IgG synthesis starts
- the most effective Ig for complement activation
- large size prevents easy exit of molecule from capillaries. Does not cross the placenta.

Immunoglobulin D (IgD)
- present in very small amounts in plasma
- often found on B lymphocytes in association with monomeric IgM
- possibly involved in control of B lymphocyte activation and suppression.

Immunoglobulin E (IgE)
- found in minute amounts in plasma
- binds via Fc portion to mast cells. Antigen binding to the Fab sites of these molecules results in activation and degranulation of the mast cell.

....

NORMAL ANATOMY OF THE IMMUNE SYSTEM

Lymph nodes

These respond to antigens within tissues reaching the nodes via lymphatics.

Functional anatomy
- two sets of channels (lymphatic and blood)
- a number of functional cell compartments
- a fibrous capsule from which septa penetrate into node.

Anatomy of lymph flow

- afferent lymphatics penetrate capsule at several points and lymph enters the marginal sinus just below the capsule
- cortical sinuses lead from the marginal sinus and penetrate into the node and break up into arborizing channels
- these small channels join to form larger sinuses (medullary sinuses)
- medullary sinuses join to form a single efferent lymphatic that leaves the node at the hilum
- sinuses are lined by endothelial cells and also by a resident population of macrophages. These act as a filter for antigens from the afferent lymph.

Anatomy of blood flow

- single artery enters node at the hilum
- this branches to form vessels of decreasing sizes and eventually a network of capillaries
- capillaries drain into high endothelial venules in which lymphocyte migration occurs
- these fuse to eventually form a single vein that leaves the node at the hilum.

Cellular compartments

B lymphocytes

- most found in cortex in rounded aggregates (**follicles**)
- unstimulated follicles are small and show no division
- stimulated follicles enlarge and show an internal paler **follicle centre** surrounded by a darker rim of smaller cells (the **mantle**)
- the follicle centre contains two main B cell types. **Centroblasts** are large actively dividing cells; **centrocytes** are smaller and have irregular nuclei
- B-cell differentiation in the follicle centre is driven by encounter with antigen. In a primary immune response small B cells transform directly into immunoblasts which differentiate into IgM secreting plasma cells. In a late primary or secondary response differentiation and proliferation of B cells occurs in the follicle centres. Small B cells transform into centroblasts. Following this centrocytes appear in the follicle centre which can differentiate into immunoblasts. From these are derived plasma cells and memory B cells.

T lymphocytes

- most found in the paracortex between the follicles
- cells are small and morphologically indistinguishable from B lymphocytes.

Antigen-presenting cells

Two variants.

- follicular dendritic cells which form a meshwork within the follicle centres. They trap immune complexes which then act as powerful immunogens and cause B cell proliferation and activation in the follicle centres.
- interdigitating reticulum cells are found in the paracortex. They stimulate T cells within the paracortex.

Spleen

- Responds to antigens within blood.
- Lymphoid tissue is concentrated in white pulp (**Malpighian corpuscles**) arranged around arterioles. Divided into B and T cell areas.
- T-cell areas are around the central arteriole and consist of 70% suppressor and 30% helper types.
- B-cell areas consist of germinal centres surrounded by a mantle zone and an outer marginal zone of slightly larger paler resting post-germinal centre B cells.

Mucosa associated lymphoid tissue (MALT)

This responds to antigens at mucosal surfaces (mostly found in the intestinal tract) and is important in the transport of immunoglobulins to luminal surfaces. It functions as a specific pool of lymphocytes that appear to home to MALT. There are three main components in the gut.

Peyer's patches

These consist of a central reactive follicle centre surrounded by a mantle zone of small lymphocytes and an outer marginal zone. These two zones are thickest and point to the luminal surface. The marginal zone B cells extend into the epithelium around epithelial cells that are modified to transport antigen from the lumen to the underlying lymphoid tissue (**M cells**).

Lamina propria cells

A mixed population of macrophages, plasma cells and small lymphocytes. Mucosal plasma cells secrete equal amounts of each class of IgA, two-thirds of which are in dimeric form which bind to secretory component and is transported across the gut epithelium into the lumen.

Intraepithelial T cells

These are essentially suppressor T cells. Their function is unknown.

Lymphocyte 'traffic'

Pathways include:

* extensive network of lymphatics
* blood.

Migration takes place by several mechanisms:

* in lymph nodes

  – across high endothelial venules (post-capillary venules lined by tall endothelium)
  – migration mediated by adhesion to endothelium by interaction between adhesion molecules on lymphocyte surface and **addressins** on endothelial cells (lymphocyte surface ligand is **L-selectin**).

* in MALT

  – migration mediated by binding of CD44 on lymphocyte to endothelial selectin.

* at sites of inflammation

  – various interactions between surface sugars, integrins, selectins and adhesion molecules are important.

....

THE IMMUNE RESPONSE

The signal

B and T cells may respond to the same antigen. B cells can recognize antigen irrespective of its form. They can bind free antigen in solution, antigens bound to membranes and antigens insolubilized in several ways.

Most T cells can only bind antigen associated with the cell surface. Helper T cells recognize antigens that have been processed and presented. A second signal is also required and this is provided by the major histocompatability complex.

The major histocompatability complex (MHC)

- A set of genes encoding cell surface glycoproteins.
- Antigen-presenting cells and macrophages chiefly express class II MHC antigens.
- MHC class I proteins are present on virtually all nucleated cells and signal to cytotoxic T cells.
- MHC class II molecules are particularly associated with antigen-presenting cells, B cells and macrophages and signal to T helper cells.

Antigen processing

Within cells expressing MHC class II:

- exogenous, soluble protein antigens are endocytosed by the antigen-presenting cell
- within the endosome these proteins undergo unfolding and limited proteolysis
- a vacuole containing a complex of class II and invariant chains fuses with the endosome.

Cathepsins B and D from the endosome degrade the invariant chain. This releases class II binding groove and allows antigen binding. The class II-antigen complex is transported to the surface.

Within cells expressing MHC class I:

Virally encoded proteins can pass through a process of proteolysis with formation of peptides some of which are recognized by T cells. These proteins are degraded to peptides after conjugation with ubiquitin by a complex of peptidases known as a proteosome. The peptides are translocated into the endoplasmic reticulum of the infected cell by a transporter mechanism TAP1 and TAP2.

In the endoplasmic reticulum the peptides co-operate with B_2-microglobulin and complex with newly formed class I heavy chains bound to membranes.

The peptide-MHC complex is transported across the Golgi apparatus where it acquires carbohydrate side chains. The complex is presented on the cell surface.

The response

Antigen recognition by T cells and T-cell activation

Antigen-specific T cell receptors
- membrane bound
- consist of two chains (usually one α and one β) linked by disulphide bonds
- less commonly the chains are γ and δ. T cells with this combination account for 5–15% of T cells.

The CD3 complex
- binding of antigen to T-cell receptor is insufficient for T-cell activation
- CD3 is closely linked to the receptor and is responsible for transduction of the signal into the interior of the T cell.
- CD3 is made up of 5 peptide chains (γ, δ, ϵ, ζ and η). Two of these (γ and ζ) are also associated with FC receptors I and III on natural killer cells and function as signal transducers in these cells.

Adhesion of T cells to antigen-presenting cell
- precedes antigen recognition
- mediated by ligand-receptor bond. Adhesion molecules on T cells are LFA-1 (binds to ICAM-1) and CD2 (binds to LFA-3).

T-cell activation
- requires co-stimulatory signals
- derives from either B7 (CD86) or IL-1
- involves phosphorylation of CD3.

Effects of T-cell activation

T helper (T_H cells)
- CD4 positive T cells
- play a dominant role in cell-mediated immunity

- select the antigens and epitopes that are recognized
- determine which effector mechanisms are used that may be:

    - cytotoxic (CD8+) T lymphocytes
    - antibody and cells such as mast cells and eosinophils
    - macrophages

- assist the proliferation of appropriate cells via cytokine release
- upregulate the functions of phagocytic cells
- divided into two main groups

    - T_{H1} cells promote macrophage activation and tend to respond well to antigens presented by macrophages. They produce IL-2 and IFNγ
    - T_{H2} cells tend to promote antibody production and stimulate mast cells and eosinophils. Produce IL-4, IL-5, IL-6 and IL-10.

T-cell-mediated cytotoxicity

- Cytotoxic CD8+ T cells also synthesize and release cytokines.
- Killing of cells by lymphocytes takes place under three separate circumstances:

    - MHC-restricted (mainly CD8+) T lymphocytes recognize specific antigens on cell surface. Binding is via the T cell receptor
    - natural killer (NK) cells recognize certain epitopes. These cells are derived from circulating large granular lymphocytes. They do not express surface CD3 but do express CD16 and CD56. Expression of MHC class I proteins on the cell surface is protective against NK cell mediated cell killing.
    - cells coated by antibody are recognized and lysed by lymphoid cells with the appropriate Fc receptor (antibody-dependent cell-mediated cytotoxicity).

- Mechanisms of cytotoxicity follow the same pathway irrespective of circumstances involved:

    - cytotoxic cell adheres to ligand on target cell
    - contents of vesicles in cytotoxic cells are released into space between the cells (calcium dependent)

— vesicle contents include **perforin** which becomes inserted into target cell membrane creating a trans-membrane channel and induces apoptosis of the cell. Vesicles also contain **granzymes** (some also thought to induce apoptosis), tumour necrosis factor β and ATP.

B-cell activation

Specific activation of B cells involves recognition of homo-specific antigen and in most cases T cell co-operation. Some antigens can trigger B cell activation in the absence of T cell help (thymus-independent antigens). These are all polymers and include pneumococcal polysaccharide. Recognition is mediated by surface immunoglobulins. Differentiation to plasma cells occurs. The type of immunoglobulin produced depends on the surface immunoglobulin present on the B cell. Plasma cells derived from cells with IgM or IgM and IgD will produce IgM. Cells which have other classes will produce plasma cells secreting the appropriate immunoglobulin that was expressed on the surface.

B- and T-cell co-operation

This occurs as a two-way process:

- a specific antigen is presented to T_H by B cells
- the same B cells receive signals from the stimulated T_H cells causing proliferation (IL-2, IL-4) and differentiation into antigen producing cells (IL-4, IL-6, IL-10 and IFN-γ).

COMPLEMENT ACTIVATION

Biological functions include

- bacterial killing by membrane lysis
- promotion of phagocytosis by opsonization
- mediation of vascular and cellular components of acute inflammation
- processing of immune complexes
- assistance in binding antigen to antigen presenting cells and B cells.

Activation occurs in a stepwise cascade where each activated component has the ability to activate several molecules of the next protein in the cascade. Activation takes place by one of two pathways:

Classical pathway

Activated by bound IgM or IgG. Occurs more easily with IgM. During activation of the pathway C3a (chemotactic to phagocytes, causes release of histamine from mast cells) and C3b (bound to surface membrane of cells to which the antibody is bound and acts as an opsonin) are formed.

The final phase is the formation of a membrane attack complex. This starts with the binding of C5 to C3b. Final binding of C8 and C9 leads to cell lysis.

Occasionally the classical pathway can be activated in the absence of immune complexes (e.g. certain polyanions, some micro-organisms including mycoplasma and certain retroviruses although not HIV).

Alternate pathway

This can be triggered by many stains of bacteria, polysaccharides of certain cell walls (e.g. bacterial endotoxins), some aggregated immunoglobulins, cells infected by viruses (including Epstein–Barr Virus), trypanomes, fungi and some miscellaneous factors including dextrans sulfate. Activation starts with the action of C3b and factor B. The eventual formation of a convertase activates more C3 in a positive feedback loop. Eventually a membrane attack protein identical to the classical pathway is formed.

....

IMMUNE RESPONSE IN DEFENCE AGAINST INFECTION

Bacteria

Antibody production may block bacterial pathogenicity at different stages of bacterial behaviour.

- bacterial attachment
- bacterial proliferation
- mechanisms for avoidance of phagocytosis in bacteria
- synthesis and release of toxins
- invasion associated with synthesis and release of bacterial spreading factors.

Cell-mediated immunity

This is particularly important aganist organisms growing inside cells such as mycobacterial species, *Salmonella typhi*, *Brucella abortus* and *Listeria* monocytogenes.

Pathways not involving lymphocytes

- triggering of alternate pathway of complement activation
- activation of natural killer cells, monocytes/macrophages and neutrophils by components of the bacterial cell wall.

Viruses

Antibody production:

- binds free viruses
- may block binding of virus to target cell, inhibit entry and uncoating of virus
- may bind free virus in association with complement and lyse viral envelope
- may bind to cells infected by virus leading to antibody-dependent cell-mediated cell lysis
- may bind to virally infected in association with complement leading to opsonization and phagocytosis or directly to cell lysis.

Cell-mediated immunity:

- causes direct destruction of the infected cell by cytotoxic T cells
- leads to release of lymphokines from activated T cells which attracts macrophages that are activated by the lymphokines and kill the infected cells
- triggers release of interferons which block viral mRNA transcription and render other cells resistant to infection and viral replication.

Non-specific mechanisms include:
- interferon production (α and β) which actives mechanisms in adjacent cells making them resistant to viral infection
- activation of natural killer cells.

Protozoa

Antibody production is important against blood-borne parasites such as in malaria and *trypanosomiasis*. Cell-mediated immunity is important against intracellular parasites such as *Leishmania*.

Helminths

Associated with production of high levels of IgE and in increased numbers of circulating eosinophils suggesting production of cytokines by T_{H2} lymphocytes. Degranulation of IgE-coated mast cells around the worm leads to release of histamine and attraction of eosinophils.

Disorders related to the immune system

....

IMMUNE DEFICIENCY

This may be defined as an inadequate response to the introduction of an antigen. It may involve the specific afferent (antigen presentation and recognition) or efferent (T-cell activation and antibody production) pathways or non-specific effector mechanisms (e.g. complement system; bacterial killing by phagocytes).

Disorders of specific immunity may arise at any point in B- and T-cell differentiation. The functional defect depends on the site of the defect. The earlier the defect in the pathway the broader the range of functions affected.

Primary immune deficiency

Stem cell deficiency

These are defects arising before lymphoid cells are processed by thymus/bursa equivalent. **Reticular dysgenesis** (its most severe form) causes complete failure of the development of B and T cells as well as other bone marrow cells. Individuals may die in the first week of life, usually as a result of overwhelming sepsis.

Severe combined immune deficiency (SCID)

This arises at the pre-thymus, pre-bursa stage giving defect of B- and T-cell systems. It is an X-linked or autosomal recessive trait.

About 50% sufferers lack the enzyme **adenosine deaminase** and are helped by blood transfusions (red cells contain this enzyme).

The thymus is usually small or absent. When present there is gross lack of thymocytes and Hassall's corpuscles.

Lymphoid tissue in gut and other peripheral sites is atrophic.

Features
- low immunoglobulin levels
- low blood lymphocytes ($<1 \times 10^9/l$)
- affected children cannot produce antibodies or mount cell-mediated immunity (against intracellular bacteria and viruses).

Treatments
- bone marrow transplant
- blood transfusion and thymic extracts may improve situation.

Outcome
- Many children die in the first year or two often due to pulmonary infections associated with agents that are not normally virulent (opportunistic infections).

Ataxia telangiectasia

An autosomal recessive trait.

Features
- Cerebellar degeneration and spinocerebellar atrophy giving choreo-athetoid movements early in life.
- Leashes of dilated blood vessels (telangiectasia) especially on flexor surfaces of forearms and conjunctiva at 5–8 years.
- Diminished resistance to infection. Lower plasma IgE and IgA and depressed cellular immunity. Leads to repeated infections of sinuses and respiratory tree leading to bronchiectasis.
- Associated with chromosome breakages and increased risk of development of neoplasia (predominantly lymphoid).

Wiskott–Aldrich syndrome

An X-linked recessive trait. Signs and symptoms develop in first few months of life.

Features
- low platelet count
- eczema
- recurrent infections
- low levels of IgM leading to poor response to polysaccharide antigen
- normal IgG levels and raised IgA and IgE

- some depression of cell mediated immunity with progressive decline in T-cell number and effectiveness
- increased risk of malignant neoplasms of lymphoreticular system.

Primary deficiencies of T-cell function

Di George and Nezelof syndromes Di George syndrome is not inherited; Nezelof syndrome is X-linked or autosomal recessive trait. Both have selective T-cell deficiency associated with failure of thymus development.

Features:
- defective cell-mediated immunity and may succumb to viral infection
- subnormal antibody response to bacteria
- Di George syndrome is associated with cardiac defects, cleft palate, abnormal facies, hypocalcaemia (lack of parathyroids).

Primary deficiencies of B-cell function

Bruton's congenital agammaglobulinaemia An X-linked trait. The defect occurs at pre-B-cell stage with failure of maturation and lack of circulating mature B cells.

Features
- very low plasma immunoglobin levels
- lack of lymphoid follicles and germinal centres in lymph nodes. Lack of plasma cells in tissues
- repeated infections (particularly *Staphylococcus aureus; Streptococcus pyogenes; Streptococcus pneumoniae; Haemophilus influenzae; Neisseria meningitidis; Pneumocystis carinii; Giardia lamblia*)
- pure cell-mediated responses are normal.

IgA deficiency Common in Caucasians (1/700) and rare in other ethnic groups. IgA lymphocytes fail to mature to plasma cells. It is associated with defect in IgG2 and IgG4 in 20%.

Features
- mostly asymptomatic
- increased pyogenic infection if associated with IgG abnormalities.

Common variable immunodeficiency

Consists of a number of different conditions. Males and females equally affected.

Features
- hypogammaglobulinaemia
- tendency to recurrent infections
- may occur with several different circumstances

    - failure of marrow pre-B cells to mature
    - failure of circulating B cells to mature to plasma cells
    - failure of T cells to respond to polyclonal activators (30% cases)
    - presence of T cells with marked B-cell suppressor activity.

Transient hypogammaglobulinaemia of infancy

The delayed synthesis of Ig by infants. Newborn infants are initially protected by maternal IgG which has crossed the placenta but this has been catabolized by 3 months. The condition usually corrects itself by 4 years.

Features
- increased infections, particularly of respiratory tract.

X-linked hyper-IgM syndrome

Failure to switch Ig class production from IgM to IgG and IgA.

Features:
- deficiency in IgG and IgA
- large amounts of IgM
- increased risk of infection
- IgM antibodies (may be cytotoxic) may form against blood cells (e.g. neutrophils; platelets).

Secondary immune deficiency

Immune deficiency may occur in postnatal life as a result of various factors.

Age

There is a relative lack of immune response effectiveness in infancy and old age.

Malnutrition

May be associated with defective B- and T-cell function.

Neoplastic disorders of immune system

Decreased antibody responses are associated with B-cell proliferations (e.g. B-cell lymphoma, myeloma, chronic lymphocytic leukaemia)

Hodgkin's disease is associated with deficiency of cell-mediated immunity and patients are susceptible to infection by mycobacteria, viruses and fungi.

Iatrogenic immune deficiency

Deliberately used in two circumstances:

- to prevent rejection of allografts
- to modify immune response in autoimmune disease.

Side-effect of other treatments (e.g. cytotoxic therapy for malignant neoplasms or corticosteroid use).

Infections

Acquired immunodeficiency syndrome (AIDS) The end result of infection by a retrovirus **human immunodeficiency virus (HIV)**. Two strains (HIV1 and HIV2) exist. Most cases are caused by HIV1.

The principal target cell is the **T helper cell**. Other targets are macrophages, dendritic cells in lymphoid tissues, skin Langerhans cells and neuroglia. All express CD4 on their surface. Infection leads to cell death and decreased numbers of those cells predisposing to opportunistic infections.

Infection occurs via:

- sexual intercourse (in the West this is usually homosexual but in Africa the common route is heterosexual intercourse)
- intravenous drug abuse
- transfusion of infected blood or blood products
- vertical transmission from mother to infant.

Characteristics of HIV Retrovirus with single stranded RNA genome containing the three genes common to these viruses:

- *gag* encodes protein that is cleaved into nucleocapsid constituents p24, p17, p9 and p7. P24 elicits antibodies that assist in diagnosis
- *pol* encodes reverse transcriptase
- *env* encodes glycoprotein with molecular weight 160 and is cleaved into envelope proteins gp120 and gp41. Gp120 binds CD4 allowing entry into cells.

Together with:

- *tat* transcriptor gene that upregulates transcription of viral genome
- *vpu* required for efficient virion budding
- *vif* controls infectivity of free virus
- *rev* acts post-transcriptionally and promotes transport of viral mRNA to cytoplasm of infected cell.

Consequences of infection   The virus enters the cell; the viral genome is uncoated. Viral reverse transcriptase makes a single stranded DNA copy of RNA genome. Complementary strand of DNA is made and the strands anneal and may be inserted into host genome as provirus: provirus may be transcribed with production of new viral RNA. This is translated in endoplasmic reticulum to form new virions which bud from the cell plasma membrane (**productive infection**).

In some cases the provirus is not transcribed (**latency**). Latency is overcome if the infected T cells are stimulated by other viruses or by cytokines (e.g. TNF-α). Immune response results in antibodies to p24 and envelope glycoproteins and CD8+ gp120 specific cytotoxic T cells are formed. This combats viraemia but the gp120 region of the viral genome mutates readily and frequently.

A pivotal event in development of serious consequences is the fall in CD4+ T cell numbers. This is because of

- increased susceptibility of HIV infected cells to apoptosis
- failure in antigen presentation leading to depleted pool of memory T cells
- direct cytopathic effect of virus.

Features of infection
- *Acute early syndrome* (occurs in 50–70%) – fever, myalgia and joint pain. Correlates with viraemia. p24 can be identified in blood.

Asymptomatic phase – antiviral antibodies present in blood. Individuals are infective. Hypergammaglobulin is usual. CD8+ T cells specific for HIV antigens can be found. Phase may continue for years.

Persistent generalized lymphadenopathy – seen in some. Mild constitutional symptoms.

AIDS related complex (ARC) – associated with CD4 cell count < 400/mm^2. Characterized by fever lasting more than 3 months, weight loss, diarrhoea, anaemia, night sweats. May develop superficial fungal infections (especially mouth and oesophagus).

AIDS – usually associated with CD4 count < 200/mm^2. Immunodeficiency predisposes to opportunistic infections (e.g. mycobacterial, cytomegalovirus, *Candida*, histoplasmosis, toxoplasma, pneumocystis, *Cryptosporidium*, isospora). Increased risk of developing tumours. Direct effects on nervous system including progressive encephalopathy associated with dementia, opportunistic infections (e.g. toxoplasmosis, cryptococcal meningitis), peripheral neuropathies, vacuolar changes in spinal cord.

HYPERSENSITIVITY

Type I hypersensitivity (immediate hypersensitivity, anaphylactic hypersensitivity, reagin-mediated allergy)

Foreign antigen reacts with IgE bound to mast cells via the Fc portion. Bridging of Fab portions of two adjacent IgE molecules results in release of contents of mast-cell granules into microenvironment and synthesis of metabolites of arachidonic acid.

It can be transferred passively by serum as it is due to a plasma component (IgE). Individuals producing an excessive reaction to antigens (usually harmless) are termed **atopic**. Examples:

- allergic rhinitis
- extrinsic allergic asthma
- atopic conjunctivitis
- atopic dermatitis

- urticarial angio-oedema
- gastrointestinal disturbances (e.g. pain, vomiting, diarrhoea).

Treatment

- avoidance of allergen
- tendency to react to allergen can be reduced by repeated small injections of allergen (**desensitization**)
- entry of calcium into mast cell (important in release of arachidonic acid) can be blocked by disodium chromoglycate (ineffective for gastrointestinal mast cells)
- contraction of microfilaments (essential to mast-cell degranulation) can be inhibited by corticosteroids
- effect of histamine can be blocked by antihistamines
- smooth muscle contraction can be inhibited by isoprenaline or adrenaline
- cAMP/cGMP ratio can be increased by theophylline. As cAMP increases the intracellular events associated with degranulation are damped down.

Type II hypersensitivity (cytotoxic hypersensitivity)

Tissue damage is due to the presence of circulating antibody to some tissue component. Binding of antibody to antigen leads to damage to and death of the cells via a number of effector mechanisms:

- lysis of cell membrane following activation of complement system
- phagocytosis of cell to which antibody is bound
- antibody-coated cell killed by killer cells (antibody-dependent cytotoxicity).

Examples:

Immune haemolysis occurs under three circumstances:

- incompatible blood transfusion
- haemolytic disease of the newborn
- autoimmune haemolytic disease

Drug induced type II hypersensitivity: several mechanisms may be involved.

- drug binds to carrier cell and acts as a hapten
  (e.g. sedormid)
- antibodies formed react with self antigens
  (e.g. α-methyldopa).

Type III hypersensitivity (immune complex-mediated hypersensitivity)

Associated with antibody and antigen complexes in finely dispersed or soluble form. It elicits inflammatory reaction by activation of complement and subsequent recruitment of neutrophils and platelets. Tissue injury is largely the result of:

- release of lysosomal enzymes by neutrophils
- vasoactive amines released by aggregated platelets
- formation of platelet aggregates which occlude the microcirculation.

The size of the complexes is important in determining the reaction. Large complexes are usually phagocytosed: phagocytosis may be preceded by inflammatory reaction if the complex is localized within the tissue.

Very small complexes may circulate in plasma and pass harmlessly through the glomerular filter into urine.

The nature of the complex is partly governed by relative proportions of antibody and antigen.

- **Antibody excess or mild antigen excess** – complexes rapidly precipitated and localized to site of antigen induction giving local tissue reaction.
- **Moderate to gross antigen excess** – complexes are soluble and circulate widely and become deposited in relation to basement membrane of small vessels (e.g. glomerular capillaries, in joints and skin).

Microscopic appearance of small blood vessels

There may be extensive necrosis of smooth muscle associated with deposition of fibrin and immunoglobulin (fibrinoid necrosis). Special stains will demonstrate presence of fibrin, immunoglobulin and C3.

Tissue reactions are influenced by whether complexes are formed locally or within the circulation.

- **local** (e.g. Arthus reaction) – associated with high concentrations of antibody. Antigen rapidly precipitated at or near point of entry. Microscopically there is intense neutrophil response. Diseases associated with this type are rheumatoid arthritis and farmer's lung.
- **formed in circulation** – soluble complexes cause disease at a wide variety of sites if they are of appropriate size. Diseases include serum sickness and various types of glomerulonephritis.

Type IV hypersensitivity (cell-mediated reactions)

This occurs when injury results from activities of sensitized T lymphocytes. It is associated with three main circumstances:

- **Microbial agents** – including bacteria (e.g. tuberculosis, leprosy); viruses (e.g. smallpox, measles, herpes); fungi (e.g. candidiasis, histoplasmosis).
- **Rejection of tissue or organ grafts.**
- **Contact dermatitis** – seen in association with chemicals, plant products and metals.

Stimulatory reactions caused by antibody (type V reactions)

An example of this is Graves' disease – thyrotoxicosis associated with enlarged thyroid gland and increased thyroid hormones in plasma. Associated with antibodies that are stimulatory to thyroid epithelial cells.

Autoimmune disease

....

Definition   Disease caused by loss of the normal unresponsiveness (**tolerance**) of the immune system to the host organism's own tissues.

Tolerance

Fundamental to the successful operation of the immune system is the ability to distinguish **self** from **non-self**.

Normally tolerance to self is induced during fetal development or very early neonatal life. Exposure of the immune system to potential antigens at this time leads to failure to respond to these antigens when the animal becomes immunologically mature. This may be due to deletion of reactive lymphoid clones after exposure of immature lymphoid cells to a specific antigen.

Induction of tolerance
Tolerance can be induced in adult animals under two sets of circumstances.

Low zone tolerance
- induced by repeated low doses of certain antigens
- easily induced by antigens that are *weakly* antigenic
- can be induced by strongly immunogenic antigens if antibody synthesis is inhibited during dosage by immunosuppression
- only T cells unresponsive
- possible to bypass tolerant T cell by change in determinants in an antigen complex.

High zone tolerance
- induced by repeated *high* doses of antigen
- easier with proteins that are soluble rather than present in macromolecular/aggregated forms

- avoidance of antigen processing by macrophages before presentation to lymphocytes is more likely to lead to tolerance
- B and T cell involved
- More certain method of maintaining immunological unresponsiveness.

Tolerance to self antigens may also be maintained by **suppressor T-cell** activity and loss or reduction of these T cells (e.g. by neonatal thymectomy) is associated with tendency to form antibodies against self components.

Tolerance does not develop to some self components although these are not associated with the formation of auto-antibodies. This is a result of the immune system never being exposed to these areas (**secluded areas**; e.g. lens of eye, sperm, myocardium). Later damage to these sites and exposure of components to the immune system elicits auto-antibody formation.

....

AUTOIMMUNITY

Effector mechanisms are essentially the same as seen in hypersensitivity. Many autoimmune diseases are associated with circulating antibody or soluble immune complexes and divide into two groups: **organ-specific** and **multi-system** (see Table 12.1).

Organ-specific autoimmune diseases are further divided:

- Specific lesion in target organ is associated with antibodies against a specific component of that organ.
- Lesions restricted to a single organ but associated with antibodies that are not organ specific (e.g. primary biliary cirrhosis which is associated with anti-mitochondrial antibodies).

Presence of antibody in an individual's serum need not indicate the presence of autoimmune disease. Auto-antibodies may also result *from* tissue damage rather than causing it.

Table 12.1 Examples of autoimmune disorders

Organ-specific with antibodies only against antigens in affected organ

Hashimoto's thyroiditis	Thyroglobulin
Primary myxoedema	Thyroid peroxidase
Thyrotoxicosis	TSH receptors on cell surface
Addison's disease	Hydoxylases in adrenal cortical cells
Pernicious anaemia	Intrinsic factor
Insulin-dependent diabetes mellitus	Islet cell cytoplasmic antigen; insulin
Goodpasture's syndrome	Basement membranes of glomeruli and lung
Myasthenia gravis	Acetylcholine receptors on muscle
Idiopathic thrombocytopaenic purpura	Platelet antigens
Pemphigus vulgaris	Desmosomes between prickle cells
Pemphigoid	Epidermal–dermal basement membranes
Autoimmune haemolytic anaemia	Red cell membrane antigens
Phacogenic uveitis	Lens
Sympathetic ophthalmia	Uveal tract antigens

Organ-specific without organ-specific antibodies

Primary biliary cirrhosis	Mitochondria
Chronic active hepatitis	Smooth muscle, nuclear lamins
Ulcerative colitis	A lipopolysaccharide

Multi-system disorders

Sjögren's syndrome	Single-stranded RNA (Ro); duct epithelium; mitochondria
Dermatomyositis	Extractable nuclear antigens
Wegener's granulomatosis	Antigen in neutrophil cytoplasm (ANCA)
Mixed connective tissue disease	DNA
Scleroderma	DNA-topoisomerase; centromeres
Rheumatoid arthritis	IgG
Discoid lupus erythematosus	Nuclear antigens
Systemic lupus erythematosus	Double stranded DNA; single stranded DNA; histones; ribonucleoprotein; Sm (Smith) antigen (extractable nuclear antigen); Ro (a small ribonucleoprotein); cardiolipin

Possible mechanisms for induction of autoimmunity

Exposure of previously secluded antigens This can certainly happen following open trauma to one eye where severe inflammation in the other eye may develop 2–3 weeks later (**phacogenic ophthalmitis**).

Alteration of self antigens to bypass tolerant T cells
Modification of self antigens can occur in association with
the use of certain drugs (e.g. haemolytic anaemia due to
antibodies against e-antigen of rhesus system following α-
methyldopa) and following certain viral infections. The
antigens may be directly modified or there may be alter-
ation/insertion in some molecules concerned in **associative
recognition** (where one component provides help for the
immune response to another).

Cross-reactions that bypass tolerance Presence of a shared
determinant on a totally different carrier may end tolerance to
the antigen (e.g. rheumatic fever following infection by
certain strains of β-haemolytic streptococci).

Idiotypic bypass As T helper cells with specificity for the
idiotype on a certain B cell receptor play a role in the
stimulation of that B cell clone, autoimmunity may follow
formation of an antibody which has an idiotype that cross-
reacts with the receptor of a potentially autoreactive B or T
cell (e.g. rheumatoid arthritis, systemic lupus erythematosus).

Inappropriate Ia expression Most organ-specific antigens
appear on the surface of the cells as class I but not class II
MHC-coded molecules and so cannot communicate with T
helper cells and cannot act as immunogens. If class II genes
could become derepressed MHC class II-coded proteins
may appear on the cell surface allowing presentation to T
helper cells (thought to occur in Graves' disease).

Impaired regulation of T cells B cells from normal individuals have potential to produce autoantibodies. If stimulated in vitro they are able to produce antibodies to a range
of widely distributed antigens (e.g. DNA; IgG phospholipids; red blood cells; lymphocytes) and this might be an
inherent property of the immune system. Regulation is a
function of T cells (either action by suppressor T cells or
lack of activity in helper-inducer T cells) and dysfunction
may result in autoimmune disease.

Possible role of anti-idiotype antibodies An idiotype is a
serologically identifiable configuration in the antigen binding
site of an antibody. An anti-idiotype specifically binds to this
site. Binding of the antibody to the anti-idiotype can be
inhibited by the antibody's specific antigen while binding of
antigen to antibody can be inhibited by the anti-idiotype. If an

antibody develops to a protein that has a specific receptor an anti-idiotype which subsequently develops will have specificity for both the antibody and the protein receptor. This may occur in **myasthenia gravis** where the protein is acetylcholine and the anti-idiotype antibody binds to the acetylcholine receptor. Other possible examples include antibodies against the insulin receptor in type I diabetes and thyroid stimulating antibodies in thyrotoxicosis.

EXAMPLES OF AUTOIMMUNE DISORDERS

Systemic lupus erythematosus (SLE)

A multi-system autoimmune disease with lesions produced by immune complexes, characterized by generalized excessive autoantibody production. Predilection for females (M:F 1:9); black females in USA particularly at risk. Associated with HLA antigens DR2, DR3, BW15.

Features
- skin – characteristic erythematous rash in 'butterfly area' of face
- joints – polyarthritis
- kidney – glomerulonephritis (see section under Kidney pages 478–488)
- heart – small warty excrescences on valves (Libman–Sacks endocarditis) in 50% cases.

Possible pathogenetic pathways
- decline in suppressor T-cell activity allowing B cells unfettered ability to produce autoantibodies
- direct polyclonal activation of B cells which bypasses need for helper T-cell signals.

Drug induced SLE
- A lupus-like syndrome (usually without significant renal involvement) has been seen with certain drugs e.g. hydralazine, procainamide, isoniazid.
- withdrawal of drug is usually followed by regression of condition
- no antibodies to double-stranded DNA. Antibodies to nucleoprotein are most prominent
- associated with HLA DR4.

Transplantation and the major histocompatibility complex

Transplantation refers to the substitution of a defective organ within one individual by a functioning organ from a donor. **Rejection** of the transplanted organ by the recipient will occur unless the donor and recipient are genetically identical or at least very similar.

Types of graft
- **autograft** – taken from the patient himself
- **isograft** – taken from a genetically identical (syngeneic) donor such as an identical twin
- **allograft** – taken from a donor of the same species but not of identical genetic make-up (allogeneic)
- **xenograft** – taken from a donor not of the same species (xenogeneic).

REJECTION

Evidence for immunological basis

Presence of second set reaction

In immune reactions the second contact with a responsible antigen results in an accelerated and increased tissue response. This second-set reaction can be demonstrated following experimental skin grafts in mice, and shows specificity that can be demonstrated by transplantation of skin from genetically different mice to the same donor where the second graft is rejected at the same rate as the first (two first-set reactions).

Cell mediated reaction

Transfer of lymphoid cells from a transplant recipient mouse to another mouse results in an accelerated rejection of an identical graft by the recipient of the lymphoid cells.

In animals that are thymectomized in the neonatal period allografts survive longer. Normal rejection time can be achieved following injection of lymphocytes from a genetically identical animal.

Antibody production

Humoral antibodies reacting with donor cells can be found in recipient animals following rejection.

Major histocompatability complex

The genes for MHC are located on the short arm of chromosome 6. The dominant group of antigens governing rejection are part of the **H**uman **L**eucocyte **A**ntigen (**HLA**) system.

Class I molecules
- coded for at 3 major loci A, B and C
- there is marked polymorphism in the major histocompatibility loci with 24 alleles for HLA-A, 42 for HLA-B and 11 for HLA-C
- HLA-A and -B readily induce formation of complement-fixing cytotoxic antibodies and act as cell surface recognition markers for cytotoxic T cells. They usually present viral antigens on the surface of infected cells which allows cytotoxic (CD8) T cells to destroy virally infected cells.

In kidney grafts class 1 antigens are present on vascular endothelium, tubular epithelium and intestitial and mesangial cells.

HLA typing is done by setting up an individual's lymphocytes against a panel of known antibodies in the presence of complement, looking for cell membrane damage in reactions containing appropriate antibodies.

Class II molecules

Originally defined as HLA-D locus and now has been split into three loci DR (20 alleles), DQ (9 alleles) and DP (6 alleles), expressed on the surface of B lymphocytes, monocytes, macrophages and other antigen presenting cells. Matching of class II antigens is the most important factor in predicting outcome of transplantation.

MECHANISMS OF ALLOGRAFT REJECTION

In humans this has been best studied in renal transplantation; this forms the paradigm for rejection reactions. Rejection can occur at different times after transplantation and this is probably associated with different mechanisms.

Hyperacute rejection

- rare (0.5% of all rejections)
- takes place within minutes of graft insertion
- characterized by the presence of small thrombi and sludged red cells in glomeruli
- classical of a type II immunological reaction where preformed antibodies (e.g. from ABO incompatability) bind to endothelial cells in the donor kidney and activate complement leading to activation of platelets and the clotting system causing occlusion of the vessels and ischaemic necrosis of the graft
- macroscopically the donor kidney rapidly becomes blue, mottled and flabby (rather than pink and firm)
- microscopically there is extensive occlusion of the small vessels by fibrin and platelets with extension into glomeruli. Immunocytochemistry shows the presence of IgG and C3 bound to the endothelial cells.

Early acute rejection

- common. Not necessarily associated with graft failure
- recipient may have several episodes during initial weeks after transplant
- takes place 7–10 days after transplant
- clinically manifest by:
  - oliguria
  - rise in serum creatinine
  - fever
  - some swelling and tenderness of kidney
  - presence of protein, lymphocytes, tubular epithelial cells and interleukin-2 in urine
- microscopically characterized by dense infiltration by cytotoxic T lymphocytes.

Mechanisms are diverse and may be the result of the following.

Cellular response mediated via recipient T cells

- Principal targets are tubules and interstitial tissues.
- Microscopy shows interstitial oedema and dense mononuclear cell infiltrate (T cells and macrophages) which extend into the tubular epithelium associated with tubular necrosis.
- Due to reaction between recipient's T cells and antigens presented on donor vascular endothelium and on dendritic cells in the interstitium.

Acute vascular response mediated by antibody

- Clinical and laboratory features similar to acute cellular rejection but with the additional feature of platelet sequestration in the transplanted kidney.
- Cell infiltrate is concentrated on vascular endothelium. If severe there may be fibrinoid necrosis in small vessels with extension into glomerular tufts with resulting thrombosis.
- Once there is fibrinoid necrosis and/or thrombosis in small blood vessels or glomerular capillaries the outlook for graft survival is bleak.

Acute late rejection

- occurs between 11 days and 6 weeks after transplantation
- occurs in patients immunosuppressed with prednisolone and azathioprine. This regimen damps down the T cell response but is not completely effective in stopping the antibody production
- characterized by florid vascular damage mediated by antibody and complement.

Chronic rejection

- responsible for about 8% of kidneys rejected in the first year after transplantation and for the vast majority of those occurring thereafter
- basically ischaemic. Most patients become hypertensive

- microscopic features include fibromuscular hyperplasia of the intimal lining of small-and medium-sized vessels in the kidney. The occlusion leads to ischaemic necrosis of the glomeruli. This is thought to be mediated by antibodies binding to HLA antigens on the vascular endothelium in the donor kidney.

Arterial changes in chronic vascular rejection

- The closer the HLA match between donor and recipient the less the risk of chronic vascular rejection.
- Mostly affects arcuate and interlobular arteries.
- Intima is grossly thickened along the whole circumference. Partly the result of connective tissue rich in mucins and partly due to cells including lipid-laden macrophages.
- As the lesion ages the collagen in the intima increases and the vessels become stiff and non-compliant.
- The intimal thickening is associated with the presence of mural thrombi on the endothelial surface of the affected vessels. This suggests that the vascular damage is due to recurrent endothelial injury and the intimal thickening is mediated by growth factors released from the thrombi.

Glomerular changes in chronic rejection

- Occurs in about 4% of all grafted kidneys.
- Clinically associated with moderately heavy proteinuria (>I g per day) which may be sufficient to cause a nephrotic syndrome.
- Microscopy shows thickening of the wall of the glomerular capillaries due in part to widening of the sub-endothelial region with interposition of mesangial cell cytoplasm giving a double contour basement membrane. There is also increase in mesangial matrix and mesangial cell numbers.

....

AVOIDING REJECTION

Ensure:

- good matching between donor and recipient
- suppression of the immune responses of the recipient.

Drugs used in suppression of immune responses

Azathioprine

- inhibits T-cell mediated rejection
- interferes with nucleic acid synthesis
- affects cells which are actively replicating which in the immediate post-transplant period will be T cells undergoing clonal expansion
- not specific and will affect all cells undergoing proliferation.

Cyclosporin A

- fungal product
- selectively penetrates antigen-sensitive T cells in G_0 and G_1 phase and inhibits RNA polymerase causing blockage of interleukin 2 production by T_H needed for clonal expansion of cytotoxic T cells
- nephrotoxic at certain doses so blood concentrations need to be monitored.

Tacrolimus (FK506)

- fungal product
- suppresses lymphokine production by T_H.

Rapamycin

- fungal macrolide
- interferes with intracellular signalling pathways of the IL-2 receptor.

Effects of immunosuppressive treatment

Nephrotoxicity

Direct acute nephrotoxicity is associated with cyclosporin treatment linked with vacuolation of tubular epithelium and hyalinization of arteriole walls. Chronic nephrotoxicity can also occur with cylosporin treatment associated with interstitial fibrosis and tubular atrophy.

Infection

Immunosuppression increases the risk of infection.

Hypertension

Seen in about 50% of post-renal transplant patients. May be associated with cyclosporin which causes vasoconstriction. This is independent of the renin–angiotensin system and is responsive to restricted salt intake.

Hyperlipidaemia

Seen in about 60% post-transplant patients. Combined type (cholesterol and triglyceride increased).

Neoplasia

Likely to be caused by decreased immunosurveillance. Tumours include:

- squamous cell carcinoma of skin
- post-transplant lymphoproliferaive disorders. These are lymphoproliferations, mostly B-cell type and associated with Epstein–Barr Virus infection, which may respond to decreased immunosuppression or may behave more aggressively, in which case they are considered to be lymphomas and treated accordingly with chemotherapy.
- Kaposi's sarcoma
- carcinoma of the cervix uteri.

Bone marrow transplantation and graft–versus–host disease

The result of competent lymphoid cells from a donor being transferred into a recipient who is unable to reject them. If these donor lymphoid cells last long enough they mount an immune response against host (recipient) cells.

- clinically characterized by fever, weight loss, a rash, splenomegaly, anaemia and diarrhoea
- may respond to cyclosporin A therapy.

HLA RELATIONSHIPS WITH DISEASE

HLA distribution and linkage disequilibrium

Prevalence of various HLA types varies between populations. Sometimes alleles of one or more loci occur together more often than expected (linkage disequilibrium) which may be the result of:

- certain combinations conferring selective evolutional advantage in the past which would be different for different population groups
- combinations have arisen recently in evolution and insufficient time has elapsed for equilibrium to return
- migration has resulted in introduction of foreign haplotypes into a population leading to disequilibrium.

HLA associations with disease

Ankylosing spondylitis

B27 antigen is found in 90% of patients with ankylosing spondylitis (compared with 5% controls) and possession of the antigen gives an 80–90 times greater risk of developing the disease. Individuals with B27 have a 5–20% chance of developing ankylosing spondylitis. Fifty per cent of first-degree relatives of spondylitics also have B27 and 30% of these develop ankylosing spondylitis or some other spondyloarthropathy. Prevalence of B27 in different populations correlates with distribution of ankylosing spondylitis (B27 virtually absent from Japan and ankylosing spondylitis is rare in Japanese). Although B27 is equally distributed between males and females ankylosing spondylitis is 5 times more common in males so other factors must be involved.

Rheumatoid arthritis

Associated with DW4 and DR4 (present in 25% of controls and 45% individuals with rheumatoid arthritis). DR4 association is strongest for those with severe erosive changes and rheumatoid factors in serum. B8 and DR3 are associated with development of immune complex nephritis in patients treated with gold or D-penicillamine.

Coeliac disease

Strong association with B8 (60–81% coeliacs; 16–22% controls), DR3 (79% coeliacs) and D7 (45% coeliacs).

Myasthenia gravis

- early onset type associated with thymic hyperplasia has association with B8 and DR3
- adult onset type (often associated with thymoma) has no strong HLA association.

Juvenile diabetes

Shows associations with B8 and DR3 or B15 and DR4. Presence of DR3 increases relative risk to 3.3. Presence of DR4 increases relative risk to 6.4. Homozygosity for these increase the relative risk to 10 for DR3 and 16 for DR4. If both DR3 and DR4 are present the relative risk is 33.

Possible mechanisms for HLA associated disease

Possibilities include:

- molecular mimicry – histocompatibility antigens might show partial homology with some determinants on certain micro-organisms leading to a cross-reaction phenomenon
- certain HLA antigens might be susceptible to alterations following viral infection, toxin exposure and neoplastic transformation leading to loss of tolerance
- genes associated with the HLA complex and which determine the degree of immune reactivity might be involved in the HLA-associated diseases and determine the immune over-reaction associated with many of the conditions.

Granulomatous inflammation

.....

Definition Type of chronic inflammatory reaction characterized by accumulation of large numbers of macrophages.

Causes Occurs when a living pathogen (e.g. tuberculosis, leprosy, schistosomiasis) or foreign material (e.g. beryllium) that cannot be eliminated from the host by phagocytosis and killing or digestion.

.....

CELL BIOLOGY OF THE MACROPHAGE

Origin Derived from the bone marrow. Pro-monocyte released into the circulation as a monocyte. After 12–32 h monocytes migrate to the tissues maturing to form a macrophage. Macrophages can undergo mitotic division.

Phagocytosis and endocytosis

The macrophage can ingest a wide range of substances which then exist within its cytoplasm in membrane-bound vesicles (phagosomes). Large particles are engulfed by phagocytosis in a process that is:

- triggered by contact with object to be engulfed
- aided by opsonization (macrophage has receptors for the commonest opsonin IgGon surface as well as other receptors).

Pseudopodia form which surround the object.

Bacterial killing

Ingestion of the particles in the phagosome is associated with a respiratory burst and fusion of the phagosome with lysosomes resulting in microbial killing. Other microbicidal mechanisms are associated with the inducible pathway for nitric oxide (NO) synthesis. NO is important in the killing of certain pathogens and is one of the pathogenetic factors involved in septic shock. Some organisms (e.g. mycobacteria, *Brucella, Listeria, Salmonella,* toxoplasma, *Leishmania, Chlamydia, Rickettsia* and *Legionella pneumoniae*) maintain symbiosis with the macrophages unless the latter become activated.

The fate of macrophages

Following migration to a site of infection or tissue injury one of the following may occur:

1. The material ingested may be toxic to the macrophage which dies with release of intralysosomal contents.
2. If the stimulus disappears the macrophages migrate from the site of the lesion.
3. Ingestion of non-toxic undegradable material leads to conversion to a long-lived form that persists in the tissue.
4. Conversion into epithelioid cells. These may fuse to form macrophage polykaryons (multi-nucleate giant cells).

Epithelioid cells

- Slight morphological resemblance to squamous epithelial cells under light microscope.
- There is elongation of the cells with indistinct cell boundaries.
- Epithelioid cells have increased rough endoplasmic reticulum, more plasma membrane and more developed Golgi than unactivated macrophages.
- They have one tenth of the phagocytic ability of a non-transformed macrophage.
- There is less surface receptor expression.
- They are seldom associated with phagocytic material in their cytoplasm.
- They contain lysosomal enzymes (e.g. muramidase) and angiotensin-converting enzyme.
- Expression of 1-α-hydroxylase may result in the formation of active vitamin D (1,25 dihydroxy

cholecalciferol). In some cases this may be associated with hypercalcaemia.

Function of the macrophage

Macrophages are associated with the production of fever, expression of mediators of acute and chronic inflammation, microbicidal activity, preferential selection of TH1 or TH2 responses, lymphocyte activation, tissue breakdown and connective tissue matrix production.

Multi-nucleated giant cells (macrophage polykaryons)

Although not in fact the case there are conventionally thought to be two distinct forms:

- Foreign body giant cell – has nuclei dispersed evenly though the cytoplasm associated with response to exogenous foreign material (e.g. sutures) or misplaced endogenous material (e.g. hair, cholesterol crystals or keratin).
- Langhans' giant cell – multiple nuclei tend to form around the periphery of the cell in a horseshoe pattern. Most commonly seen in chronic infective granulomas (e.g. tuberculosis).

Giant cells are formed by macrophage fusion which may be stimulated by the attempt of two or more cells to endocytose the same material.

CLASSIFICATION OF THE GRANULOMATOUS RESPONSE

Cell kinetics

Low turnover Macrophages remain for a long time with little migration of new cells and little mitotic activity. The irritant is typically non-toxic and non-degradable and persists within the cells. Epithelioid cells are usually not present. Lymphoid cells are unusual.

High turnover   Constant recruitment of macrophages to compensate for high death rate. Irritant is usually highly toxic and present in a small proportion of the cells. Epithelioid cells are common.

Involvement of immunological mechanisms

Without evidence of immunological mechanisms

A major feature is the lack of specific recognition of the irritant by the immune system and therefore no enhanced response on second exposure to the agent. Lesions appear at the same time after exposure and are of the same size. Immunosuppression has no effect on granuloma formation. It is impossible to transfer reactivity from animal to animal.

With evidence of immunological mechanisms

First exposure to the irritant results in an altered state of reactivity with an accelerated and more severe response to subsequent exposure. Immunosuppressive agents can modify the granulomatous response. Altered reactivity can be transferred from animal to animal by cells, serum or both.

Scar tissue formation on granulomas

Results from a balance of factors secreted by the cells of the granulomas that on one hand promote fibroblast chemotaxis, division and activity, and on the other hand lead to collagen breakdown.

Some specific granulomatous disorders

TUBERCULOSIS

Epidemiology

Incidence decreased in Western countries dropping from causing 200 deaths per 100 000 per year in the USA at the beginning of the twentieth century to 4.1 per 100 000 per year in 1965. In less privileged countries the prevalence remains high and worldwide approximately 3–5 million people die from tuberculosis each year. More recently emergence of multi-drug-resistant organisms in developed countries and the appearance of the acquired immunodeficiency syndrome (AIDS) has lead to a resurgence of the disease.

Decline in mortality from tuberculosis has been associated with better socio-economic factors including improved housing, nutrition and sanitation, effective chemotherapy, enhanced detection by mass miniature radiograph screening, pasteurization of milk and tuberculin testing of dairy cattle.

Associations

Increased risk of developing tuberculosis is associated with diabetes, immunosuppressive treatment, AIDS and silicosis.

Bacteriology

Caused by *Mycobacterium tuberculosis* a slender slightly curved rod-shaped aerobic bacterium. Staining characteristics include resistance to decolourization by acid and alcohol (acid-fast) associated with long-chain fatty acids in the capsule. The organism stains red with a Ziehl–Neelsen stain and can be stained with auramine (giving yellow fluorescence under UV light). The organism grows slowly (colonies may only be visible after 4 weeks) on the egg-based Löwenstein–Jensen medium or the agar-based Middlebrook 7H10 and 7H11. Direct examination of smeared material (e.g.

sputum) gives a sensitivity of detection of only 22–80% (mean 55%). Newer DNA based detection has reduced the time and increased the sensitivity of tests compared to conventional staining.

Pathogenesis

Five strains are recognized (human, bovine, murine, avian and reptilian) and infection can occur by inhalation, ingestion (rare following testing of cattle and pasteurization) and inoculation. The tissue damage associated with tuberculosis is due to the specific reactivity of the immune system occurring as a result of the presence of the bacterium. This expresses itself in two ways:

1. Enhanced resistance to infection and more effective clearing of the bacterium.
2. Appearance of hypersensitivity causing most of the damage.

Virulence of mycobacteria   No exotoxin is secreted. Different strains exhibit differences in their power to cause disease.

Increased virulence is associated with components that protect the organism from intracellular killing:

- 'Cord' factor – a surface glycolipid. When present causes the organism to grow in cords. Associated with the ability to induce granuloma formation and inhibits neutrophil chemotaxis.
- Sulfatides – surface glycoproteins. Inhibit fusion between lysosomes and phagosomes.
- Lipoarabinomannan (LAM). A lipopolysaccharide resembling endotoxin. Inhibits upregulation of macrophage killing by interferon, increases output of TNF (associated with fever, weight loss and tissue destruction) and increases IL-10 secretion which inhibits induced T cell proliferation.

Tuberculous granuloma

Evolution of granuloma from first introduction of bacterium:

1. Initial mild and transient acute inflammatory reaction.
2. Organisms are engulfed by local macrophages and presented to appropriate T-helper cells.

3. This interaction leads to a proliferation of specifically coded T cells and the release of cytokines.
4. Next there is infiltration by macrophages which accumulate at the site of infection and become immobilized.
5. Many macrophages undergo epithelioid change. Some fuse to form multi-nucleate giant cells. The clusters of epithelioid cells acquire a mantle of T lymphocytes.
6. Within 10–14 days evidence of coagulative necrosis begins to appear, characterized by firm 'cheesy' material (caseation).

Natural history of the tissue response

Different tissues and different individuals may react differently to the presence of *Mycobacterium tuberculosis*. These differences are probably accounted for by:

- organism virulence
- dose of bacterium
- degree of local and general resistance
- type and degree of hypersensitivity
- innate immunity – some races appear inherently more susceptible to tuberculosis (e.g. North American Indians and black races)
- age – the very young (under 5 years) and elderly appear more at risk of developing tuberculosis
- immunosuppression associated with disease (e.g. AIDS) or treatments (e.g. prolonged high-dose corticosteroids) increases the risk of tuberculosis
- previous exposure to mycobacteria – one of the most important factors modulating the natural history of tuberculosis as illustrated by the Koch phenomenon.

The Koch phenomenon This describes the results of subcutaneous injection of *M. tuberculosis* into a guinea pig not previously exposed to the organism.

No reaction for first 10–14 days followed by appearance of a nodule containing tuberculous granulomas. Mycobacteria have been transported to regional lymph nodes which become enlarged and show caseous necrosis. In time there is dissemination of the disease followed by death. If the dose is such that the animal survives at least 4 weeks a second subcutaneous injection results in rapid (within a few days) development of a nodule which ulcerates and heals without regional lyph node enlargement.

These findings indicate that:

- local tissue response to second infection is more rapid than the first
- local clearance of organisms by macrophages is more rapid with the second exposure
- macrophages containing viable organisms are immobilized at the site with the second infection
- local hypersensitivity is increased after the second infection causing rapid necrosis.

Hypersensitivity in tuberculosis

The chief factor in the modulation of the degree of tissue destruction in tuberculosis is hypersensitivity to some antigenic components of the bacillus. This causes caseation necrosis and is associated with the severe constitutional effects associated with large bacterial doses. Liquefactive necrosis may occur with active local proliferation of baceria. This liquefied tissue usually contains large numbers of bacteria and may rupture along tissue plains or into bronchi, lymphatics and blood vessels.

The balance between cell-mediated immunity (as manifested by an enhanced ability to clear mycobacteria from host tissues) and the tissue damage related to hypersensitivity determines the natural history of tuberculous infections. The tissue-damaging component is the major contributor to the clinical expressions of tuberculosis.

Patterns of tuberculosis

First infection type (childhood tuberculosis)

Lodgement of of *M. tuberculosis* is usually followed by development to a small lesion often less than 1 cm in greatest dimension. This lesion is almost always situated just below the pleura either in the basal segment of the upper lobe or the apical segment of the lower lobe (Ghon focus).

Macrophages laden with the organism travel to the draining hilar lymph nodes which enlarge and show caseation necrosis. The combination of the rather inconspicuous parenchymal lesion and the prominent lymphadenopathy is known as the primary or Ghon complex.

Most primary lesions both in the lung parenchyma and in the lymph node heal with complete replacement of the caseous necrosis by fibrous tissue or (more often) by walling off of the necrotic area by scar tissue followed by dystrophic calcification in the caseous material. In the latter case organisms can survive in the calcified foci for many years. If high grade hypersensitivity develops there may be an outpouring of fibrin-rich exudate. Spread may take place via the bronchi or bloodstream, usually after softening of the necrotic material.

Miliary tuberculosis   If the number of organisms in the circulation is large and host resistance low spread is characterized by very large numbers of small granulomas of almost equal size which stud the kidneys, spleen, brain, meninges, adrenals and liver. This type of spread may also be seen in the elderly receiving immunosuppressive therapy and in patients with AIDS.

'Organ' tuberculosis   If the dose of organism in the bloodstream is small a different distribution is seen with a single organ the dominant site.

Adult-type pulmonary tuberculosis
In the adult the parenchymal lesions usually start in the sub-apical region of the upper lobe (Assman foci). No prominant lymph node involvement is seen although microscopic involvement may be present.

The lesions are thought to arise from:

* primary infection with different response from that in childhood
* secondary infection in someone who has a degree of immunity
* reactivation of previous infection due to decline in efficacy of cell-mediated immunity.

Natural history of adult-type pulmonary tuberculosis
* healing: If there is a high degree of immunity lesions may heal with scarring and calcification
* softening and cavitation: Softening with caseous necrosis may occur and if this is associated with erosion into a bronchus there may be cavitation. Communication with an airway increases oxygen tension and favours bacterial multiplication. The patient will cough up potentially infectious material. Blood vessels in the wall of the cavity may show thombotic occlusion or may be eroded

with resultant massive haemorrhage. Involvement of overlying pleura may be associated with a serous pleural effusion, a persistent fibrinous exudate or tuberculous empyema (pleural space containing partly liquefied caseous material)

- spread: Spread may be via the bloodstream or by natural anatomical pathways such as through the bronchial system, up into the larynx and subsequently into the bowel.

·····································

LEPROSY

Definition   Chronic infectious disease of humans caused by *Mycobacterium leprae*.

Sites   Principally the skin, nasal mucosa, peripheral nerves and testis.

Bacteriology   Same morphological features as other mycobacteria but more easily decolourized by acid necessitating a modification of the Ziehl–Neelsen stain for identification (Wade–Fite stain). Organism is an obligate intracellular parasite and cannot be cultured but can proliferate in the footpad of the mouse and nine-banded armadillo.

Epidemiology   Rare disease in Western communities. Most sufferers are found in Asia.

Transmission   Person to person with low infectivity rates. The incubation period is about 3–6 years before tuberculoid lesions are seen but 10–20 years for the lepromatous form.

Pathology   Response to infection by *Mycobacterium leprae* is variable depending on the degree of cell-mediated response. The two extremes are termed lepromatous and tuberculoid leprosy.

Lepromatous leprosy

Widespread lesions are present in the skin and mucous membranes. These lesions contain large numbers of foamy macrophages, some lymphocytes, plasma cells and mast cells. Enormous numbers of organisms are present in the macrophages. There is no cutaneous hypersensitivity suggesting poor or absent cell-mediated immunity. However the patients are able to produce antibody to bacterial determinants and in some people this may result in immune complexes being deposited in small subcutaneous blood vessel walls causing painful nodules (erythema nodosum leprosum).

Tuberculous leprosy

Scantier lesions but peripheral nerve involvement is common. Histologically there are tightly packed organized granulomas without caseation. Lymphocytes are numerous. Bacteria are very difficult to identify. Cutaneous hypersensitivity can be demonstrated showing that there is some cell-mediated immunity.

Intermediate forms

Intermediate forms of tissue response exist with those more closely resembling the lepromatous form containing more bacteria.

....

SARCOIDOSIS

Epidemiology Fairly common in Northern Europe. Highest incidence in Sweden.

Aetiology   Unknown. Suggestions include:
- mycobacterial infection with altered cell-mediated immunity
- non-specific reaction to a variety of irritants
- infective agent that is as yet unrecognized. This is supported by the observation that development of granulomas can be induced by the transfer of material from the lesion from one animal to another immunologically deficient animal.

Sites Most organs and tissue may be involved but the lung is most frequently involved. Lymph nodes, spleen and liver may also be involved. In the skeleton the small bones of the fingers are most conspicuously affected. Skin, uveal tract, lacrimal and salivary glands may be involved. Occasionally sarcoidosis may affect the neurohypothesis causing diabetes incipidus. Hypercalcaemia is not uncommon as a result of activation of 1-α-hydroxylase in epithelioid cells.

Histopathology   Well-formed epithelioid granulomas with little or no central necrosis. Multi-nucleated cells may contain calcified bodies which in some cases are star-shaped (asteroid bodies). The granulomas are cuffed by small lymphocytes.

SYPHILIS

Bacteriology   Caused by the spirochaete *Treponema pallidum*, a corkscrew-shaped bacillus. The organism cannot be cultured but can be maintained in the tissues of living animals such as rabbit testis. The organism can be visualized in fluid taken from ulcerated lesions either by silver impregnation techniques or by using dark-field microscopy. There is an anti-phagocytic mucopolysaccharide capsule and the organism can down-regulate the T cell response.

Transmission   Sexually transmitted disease requiring direct contact. Entry of the organism is facilitated by the presence of minute abrasions in the skin and mucous membranes. The organism is sensitive to heat and drying so transmission on inanimate objects (e.g. tea cups) is unlikely. Transplacental infection can occur.

Immunology   Within 1–3 weeks of the first lesion appearing antibodies can be detected. Two groups of antibodies have been identified, one of which forms the basis of diagnostic tests: the VDRL (Venereal Disease Research Laboratory) and Wassermann reactions.

Wassermann antibodies (anti-cardiolipin)
An IgM molecule reacting to cardiolipin. Not specific for syphilis and may be seen in association with malaria, leprosy, glandular fever, trypanosomiasis, other treponemal infections (yaws, pinta, bejel), mycoplasma pneumonia, some autoimmune haemolyic anaemias, sytemic lupus erythematosus, and after Coxsackie B infection. Cardiolipin has been shown to be present in *Treponema* which may act as the antigen but the antibodies do not react with the intact organism.

Antibodies binding specifically to intact Treponema pallidum

These can be detected in two ways:

- by immobilization of organisms in suspension
- by fluorescent antibody technique.

Natural history In many patients the disease will pursue a course lasting many years if untreated and falls into three clearly defined stages.

Primary syphilis

An indurated papule which is usually painless and often ulcerates (chancre) occurs usually within a month of infection. Microscopically there is an inflammatory infiltrate that is rich in plasma cells, lymphocytes and macrophages. Endothelial cells lining blood vessels in the area swell and may occlude the lumen. The draining lymph nodes may be enlarged. Organisms are usually plentiful and may be found in the fluid that oozes from the ulcerated chancre. The chancres heal spontaneously. In about 50% the disease progesses no further but in the other half widespread dissemination of the treponema occurs leading to the secondary stage.

Secondary syphilis

Occurs within 2–3 months of exposure. There is a generalized rash (particularly face, palms and soles) usually with red or copper-coloured papules. The mucous membranes of the mouth show white patches that break down to form lesions known as 'snail-track ulcers'. Flat papules (condylomata lata) occur at moist cutaneous/mucocutaneous areas (e.g. anus, vulva and perineum) which contain large numbers of organisms and are very infectious. Generalized, slightly tender lymph-node enlargement is common. Immune complexes may cause lesions in the kidney. Fever, myalgia and general malaise are common. The symptoms and the lesions disappear spontaneously over a few months and the patients are then no longer infectious. Complete clearance of the organism is rare and the treponemas appear to enter a latent phase which may last many years and is brought to an end when there is some diminution of cell-mediated immunity.

Tertiary syphilis

These lesions are very destructive. There are two basic tissue responses.

Gummatous necrosis   A gumma may occur anywhere in the body with predilection for the liver, testis, subcutaneous tissue and bone The clinical features will depend on the location. The gumma is an area of rubbery coagulative necrosis. Microscopically the gumma is surrounded by plump fibroblasts. Blood vessels in the periphery show narrowing of the lumen. Treponemas are very scanty. Healing occurs with criss-crossing fibrous bands and coarse scarring.

Small blood vessel disease   There is periadventitial cuffing by lymphocytes and plasma cells. Endothelial cells swell and may proliferate and can lead to obliteration of the lumen. In the cardiovascular system the ascending and thoracic parts of the aorta are the chief targets. Involvement of the vasa vasorum and their extensions into the aortic wall leads to destruction of the elastic laminae and smooth muscle of the media and thus to aneurysm formation. The intimal surface shows a wrinkled appearance likened to tree-bark. Neither of these changes are specific for syphilis.

Syphilis and the central nervous system

Tertiary syphilis in the central nervous system falls into two groups.

Meningovascular syphilis   Involving either the leptomeninges (more frequently) or pachymeninges. Leptomeningitis occurs mostly at the base of the brain with swelling and thickening. Gummatous necrosis may occasionally be seen. Cranial nerve involvement is not uncommon and there may be obstruction of the 4th ventricle causing hydrocephalus. Pachymeningitis may occur over the surface and in relation to the spinal cord.

Parenchymatous neurosyphilis

1. Tabes dorsalis: Characterized by degeneration of certain sensory fibres in the posterior nerve roots and posterior columns of the spinal cord. The posterior columns atrophy and become grey. This is associated with fibre loss and demyelination. The degeneration leads to loss of function especially in respect to deep pressure sensation,

vibration and position sense and co-ordination leading to a stamping gait. There may be severe shooting pains in the limbs (lightning pains). The lack of sensation may lead to disorganization of joints (Charcot's joints).

2. General paresis of the insane: The brain becomes shrunken and the cerebral cortex is disorganized with degeneration of nerve cells and fibres especially in the grey matter which is associated with proliferation of astrocytes. Intracerebral blood vessels show perivascular plasma cells cuffing and endothelial swelling. Organisms are relatively easy to find. Clinically there is deterioration in personality and changes in mental function which may express themselves in bizarre and grandiose delusions. If untreated there is dementia.

Congenital syphilis

Transplacental spread usually occurs in the fifth month of pregnancy. This may lead to abortion, stillbirth, development of congenital syphilis in the neonatal period or latent infection. If the infection causes lesions in the perinatal period these are dominated by skin and mucous membrane involvement. These lesions are highly infective and contain large numbers of organisms. Severe deformities of bone may occur including formation of new bone over the surface of the tibia giving a sabre-like appearance. The liver may be diffusely affected, there may be interstitial fibrosis in the lung and the cornea may show inflammation. The teeth can show characteristic changes with screw-driver or peg-shaped incisors (Hutchinson's teeth).

Congenital infection with a prolonged latent period shows similar manifestations to the tertiary stage of acquired infection.

16

Amyloid and amyloidoses

....

Definition Disparate set of disorders characterized by extracellular deposition of proteins with fibrils arranged in the form of a β-pleated sheet.

Synonyms Waxy or lardaceous degeneration.

Macroscopy Organs in which large amounts of amyloid are deposited become larger, firmer and paler than normal. Amyloid may stain a rich brown colour with Lugol's iodine.

Microscopy
- eosinophilic and lacks structure
- binds the dye **Congo red** staining orange-red and shows characteristic green/yellow birefringence in polarized light. This is a fairly sensitive method of detection and the most reliable everyday diagnostic method. If the sections are treated with potassium permanganate staining with Congo red is abolished for amyloid derived from cleavage of the acute phase protein SAA (amyloid A) but retained for amyloid derived from immunoglobulin light chain
- shows metachromasia when stained with **methyl violet** (stains red)
- electron microscopy shows bundles of fibrils of variable width (**7–14 nm**) measuring up to **1600 nm** in length. Pentagonal sub-units are seen along the fibrils consisting of **amyloid P component** (coded on chromosome 1).

P component Belongs to family of pentameric glycoproteins called pentraxins which include acute phase proteins such as C reactive protein. Blood concentrations of amyloid P component increases under the same circumstances as other acute phase proteins.

CLASSIFICATION

Older classifications relied on clinical and pathological criteria but contained inconsistences.

1. **Primary amyloidosis**: presence of a tendency to nodular deposition with predilection for mesenchymal tissues. Absence of preceding or concurrent disease. Differs from amyloidosis associated with myelomatosis only by the presence of osteolytic lesions in the latter.
2. **Secondary amyloidosis**: followed or associated with a wide range of identifiable diseases (mainly chronic inflammatory disorders).

Newer classifications are based on assessment of three characteristic properties:

- nature of the amyloid protein
- whether the amyloidosis is acquired or inherited
- distribution of the amyloid deposits.

SYSTEMIC AMYLOIDOSIS
Amyloidosis of immune origin (AL type)

Acquired disorder, systemically distributed with immunoglobulin light chain (or homologous N-terminal fragment) as precursor.

Associations Monoclonal proliferations of B lymphocytes or plasma cells. Twenty per cent associated with myeloma but others associated with Waldenstrom's macroglobulinaemia, heavy chain disease and agammaglobulinaemia.

Chemistry Composed of intact immunoglobulin light chains, amino-terminal fragment of light chain or occasionally a combination of these. Most are λ light chain. Deposition is associated with conversion from an α-helical structure to a β-pleated sheet. Not all light chains can undergo this change.

Cellular source Most are due to a single clone of B-lymphocyte derived cells whose product circulates in the blood in the form of Bence Jones protein.

Epidemiology   Disease of middle life and old age. M>F.

Clinical features   May be associated with neuropathy (peripheral or autonomic), restrictive cardiomyopathy (with exquisite sensitivity to digitalis, increased risk of arrhythmias, conduction defects and sudden death), skin manifestations (pinch purpura, nodules on skin resembling drops of candle wax and changes similar to scleroderma), polyarthropathy, enlargement of the tongue (macroglossia), isolated deficiency of clotting factor X and carpal tunnel syndrome. Amyloidosis may be associated with long-term haemodialysis when the protein involved is β-2-microglobulin which shows some homology to the constant region of immunoglobulin heavy and light chains.

Laboratory findings   Plasma or urinary monoclonal immunoglobulin in 90%. Bone marrow contains increased numbers of plasma cells.

Reactive systemic amyloidosis (AA type)

In most cases this is acquired but may be associated with the inherited familial Mediterranean fever (autosomal recessive), systemically distributed (kidney, liver, spleen and adrenals are sites of predilection) with serum amyloid A (SAA) as the precursor protein.

Chemistry   SAA is an acute phase protein (12.5 kilodaltons) produced chiefly by the liver, production of which is upregulated by IL-1, TNF-α and probably IL-6. Amyloid A appears to be a cleavage product of SAA from which 28 amino-acid residues have been removed from the carboxy-terminal end. The pathogenesis remains unclear.

Associations   Chronic inflammatory diseases associated with infections (e.g. tuberculosis, leprosy, syphilis, chronic oseomyelitis and bronchietasis), other chronic inflammations of unknown aetiology (e.g. rheumatoid arthritis and other connective conditions, ulcerative colitis and Crohn's disease) or where infection may be implicated (e.g. Reiter's syndrome, Whipple's disease), long-standing paraplegia (possibly associated with recurrent urinary tract infections) and some neoplasms (especially renal adenocarcinoma and Hodgkin's disease).

Clinical features and pathology The liver is enlarged, firm and pale with amyloid deposited in the space of Disse. The liver cell cords become atrophic but clinical effects may not be apparent due to hepatic reserve. In the kidney the amyloid is deposited in the walls of the glomerular capillaries and in relation to the basement membranes of arterioles and tubules. The kidney is either enlarged and pale or if there has been secondary ischaemic changes may be scarred and shrunken. Involvement of glomeruli leads to the nephrotic syndrome and eventually chronic renal failure. Involvement of the spleen is discussed elsewhere.

Hereditary systemic amyloidosis
Collection of hereditary syndromes with systemic distribution associated with transthyretin (previously prealbumin) as the precursor except in the Finnish variety of familial amyloid polyneuropathy where gelsolin is the precursor and familial Mediterranean fever (SAA).

Chemistry Transthyretin transports about 25% of plasma thyroxine and transports retinol (vitamin A). Hereditary amyloidosis is associated with mutations in the gene encoding this protein. The tertiary structure of transthyretin is normally β-pleated with the molecule forming first dimers and then tetramers by the fusion of two dimers. The presence of a mixture of normal and mutated transthyretin in a tetramer appears to promote the joining of several hundred tetramers to form amyloid fibrils.

Epidemiology Rare disorders (fewer than 1 per 100 000 per year in the USA). With the exception of familial Mediterranean fever (autosomal recessive) all have autosomal dominant inheritance.

Clinical features Three syndromes:
- *Neuropathic* characterized by progressive systemic polyneuropathy which occurs in three forms:
  A group in which lower limbs are affected first and predominantly. Found in Portugal, Sweden and Japan.
  B group in which upper limbs are particularly affected. Found in Germany and Switzerland.
  C group in which the face is affected. Reported only in Finland.

- *Cardiopathic* found in one Danish family and a kindred in the Appalachian region of the USA of German–Irish–English origin.
- *Nephropathic* with two forms:

  1. Familial Mediteranean fever.

     Epidemiology Commonest form of hereditary systemic amyloidosis. Autosomal recessive inheritance. High incidence in Sephardic Jews, Anatolian Turks, Armenians and Middle Eastern Arabs.

     Chemistry AA amyloid. Plasma concentrations of SAA are raised between attacks but rise steeply during febrile bouts.

     Clinical features Expressed in one or both of
     - short-lived self-limiting febrile attacks associated with pain
     - amyloidosis which may manifest itself early in life.

     Early diagnosis before the development of the nephrotic syndrome is important as development of amyloid can be inhibited in 90% by administration of colchicine.

  2. Familial neuropathic amyloidosis with febrile urticaria and nerve deafness.

     Clinical features Febrile attacks associated with urticarial skin rash and malaise, rigors and limb pains. Progressive nerve deafness followed in some patients by development of proteinuria leading to nephrotic syndrome and chronic renal failure.

Senile cardiovascular amyloid (transthyretin)

Epidemiology Non-familial. Occurs in elderly people. About 25% people over 80 years of age are affected

Clinical features Present with cardiac failure. Systemic sites may be effected. Other forms of amyloid in the elderly involving only the cardiovascular system include **isolated atrial amyloidosis** and **aortic amyloidosis**.

LOCALIZED AMYLOIDOSIS

Endocrine related amyloid

Certain endocrine organs can be infiltrated with amyloid. In the pituitary this is age-related but in the pancreatic islets this is associated with non-insulin dependent diabetes mellitus. Certain tumours are associated with amyloid deposition locally but not systemically, including medullary carcinoma of the thyroid (precursor protein is the 9–19 amino acid portion of the calcitonin molecule).

Intracerebral amyloidosis

Central nervous system amyloidosis is the commonest localized form. Occurs in Alzheimer's disease, in some spongiform encephalopathies, in the dementia occurring in boxers and in some hereditary haemorrhagic syndromes.

General pathology of viral infection

··

GENERAL CHARACTERISTICS

Size

- smallest infective agents known (20–300 nm diameter)
- majority can only be visualized by electron microscopy.

Genome

- each virus contains one nucleic acid type (DNA or RNA) which forms the basis of virus classification
- nucleic acid is covered by a symmetrically arranged protein shell (**capsid**) containing clusters of polypeptides that form recognizable units (**capsomeres**)
- arrangement of the capsid falls into two structural patterns
  - **icosahedral** (20 sided)
  - **helical**
- DNA viruses (except poxviruses) have icosahedral capsid
- RNA virus capsid may be icosahedral or helical
- the mature infective virus particle (**virion**) may be the genome and the capsid only (most DNA viruses except herpes viruses) or this may be surrounded by a glycoprotein envelope (most RNA viruses except picornaviruses and reoviruses).

··

INTERACTION BETWEEN VIRUS AND HOST

Viruses and the target cell

Effects of a disease-causing virus may stem from:

- changes produced by virus on host cell:
  - damage or death of cell
  - persistence of virus in cell without injury (**persistent infection**)

129

    – transformation of cell allowing indefinite numbers of passages in culture and making it susceptible to tumour formation in vivo (**tumourgenicity**)

- host tissue reaction to these changes
- response of the immune system to virus and/or tissue changes.

Transmission of viral infections

This may be:

- **vertical**: mother to child in utero or perinatally
- **horizontal**: person to person via respiratory (aerosols), gastrointestinal (faecal–oral), genitourinary (sexual) or percutaneous routes, or it may be accomplished by a sequence of steps.

1. Attachment to cell surface membrane

This mostly requires the presence of a receptor on the surface membrane of cell e.g.

- poliovirus – specific lipoprotein receptor on neurones and intestinal tract lining cells
- influenza virus – specific glycoprotein receptor (N-acetylneuraminic acid, NANA)
- Epstein–Barr virus – receptor for C3
- rabies virus – acetylcholine receptor
- human immunodeficiency virus – CD4 receptor.

Not all viral attachment is specific. Ortho and paramyxo-viruses attach to sialic acid residues on host cell surfaces of most cells including those not susceptible to infection.

2. Penetration of cell

Following attachment the virion becomes engulfed within the cell by a process akin to receptor mediated endocytosis, which is temperature and energy dependent. In some cases the viral envelope and plasma membranes fuse to release nucleoplasmid into the cell cytoplasm.

3. Uncoating of viral nucleic acid

The physical separation of viral nucleic acid from outer structural proteins is associated with loss of infectivity and usually occurs within cytoplasm.

It sometimes starts during the attachment stage. In a few viruses of reovirus group uncoating is never completed.

4. Viral replication

DNA viral replication   Transcribed in two stages giving rise to mRNA at two points: **early** and **late**.

Early transcription occurs in host cell nucleus. The mRNA reaches the cytoplasm and is translated on host ribosomes to **early proteins**. These are required for the formation of new viral DNA which takes place in the host nucleus.

Late mRNA is then transcribed. This leaves the nucleus and is translated into **late proteins** which constitute material for capsomeres. These enter the nucleus and the virions are assembled; the virions are released by bursting of the cell.

All DNA viruses replicate in this way using host cell polymerases *except* poxviruses which replicate in the cytoplasm and use their own DNA-dependent RNA polymerase.

RNA viral replication   All RNA viruses replicate in the cytoplasm *except* orthomyxoviruses and retroviruses which replicate in the cell nucleus. RNA viruses carry their own RNA-dependent polymerase; after uncoating the viral RNA may act as its own messenger and this is translated to form the RNA polymerase used to create the intermediate replicative viral RNA which is double stranded (one strand is parent; the other strand being complementary). At this time inhibitors are formed which effectively switch off normal cell synthetic processes.

From double stranded replicative RNA single stranded viral RNA molecules are formed which may:

- serve as templates for further viral RNA synthesis
- serve as mRNA for capsid protein synthesis
- become encapsulated to form mature virions.

Retroviral replication   Viral genetic information is inserted into the host genome. First, viral RNA must be copied to DNA by action of RNA-dependent DNA polymerase (reverse transcriptase). The DNA replica (provirus) is then inserted into the host DNA.

Transcription of the provirus is mediated by host-cell RNA polymerases, and transcribed RNA serves both as mRNA for the synthesis of viral antigens and as genomic viral DNA to be packaged into new virions.

5. Release of virus

This may occur by:

- bursting or lysis of the host cell
- budding from the host cell membrane (host cell not destroyed).

Morphological and functional effects of viruses on host cells

No change   Cells in which the viral infection is **latent** show no structural abnormality.

Cell death   Common outcome of viral infections. Cell type affected plays dominant role in determining patterns of disease. In cell culture the changes leading to cell death help in viral identification. Cell death is not always obvious but may be the result of:

- cell lysis
- cessation of normal synthetic activity of host cell
- destruction by immune system which recognizes viral proteins on host cell surface as foreign.

Alterations to cell surface membranes   Some viruses (e.g. some paramyxoviruses) cause fusion between infected and non-infected cells.

Formation of inclusion bodies   Inclusion bodies are localized changes in the staining properties of nucleus or cytoplasm of cells infected by certain viruses, and may be detected by light microscopy. Appearing as rounded, sharply demarcated areas with affinity to acid dyes (eosinophilic), they may be:

- intracytoplasmic e.g. poxviruses; paramyxoviruses, reoviruses
- intranuclear e.g. herpes viruses; adenoviruses.

Cell proliferation   Independent of oncogenic effect, certain viral infections cause cell proliferation (e.g. B lymphocyte proliferation associated with Epstein–Barr virus causing infectious mononucleosis).

Neoplastic transformation   Some viruses are directly implicated in tumourgenesis.

NATURAL HISTORY OF VIRAL INFECTIONS

Acute productive infections

Virus replicates in infected cells with viruses produced and released. This may lead to clinical symptoms or may be sub-clinical.

Failure of viral elimination

If this occurs there may several consequences. Such infection may be:

latent – viruses not normally detected. Infection persists in occult, quiescent form. Episodes of reactivation occur with acute self-limiting illnesses. Often occurs with viruses of the herpes group (e.g. herpes simplex; varicella zoster virus).

chronic – viruses continually detected. Symptoms may be mild or absent.

persistent and slow – infection persists causing prolonged disease with slow development and often inexorable progress. Persistent infections are associated with infected individuals 'carrying' the virus (e.g. hepatitis B, cytomegalovirus, Epstein–Barr virus, virus causing lymphocytic choriomeningitis [an arenavirus], measles virus associated with sub-acute sclerosing panencephalitis). Slow progressive infections are associated with lentiviruses in sheep. Slow infections in humans include sub-acute sclerosing panencephalitis and progressive multi-focal leucoencephalopathy (caused by member of the papovavirus group, the JC virus).

oncogenic – part of viral genome incorporated into host genome causing malignant transformation.

PROTECTIVE RESPONSES OF HOST CELLS AGAINST VIRAL INFECTIONS

Interferons

These are divided into three groups, and associated with particular cell types although it is likely that all cells can produce each type when suitably stimulated.

- α interferon (IFN-α): released chiefly from leucocytes
- β interferon (IFN-β): released chiefly from fibroblasts
- γ interferon (IFN-γ) released by activated T lymphocytes.

Most important inducers of release of IFN-α and IFN-β are:

- viral infections
- infections caused by rickettsiae, protozoa
- bacterial endotoxins
- some synthetic polynucleotides.

Interferons produced by viral infections are species specific (e.g. chick interferon will not protect monkey cells) but are not virus specific. They appear 12–48 h after infection and at that time viral replication starts to decline.

Interferon secreted by an infected cell diffuses from that cell and binds to a membrane receptor on the surface of a neighbouring uninfected cell. IFN-α and IFN-β bind to the same receptor but IFN-γ is distinct. IFN binding triggers tyrosine kinase activity leading to transcription of genes encoding enzymes that block viral replication. Protection is mediated by blocking translation of viral mRNA – viral attachment and penetration is unaffected.

Other effects of interferon include inhibition of cell proliferation (at high doses); modification of some immune responses with increased T- and NK-cell activity and decreased antibody formation.

CLASSIFICATION OF VIRUSES

Most viruses can be separated into clearly defined groups on the basis of:

- type and form of nucleic acid genome
- size and morphology of virus
- method of transmission from host to host
- susceptibility to a variety of chemical/physical agents
- preference for certain hosts, tissues and cells
- diseases caused.

DNA-containing viruses

Poxviruses

- largest and most complicated viruses known

- double-stranded DNA genome
- brick-shaped or elliptical
- nucleocapsid enveloped by double membrane
- replicate solely within cytoplasm. May be associated with inclusion bodies
- diseases caused: **smallpox** and **molluscum contagiosum** in humans; **vaccinia** (cowpox), **monkeypox** and **orf** in animals (which may be transmitted to humans).

Herpes viruses

- large (nucleocapsid 90–110 nm; enveloped forms 120–200 nm diameter)
- double-stranded DNA genome
- capsid possesses icosahedral symmetry
- capsid enveloped by lipid containing envelope
- form intranuclear inclusion bodies (Cowdry type A bodies) rich in DNA, that virtually fill nucleus
- three types:

  - α herpes viruses: grow fast; cytolytic; tend to establish latent infection in neurones
  - β herpes viruses: slow growing; cause cellular enlargement (cytomegaly); become latent in secretory and renal tubular epithelia
  - γ herpes viruses: infect lymphoid cells.

Diseases caused:

- **herpes simplex virus** – cold sores; genital blistering
- **varicella zoster** – chickenpox; shingles
- **Epstein–Barr virus** (a γ herpes virus) – infectious mononucleosis; role in induction of Burkitt's lymphoma and nasopharyngeal carcinoma
- **herpes virus type 1** – an encephalitis; a keratoconjunctivitis; Kaposi's varicelliform eruption
- **cytomegalovirus**
- **human herpes virus 8** – implicated in development of Kaposi's sarcoma, some lymphomas and other malignancies.

Adenoviruses

- medium-sized (70–90 nm)
- double-stranded DNA genome
- icosahedral

- most of the 252 capsomeres are hexons but 12 are pentons in which the cytotoxic potential resides. From the pentons that form the corners of the virion fine fibres project, ending in a knob-like structure. These terminal knobs are responsible for red cell agglutination and adhesion to host cells
- nucleocapsid is not enveloped. Virus resists treatment with ether
- viral replication in nucleus
- seven main groups divided on basis of animal red cells that are agglutinated. 33 sub-types divided on basis of antigenic differences in hexon and fibre proteins
- of viruses infective to humans many exhibit latency and may survive in lymphoid tissue for many years.

Diseases caused:

- **Acute febrile pharyngitis** – affects infants and children most commonly. Usually caused by group C viruses. Symptoms are stuffy nose, cough, sore throat, fever.
- **Pharyngoconjunctival fever** – tends to occur in outbreaks in enclosed communities. Usually caused by group B viruses. Symptoms similar to acute febrile pharyngitis but with conjunctivitis.
- **Acute respiratory disease** – tends to occur in young military recruits. Associated with overcrowding and fatigue. Usually caused by group B viruses. Symptoms of fever, pharyngitis, cough, malaise.
- **Pneumonia** – complication of acute respiratory disease. May affect children and young adults. Mortality in children is high (8–10%). May occur in immunocompromised and bone marrow transplant recipients.
- **Mild self-limiting conjunctivitis** – associated with respiratory and pharyngeal syndromes
- **Follicular conjunctivitis** – self-limiting. Similar to that seen with chlamydial infection.
- **Epidemic keratoconjunctivitis** – acute conjunctivitis associated with enlargement of the pre-auricular nodes. Followed by corneal inflammation and formation of sub-corneal opacities which last up to 2 years.
- **Infantile gastroenteritis** – associated with serotypes 40 and 41.

- **Acute haemorrhagic cystitis** – occurs in male children. Associated with types 11 and 21.

Papovaviruses

- name derived from three members – papilloma virus, polyoma virus and vacuolating virus in monkeys
- small (43–53 nm)
- double-stranded DNA genome with circular pattern
- disease caused: in humans papilloma viruses cause common warts and almost certainly have a role in pathogenesis of cervical neoplasia and other squamous neoplasms of the genital region. Polyoma virus infection (**JC virus**) is associated with progressive multi-focal leucoencephalopathy.

Parvoviruses

- small (diameter about 20 nm)
- single-stranded DNA genome
- replicates in nucleus.

Diseases caused: **temporary erythroid aplasia** in patients with haemolytic anaemia (e.g. sickle cell anaemia), a common rash illness of childhood (erythema infectiosum, also known as fifth disease), a variety of gastroenteritis occurring particularly in cold weather (winter vomiting disease).

Hepadnaviruses

Many types that cause hepatitis in animals but only one virus causing disease in humans (**hepatitis B virus**). See liver section (page 416) for more details.

RNA-containing viruses

Picornaviruses

- very small (20–30 nm)
- single-stranded RNA as genome
- resistant to ether treatment
- divided into two genera.

Enteroviruses   These include:
- 3 types of poliovirus
- 29 types of Coxsackie virus
- 32 types of ECHO virus (enteric cytopathic human orphan virus).

They cause a variety of diseases including poliomyelitis, aseptic meningitis, myocarditis, myositis, herpangina and upper respiratory tract infections. Infection occurs via alimentary and respiratory tracts. There is no natural animal host, implying that eradication of disease in humans would eliminate the disease completely (e.g. for polio).

Rhinoviruses   113 types of this virus cause the common cold.

Orthomyxoviruses

- medium-sized
- pleomorphic: some spherical, some filamentous
- single-stranded RNA as genome. Exists in form of eight segments each representing a single gene. The eight gene segments code for 10–11 viral proteins
- viral genome continually changes. Minor changes in haemagglutinins through a series of point mutations over a long peiod is termed **antigenic drift**. From time to time a more fundamental change occurs, probably as a result of recombination of genome segments which is termed **antigenic shift**
- helically arranged capsid
- enveloped. Lipid envelope is studded with spike-like projections (peplomers) of two varieties – one a viral haemagglutinin (binds N-acetylneuraminic acid on surface membrane of most cells) the other a neuraminidase.

Diseases caused: **influenza**. Three types of influenza virus (A, B and C). Type A is most likely to undergo antigenic shift and causes most epidemics. Types B and C do not undergo antigenic shift. Type C is most stable.

Paramyxoviruses

- share some morphological features with orthomyxoviruses but are larger. Have haemagglutinins and neuraminidase which co-exist on the same spike on the envelope
- roughly cubical shape
- single-stranded RNA genome
- promote cell fusion with formation of multi-nucleate cells. This is due to a spike on the envelope glycoprotein

which is also necessary for penetration into cells (**F glycoprotein**).

Diseases caused:

- **sore throats and croup** (parainfluenza virus)
- **measles**
- **mumps**
- **infections of lower respiratory tract** (respiratory syncytial virus).

Rhabdoviruses

- curious shape-flattened at one end, rounded at the other
- single-stranded RNA genome
- nucleocapsid is enclosed in an envelope bearing spikes 10 nm in length.

Diseases caused: **rabies**.

Arenaviruses

- single-stranded RNA genome
- possess electron-dense granules in the virion.

Diseases caused:

- **Argentinian** and **Bolivian haemorrhagic fevers**
- **Lassa fever**
- **lymphocytic choriomeningitis** in mice.

Coronaviruses

- medium-sized
- pleomorphic with widely spaced club-shaped peplomers in lipoprotein envelope
- single-stranded RNA genome.

Togaviruses

- spherical, closely enveloped virus
- single-stranded RNA genome
- multiply in cell cytoplasm
- mature by budding from cytoplasmic membranes
- all, except rubella virus, belong to **arbovirus** group (**AR**thropod **BOR**ne viruses) in which arthropods are both the vector and the natural host. Viral multiplication

occurs before transmission to secondary vertebrate hosts. The vertebrates act as a reservoir. When humans, unnatural hosts, are infected there is serious illness.

Diseases caused:

- **yellow fever**
- **rubella** – not transmitted by insect. Classified as rubivirus.

Reoviruses

- single-stranded RNA genome.

Diseases caused:

- **orbivirus** – an arbovirus. Causes Colorado tick fever
- **rotavirus** – has double-layered capsid (outer layer smooth, inner layer roughened) giving wheel-like appearance to virion. Important cause of gastroenteritis.

Retroviruses

- diploid RNA genome which encodes reverse transcriptase (RNA-dependent DNA polymerase)
- genome contains at least 3 genes – *gag; pol; env.*

Three sub-families:

- **oncovirinae** – includes tumour-producing viruses
- **lentivirinae** – includes HIV
- **spumavirinae**.

Disorders of blood flow: a basis

....

THROMBOSIS

Definition A thrombus is a solid mass or plug formed within the heart, arteries, veins or capillaries from the components of streaming blood. In contrast to **clotting**, which is the activation of a protein cascade resulting in the formation of thrombin and the conversion of fibrinogen to fibrin polymer, **thrombosis** is characterized by a series of events involving the platelets of the blood.

Platelets and haemostasis

The contributiuon of platelets to haemostasis is mediated via a number of steps.

Adhesion

The platelet adheres to damaged endothelium or to exposed sub-endothelial tissues. This requires the binding of vessel wall-derived ligands to glycoprotein receptors on the platelet. Collagen in subendothelial tissue binds to the glycoprotein receptor GP Ia and von Willebrand's factor (**vWf**; exposed on damaged endothelial cells) to GP Ib. Deficient vWf (as in von Willebrand's disease) or of lack of GP Ib receptor (as in Bernard–Soulier syndrome) will result in a prolonged bleeding time. Adhesion is associated with a change in shape from the normal disc shape to a rounded shape.

Release

As a result of the shape change there is release of pre-formed and newly formed molecules that affect both the haemostatic process and the metabolism of the underlying vessel wall. Platelets contain two types of storage granules: α-granules contain e.g. **platelet derived growth factor,** thrombospondin, platelet factor 4, β-thromboglobulin, fibrinogen, fibronectin and vWf, while dense bodies contain ATP, ADP, GDP, GTP, serotonin and calcium. Release of the chemicals is usually triggered by exposure to collagen or thrombin. In addition to the release of these stored compounds collagen and thrombin initiate the release of arachidonate from the platelet membrane. This is the first step in the synthesis of prostaglandins including prostacyclin (anti-aggregatory) and thromboxane A_2 (pro-aggregatory). Stimulated endothelial cells also produce factors with the oposite effect to thromboxane A_2 the most potent of which is prostaglandin I_2.

Aggregation

This is the adhesion of platelets to other platelets to form a mass of activated cells associated with the formation of interplatelet fibrinogen bridges. Stimuli for aggregation are ADP and thromboxane A_2. These also activate more platelets giving a positive feedback and a rapid accumulation of platelets at a site of injury.

Provision of co-factors for clotting

Platelets also interact with clotting proteins playing an important part in the activation of prothrombin by Factor Xa and the activation of Factor X by the Factor IXa–VIIa complex.

Factors promoting thrombosis

Thrombosis can be likened to haemostasis occuring in the wrong place or at the wrong time and is therefore harmful rather than beneficial. Factors that promote thrombosis fall into three groups first recognised by Virchow (**Virchow's triad**).

Changes in the intimal surface of the vessel

The most important of these is atherosclerosis but injury, inflammation and neoplasms may be associated with thrombosis. When there is loss of the endothelial cell and exposure of subendothelial collagen platelet adhesion is inevitable. This happens in complicated atherosclerotic plaques when there is splitting (deep injury) or fraying (superficial injury) of the connective tissue 'cap'. Endothelial desquamation can also take place in the rare inhertied metabolic disorder homocystinuria and possibly in people who smoke.

Trauma to the endothelium can occur in certain circumstances e.g. following burning or freezing (frostbite) and may be associated with indwelling cannulas. **Chemical injury** is seen associated with infusion of certain compounds into veins and may be used therapeutically in the treatment of haemorrhoids and varicose veins. **Inflammation** such as seen on heart valves in patients with rheumatic or infective endocarditis may induce thrombosis. Arteries involved in an immune complex mediated inflammatory reaction (e.g. polyarteritis nodosa or temporal arteritis) may become thrombosed. **Neoplastic involvement** of small venules with invasion by malignant cells may be associated with thrombosis.

Changes in the pattern of blood flow

The important changes associated with thrombosis are change in the **speed** of normal laminar flow (particularly is relation to thrombosis in veins) and **loss of the normal laminar flow** by a **turbulent flow pattern** (particularly in the heart and arteries).

Reduction of the speed of blood flow may be general or local. Generalized slowing is seen in patients with severe congestive cardiac failure. Local slowing tends to occur particularly in the veins of the leg in association with prolonged dependence of the limb, reduced muscle pump activity and proximal occlusion of venous drainage. These are most likely to occur when a patient is immobilized in bed, especially after surgery so that deep venous thrombosis can be seen at autopsy in up to 30% of all patients and 60% of surgical patients. Prevention relates to minimizing changes in blood flow and should include exercises emphasizing calf and thigh muscle contraction, early postoperative ambulation and avoidance of prolonged dependency of lower limbs. **Stasis** of blood can occur in the heart and large vessels if segments become abnormally dilated (aneurysm), in dilated heart chamber associated with congestive cardiomyopathy and in the dilated atria of patients with mitral valve disease (particularly in association with atrial fibrillation). Intraventricular thrombosis may also occur following myocardial infarction because of local disturbances in blood flow.

Turbulent flow is of importance where arteries branch and in narrowed areas of arteries (chiefly due to atherosclerosis) where platelets tend to occur on the outer walls of the branches.

Changes in the constituents of the blood

Platelets   An abnormally low platelet count or impaired platelet function is associated with an abnormally long bleeding time. Increased risk of thrombosis may be associated with upregulation of platelet/vessel wall interactions (e.g. associated with injury to atherosclerotic plaque cap, prosthetic valves or synthetic grafts), an increase (usually local) of pro-coagulant factors, a decrease in natural anticoagulant factors, increased blood viscosity (e.g. associated with increased immunoglobulins in myeloma or with polycythaemia), the presence of anti-cardiolipin antibodies (lupus anti-coagulants), release of pro-coagulants by tumours, an increase in platelet count (thrombocytosis) or an increase in platelet adhesiveness or aggregatability.

Inherited disorders that increase risk of thrombosis

Abnormalities of anti-thrombin III

Genetics   Autosomal dominant inheritance. Most are heterozygotes with 50% decrease in normal AT III plasma concentrations.

Clinical features   Recurrent episodes of mainly venous thrombosis mostly affecting leg veins. Commonly complicated by pulmonary embolus. In women thrombi may be seen for the first time associated with pregnancy or oral contraceptive use; in men thrombus may develop following injury or surgery. Episodes increase with advancing age.

Protein C deficiency

Genetics   Autosomal dominant inheritance.

Laboratory findings Occurs in two forms. In the first the amount of plasma protein C is decreased while in the second type the concentrations are normal but there is a functional defect.

Clinical features Heterozygotes suffer from deep vein thrombosis and recurrent thrombophlebitis. Rarely the disease is homozygous when children have a devastating thrombo-embolic diathesis starting in infancy.

Protein S deficiency

Genetics Autosomal dominant inheritance.

Clinical features Similar to protein C deficiency.

Protein C resistance

Genetics Autosomal dominant inheritance.

Laboratory findings All natural anti-coagulant factors present in normal concentrations but there is an abnormal resistance to the normal biological effect of protein C.

Clinical features A syndrome associated with familial recurrent venous thrombosis.

Acquired disorders and environmental factors and thrombosis

Oral contraceptives

Confers 3–5 times increased risk of developing myocardial infarction or stroke. Risk correlates to amount of oestrogen in the compound. Contraceptives increase the plasma concentrations of fibrinogen and vitamin K-dependent factors by 10–20% and decrease levels of anti-thrombin III. Factor XII and pre-kallikrein are also increased.

Malignancy

In addition to disseminated intravascular coagulation patients with certain malignancies are prone to thrombosis. This is particularly true for mucin-secreting adenocarcinomas (especially pancreatic) and thrombosis (usually venous) may predate the presentation of the tumour. Malignant cells may release tissue thromboplastin and mucins or proteases from malignant cells may activate the extrinsic clotting pathway.

Nephrotic syndrome

Venous thrombosis (particularly renal vein) complicates up to 35% of cases. Arterial thrombosis occurs but is much rarer. The cause is unknown but antithrombin II levels fall proportionally with decline in serum albumin.

Evolution of venous thrombi

The process of thrombus formation in a non-inflamed vein is termed **phlebothrombosis**. When thrombosis occurs in an inflamed vein it is **thrombophlebitis**.

The site of initiation is usually the valve pocket with platelet adhesion. Once platelets are aggregated clotting factors are activated locally and fibrin strands stabilize the platelet aggregate and help to anchor it to the underlying vessel wall. A second phase begins in which a further batch of platelets is laid down over the original aggregate. At this stage the platelets can be seen to have aggregated in the form of laminae which project from the surface of the initial aggregate and lie across the stream of blood. The forces of the stream of blood bend the laminae in the direction of flow and form a somewhat coralline structure. Between the platelet laminae there are large numbers of red cells, some fibrin strands and a moderate number of leucocytes. This arrangement gives a rippled appearance when viewed from above. The elevated ridges on the surface of the thrombi are known as the **lines of Zahn**. The more rapid the blood flow the more prominent are the lines of Zahn. At this stage the process may terminate and the thrombus will become covered by endothelium and become incorporated into the underlying wall. If the process continues the mass continues to grow and the stream of blood slows further. Occlusion may ultimately occur. This phase is mediated predominantly via the clotting pathways rather than platelet adhesion and aggregation.

Once a segment is occluded the flow of blood cephalad to the occlusion becomes stagnant, up to the point at which the next venous tributary enters. The stagnant column clots (**consecutive clot**). This is the first step in the **propagation** of the thrombus. Propagation may proceed in one of two ways:

1. At the point at which blood enters from a tributary platelets adhere to the fibrin meshwork on the clot surface forming a small platelet thrombus and the process then proceeds as before.
2. If the venous return from the limb as a whole is slowed, propagation may proceed by formation of a consecutive clot on a massive scale.

Natural history of thrombi

Lysis   Some thrombi undergo lysis mediated by **plasmin**. Lysis can be initiated by treating patients with lytic agents such as streptokinase or genetically engineered plasminogen activator.

Embolization   Thrombi may become detached from the underlying wall and travel along the vascular path in the direction of normal flow. At some stage a vessel will be reached whose calibre is less than the diameter of the thrombotic material and impaction occurs.

Recanalization   Quite early on clefts may occur within the thrombotic material. These often lie along the long axis of the thrombus and may link up to form new channels. Within a few days these channels become lined by flattened cells of mesenchymal origin that differentiate into endothelial cells.

Organization of an occlusive thrombus   New capillary vessels of granulation tissue-type grow from the vasa vasorum in the adventitia, across the media, into and across the intima and into the thrombus. At the same time removal of the thrombotic material, largely by macrophage activity, is proceeding. Eventually the occlusive thrombus may be replaced by a solid plug of collagenous tissue.

Organization of mural thrombus   As oxygenated plasma enters from the luminal surface (from the blood) granulation-type capillaries from the vasa vasorum grow very slowly if at all, into the thrombus. Many platelets disaggregate and are washed away. Within a few days the surface is covered by flattened cells (possibly smooth-muscle derived). The mass becomes vascularized from the luminal surface and the proliferation of smooth muscle that ensues tends to be on the luminal side of the thrombus which appears to lie deep to the new intima. This may play a part in the formation of atherosclerotic plaque.

....

EMBOLISM

Definition An embolus is an abnormal mass of material, either solid or gaseous, which is transported in the blood-stream from one part of the circulation to another and which finally impacts in the lumen of a vessel whose lumen is too small to allow passage of the material.

Emboli may consist of:

* thrombus
* mixed thrombus and clot
* air
* nitrogen
* fat
* small pieces of bone marrow
* debris from an atherosclerotic plaque
* groups of tumour cells.

Thrombus-derived emboli

About 99% of emboli are thrombus/thrombus-plus-blood clot derived.

Pulmonary emboli When the origin of the embolus is a venous thrombus and impaction occurs in the pulmonary arterial tree.

Systemic emboli Most are derived from the left side of the heart. Intraventricular thrombosis may complicate trans-mural myocardial infarction or congestive cardiomyopathy. Thrombi affecting the heart valves that are sufficiently big to be clinially important are usually associated with **infective endocarditis** in the form of bulky and friable **vegetations**. Portions of vegetations break off and impact at any peripheral site but favoured sites include brain, lower limbs, spleen and kidney. When an infected thrombus impacts there is a local inflammatory reaction and this leads to destruction of part of the wall and dilation of a segment of the artery (**mycotic aneurysm**) which may result in rupture and haemorrhage.

Gaseous emboli

Air May be introduced by operations on the head and neck (following inadvertent opening of a large vein), mismanagement of blood transfusions where positive pressure is used to speed up the rate of transfusion, during haemodialysis, following insufflation of Fallopian tubes (during investigation of sterility) and following interference of the placental site during criminal abortion. Air enters the right side of the heart where it is whipped up into a frothy mass in the right ventricle. In some cases the gas may enter the systemic arterial circulation and impact there. As little as 40 ml of air can give serious results and 100 ml can be fatal although up to 200 ml have been tolerated.

Nitrogen Occurs in decompression sickness (caisson disease) and occurs in people who are at high pressure and return to normal pressure too quickly (e.g. deep-sea divers). At high pressure inert gases (of which nitrogen is the most important) are dissolved in plasma and interstitial tissue, particularly adipose tissue. If return to normal pressure is too quick the gas comes out of solution and small bubbles are formed. These may coalesce to form large masses. Symptoms relate to the presence of bubbles in tendons, joints and ligaments giving pain (the bends) and the brain. The symptoms may be relieved by forcing the nitrogen back into solution in a decompression chamber.

Fat emboli

Occurs in 90% of patients with significant trauma and is associated with fracture of long bones, severe burns, severe soft tissue trauma, hyperlipidaemia, ischaemic bone marrow necrosis (in patients with sickle cell disease), joint reconstruction, cardiopulmonary by-pass, acute pancreatitis and intramedullary nailing associated with orthopaedic procedures.

The pathogenesis may be related either to lodging of bone marrow-derived fat globules in the pulmonary vasculature or, if less than 7–10 μm, in the sysemic circulation, or to the effect of circulating free fatty acids on gas exchange.

Bone marrow emboli

These may be seen in the lungs of patients following unsuccessful resuscitation for cardiac arrest when bone marrow is squeezed from fractured ribs into veins. The significance of this finding is unknown.

Emboli derived form atheromatous plaques

These only occur in the arterial system. The emboli are usually found incidentally and can be recognized as they consist of thrombotic material and lipid-rich debris in which there are cholesterol crystals present.

19 Ischaemia and infarction

Definition The state existing when arterial perfusion is lowered relative to metabolic needs. This is most often localized to an area of tissue or a whole organ. Occasionally the ischaemic state may be generalized due to a fall in cardiac output.

ISCHAEMIA

Causes of ischaemia

Local causes of ischaemia:

- atherosclerosis
- thrombosis
- embolus
- venous occlusion: Occurs in areas where venous drainage cannot bypass the obstruction via collateral channels. Affected tissues become intensely congested, possibly haemorrhagic. Situations in which it is likely include:

  1. Extensive mesenteric venous thrombosis affecting the small bowel.
  2. Strangulation of hernias. Entrapment of contents leads to oedema and thus to pressure on veins.
  3. Cavernous sinus thrombosis may lead to thrombosis of the retinal vein and ultimately to blindness.
  4. Thrombosis of the superior longitudinal sinus in the dura. Occurs in severely dehydrated children. Leads to patchy necrosis of cerebral cortex.

- capillary obstruction: due to physical damage to capillaries e.g. frostbite, parasites (cerebral malaria), abnormal cells (sickle cell disease, some autoimmune

haemolytic anaemias), fibrin (disseminated intravascular coagulation), antigen/antibody complexes, fat or gas emboli or external pressure (as in bed sores)
• arterial obstruction causes ischaemia if there is no or insufficient collateral arterial supply.

Changes associated with ischaemia

Functional disturbances are noted when the collateral supply is only good enough to maintain perfusion if the metabolic demands are at a basal level. For example in a heart with compromised blood flow exercise may produce ischaemia and the patient will experience sub-sternal pain (**angina pectoris**). The eventual functional changes of tissue or an organ which is ischaemic may result either from loss of cells or deficient behaviour in surviving cells.

Structural changes may take the form either of patchy loss of parenchymal cells or of massive necrosis. If the patient survives the lost cells/tissue are replaced by fibrous tissue – with the exception of the brain – in an identical manner to repair. The degree of post-ischaemic necrosis is proportional to the degree of ischaemia.

When ischaemia is slow in onset and long in duration the death characteristically affects single or small groups of cells. Initially the changes may be intracellular oedema or fatty change but eventually the cells die and are replaced by small foci of fibrous tissue.

Degree of ischaemia

Depends on an interaction between:

• Metabolic needs of affected tissue: Tissues vary in their ability to withstand ischaemia. The brain is the most sensitive with deprivation of oxygen for more than 3–4 min resulting in irreversible damage to nerve cells. The myocardium is also susceptible to underperfusion.
• Speed of onset of arterial perfusion: a rapid onset gives more severe effects as there is no time for collateral vessels to open.
• The completeness of the arterial block. Complete occlusion will give more severe effects than stenosis. The

more proximal the occulsion the greater the area affected.

- Anatomy of local blood supply: Some organs or tissues have no collateral arterial supply and are therefore supplied by `end-arteries' (e.g. retina). The smaller arteries in the cerebral cortex also act as end-arteries. Other organs (e.g. the lung) have a double arterial supply making necrosis due to occlusion of one part very rare.
- State of collateral circulation.

···

INFARCTION

Definition A large localized area of tissue necrosis (usually coagulative) brought about by ischaemia.

Appearance

Blood may seep into an ischaemic area as a result of back flow from venules or escape through damaged vessel walls so that infarcts may contain blood in the early stages. Later the dying cells swell, which squeezes the blood out of the interstitial tissue and the infarct becomes paler. However in the brain infarcts other than those caused by emboli are pale from the start, while in the lung infarcts remain red and undergo repair when still at this stage. The dead parenchymal cells undergo autolysis and the dispersed red cells haemolyse. At the margins of the infarct there is an acute inflammatory reaction which is followed by infiltration of the necrotic tissue by macrophages. Breakdown products of haemoglobin (haematoidin) and ferritin (haemosiderin) may be seen in the area and are ingested by macrophages. At this stage (about 1 week) the infarct is solid and firm, yellow in colour and has a red zone at the margins. In some tissues (e.g. heart) dead cells are removed rapidly with equally rapid replacement by granulation tissue followed by scar tissue. In other organs (e.g. kidney) the infarcted area persists for months.

Abnormal accumulations of fluid and disturbances of blood distribution

OEDEMA

Definition Abnormal accumulation of fluid in the extracellular space.

Physiology Total body water is about 49 litres distributed between the intracellular (about 35 litres with little variation), intravascular (about 3 litres) and extracellular (about 11 litres) compartments. The intra/extravascular water distribution depends on a number of factors:

1. Factors causing fluid to leave the vasculature:

   - increased intravascular hydrostatic pressure
   - increased colloid osmotic pressure in the extravascular compartment.

2. Factors normally keeping fluid within vessels:

   - osmotic pressure of plasma proteins (particularly albumin)
   - selective permeability of endothelium
   - tissue tension.

Under normal circumstances there is a net loss of fluid from the vascular compartment but no oedema develops as the excess fluid enters the lymphatic channels and is drained from the site eventually re-entering the bloodstream via the thoracic duct. If the lymphatic drainage is obstructed oedema will supervene (lymphoedema).

Types of oedema fluid: If the collection of interstitial fluid is associated with increased vascular permeability the fluid will contain a large amount of protein (including fibrinogen) and is termed an **exudate**. If the mechanisms are mainly hydrostatic there will be a low protein content and the fluid is termed a **transudate**.

Causes of oedema

The most important causes are:

- raised intracapillary pressure
- low plasma oncotic pressure
- retention of salt and water.

Systemic oedema

Cardiac oedema

Congestive cardiac failure is associated with both a redistribution and a retention of fluid. The oedematous areas readily pit on finger pressure.

Sites Determined by gravity. In ambulant patients this involves the ankles and legs. In those confined to bed, swelling is in the sacral or less commonly genital regions.

Mechanism The oedema is not purely caused by a failure of the pumping function of the heart. Evidence for this includes:

- increased plasma volume (which may occur before there is a rise in central venous pressure)
- oedema frequently occurs before there is a rise in central venous pressure
- degree of oedema is not proportional to the height of central venous pressure.

The most important mechanism is **excess retention of salt and water by the renal tubules**. Failure of the heart pump leads to decreased mean capillary pressure and so reduced renal perfusion. This in association with vasoconstriction mediated by the sympathetic nervous system leads to relative renal ischaemia causing an increase in production of renin and thus angiotensin I. The rise in angiotensin causes increased release of aldosterone from the adrenal cortex and retention of salt and water. Initially this is beneficial as it allows increased mean filling pressure in the circulation which, in the heart, leads to stretching of cardiac muscle fibres and increased force of contraction (Starling's law) but in time this advantage is lost.

Renal oedema

Occurs in two circumstances:

1. Associated with glomerulonephritis (nephritic syndrome). Face and eyelids predominantly affected. No entirely satisfactory explanation for the cause or distribution of the oedema. Possibly related to fall in glomerular filtration rate associated with normal tubular reabsorption of sodium.

2. Associated with the nephrotic syndrome.
   This syndrome includes heavy proteinuria leading to hypoalbuminaemia and decreased plasma oncotic pressure. Sodium retention partly due to increased aldosterone production is also important.

Nutritional oedema

Associated with prolonged starvation. No correlation between degree of oedema and blood concentrations of protein. Oedema associated with starvation can be seen with normal protein levels. The explanation for this may lie in the loss of subcutaneous fatty tissue leading to reduced tissue tension. **Kwashiorkor** is a type of nutritional oedema resulting from protein and calorie undernutrition in young children. These children fail to grow normally, are anaemic and have fatty livers. They have oedema (associated with hypoalbuminaemia), mucocutaneous ulceration and depigmentation of hair.

Oedema due to chronic liver disease

(See page 449)

Pulmonary oedema

(See page 306)

Local oedema

Causes:

- local increase in hydrostatic pressure in the microcirculation (e.g. pregnancy, occlusive venous embolism, varicose veins with incompetent valves
- increased local vascular permeability

- lymphoedema. Obstruction to the lymphatic drainage system may result from surgical intervention (e.g. axillary lymph node dissection in patients with breast carcinoma), inflammation (e.g. infection with *Wuchereria bancrofti* [filariasis] which may lead to the obstruction of inguinal lymphatics and gross oedema of lower limbs and genitalia termed elephantiasis) or as part of a congenital malformation of lymphatic drainage (Milroy's disease).

··

HYPERAEMIA AND CONGESTION

Definition   Greater amount of blood than normal in organ or tissue.

Causes

1. Increased inflow (active hyperaemia): Associated with arteriolar dilatation (e.g. in acute inflammation, after exposure to heat, in flushing and at the margins of ischaemic necrosis).
2. Decreased outflow (passive hyperaemia): Obstruction may be structural or functional. May be generalized or localized.

Generalized venous congestion

In the acute form this may be present in patients dying suddenly from a variety of causes. The commonest cause of chronic venous congestion is ventricular failure. It results from a rise in pressure in pulmonary and systemic veins and in the pulmonary veins from the additional shift from systemic to pulmonary circulation associated with peripheral vasoconstriction. Generalized venous congestion also arises in a variety of pulmonary disorders associated with a rise in pulmonary arterial pressure. This leads to an increase in right ventricular muscle mass. In time this fails to maintain normal output leading to a rise in systemic venous pressure and congestion in peripheral organs such as the liver and spleen. This form of cardiac failure is known as **cor pulmonale** and may be the result of diseases affecting the bronchioles, alveoli, thoracic movement or pulmonary vasculature.

Morphological changes Generally the organs become swollen, firmer and darker in colour.

- lung – each capillary is stuffed with blood. Small intra-alveolar haemorrhages are seen, clinically associated with the patient coughing blood (haemoptysis). Haemosiderin is produced by the breakdown of haemoglobin and is phagocytosed by macrophages (siderophages). In time the alveolar septae become thickened and there may be interstitial fibrosis
- liver – there is a rise in pressure in the hepatic veins, central veins and sinusoids associated with poor perfusion of part of the hepatic lobule furthest from the arterial supply (see page 411)
- spleen – this becomes enlarged (up to 250 g) and is firm with a deep red/purple cut surface. There is distension of the sinusoids which are packed by red cells and an increase in reticulin in the sinusoid wall and in the connective tissue of the septae.

Localized venous congestion

Results from obstruction of flow to venous blood. Usually due to thrombosis or external pressure occluding the vein from outside (e.g. tumour). The effects depend on the speed of onset of the obstruction and the presence of collateral draining veins. If the onset is acute then the presence of collateral veins is vital to avoid local oedema and haemorrhage. In the brain collateral vessels are absent and venous occlusion not uncommonly results in haemor-rhages. When venous obstruction is chronic the collateral system, if present, will become distended and may them-selves rupture (e.g. bleeding oesophageal veins in portal hypertension).

Pigmentation and heterotropic calcification

··

PIGMENTATION

Melanin

Normal location Constitutes the colouring of hair, skin and eyes. Also normally present in the leptomeninges, nerve cells of the substantia nigra and adrenal medulla. Small numbers of melanin-producing cells may also be found in the ovary, gastrointestinal tract and urinary bladder

Demonstration in tissues Usually produces a yellow-brown colour. If present in large amounts appears black. Has ability to reduce solutions of ammoniacal silver with deposition of black silver granules on the melanin granules (**argentaffin** reaction). Melanin pigment can be bleached from tissues by hydrogen peroxide.

Site of production Produced by **melanocytes**. These are thought to be of neural crest origin. The average number of melanocytes is roughly constant irrespective of race (average 1500/mm^2; range 2000/mm^2 [forehead and cheeks] – 800/mm^2 [abdomen]). The darker skin of some races is due to increased activity rather than numbers. Melanin is produced in **melanosomes** found in the Golgi apparatus. Melanin granules are transferred into adjacent epidermal cells.

Formation Produced from tyrosine. Absence of tyrosinase results in albinism. Melanocyte-stimulating hormone (MSH) affects the activity of melanin-producing cells.

Abnormalities of melanin production

Generalized hyperpigmentation May be due to:
• Addison's disease – loss of normal feedback mechanisms controlling the adrenal gland results in increased ACTH and MSH secretion

- acromegaly
- increased oestrogen levels – as treatment for prostatic cancer, in chronic liver disease and in pregnancy
- chronic arsenical poisoning
- haemochromatosis (excess storage of iron in parenchymal cells)
- in association with chlorpromazine administration.

Focal hyperpigmentation

- freckles
- café-au-lait spots – large pigmented macules associated with increased melanocyte numbers and seen in neurofibromatosis and Albright's syndrome (polyostotic fibrous dysplasia, hyperpigmentation and sexual and skeletal precocity)
- Peutz–Jeghers syndrome – autosomal dominant condition with focal hyperpigmentation around the lips associated with multiple polyps in the gastrointestinal tract
- lentiginosis – multiple hyperpigmented spots (increased melanocyte numbers) associated with hypertrophic cardiomyopathy in a few cases
- associated with localized exposure to ionizing radiation, ultraviolet light, heat (erythema ab igne) or chronic irritation
- tumours arising from melanocytes
- other skin tumours that accumulate melanin e.g. seborrhoeic keratoses and basal cell carcinomas.

Hypopigmentation

- albinism – due to tyrosinase deficiency. In classic cases the skin is very white, the hair pale, the irides transparent and the pupils pink. The individuals are prone to skin cancers
- vitiligo – well-demarcated areas of localized hypopigmentation associated with paucity or absence of melanocytes.

Pigments derived from haemoglobin

Mostly associated with the iron-containing pigments. Initially excess iron is stored as ferritin (not seen under light microscope or with special stains) but with increased intracellular levels the ferritin molecules merge to form haemosiderin. These are 36% iron and may be identified by Prussian blue stains (Perl's or Turnbull's reaction).

Localized haemosiderin deposition

Always implies previous haemorrhage (bruise, haematoma, fracture sites, haemorrhagic infarcts and some tumours) and is frequently seen in the lungs associated with left ventricular failure. Renal tubular cells can convert haemoglobin to haemosiderin (haemosiderinuria may therefore follow haemoglobinuria).

Generalized haemosiderosis

Haemosiderin is formed in excessive amounts when the body is overloaded with iron (normal quantity in body 4–5 g; normal intake in Western-style diet 10–15 mg of which 10% is absorbed; normal loss about 1 mg/day through cells lost in gastrointestinal tract/skin/etc. and 200–300 mg/year through menstruation in females). Excess haemosiderin may be deposited in parenchymal cells or in cells of the reticuloendothelial system (seen following parenteral iron administration or repeated transfusion).

Causes of iron accumulation:

- increased iron absorption
- decreased excretion
- impaired utilization
- excess breakdown of haemoglobin.

Haemochromatosis

See page 433.

Pigments associated with fats

This group of pigments are termed **lipofuscins**. They are yellowish-brown granular pigments appearing in atrophic parenchymal cells (particularly the heart and liver of the elderly) and when present in large amounts give brown colour to tissues (brown atrophy). The pigments are thought to be derived from breakdown products of organelle membranes.

Exogenous pigments

The commonest is tattoo marks. Can occasionally be pigmentation-associated, with long-term use of medications e.g. ear-drops containing silver.

....

HETEROTROPIC CALCIFICATION

Definition Deposition of calcium salts in tissues other than osteoid or enamel.

Two main types: dystrophic and metastatic calcification.

Dystrophic calcification

Characteristics Serum calcium is normal. Calcium salts deposited in dead/degenerate tissues.

Associations
- caseous necrosis
- fat necrosis
- thrombosis
- haematomas
- atherosclerotic plaques
- chronic inflammatory granulation tissue (e.g. constrictive pericarditis)
- Mönckeberg's sclerosis of the medial coat of muscular arteries
- degenerate colliod goitres
- cysts of various types
- degenerate tumours (e.g. uterine leiomyomas).

Metastatic calcification

Characteristics Elevated blood calcium level. Deposition occurs in a variety of sites.

- kidney – around tubules causing damage and eventual renal failure. Patients are unable to acidify urine. Stone formation occurs in renal pelvis and ureter often associated with nephrocalcinosis
- lung – in alveolar wall
- stomach – around the fundal glands

- blood vessels – coronary arteries most affected
- cornea.

Causes May be associated with primary hyperparathyroidism, excessive absorption of calcium from the gut (associated with hypervitaminosis D, vitamin D sensitive states or even excessive milk drinking), hypophosphataemia, destructive bone lesions (e.g. osteolytic secondary deposits of malignant tumours or humoral hypercalcaemia in malignancy without bony secondaries) or renal tubular acidosis.

Demonstration in sections Calcium salts stain deep blue with haematoxylin. May be stained with alizarin red (magenta) or von Kossa method.

Neoplasia: disorders of cell proliferation and differentiation

. . . .

Definitions Neoplasia may be roughly translated as new growth (Greek: *neos* = new; *plassein* = to mould). Defined by Willis as 'an abnormal mass of tissue, the growth of which exceeds and is unco-ordinated with that of normal tissues, and which persists in the same excessive manner after cessation of the stimulus which has evoked the change'.

Components of neoplasia

Disturbances in cell proliferation

Escape from normal proliferative control gives rise to a populations of cells which could be considered to be immortal. The end result is a focus made up of a single cell type in numbers that are inappropriate for the location. This will lead to the formation of a mass or **tumour**.

Disturbances in cell differentiation

Differentiation is the process by which cells achieve their specific set of functional and morphological characteristics. As all cells possess the same genetic information this must involve restriction of genomic expression. Impairment of differentiation is common in neoplasms. Loss of the ability to differentiate leads to the aquisition of characteristics foreign to the normal counterpart. In general, the poorer the degree of differentiation (i.e. poor similarity to normal cell) the worse the behaviour of the tumour.

Disturbances in relationship between cell and stroma

In some instances a tumour will grow in an expansile fashion (**benign neoplasm**). In others the constituent cells invade the surrounding tissues and may spread to distant sites (**malignant neoplasm**).

CLASSIFICATION OF NEOPLASMS

The most useful criteria for tumour classification is the tissue of origin and biological behaviour. At the simplest level tissues can be divided into **epithelia** and **connective tissue** but greater sub-division is possible and desirable. Tumours are also divided on the basis of behaviour into two main groups: **benign** and **malignant**. Malignant tumours of epithelia are called **carcinomas** and malignant tumours of connective tissue are called **sarcomas**.

Benign tumours may constitute a serious hazard but show no tendency to invade surrounding tissues and never spread to distant sites. Usually they are clearly demarcated and surrounded by a thin fibrous capsule with compressed normal tissue around it. Benign epithelial neoplasms may grow in sheets covering a surface (**papilloma**) or as solid islands or masses separated by stroma (**adenoma**). These latter tend to arise from gland or duct epithelium. Occasionally accumulation of secretions from the cells cause dilation of the lumen causing formation of a **cyst**. A neoplastic cyst derived from acinar or ductal epithelium is called a **cystadenoma** and if the lining has papillary infoldings it is termed a **papillary cystadenoma**.

Malignant tumours show invasion of surrounding tissue and cells may gain access to vascular channels (lymphatic or blood vessels) and spread to a distant site where they impact, emigrate to the extravascular space and form new deposits of neoplastic tumour (**secondary deposits** or **metastases**). Malignant tumours tend to show evidence of increased cell proliferation, frequently with abnormal mitoses and poor differentiation with the cells frequently being larger than normal with greater degrees of variation in size and shape and larger nuclei which occupy a greater proportion of the cell (increased nuclear: cytoplasmic ratio). Many of the orderly cell arrangements and intercellular relationships (e.g. ductules, glands etc.) are lost or differ from normal. Very poorly differentiated tumours grow in disorganized sheets of cells.

DYSPLASIA

Definition Morphological features of malignancy at a stage when invasion of surrounding tissue is not evident (Greek: *dys* = bad).

Implication The finding of dysplasia implies some irreversible genomic alteration within the cells suggesting that invasive malignancy may develop at the site in the future. Epithelial dysplasia (also known as intra-epithelial neoplasia) of the uterine cervix (cervical intraepithelial neoplasia – CIN) can be assessed by microscopic examination of exfoliated cells collected on a spatula. This is the basis of the 'cervical smear' used to screen for cervical carcinoma. CIN is graded I–III with CIN III being the most severe change (**carcinoma in situ**).

Lesions which may be confused with true neoplasms

Hamartoma

Definition Tumour-like masses which lack autonomy in which the elements are fully differentiated and are normally found in the organ of origin but in which the constituent parts are abnormally organized (Greek: *hamartanein* = to make a mistake).

Occurrence May be found at a variety of sites most commonly in the lung. Vascular hamartomas range from the flat 'port wine stain' to large complex masses of vascular spaces. Hamartomas may also form part of an inherited syndrome (e.g. intestinal hamartomas in Peutz–Jegher's syndrome).

Heteroplasia

Definition Differentiation of a part of an organ/tissue in a way that is foreign to the part. The anomalous differentiation takes place at the stem cell stage.

Occurrence Examples include the finding of gastric mucosa in a Meckel's diverticulum of the ileum or exocrine pancreatic tissue in the wall of the ileum.

Non-neoplastic disturbances in cell growth and proliferation

....

THE CELL CYCLE

- Cells proliferate by undergoing **mitosis**.
- Mitosis is only a small part of the cell cycle.
- The length of the cell cycle determines the cell kinetic characteristics of a tissue.
- The phases of the cell cycle are:

  - **M phase (mitosis):** 1–2 h
  - **G1 phase (gap):** duration varies greatly between cell types. May last days or even years
  - **S phase:** 7–12 h phase in which DNA synthesis occurs
  - **G2 phase (second gap):** 1–6 h.

- M, S and G2 phases have relatively constant duration between tissues.
- Differences in cell cycle times that characterize different tissues is related to G1 duration.
- Once cell has passed out of G1 the cell cycle proceeds to completion. A point of no return occurs late in G1 (**restriction point**).
- In any tissue not all the cells are in cell cycle. Most fully differentiated cells leave cell cycle and progress down a pathway of differentiation ending in obsolescence.
- Cells can leave the cell cycle temporarily and re-enter later. These cells are said to be in **GO phase**.
- The proportion of a cell population in cell cycle is the **growth fraction (stem cell compartment)**.
- The proliferative activity of the cell population is a function of the growth fraction and length of the cell cycle for that tissue.

HYPERTROPHY AND HYPERPLASIA

Excess growth with maintained normal controls as an adaption phenomenon.

Usually associated with a recognizable stimulus (often physiological). Once the stimulus is removed there is reversion to normal.

Hypertrophy

- Increase in bulk is due to **increase in cell-size, cell numbers remain constant**.
- Isolated hypertrophy occurs only in muscle and is associated with increased workload.

Examples:

Urinary bladder

Increase in size of bladder smooth muscle fibres giving a trabeculated pattern to the mucosa is associated with urinary obstruction e.g. post-inflammatory urethral strictures or prostate enlargement.

Gastrointestinal tract

Muscular hypertrophy occurs proximal to obstruction from any cause e.g. oesophagus – post-inflammatory scarring, carcinoma, disorders of innervation.

In the stomach hypertrophy may also cause obstruction e.g. congenital hypertrophic pyloric stenosis.

Heart

High-pressure overload e.g. aortic valve stenosis, systemic hypertension or aortic coarctation gives left ventricular hypertrophy associated with ventricular lumen of normal or smaller size.

High-volume overload as a result of increased end-diastolic volume e.g. aortic or mitral valve incompetence is associated with larger ventricular cavity.

Hyperplasia

Increased bulk due to **increased cell number**; increased cell size may be an accompanying feature.

Mostly constitutes a demand-led event responding to increased functional need.

Examples:

Congenital adrenal hyperplasia

Characterized by masculinization of females; precocious puberty in males; salt-losing state.

Due to enzyme (C21 or C11 hydroxylase) deficiency in adrenal cortical cells responsible for production of cortisol and aldosterone. Resultant lack of cortisol and aldosterone stimulates ACTH production by pituitary. Adrenal responds by increasing the number of functional cells. The block in hormone production results in excess precursors being diverted to production of androgenic steroids.

Thyroid hyperplasia

May occur due to:

Operation of normal feedback mechanisms controlling TSH production Associated with lack of secreting tissue (cretinism); lack of substrate (iodine deficiency); lack of enzymes in synthesis pathway (dyshormonogenetic goitre).

Abnormal stimuli Associated with thyroid stimulating immunoglobulin (Graves' disease).

Hyperplasia in target organs of hormones

Breast Associated with puberty in females. Hormone induced. Increase in both epithelial and stromal components. In adult life breast hyperplasia may develop associated with mixture of hyperplastic and involutionary changes leading to lumps (localized or generalized). Pathological changes are increased number of ducts in a lobule (adenosis) or heaping up of epithelial cells in ducts (epitheliosis).

Prostate Common in males over 60 years. Fibromuscular and ductal elements involved.

Non-specific reactive epithelial hyperplasia

Occurs in skin, mouth, alimentary and respiratory tracts; associated with persistent irritation.

....

ATROPHY

Definition   Decrease in bulk of tissue.

Physiological atrophy

In the fetus many structures formed during embryogenesis undergo regression during later stages (e.g. notochord, branchial clefts, thyroglossal duct). In adults atrophy of the thymus occurs normally. Atrophy may result from decrease in demand.

Examples:

Muscle atrophy

Following immobilization for treatment of a fracture.

Atrophy of gut

With starvation.

Osteoporosis

Condition in which the mass of bone tissue per unit volume of anatomical bone is reduced. No defect in mineralization.

Localized atrophy

Occurs following:

* ischaemia
* external pressure
* denervation.

Cell proliferation and differentiation in relation to neoplasia

···

In neoplasia the proliferation of cells is generally thought to be **autonomous**, in contrast to non-neoplastic which is demand-driven, proliferation ceasing with the withdrawal of demand.

···

TRANSFORMED CELLS IN CULTURE

Much of the data on the growth of tumour cells is derived from extrapolation of observations of the behaviour of transformed cells in culture.

Loss of contact inhibition

When normal cells are grown in a monolayer growth stops when the cells reach confluence and each cell is in contact with a neighbour (**contact inhibition**). This is thought to be mediated by:

1. cells recognizing each other
2. exchange of information regulating proliferation
3. adherence to each other (homotypic adhesion).

In monolayer cultures neoplastic cells continue to grow after reaching confluence and become heaped up in a multi-layer fashion.

Differences in surface membrane

Neoplastic change is associated in most instances with changes in surface membrane glycoproteins. This can be demonstrated by increased binding of proteins known as **lectins**. This is thought to be caused by loss of cell surface components leading to exposure of lectin-binding sites. This allows lectins to agglutinate neoplastic cells in suspension.

Autonomous growth

This may be through one of two pathways:

1. Failure of an inhibiting mechanism which normally restrains excessive growth.
2. Abnormal response to growth factors. This may be the result of excessive amounts of the growth factor, excess expression of the growth factor receptor or to abnormal signal transduction following binding of factor to receptor.

It has been suggested that autonomous growth may be due to production of polypeptide growth factors by the neoplastic cell which also has the appropriate receptor on the cell surface, a situation termed **autocrine secretion**. Peptides identified as functioning in this way include:

Transforming growth factor α. Structurally related to epidermal growth factor (EGF).

Platelet derived growth factor (PDGF). Molecules showing homology to PDGF are released by some tumours in humans including malignant neoplasms of bone (osteosarcomas), malignant tumours of brain glial cells and a cell line derived from bladder carcinoma.

Bombesin (gastrin releasing peptide). A peptide produced by most small cell carcinomas of the lung. Prevention of the binding of bombesin to its receptor inhibits small cell carcinoma proliferation in culture and in mouse xenografts.

Autocrine peptides can also inhibit growth

Transforming growth factor β (TGF-β). A family of proteins secreted in an inactive form. It is widely distributed in adult tissues and binds to receptors on many cell types with different effects:

- stimulation of fibroblast growth in culture in the presence of PDGF
- inhibition of fibroblast growth in culture in the presence of EGF
- stimulation of osteoblast growth but with reversal of this effect by EGF, PDGF and tumour necrosis factor α

- inhibition of most epithelial cell lines in culture
- promotion of growth of fibrous tissue matrix in wound healing and atherogenesis.

....

DIFFERENTIATION

Neoplasia and disordered cell differentiation

Since one of the cardinal features of neoplasia is the ability of the cell population to proliferate in a relatively autonomous manner the cells from which the neoplasm arises must have the capacity to respond to mitogenic stimuli and to divide. In most cell populations these cells reside in the stem cell compartment. When a stem cell divides one of the daughter cells may retain the ability to divide. The other becomes committed to differentiation and ultimately to death. For a differentiated cell there must be a heritable pattern of read-out of the genome such that some genes are expressed while others are not. This will allow cells to have different characteristics even though each cell in the body possesses the same genetic information. Control of gene expression and protein synthesis can occur at several levels:

- transcriptional control – usually the most potent mechanism. Controlled by a number of gene regulatory proteins with structural motifs such as zinc finger motifs, leucine zipper motifs and helix loop motifs.
- RNA-processing control
- RNA-transport control
- translational control
- degradation control
- control of protein activity.

Differentiation is also affected by other mechanisms. For many organ systems this would include the interaction between mesenchymal and epithelial elements. Cell–cell interactions also appear to play a role in differentiation and growth factors (including epidermal growth factor) may also be involved.

METAPLASIA

Definition A complete change in differentiation from one fully differentiated form to another fully differentiated form. This transformation is therefore **not** neoplastic.

Examples: The commonest form involves the transformation of cuboidal or columnar epithelium to souamous epithelium (**squamous metaplasia**) mostly associated with inflammation or irritation of the tissue.

- Transformation of bronchial pseudo-stratified cilliated columnar epithelium to squamous epithelium. Associated with cigarette smoking and chronic bronchitis.
- Transformation of cervical glandular epithelium to squamous epithelium. Associated with chronic cervicitis.
- Transformation of transitional epithelium of the renal pelvis to squamous epithelium in the presence of chronic inflammation.
- Transformation of the columnar lining of the gall bladder to squamous epithelium in the presence of gallstones and chronic inflammation.
- Transformation of columnar epithelial lining of prostatic ducts to squamous epithelium associated with oestrogen treatment for prostatic carcinoma.
- Squamous metaplasia in the nose, bronchi and urinary tract associated with vitamin A deficiency.

Cellular differentiation in malignant neoplasms

Cancer cells are not fully differentiated. As fully differentiated cells are unlikely to regress to a partially differentiated stage this implies that there is a block in the normal maturation process. These neoplastic cells have also retained the ability to divide. The degree of differentiation in neoplasms may be related to the precise point at which transformation occurred.

Relationship of neoplastic cells with their environment: tumour spread

··

The only absolute criterion for distinguishing between benign and malignant tumours is the ability of malignant tumours to invade surrounding tissues and to colonize distant sites (**metastasize**).

··

ROUTES OF SPREAD

Direct spread

This involves the invasion of tissues adjacent to the original lesion and is thought to involve the following processes.

Acquisition of new and adequate blood supply (angiogenesis)

Without new capillary formation the tumour will be unable to grow more than a few millimetres in any direction. The greater the new blood supply the greater the risk of metastatic spread. The new blood vessels are derived from adjacent venules and capillaries and are stimulated by chemical signals (e.g. **basic fibroblast growth factor, transforming growth factor-α and angiogenin**) and is inhibited by **transforming growth factor $\beta 1$**. Stimulation causes the resting endothelial cells to:

- degrade their own basement membrane
- migrate into and through the extravascular stroma
- form capillary sprouts which become luminated.

Proteolysis is pivotal to migration and to the formation of lumens within the vessel sprouts. Inhibitors of proteolysis (e.g. tissue inhibitors of metalloproteases) block angiogenesis.

Decrease in adhesion of tumour cells to one another (loss of homotypic cell adhesion)

Infiltrating cells are shed from the main tumour bulk which implies a reduction in the adhesiveness compared with normal cells of the same type.

Mechanisms involved in the decreased adhesion are thought to include:

- total or partial loss of the normal anchorage points found in epithelial cells (desmosomes)
- increase in the net negative surface charge of tumour cells
- alteration in the expression of cadherins.

Cadherins are calcium-dependent cell–cell adhesion molecules. They are divided into a number of sub-classes of which E-cadherins (epithelial cadherins) are most relevant to tumour invasion. Carcinoma cell lines with loss of E-cadherin are highly invasive. If DNA encoding for E-cadherin is inserted into highly invasive cells they revert to a non-invasive form while treatment of cells with anti-sense RNA specific for E-cadherin or antibodies to E-cadherin increases invasiveness. There is an inverse relationship between E-cadherin expression and differentiation and invasiveness in some human tumours.

Adhesion of malignant cells to basement membranes and extracellular matrix

Transition from in situ (intraepithelial) to invasive carcinoma is marked by the malignant cells crossing the basement membrane and reaching the stromal compartment. Crossing the basement membrane must be accompanied by focal destruction of the basement membrane matrix (proteins and glycoproteins). This requires three steps: **attachment** of tumour cells to basement membrane, **lysis** of the basement membrane matrix and **movement** of the cells through the membrane.

Attachment involves adhesion to matrix components such as collagen, fibronectin and laminin (Table 25.1). **Integrins** have a fundamental role in this process as they bind to adhesion molecules by recognizing specific RGD (Arg-Gly-Asp) sequences.

Table 25.1 Interaction between matrix proteins and tumour cell receptors

Binding molecule on cell	Matrix protein/glycoprotein
VLA-2 ($\alpha_2\beta_2$)	Collagen and laminin
VLA-4 ($\alpha_4\beta_1$)	Variant of fibronectin
VLA-5 ($\alpha_5\beta_1$)	Fibronectin
VLA-6 ($\alpha_6\beta_1$)	Laminin
$\alpha_6\beta_4$	Laminin
$\alpha_v\beta_3$	Vitronectin

In normal cells laminin receptors are only found on the aspect of the cell opposed to the basement membrane. Invasive cells have laminin receptors diffusely distributed over the entire cell surface. If these tumour cells are treated with the receptor-binding fragment of laminin their capacity to invade is greatly reduced.

Lysis of the basement membrane and interstitial stroma matrix

This requires dissolution of the proteins by enzymes derived from the tumour cells. This is carried out in a well-organized manner as cell migration requires sequential attachment to and detachment of the matrix as the cell moves. Antibodies to the enzymes or inhibitors of protease activities block invasion while expression of several classes of proteinase by tumour cells are correlated to aggressive behaviour.

Classes of proteolytic enzymes so far found to be important in connective tissue lysis include:

• Metal ion-dependent proteases (metalloproteases).

This has been the most studied group and is divided into three main groups based on their substrate – **interstitial collagenases, gelatinases** and **stromelysins**. All are secreted in inactive forms and their activation is an important control step.

• Heperanases.
• Serine-dependent proteases.
• Thiol-dependent proteases.

Tumours have also been shown to have fibrinolytic activity. This is due to the production of plasminogen activator and it has been suggested that acquisition of the ability to secrete this is associated with an ability to invade extra-cellular matrix.

Active movement of malignant cells

This is essential to invasion and metastasis but whether this is random (kinesis), directed (taxis) or both is uncertain. Factors important in movement include:

- Intact and fragmented molecules of the extracellular matrix.
- Tumour autocrine motility factor (AMF). This binds to a glycoprotein receptor on the cell and is followed by activation of a G-protein mediated signalling system. Movement is associated with phosphorylation of the receptor.
- Scatter factor. This is synthesized and secreted by fibroblasts and exerts a scattering effect on many epithelial cells. It is similar to plasminogen and identical to hepatocyte growth factor. It has a multi-functional role including induction of motility in tumour cells, induction of proliferation in epithelial cells and being a morphogen being able to induce tubule formation in some epithelial cell lines. A receptor for scatter factor is the product of the proto-oncogene *c-met*.

Role of mechanical pressure in direct tumour spread
Invading cells tend to follow the path of least resistance and spread along natural clefts and tissue planes, but this does not explain the rapid invasive behaviour of some maligant tumours. Additionally in cell culture systems invasion can be seen in the absence of significant mechanical pressure.

Changes in extracellular matrix associated with neoplasia

Malignant cells can alter the extracellular matrix in three ways:

- destruction of matrix (see above)
- increased production of matrix by the host (desmoplasia)

This determines the consistency of the tumour. Desmoplasia is not essential to tumour invasiveness. Some tumours such as breast and bile duct carcinomas show marked desmoplasia.

• synthesis of matrix by the tumour.

There is controversy as to the origin of the fibrous tissue related to malignant tumours. Some workers maintain that the collagen associated with invasive breast carcinomas is synthesized and secreted by the tumour cells while other studies support the role of the host cells. Recently it has been suggested that the tumour cells recruit or stimulate myo-fibroblasts that produce the extra connective tissue.

Loss of anchorage dependence With the exception of haemopoietic cells and lymphocytes normal cells will only grow on a firm surface. This is termed anchorage-dependent growth. Many cell lines derived from malignant tumours can grow in suspension or in semi-solid media. This feature is highly associated with tumourigenicity when cells are injected into animals.

Loss of fibronectin from the cell surface Fibronectin can be found on the external surface of many cells and it acts as an adhesive protein in cell–cell binding and in the binding of cells to the sub-stratum. Malignant transformation is associated with loss or marked down-regulation of this protein which may be associated with an increase in degradative proteins on the surface of the cells or a disturbance in the cytoskeleton.

Lymphatic spread

Invasion of lymphatic channels at an early stage of the infiltrative process is a characteristic of carcinomas, while sarcomas show a greater tendency to invade small blood vessels. Invasion of lymphatics may be easier because of a lack of type IV collagen and laminin in their basement membrane.

Little is known about the mechanism of lymphatic invasion but in some experimental models the cells first enter the channel by pushing cytoplasmic processes between the endothelial cells. Once the malignant cells have gained access to the lymphatic channel they can grow along the lumen as a continuous cord. Presence of lymphatic invasion is an indicator of possible spread to local lymph nodes but in some instances (e.g. breast carcinoma) there is some evidence that lymphatic invasion in the absence of lymph node mestastasis is associated with an increased risk of distant metastasis. In breast carcinoma lymphatic blockage is prominent and may be associated with blockage. This causes diversion of lymph flow and may be associated with diversion of groups of malignant cells resulting in the production of satellite tumour nodules. Lymphatic blockage also causes lymphoedema of the tissues distal to the blockage and in the breast is associated with the skin change **peu d'orange**. In the lung extensive lymphatic permeation often associated with a breast or gastric primary produces **lymphangitis carcinomatosa**. Melanomas also permeate along lymphatics and may produce a black streak in the subcutaneous tissue.

Tumour cells enter the lymph node and gain access to the sub-capsular sinus. From there they extend to involve the sinuses of the centre of the node. Within the node the tumour cells may be destroyed, may remain dormant or may establish a growing focus with partial or total replacement of the node. In the last of these acquisition of an adequate blood supply is important. Tumour cells within lymph nodes may gain access to the bloodstream by invasion of intranodal vessels, invasion of extranodal vessels, by the opening up of small lymphaticovenous channels or via the thoracic duct.

Blood spread

Malignant cells may enter the bloodstream either by invading new vessels or by invading host vessels near the growing edge of the tumour. The new vessels have a defective basement membrane and may lack normal perivascular connective tissue. Sarcomas often contain large irregular blood-filled channels, the linings of which are entirely or partly composed of malignant cells which can be shed into the lumen. Permeation in continuity may be seen in certain tumours (e.g. tumours of the renal tubular epithelium and carcinoma of the bronchus).

This is the sequence of events following invasion of the serosal lining of an organ by malignant cells: there is usually a local inflammatory response with tumour cells becoming incorporated in the inflammatory exudate. These small groups of cells become detached, float in the fluid portion of the exudate and settle on the walls of the cavity at a distant site. This type of spread is commonly seen in the peritoneal cavity associated with tumours arising in the stomach, colon or ovary.

....

METASTASIS

Definition   A growing colony established at a point distant from the primary tumour with no continuity between primary and new deposit.

Pathogenesis   Most are the consequence of lymphatic or blood vessel invasion. Metastasis is primarily an embolic process which follows a series of events:

- Liberation of cells from the primary tumour.
- Invasion of blood vessels or lymphatics.
- Transfer of tumour cells as emboli to a distant site.

While in the bloodstream malignant cells form clumps. The greater the degree of clumping the more likely is impaction and the greater the chances of a secondary deposit forming. After impaction some tumour cells stimulate fibrin production, which has been suggested as protecting the clump and allowing proliferation.

- Adhesion to endothelium in the vascular bed of new site.
- Migration from vessel in which the embolus has impacted. After impaction the cells emigrate through spaces created by endothelial cell retraction.
- Survival of cells at the new site.
- Multiplication and growth to form secondary tumour.

For this to occur a new and suitable microenvironment must be established, including the acquisition of a new blood supply.

Only a small fraction of cells released from a primary tumour will survive to establish metastatic deposits. This suggests that the original tumour cell population is not homogeneous in respect of the qualities needed to establish metastases. It has also been suggested that the different patterns of metastasis seen in different tumours are due to different tumour cells thriving in certain 'biological soils' but not in others. Experimental evidence suggests that tumour cells destined to form secondary deposits may home into favoured tissue sites.

Certain genes may be associated with a metastatic phenotype. Currently the most interesting of these is a suppressor gene for metastasis **NM23** which is coded for on the long arm of chromosome 17. In human breast cancer poor survival is correlated to loss of expression of NM23. In a variety of human malignancies mutations or abnormal expression of the *ras* and *myc* oncogenes have been associated with aggressive behaviour.

Sites of metastasis

Liver This is the site at which blood-borne metastases occur most frequently, particularly for gastrointestinal and pancreatic primaries (associated with portal drainage system). Other tumours commonly spreading to the liver include carcinomas of the lung, breast and genitourinary system, malignant melanoma and various sarcomas. Rare cases of transplacental metastases have been recorded in the liver.

Lung These include carcinoma of the breast, stomach and sarcomas. Blood-borne metastases may be single or multiple and tend to form well-demarcated round masses.

Skeleton After the liver and lungs this is the third most frequent site. The primary is frequently carcinoma of the lung, breast, prostate, kidney or thyroid. Bony metastases may be associated with production of new bone (osteosclerotic) or destruction of bone (osteolytic). Osteosclerotic deposits are hard and appear as radio-opaque lesions on X-rays. They are associated with high plasma alkaline phosphatase and are commonly seen in association with metastatic prostatic carcinoma. Osteolytic lesions are radiolucent and may present with a pathological fracture. If bone destruction is extensive plasma calcium levels may be elevated.

Brain Secondary deposits occur quite frequently in the brain, with the lung as a common primary site.

Adrenal This is the most commonly affected endocrine site. The medulla is more frequently involved than the cortex. Common primary sites are the lung and breast.

Clinical importance

Determination of the extent of spread (staging) of a tumour gives important prognostic information. The occurrence of blood-borne metastases is the feature of malignant disease which is responsible for death in most fatal cases.

Effects of neoplasms on the host

....

LOCAL EFFECTS

Mechanical pressure or obstruction

Effects of the neoplasm on the host will in many cases depend on the size of the tumour and its site. In the gastrointestinal tract clinical presentation often relates to the presence of obstruction caused by the tumour. This obstruction may be due to the actual bulk of the neoplasm or to the presence of a dense fibrous stroma induced by the tumour (desmoplasia). Occasionally polypoid tumours cause intestinal intussusception leading to obstruction.

The anatomical site of the neoplasm will determine how early obstruction occurs and its severity. A small neoplasm in an unfavourable location (such as the bile duct or head of the pancreas) will produce severe obstruction.

Obstruction can occur in structures adjacent to the site of origin of the tumour as a result of infiltration. In carcinoma of the cervix direct spread through the pelvis may result in ureteric obstruction.

Mechanical disturbances can be the result of local disturbances due to the tumour. One example of this is the serious consequences that can develop due to the usually benign tumour or the meninges (meningioma) which can cause serious or fatal consequences as a result of increased intracranial pressure.

Destruction of tissue

This may occur as a result of:

- Pressure e.g. erosion of the pituitary fossa associated with pituitary adenomas.
- Aggressive properties of the tumour.

Haemorrhage

Neoplasms involving surfaces or underlying tissue usually undergo a certain degree of ulceration and haemorrhage. Mostly this is chronic and may lead to iron deficiency anaemia.

Infection

Local infection may be the result of obstruction to a drainage system and retention of secretions (e.g. broncho-pneumonia associated with bronchial carcinoma). Malignant disease may also lead to immunosuppression predisposing to infections.

....

SYSTEMIC MANIFESTATIONS

Fever

Fever is very common in patients with malignant disease (particularly lymphoma, leukaemia and Hodgkin's disease), possibly as an effect of release of IL-1 or TNF-α by tumour cells or infiltrating macrophages.

Cachexia

Marked weight loss and tissue wasting are well-recognized features of the later stage of malignant disease and may be due to:

- anorexia
- malabsorption e.g. medullary carcinomas of thyroid that secrete products increasing gastrointestinal motility
- metabolic processes of the tumour
- the possibility of a cachexia-inducing product secreted by tumour cells e.g. TNF-α (also known as cachectin).

Depression of immune system

Both humoral and cellular immunity can be affected leading to increased susceptibility to infections. Most commonly associated with tumours of the lymphoid system. There may also be development of associated autoimmune disease e.g. immune complex mediated nephrotic syndrome.

Haematological effects of neoplasms

Anaemia

May be due to:

- occult blood loss (iron deficiency)
- poor nutritional state associated with folate deficiency and macrocytic anaemia
- malabsorption may result in folate deficiency
- red-cell destruction causing autoimmune haemolytic anaemia. May be associated with malignancies of the lymphoreticular system. Mechanism is poorly understood
- associated with decreased erythropoietin production.

Increased red cell production

Seems to be caused by ectopic production of erythropoietic factors. Most seen in association with

- renal adenocarcinoma
- cerebellar haemangioblastoma
- uterine fibroleiomyoma
- liver cell carcinoma
- less often with ovarian carcinoma, adrenal tumours and carcinoma of the lung.

Effects on platelets and clotting

There may be decreased platelet numbers sometimes associated with autoimmune destruction. More frequently there is an increased clotting tendency associated with increased fibrin-degradation products associated with intravascular coagulation. Some malignant tumours (e.g. carcinomas of the bronchus, pancreas, stomach and female genital tract) are associated with recurrent migratory thrombophlebitis.

Endocrine effects of neoplasms

Appropriate hormone production

Neoplasms (benign or malignant) produce hormones appropriate to the location of the tumour (e.g. adenomas of the β cells of the pancreas producing insulin) but without normal feedback controls.

Ectopic hormone production

Hormones secreted by tumours arising from cells not normally associated with hormone production.

Non-metastatic hypercalcaemia

Some tumours may secrete a parathyroid hormone-related peptide (PTHRP); this is especially associated with tumours of the lung and kidney. Occasionally tumour-related hypercalcaemia may be seen in the absence of increased levels of PTHRP. Part of this effect is thought to be associated with prostaglandin production either by the tumour cells or other cells associated with the tumour. In other tumours TNF β may be produced which stimulate osteoclasts to resorb bones.

Non-metastatic osseous and soft tissue changes

Clubbing

Changes that result in the the angle between the nail and the cuticle becoming filled. The nail is curved from front to back. In severe cases the periosteum over the terminal phalanges, wrists and ankles thicken and new bone is formed (hypertrophic pulmonary osteoarthropathy). Clubbing may occur in association with a number of non-neoplastic diseases (e.g. cyanotic congenital heart disease, chronic pulmonary sepsis and infective endocarditis) as well as with mesothelioma of the pleura and carcinoma of the bronchus. The pathogenesis is obscure but increased blood flow and ectopic secretion of growth hormone have been suggested.

Non-metastatic changes in nerve and muscle

Three groups of changes exist: an encephalomyeloneuropathy (degeneration of the ganglion cells is the dominant pathological feature) and myelopathy (with or without features of myasthenia) both of which are related to the progression of the disease and demyelinating disorders which are not. Tumours most commonly associated with these changes include carcinomas of the bronchus (seen in 14% cases, mostly small cell variety), breast, ovary, uterine cervix and colon. The cause is unknown.

Cutaneous manifestations of malignancy

Polymyositis and dermatomyositis

Associated with malignancy in 25–30% of cases. Muscular symptoms include pain and weakness particularly around hip and shoulder. The rash varies from a barely perceptible rash to red or violaceous eruption. Most associated with carcinoma of the gastrointestinal tract, bladder or bronchus.

Acanthosis nigricans

Increased pigmentation of the skin (particularly axilla, back of neck and periareolar region of breast). The skin may become thick in later stages. About two-thirds of tumours associated with acanthosis nigricans are carcinomas of the stomach.

Erythema gyratum repens

Irregular wavy bands of red maculopapules. Reported with adenocarcinoma and small cell carcinoma of bronchus and carcinomas of the gastrointestinal tract, breast, uterine cervix and tongue.

....

SOME BIOLOGICAL MARKERS OF MALIGNANCY

Three groups of 'biological markers' exist:

- hormones
- iso-enzymes
- tumour-associated antigens.

Isoenzymes

Acid phosphatase

Associated with carcinoma of the prostate. High levels found in patients in whom metastases have occurred.

Carcinoplacental alkaline phosphatase

May appear in 3–15% patients with malignancy particularly carcinoma of the bronchus, colon, pancreas and liver and in germ cell tumours. Increased levels are also seen in non-neoplastic conditions such as ulcerative colitis and cirrhosis.

Tumour associated antigens

α-fetoprotein   Normally secreted by the yolk sac and fetal liver but falling to virtually undetectable levels in adults. Raised levels are seen in liver cell carcinoma and in up to 50% of malignant germ cell tumours (particularly with yolk sac elements).

Carcinoembryonic antigen (CEA)   Normally found in gatrointestinal tract, liver and pancreas in first 6 months of embryonic life. Increased levels are found in a variety of neoplasms and some non-neoplastic conditions. The main role for CEA measurement is in following up patients after surgery and in monitoring effects of therapy.

Tumour regression

Noted most frequently in neuroblastoma and malignant melanoma.

Features suggesting immune response to tumour

- Infiltration by lymphocytes and plasma cells.
- Histiocyte proliferation and epithelioid granulomas in lymph nodes draining tumour sites.

Immune deficiency and malignancy

Some increase in malignancies is seen in patients with inborn deficiency states (e.g. ataxia telangectasia, Wiskott–Aldrich syndrome and Chediak–Higashi syndrome) and in cases with iatrogenic immunosuppression suggesting the immune system may inhibit tumour formation.

Tumours in animal hosts

Adult mice appear to be protected against the oncogenic effect of certain viruses (e.g. polyoma virus) but tumours can be induced in newborn mice or mice thymectomized at birth suggesting a role for cell-mediated immunity.

Tumour-associated transplantation antigens

Tumour rejection can occur following expression of certain antigenic determinants on the surface of tumour cells (tumour associated transplantation antigens) which are especially associated with tumours induced by chemical carcinogens or viruses but may be seen in some spontaneous tumours (e.g. melanoma, renal cell carcinoma and astrocytomas).

27

Mechanisms by which the immune system can combat tumour growth

MECHANISMS BY WHICH THE IMMUNE SYSTEM CAN COMBAT TUMOUR GROWTH

Macrophages

- Destroy tumour cells in culture.
- Activated by contact with tumour antigen and due to release of activating factors from T cell activated by contact with tumour antigens.

Effector T cells

In certain transplantable tumours in animals tumour growth is increased if there is a large population of suppressor T cells.

Antibodies

Two possible modes of action:

1. Bind to tumour cells and initiate complement mediated cell lysis but evidence suggests that this is not a significant pathway.
2. Adhere to tumour cells and attract cytotoxic cells e.g. macrophages, T lymphocytes and natural killer cells.

Natural killer cells

Ability to kill tumour cells is independent of prior immunization with tumour cell determinants. Activity is stimulated by γ interferon released by T cells and natural killer cells themselves.

Immune surveillance

The original concept was that malignant transformation of cells occurs frequently but that clonal expansion was inhibited by immune mechanisms. In spontaneously arising tumours it was assumed that this mechanism failed. It has been shown that in virus and chemical-induced tumours the immune mechanisms remain intact. It is possible that many malignant cells are poor immunogens or that some tumour cells constantly shed surface antigens which form complexes and bind to killer cells preventing them from acting directly against tumour cells. A further factor is tumour bulk with small tumours more likely to yield to efforts to improve the host's immune system.

Oncogenesis and the molecular biology of cancer

Cancer may be considered to be a set of disorders characterized by disturbance in:

- mechanisms controlling cell proliferation
- cell differentiation
- normal relationship between proliferating cells and surrounding stroma.

Although there are many factors important in the development of cancer it is likely that the number of mechanisms operating at the cellular level is small and that these are mediated through abnormalities of three classes of gene:

- oncogenes
- tumour suppressor genes
- mutator genes.

The homeostatic control of growth relies on a balance between growth promoting genes (proto-oncogenes) and growth restraining genes (tumour suppressor genes).

DOMINANTLY ACTING ONCOGENES

Proto-oncogenes form part of the normal genome and contribute to neoplastic transformation only if qualitatively or quantitatively altered (becoming oncogenes) which might result in:

- The encoding of abnormal gene products as a result of point mutations.
- Over-expression of an unaltered proto-oncogene following amplification or translocation of the gene.
- Formation of new genes and the expression of chimeric gene products as a result of the fusion of a proto-oncogene with parts of other genes.

Proto-oncogenes are concerned with processes involved with division and proliferation. Thus they encode for:

- growth factors (*sis, int-2, IGF-1*)
- growth factor receptors and protein kinase (*erb-2, fms, met, trk, ret*)
- abnormally functioning growth factor receptors (*neu*)
- factors acting in transduction of signals arising from ligand receptor interactions

  - G proteins (*ras*)
  - GTPase activators (*gap, krev*)
  - membrane associated cytoplasmic kinases (*src, yes, fgr*)
  - non-membrane associated cytoplasmic kinases (*raf, mos, pim-1, fps*)

- DNA-binding proteins concerned with transcription
  - hetero-dimeric transcription factors (*fos/jun, myc/max*)
  - transcription factors (*myb, rel, ets*)
- cell cycle proteins.

Enzymes known as cyclin-dependent kinases drive the cell through the cell cycle. Cyclins are proteins whose concentration changes in a regular pattern during the cell cycle and which turn these kinases on appropriately. Production of cyclins at inappropriate times or in inappropriate quantity may stimulate abnormal cell division. Cyclin D1 (active during G1 phase) is now regarded as a proto-oncogene and is implicated in oesophageal and breast carcinoma, parathyroid adenoma and mantle cell lymphoma.

Oncogenic retroviruses

There is a group of RNA viruses capable of producing tumours in their host. These are the **oncornaviruses** or **oncogenic retroviruses**. The genome of these viruses is composed of RNA enclosed in a capsid which is in turn wrapped in an envelope. When the virus enters the cell the capsid is removed and the RNA is copied by viral **reverse transcriptase** to a portion of DNA – the **provirus**. This is incorporated into the host genome. Transcription of these sequences can act as mRNA for viral proteins or form the RNA genome of new viruses which can bud off from the cell.

Oncogenic viruses are divided into two groups:

1. A group which induces tumours slowly and irregularly but replicates well. The genome contains three genes:

   - *gag* – codes for a group specific antigen
   - *pol* – codes for reverse transcriptase
   - *env* – codes for envelope glycoprotein

   with non-coding sequences (**long terminal repeats**) at either end which promote gene expression and replication. This group typically produce lymphomas/ leukaemias in poultry, mice and cats.

2. A group which produces tumours in the appropriate host very quickly (days/weeks). These are not common in the wild. Inoculation is usually required as the viruses do not infect cells by natural pathways. Most lack the full complement of genes required for replication with the exception of the *Rous sarcoma virus*. This virus has a portion of the genome containing *gag, pol* and *env* genes necessary for replication. A second part contains a gene called *src* which is both necessary and sufficient to cause sarcomas in the appropriate host (poultry) and transform fibroblasts in culture. The viral gene (*v-src*) is now recognized as belonging to a family of about 20 transforming oncogenes known as viral oncogenes (*v-oncs*) which also include *erb b* (from avian erythroblastosis virus) and *sis* (from simian sarcoma virus).

It has been shown that there are complementary sequences to all retroviral v-oncs in DNA of many disparate species (e.g. human, yeast, fruit fly) as the proto-oncogenes. These constituents of the normal cell have the potential for being converted into active genes capable of contributing to malignant transformation.

Several facts suggest that the viral genes are derived from the cellular genes rather than vice versa. These include:

- High degree of conservation of cellular oncogenes through evolution (from yeasts to humans).
- The proto-oncogenes contain protein-coding sequences (exons) alternating with intervening sequences (introns) while in the virus the coding sequences occur in blocks.

After transcription of the proto-oncogenes the mRNA corresponding to the introns is removed and the resulting mRNA is almost identical to the viral mRNA.

Transformation by transfection of tumour cell DNA

When DNA is extracted from transformed cells and introduced into cultures of untransformed mouse fibroblasts (**transfection**), foci of transformed cells appear. These cells can produce tumours after inoculation into young mice. Transfected DNA from biopsies of some human tumours produce the same effect. Some of the active oncogenes derived from human tumours have been isolated and cloned. In each case the DNA sequence is closely related to sequences in the normal genome. Successful transfection/ transformation has been reported with the following oncogenes:

Ki-ras	carcinoma of thyroid; melanoma; acute myeloid leukaemia
Ha-ras	carcinomas of colon, pancreas and lung
N-ras	carcinomas of the thyroid and genitourinary tract; melanoma
fos	carcinomas of kidney, colon, lung and ovary
met	osteosarcoma
mos	carcinoma of breast
myc	Burkitt's lymphoma; carcinomas of breast, colon, lung and ovary
sis	glial tumours
ret	carcinoma of thyroid
raf	carcinoma of lung
int-1	carcinoma of breast
trk	carcinoma of thyroid
db1/mcf2	carcinoma of breast; some B cell lymphomas.

Activation of cellular oncogenes

Over-expression following acquisition of novel transcriptional promoter

Some proto-oncogenes can be activated by insertion of a strong transcriptional promoter very near to the proto-oncogene resulting in its strong activation (**insertional mutagenesis**).

Amplification of proto-oncogene or oncogene

In some tumours proto-oncogenes have been found to be amplified many times normal. The increased number of copies of the gene is assumed to result in a significant increase in transcription and hence the amount of the gene product.

Alteration of structure of oncogene protein

Point mutations in proto-oncogenes may convert them into potent oncogenes. Single point mutations in *Ha-ras* has been seen in some cases of bladder and lung carcinoma encoding codons specifying residues 12 and 61 respectively.

Increased activity of transcriptional promoters by 'enhancer sequences'

'Enhancer sequencers' increase the utilization of transcriptional promoters and can therefore increase the level of transcription and hence the amount of gene product. The linked promoter may be a considerable distance from the enhancer sequence which may be either up- or downstream of the promoter.

Chromosome translocation

Chromosome translocation may result in the movement of a proto-oncogene to a different site in the genome which may lead to activation. Translocations may also be associated with the formation of novel genes as a result of the fusion of proto-oncogenes and gene on the chromosome to which it has been translocated.

···

TUMOUR SUPPRESSOR GENES

Tumour suppressor genes normally inhibit excessive cell proliferation. Mutations in or loss of these genes results in loss of their growth-inhibiting functions and unfettered cell proliferation.

Detection of tumour suppressor genes

The existence of tumour suppressor genes may be inferred from:

- Suppression of tumour formation by hybrid cells derived from the fusion of malignant cells and their normal counterparts.
- Association of certain hereditary tumours with alteration or deletion of specific genes.
- Detection of loss of certain alleles identified in specific tumours and some pre-tumorous states.
- Ex vivo analysis of the activity of certain suppressor genes that have been successfully cloned.
- Restoration of suppressed, non-tumorigenic phenotype to certain tumour cells in culture following transmission of wild-type tumour (normal, unmutated) suppressor gene.

The reversion of tumour cells to normal when fused with their normal counterparts and the subsequent reversion to a malignant phenotype over a period of time in culture (associated with loss segments of genetic material) suggests that the transformed state correlates with *loss* of certain genetic material.

Retinoblastoma

This is the paradigm for the hypothesis of tumour suppressor genes. Retinoblastoma is a rare malignant tumour (1/20 000 infants and young children affected) which arises from the precursor cell (retinoblast) of the photoreceptor cells in the eye. Epidemiological data suggest that the tumour has two patterns, **sporadic** and **familial**.

The familial form occurs early (mean age 14 months), is often bilateral, may be associated with a family history and is usually multiple. Survivors have an increased risk of developing second tumours (especially osteosarcoma). Epidemiological data suggest that the gene is transmitted in an autosomal fashion. In the sporadic form (affecting about 1/100 000 children) the mean age is 30 months and the tumours are usually unilateral. Survivors show no increased risk of developing second tumours.

These observations lead Knudson to suggest that the abnormal gene could be acquired by two routes:

- inherited from a parent
- from mutation within the gene.

The differences between somatic and familial retinoblastoma could then be explained in the following way:

- All retinoblastoma genes carry two (rather than one) mutated alleles of the same gene.
- In **familial retinoblastoma** one of the mutated alleles is inherited and is therefore present in *all* cells in the body. The second mutation occurs locally as a somatic mutation in one of the already genetically abnormal retinoblasts.
- In **sporadic retinoblastoma** both mutations occur as somatic mutations occurring locally in retinoblasts. The risk of this happening would be less than the case for a single mutation which would be reflected in this variant being less common.

The retinoblastoma (RB) gene has now been mapped to the long arm of chromosome 13 (13q14) and has been associated with tumour suppressor function. Abnormalities in the gene are also found in osteosarcoma as well as breast, prostate, bladder and lung cancers.

Wilm's tumour

This is a malignant tumour with elements that resemble embryonic kidney. Three genomic abnormalities appear to be associated with this lesion in a non-random fashion.

- In WAGR syndrome (Wilm's tumour, aniridia, genitourinary tract anomalies and mental retardation) there is a deletion on chromosome 11 (11p13) encoding the gene WT-1 (coding for a protein with suppressor function related to regulation of transcription).
- In 15–20% of sporadic Wilm's tumours and in Wilm's tumours associated with Beckwith–Wiedmann syndrome there is deletion in the region of 11p15.
- In some familial Wilm's tumours there is a deletion which does not map to either of these loci.

Neurofibromatosis type 1 (NF-1)

All cases are associated with inheritance of a mutated allele (most arise from the father). The NF-1 suppressor gene appears to be on the long arm of chromosome 17 (17q11.2). The gene product is neurofibromin.

Familial adenomatous polyposis coli (FAPC)

This is an inherited disorder (autosomal dominant) associated with the development of multiple colonic adenomatous polyps in the second and third decade. One or more polyps inevitably develops a malignant phenotype. There is an FAP locus on chromosome 5 (5q15–22) which is deleted in these lesions. This locus appears to be involved in the genesis of non-familial colonic adenomas and non-familial rectal cancers.

MECHANISM OF ACTION OF TUMOUR SUPPRESSOR GENES

Tumour suppressor genes may function as:

Nuclear proteins   The gene products of some tumour suppressor genes (*RB, p53, WT-1*) are nuclear proteins. These presumably act normally in one of two ways:

1. Regulating expression of genes/gene products involved in cell proliferation or differentiation.
2. Controlling biochemical mechanisms regulating initiation of DNA synthesis.

Cytoplasmic proteins   The product of the *NF-1* gene is thought to be GTPase-activating and to interact with the p21 *ras* product thus regulating signal transduction pathways associated with cell proliferation.

Cell surface proteins   The gene *DCC* (deleted in colon cancer) is located on chromosome 18 and is thought to encode a member of the immunoglobulin gene superfamily which shows homology with neural adhesion molecules. This may influence cell–cell interactions.

Retinoblastoma gene product

In the normal cell the product of the *RB* gene (a 105Kd protein; p105-RB) forms a complex with transcription factors

(E2F and DP-1) in the G1 or G0 phase. As long as this complex exists transcription of S-phase genes cannot occur and the cell cycle cannot proceed. The ability of the RB protein to maintain this complex depends on its phosphorylation which is mediated by the cyclin dependant kinases cdk-2 and 4 which are linked with cyclins D and E.

Antigens of some DNA viruses (particularly E1A transforming protein of adenovirus, large T antigen of SV40 and E7 protein of oncogenic human papilloma viruses) bind and inactivate the *RB* protein.

p53 *gene*

Mutations in this gene appear to be the commonest abnormality related to tumour suppressor genes in human tumours. The gene encodes a nuclear phosphoprotein with 275 amino acids. It binds with transforming proteins of some oncogenic viruses (e.g. large T antigen of SV40). The activity of *p53* appears to be controlled by:

1. The level of *p53* protein which is low after mitosis but increases in G1.
2. The degree of phosphorylation. Phosphorylation occurs in S phase and may block its suppressor effect.

Alterations in *p53* may result from either complete loss of the gene or mutation within the gene associated with production of an abnormal protein. Most of the mutations are somatic but some may be found in the germline of families. The latter are associated with familial neoplastic syndromes such as the **Li-Fraumeni syndrome**.

p53 protein acts as a transcription factor which switches on the gene encoding another protein known as Cip-1 (CDK-interacting protein-1) or *WAF-1*. This in turn inhibits the activity of enzymes that drive cell cycle and cyclin-dependent kinases (CDKs) which phosphorylates the RB protein maintaining its complex with E2F and DP1. It appears that *p53* plays little part in routine growth regulation as it is not required for viability, either in fetal or in adult life. It is, however, important in the regulation of uncontrolled growth such as occurs in malignancy. It has been suggested that the major function of *p53* is to prevent chromosomal replication when DNA has been damaged This is supported by the observation that *p53* protein levels rise after irradiation leading to arrest of cells with damaged DNA in G phase and induction of apoptosis in cells harbouring genomic abnormalities.

Regulation of *p53* is by the protein product of another gene *mdm-2* (mouse double minute gene-2) which is a dominant oncogene which enhances tumour production when over expressed. The product of *mdm-2* binds *p53* and inactivates it so that the *Cip-1/WAF-1* gene is not expressed.

p16 gene

This gene is found on the short arm of chromosome 9 and appears to be important in the genesis of familial malignant melanoma although abnormalities have been reported in many other tumour types. The protein binds to a cyclin-dependent kinase (CDK 4) and thus inhibits its activation by cyclin D1.

Tumour suppressor genes in breast cancer

About 5% of breast cancers are familial and two thirds of these are thought to be associated with germline mutations in either the *BRCA-1* (on the long arm of chromosome 17) or *BRCA-2* (on the long arm of chromosome 13) gene. The *BRCA-1* is associated with one-third of familial breast cancers and over 80% of families with breast and ovarian cancers occurring together. The presence of a zinc-finger domain suggests that the protein might be a transcription factor.

··

MUTATOR GENES

The products of normal mutator genes are associated with DNA repair. They were first discovered in hereditary non-polyposis colorectal cancer. The first such gene, *MSH2*, is located on the short arm of chromosome 2 and has strong homology with the mut2 gene occurring in bacteria. A second gene, *MLH1*, is on the short arm of chromosome 3.

Oncogenesis

....

GENETIC FACTORS

An increase in the liability of an individual to develop a malignant neoplasm may be inherited as:

- part of a clinical syndrome with other diagnostic features apart from an increased risk of malignancy
- an increased likelihood of tumours developing as the only manifestation.

Inherited syndromes associated with increased risk of malignancy are:

- syndromes with a major chromosome abnormality
- syndromes apparently determined by single gene defects.

Chromosomally determined syndromes

Down's syndrome Increased risk of developing acute leukaemia (myeloblastic:lymphoblastic 1:2) as an integral part of the syndrome.

Klinefelter's syndrome Increased risk of developing tumours of the breast.

Gonadal dysgenesis in patients with female phenotype and male genotype Increased risk of gonadal tumours.

Single gene defects

May or may not be associated with immune deficiencies. These defects are not associated with immune deficiency:

Xeroderma pigmentosa
- autosomal recessive
- estimated frequency 1:65 000–250 000
- most common in North Africans

- defect is lack of enzymes responsible for excision and repair of DNA
- clinical features:

  - hypersensitivity to ultraviolet light
  - repeated exposure to sunlight gives dry scaly skin and areas of hyperpigmentation
  - unexposed skin remains normal
  - tendency to develop skin tumours in childhood and adolescence. Some are malignant including squamous cell carcinoma.

Other syndromes

Other syndromes in which DNA repair appears defective include *ataxia telangectasia* and *Fanconi's anaemia* (both associated with leukaemia) and *Bloom's syndrome* (characterized by hypersensitivity to sunlight.

Familial adenomatous polyposis coli and related disorders

- autosomal dominant with about 80% penetrance
- abnormal APC gene (a tumour suppressor gene) on long arm of chromosome 5
- clinical features:

  - multiple polyps appear in large gut
  - these are not present at birth and appear between the ages of 10–20 years
  - polyps are fairly evenly distributed through large gut but highest concentration in rectum (which is always involved)
  - carcinoma diagnosed at average age of 40 years. By 80 years almost all will develop carcinoma.

Gardner's syndrome

- autosomal dominant
- clinical features:

  - multiple colonic polyps
  - associated with tumours of the skin, subcutaneous tissue and bone
  - colorectal carcinoma develops in nearly 100% of cases.

Turcot syndrome

- autosomal dominant
- clinical features:

  - combination of colonic polyps and brain tumours
  - increased risk of colorectal carcinoma (magnitude unknown).

Increased risk of neoplasia with no precursor syndrome

Retinoblastoma

See page 949.

Phaeochromocytoma

Most are sporadic but 10–20% are thought to be familial. Occurs as part of a number of syndromes:

- Autosomal dominant tendency

  - often occur in childhood
  - more than 50% bilateral.

- Multiple endocrine neoplasia syndrome type IIa (MEN IIa, Sipple's syndrome)

  - combination of phaeochromocytoma, medullary carcinoma of the thyroid and parathyroid adenoma or hyperplasia
  - thought to be autosomal dominant with high penetrance
  - phaeochromocytoma occurs at 30–40 years
  - may be increased likelihood of malignant phaeochromocytomas.

- Multiple endocrine neoplasia type IIb (MEN IIb)

  - combination of phaeochromocytoma, medullary thyroid carcinoma and neuromas of mucosal surfaces
  - autosomal dominant.

- Neurofibromatosis

  - arises wherever chromaffin cells are present. Most common in adrenal medulla.
  - 5–10% are malignant

— tumours secrete noradrenaline and adrenaline
— patients may present with hypertension.

....

CHEMICAL CARCINOGENESIS

Historical perspective

The first observation of chemical carcinogenesis was in 1775 by Percival Pott, who noted a high incidence of cancer of scrotal skin in chimney-sweeps' boys. In 1778 the Danish Chimney Sweeps' Guild ruled that its members should bathe daily; this and the use of protective clothing was effective in decreasing the incidence of cancer.

Skin cancer was also seen in the early part of the industrial revolution in mule spinners – it was associated with lubricating oil, and it was suggested that coal tar could induce skin cancer. This led to the recognition that polycyclic hydrocarbons have high carcinogenic potential. In 1915 it was demonstrated that repeated applications of coal tar to the inside of rabbits' ears produced skin cancer. Further distillation of coal tar led to the demonstration of 3.4 benzpyrine as a powerful carcinogen.

Definitions

Remote carcinogen   Parent compound.

Proximate carcinogen   Metabolites of parent compound with greater carcinogenic potential.

Ultimate carcinogen   Final molecular species that interacts with the DNA.

Mechanisms

Transformed cells show permanent alterations in phenotype that is inherited between cellular generations implying genomic alteration (mutagenic agents).

Examples of chemical carcinogenesis

Polycyclic hydrocarbons

Moderate or powerful carcinogens include:

- 3.4 benzpyrene
- 7.12 dimethylbenzanthracine

- 1.2.5.6 dibenanthracine
- 3 methylecholanthrene.

Mechanisms
- binding to host macromolecules within the cytoplasm and the nucleus
- activated by oxidases to form epoxides
- these appear to have ability to bind DNA as well as macromolecules.

Cigarette smoking

The most important compound is probably 3.4 benzpyrene. It is associated principally with lung cancer but also with carcinoma of oesophagus, pancreas, kidney and urinary bladder. Smoking 20+ cigarettes a day confers a relative risk of developing lung cancer 32 times higher than in non-smokers. Giving up smoking reduces the risk. The longer the smoking-free time the lower the risk. About 10% of smokers develop lung cancer.

Mechanism Possible genetic contribution related to different inducibility of the enzyme **aryl hydrocarbon hydrolase (AHH)** by the hydrocarbon substrate.

Aromatic amines and azo dyes

2-naphthylamine was first observed as an increased rate of bladder cancer in workers with aniline dyes. Other occupations at risk of bladder cancer include the rubber and cable industry and those associated with the manufacture of certain paints, textile dyeing and printing. Only humans and dogs are susceptible to the urothelial effects of naphthylamine. In humans cancers develop an average of 15 years earlier than in the non-exposed population. The average latent period is 16 years.

Aromatic amines are remote carcinogens with the effect mediated by 2-amino-1-naphthol produced by hydroxylation in the liver. This is detoxified in the liver by conjugation with glucuronic acid. Human and dog urothelium produce a β-glucuronidase that splits this and releases the carcinogen.

2-Actely-aminofluorine

Developed as an insecticide but found to be carcinogenic before marketing. It produces neoplasms in liver, breast, lung and intestine. It is a remote carcinogen whose active compound is probably N-sulphate ester.

Nitrosamines and nitrosamides

Nitrosamines are remote carcinogens; they can be formed in the intestinal tract by interaction of nitrous acid (derived from nitrites) and secondary amines. It is suggested that gastric carcinoma may be associated with dietary nitrites which are found in pickled, salted and smoked foods. Nitrosamides do not require activation for their carcinogenic effect.

Direct acting alkylating agents

These bind DNA without need for prior activation and include:

- mustard gas
- β-propiolactone
- chemotherapeutic agents used in the treatment of neoplastic disease including cyclophosphamide, melphalan and busulphan.

Naturally occurring chemical carcinogens

Aflatoxin

- derived from *Aspergillus flavus* which may contaminate cereal and ground nut crops
- associated with liver carcinoma
- strong synergy with hepatitis B virus infection
- produces point mutation in codon 249 of the *p53* gene.

Occupational carcinogens

Table 29.1 lists known occupational carcinogens

Generally the neoplasm does not differ from that seen in the unexposed patient. The age at which tumours develop is related to duration of exposure and latent period for carcinogen action.

....

TUMOUR INITIATION AND PROMOTION

Initiation

- involves change in genome
- high doses of an initiator can cause tumours

Table 29.1 Occupational carcinogens

2-Naphthylamine	Urothelial malignancy (bladder, ureter, renal pelvis)
Arsenic	Skin and lung
Asbestos	Mesothelioma, squamous cell carcinoma of lung
Ionizing radiation	Lung, bone and leukaemia
Bischlormethylether	Small cell carcinoma of lung
Nickel	Lung, paranasal sinuses and larynx
Vinyl chloride monomer	Angiosarcoma of liver
Hardwood	Adenocarcinoma of paranasal sinuses
Benzene	Leukaemia

- low doses of an initiator cause damage to the genome without phenotypic alteration to cell
- initiation is a very rapid event
- is dose related
- occurs in a small proportion of the target cell population
- unless the DNA damage is quickly repaired the damage becomes permanent and is passed on in subsequent cell divisions.

Promotion

Promotors are usually agents which catalyse biochemical events leading to an altered pattern of gene expression. In an initiated cell this leads to a phenotype that is considered to be pre-neoplastic.

If exposure to a promotor is short then only a few cells will be effected; if exposure is prolonged or is replaced by a factor that increases cell turnover the effect will be present in many cells.

There are two phases:

Stage 1 promotion
- target is the cell surface membrane where there are high affinity receptors for the agent
- binding of the agent to the receptor causes alteration in the membrane phospholipid metabolism and alteration in the structure and function of the membrane.

Stage 2 promotion
- dependent on prolonged exposure to the promoting compound and sustained cell proliferation

• these agents induce enzymes whose products enhance speed of cell division (e.g. orthithine decarboxylase).

....

HORMONES AND NEOPLASIA

The link was first suggested after observation that oöphorectomy resulted in regression of some breast cancers (1895). This may partly be explained by the presence of oestrogen receptors on the cell surface of breast tumour cells. An association between oestrogens and endometrial carcinoma has been suggested following observations that:

• Oestrogen-secreting ovarian tumours are associated with endometrial hyperplasia upon which carcinoma can supervene.
• Carcinomas of the breast and endometrium may be seen in the same patient.
• There is an increased incidence of endometrial carcinoma in post-menopausal women treated with oestrogen-containing compounds.
• There is an increased risk of endometrial carcinoma in obese and diabetic women who have increased conversion of δ-4-androstenedione to oestrone.

....

PHYSICAL AGENTS AND CARCINOGENESIS

Ultraviolet light

This is low energy emission that does not penetrate deeply. The skin is the primary target. Most skin cancers occur in sun-exposed areas and are relatively rare in dark-skinned individuals. The mechanism may be associated with formation of thymine dimers in the DNA.

Most common sunlight-associated cancers include:

• basal cell carcinoma
• squamous cell carcinoma.

Ionizing radiation

An increased prevalence of leukaemia and skin cancer was seen in the early days of diagnostic radiology and associated with inadequate protection.

Increased incidence of leukaemia and carcinomas of the thyroid, breast and lung was found among survivors of the nuclear explosions in Hiroshima and Nagasaki at the end of the Second World War.

Increased risk of carcinoma of the thyroid following childhood irradiation of the neck.

Heightened risk of the following has also been noted:

- osteosarcoma following ingestion of bone-seeking radioactive substances
- leukaemia and liver neoplasms following use of thorium-containing contrast medium (thorotrast)

The mechanism is unknown but irradiation causes generation of free radicals that might react with the genome.

....

VIRUSES AND NEOPLASIA

Papilloma virus

The first virally induced mammalian neoplasm was the Shope papilloma on Kentucky cotton-tailed rabbits. In humans the papilloma viruses are the only ones proved to cause neoplasia. They are associated with common skin warts and anal and genital warts.

Human papilloma virus (HPV)

HPV is associated with carcinoma of the uterine cervix: Certain strains (types 16 and 18) are associated with considerable risk of malignancy. HPV genome encodes eight major open reading frames. Three of these (E5, E6 and E7) encode proteins with transforming properties in cell culture systems.

E6 and E7 complex with and inactivate *p53* and retinoblastoma proteins respectively and have the same effect as mutations in these tumour suppressor genes.

Polyoma virus

A large DNA virus that causes a variety of neoplasms in a variety of small animals when they are infected in the neonatal period.

Adult animals are immune unless they have been thymectomized neonatally, suggesting a link with inadequate immune surveillance.

No link with human neoplasia has been found.

Simian vacuolating virus (SV40)

Found to produce tumours in newborn hamsters, SV40 causes transformation of cultured human cells. It enters the cell through the action of its coating proteins.

After uncoating whole or part of the viral DNA it integrates with the host genome.

Herpes viruses

These cause malignant lymphoma in chickens (Marek's disease) and may be involved with human tumour formation.

Mouse mammary tumour virus

In 1936 Bittner found that a tendency for tumour development in strains of mouse with high prevalence of breast carcinoma was not entirely genetic. This suggested a factor present in the maternal milk might be responsible for the increased risk, and this was later found to be a virus.

Involvement in human breast carcinogenesis is not yet proven.

Epstein–Barr virus

This is found in 90% of world's population. It binds to the CD21 receptor on B lymphocytes but also infects epithelial cells. It is implicated in several human tumours:

- nasopharyngeal carcinoma
- Burkitt's lymphoma
- B-cell lymphomas in the immunosuppressed/immunocompromised
- Hodgkin's disease
- certain rare T-cell lymphomas.

Hepatitis B virus (HBV)

Positive correlation in humans between prevalence of carrier state of HBV and the frequency of liver cell carcinomas has been established.

Similar correlation has been seen in woodchucks carrying a virus resembling HBV in whom the viral DNA is incorporated into the host genome; similar observations have been found with HBV DNA in humans.

Human T-cell leukaemia virus 1 (HTLV-1)

This is rare in most parts of the world (e.g. 0.025% carriage rate in USA) but infection is common in Southern Japan, the Caribbean, parts of Africa and South America.

It is linked to adult T-cell leukaemia/lymphoma.

Genetic disorders

Definition: Diseases either wholly or partly due to abnormalities within the genetic material.

THE NORMAL KARYOTYPE

Normal cells contain

- 46 chromosomes
- 44 autosomes
- 2 sex chromosomes (X and Y).

The possession of an X chromosome confers male gender.

Chromosome structure

Chromosomes have a constricted centre (**centromere**). Material above the centromere is known as the **p** or **short arm** and material below the centromere as the **q** or **long arm**. The region at the end of each arm is the **telomere**. The position of the centromere divides the chromosomes into 3 groups:

- **metacentric**   chromosomes 1, 3, 16, 19, 20
- **sub-metacentric**   chromosomes 2, 4, 5–12, 17, 18, X
- **acrocentric**   chromosomes 13, 14, 15, 21, 22, Y.

Cell division

Mitosis   Each chromosome replicates with each daughter cell possessing a diploid number (46) of chromosomes.

Meiosis   Occurs in germ cells. Daughter cells possess half the normal number (haploid; 23) of chromosomes. Thus ova contain 22 autosomes and the X sex chromosome; sperm contain 23 autosomes and an X or Y sex chromosome.

Chromosome analysis (karyotyping)

Chromosome number and morphology may be determined by studying any tissue that can be grown in cell/tissue culture but common tissues used for analysis include lymphocytes, amniotic fluid cells, chorionic villus cells, bone marrow and fibroblasts (from skin biopsies). Chromosome abnormalities are described by referring to the chromosome affected (chromosome number), the arm involved and the region of that arm in terms of the group of the band and the actual band within the group.

....

MAJOR CHROMOSOMAL ABNORMALITIES

These cause some well-recognized syndromes but are also associated with spontaneous abortions; 50% of spontaneous abortions are due to chromosome abnormalities.

Abnormalities in chromosome structure

Deletions

Chromosomal break is followed by loss of genetic material. Ring chromosome formation is considered to be a form of deletion resulting from breakages at the extremes of chromosomes with fusion of truncated ends and usually associated with significant loss of material. An example is **cri du chat**, where there is deletion of the short arm of chromosome 5. This results in round facies, small head, mental retardation and a typical kitten-like cry.

Translocations

A segment is broken from one chromosome and transferred to another. These are usually **balanced** where segments break from two separate chromosomes and are reciprocally transferred. Although there is no loss of genetic material and the individual is phenotypically normal there is an increased risk of producing abnormal offspring due to the formation of abnormal gametes in meiosis. **Robertsonian translocations** are when a balanced translocation occurs between 2 acrocentric chromosomes and the breaks usually involve the long arm of one and the short arm of the other chromosome resulting in one very large and one very small chromosome.

Isochromosomes
Loss of either short or long arm with duplication of the surviving material.

Inversions
Break in a single chromosome is followed by 180° rotation of the segment and reincorporation into the parent chromosome. Inversions may involve only one arm (**paracentric**) or be on either side of the centromere (**pericentric**).

Abnormalities of autosome number

These fall into two groups in which either the chromosome number is not an exact multiple of 23 (**aneuploidy**) and which may be associated with one extra chromosome (**trisomy**) or loss of one of a pair of chromosomes (**monosomy**) or in which there is additional sets of chromosomes (**polyploidy**). Monosomy affecting an autosome is rare in live births and surviving children are usually severely handicapped and do not survive for long.

Examples of syndromes associated with aneuploidy

Monosomy 21   This is an exception and is compatible with survival. Patients develop severe difficulties when given oxygen during anaesthesia possibly due to the fact that the gene encoding the enzyme superoxide dismutase is encoded on chromosome 21.

Trisomy 21 (Down's syndrome)   Commonest numerical abnormality occurring in newborns. Frequency 1:800 live births. Commonest genetic cause of mental retardation. Risk is related to maternal age with steep increase in risk after 35 years.

Maternal age	< 20 years	Risk 1:1550
	> 45 years	Risk 1:28

Ninety five per cent of Down's syndrome children show full trisomy 21 due to non-disjunction of the chromosome at either the first or second meiotic division (in 95% of cases the non-disjunction occurs in the maternal chromosome 21), 4% show Robertsonian translocation within the maternal or paternal germ cell line usually to chromosome 22 or 14 (this is associated with increased risk of recurrence in further offspring); 1% result from non-disjunction of chromosome 21 in the zygote resulting in **mosaicism** where not all the cells show trisomy (usually less severely affected individuals).

Table 30.1 lists phenotype abnormalities in Down's syndrome.

Trisomy 13 (Patau syndrome)
- 1/10 000 live births
- 80% non-disjunction; 10% translocation in germ line; 10% mosaicism
- associated with: small head; mental retardation; small eye cavities (microphthalmia); cleft palate and hare lip; polydactyly; dextrocardia and ventricular septal defects; other visceral defects.

Table 30.1 Characteristics of Down's syndrome

Face	Tends to be flat with low bridged nose and oblique palpebral fissure and prominent epicanthic folds. The mouth is often large due to an enlarged protruding tongue which is coarsely furrowed and lacks a central groove.
Hands	Horizontal palmar crease (simian crease). Middle phalanx of little finger is short resulting in inward curvature (clinodactyly).
Long bones	Shorter than normal. Individuals have short stature. Abnormalities of rib cage and pelvis may be seen.
Cardiovascular	About 40% cases. Includes endocardial cushion defects, atrial septal and ventricular septal defects.
Haematological	10–20-fold increased risk for developing acute leukaemia (lymphoblastic or non-lymphoblastic).
Immune	Increased susceptibility to infections (especially pulmonary).
CNS	Most show mental retardation (IQ about 50). Cases surviving over 40 years almost all develop features of Alzheimer's disease (possibility related to presence of gene-coding amyloid precursor protein found in neuritic plaques in Alzheimer's disease and is on chromosome 21).

Trisomy 18 (Edwards' syndrome)
- 1/10 000 live births
- 90% non-disjunction; 10% mosaicism
- associated with: mental retardation; prominent occiput; small lower jaw (micrognathia); low-set ears; short neck; overlapping fingers; heart, kidney and intestinal defects; 'rocker-bottom feet'; hypertonicity.

Syndromes associated with aneuploidy of the sex chromosomes

Aneuploidy of sex chromosomes is commoner than aneuploidy of autosomes.

Y chromosome carries little genetic material; X chromosome carries abundant genetic information. Monosomy in respect of X chromosome (XO – Turner syndrome) is compatible with life while YO is non-viable.

In the female one X chromosome is randomly inactivated at about day 16 of embryonic life (**lyonization**) giving a mosaic population in the body with some cells having an active maternally derived X chromosome while in others the X chromosome is paternally derived. This in activation is not complete and some genes are spared and continue to function. This explains why patients with Turner syndrome (XO) and those with additional X chromosomes have abnormalities.

Turner syndrome
- 1/3000 live births
- 50% loss of entire X chromosome; 17% complete deletion of short (p) arm with isochromosome of long arm; 10% partial deletion of short arm; 20% mosaicism
- associated with short stature; webbed neck; broad chest with widely spaced nipples; increased carrying angle of forearm (cubitus valgus); pigmented naevi; low posterior hairline; increased risk of coarctation of the aorta, bicuspid aortic valve and subsequent aortic stenosis; poorly developed secondary sex characteristics; ammenorrhoea; small (streak) ovaries with few oocytes and virtually no oocytes left by 2 years.

Klinefelter syndrome
- presence of more than one X chromosome in phenotypic male

- mostly non-disjunction of X chromosome giving karyotype 47XXY
- 1/600–850 live births
- associated with male hypogonadism (atrophic testes, small penis); tall stature associated with disproportionately long lower limbs; eunuchoid appearance with wide pelvis, female pattern hair distribution; gynaecomastia; mental retardation in a minority.

XYY syndrome
- about 1/1000 male live births
- associated with tall stature; predisposition to severe acne.

'Superfemale' (more than two X chromosomes in female)
- about 1/1200 female live births
- commonest karyotype is 47XXX
- risk of mental retardation increases with increased numbers of X chromosomes.

Single gene defects

These are caused by mutation in either single or both alleles. Single allele mutations expressed clinically are **dominant**; mutations requiring both alleles mutated for clinical expression are **recessive**. They may affect autosomes or sex chromosomes.

Multifactorial disorders

These are associated with certain congenital developmental disorders and other conditions e.g. diabetes mellitus, atherosclerosis and cancer. Many involve interaction between inherited and environmental factors.

Somatic genetic disorders

These arise from mutations in certain somatic cells: as these arise in somatic cells and not germ line they cannot be inherited. They are commonly associated with tumour formation. Often involve interaction between genetic and environmental factors.

Genetic disorders

Mitochondrial genetic disorders

Mitochondrial disorders are rare and result from mutations in mitochondrial DNA. They are transmitted only through the maternal cell line with all offspring of an affected mother affected.

Single gene defects

AUTOSOMAL DOMINANT DISORDERS

- estimated to occur in 2–9/1000 live births
- single allele expressed despite presence of normal second allele
- affected individual normally has one affected parent (exception = new mutation in germ cell of one parent)
- both heterozygtes and homozygotes show abnormality. Usually much more severe in homozygotes
- males and females equally affected
- disorder present in every generation
- offspring from pairing between normal and affected individuals have 1:2 risk of showing the abnormality.

Table 31.1 gives examples of these disorders.

Penetrance and expressivity

An individual inheriting a dominant mutation may be phenotypically normal if the gene shows **incomplete penetrance**. If all individuals who inhibit the mutant dominant gene are phenotypically normal with different severity there is **variable expressivity**.

AUTOSOMAL RECESSIVE DISORDERS

- disorder manifested only when both alleles are mutated
- affected individual may have phenotypically normal parents but each parent must be a carrier (heterozygous for mutant gene)
- males and females equally affected
- disorder does not occur in every generation
- offspring of pairing between two parent carriers have 1:4 risk of showing abnormality

221

Table 31.1 Disorders caused by autosomal dominant gene defects

Disorder	Frequency (per 1000 live births)	Features
Hereditary spherocytosis	0.2	Anaemia
Familial hypercholesterolaemia	2.0	Premature atherosclerosis
Familial polyposis coli	0.1	Multiple adenomatous polyps in colon; inevitable progression to cancer
Polycystic kidney disease	1.0	Massive kidney with multiple cysts; progressive renal failure
Huntington's disease	0.2	Dementia in middle life with involuntary choreiform movements
Neurofibromatosis	0.08	Tumours of nerve sheaths; abnormal skin pigmentation
Tuberous sclerosis	0.08	Skin lesions (sebaceous adenoma); learning disability; epilepsy; hamartomas in brain and heart
Myotonic dystrophy	0.05	Delayed muscle relaxation, cardiomyopathy; cataract; diabetes mellitus; etc.
Diaphyseal aclasis	0.5	Numerous cartilagenous exostoses at ends of long bones
Osteogenesis imperfecta	0.1	Fragile bones with increased risk of fractures
Achondroplasia	0.04	Dwarfism; deformity of bone; increased risk of fractures
Thanatophoric dwarfism	0.08	Severe skeletal deformities; early death
Marfan's syndrome	0.1	Long thin limbs; increased or aortic dissection
Ehlers–Danlos syndromes	0.05	Hyperextensible joints and increased fragility of tissues
Otosclerosis	3.0	Deafness from adolescence onwards; changes in ossicles in middle ear
Dominant early childhood deafness	0.1	Deafness from childhood
Dominant blindness	0.1	Blindness
Dentinogenesis imperfecta	0.1	Abnormal development of teeth
Acute intermittent porphyria	0.01	Acute abdominal pain and neurological disturbances; dark urine (porphobilinogenuria)

- enzyme proteins are frequently affected
- penetrance is commonly complete.

Table 31.2 gives examples of these disorders.

....

X-LINKED DISORDERS

With few exceptions inheritance is recessive. Examples of X-linked dominant conditions include vitamin D-resistant rickets in which fathers only transmit the disease to their daughters.

In males there is only one X chromosome; thus recessive genes are always expressed. Only males are affected. Unaffected males do not carry the gene and cannot transmit the abnormality.

If an affected male has children all his female offspring will be carriers of a mutant gene; male offspring will be genotypically normal (X gene is inherited from the mother).

If female carrier has children male offspring have 1:2 risk of being affected; female offspring have 1:2 risk of being a carrier.

Table 31.3 lists these disorders.

....

MUTATIONS IN SINGLE GENE DEFECTS
Gene deletions

An example is α-thalassaemia. Normally there are 2 α-globin genes; if one is deleted there is excess of haemoglobin of β-globin chains (HbH). If both α-globin chains are deleted the fetus cannot make fetal haemoglobin and makes Hb Barts which has no oxygen-carrying capacity and results in stillbirth or neonatal death.

Partial gene deletion

Deletion of part of a gene means some protein may be encoded by the remnant gene but this protein is grossly abnormal.

Table 31.2 Disorders caused by autosomal recessive gene defects

Disorder	Frequency (per 1000 live births)	Features
Cystis fibrosis	0.5–0.6	Viscid secretions, recurrent lung infections; failure to thrive
Congenital deafness	0.5	Deafness from infancy
Sickle cell disease	0.1	Haemolytic anaemia
Adrenal hyperplasia	0.1	Precocious development of genitalia in males; virilism in females; may have Addisonian crisis
Phenylketonuria	0.2–0.5	Learning disability
α_1-antitrypsin deficiency	0.1–0.5	Chronic liver disease which may present in infancy; emphysema
Recessive blindness	0.1	Blindness
Cysteinuria	0.06	Recurrent renal calculi
Tay–Sachs disease	0.004	Learning disability; blindness
Mucopolysaccharidoses	0.03	Visceromegaly; mental retardation in some varieties
β-thalassaemia	0.05	Anaemia; bone deformities; enlarged spleen
Galactosaemia	0.02	Chronic liver disease starting in infancy; cirrhosis; liver failure
Homocystinuria	0.01	Learning disability; eye, bone and blood vessel abnormalities
Metachromatic leucodystrophy	0.02	Blindness; intellectual deterioration
Friedreich's ataxia	0.02	Early onset of progressive unsteadiness and dysarthria; skeletal deformities; cardiomyopathy in some cases
Spinal muscular atrophy	0.04	Progressive muscle weakness
Wilson's disease		Involuntary athetoid movements; chronic liver disease
Some varieties of Ehlers–Danlos syndrome		Hyperextensible joints; fragility of connective tissues
Neurogenic muscular atrophy	0.01	Progressive muscle weakness

Table 31.3 X-linked disorders

Disorder	Frequency (per 1000 live births)	Features
Fragile X syndrome	0.9	Learning disability; characteristic facies; large testes
Muscular dystrophy (Duchenne and Becker types)	0.3	Progressive muscle weakness (more severe in Duchenne type) leading to death in 3rd decade
Haemophilia A and B	0.1	Excessive post-traumatic bleeding
Ichthyosis	0.1	Thick skin with excessive keratin
Glucose-6-phosphatase deficiency		Haemolysis following ingestion of certain drugs
X-linked agamma-globulinaemia		Increased susceptibility to infection
Red–green colour blindness	8	

Examples include Duchenne and Becker types of muscular dystrophy with mutations in the dystrophin gene.

Codon deletion

Deletion of a codon or small set of codons means the reading frame is not altered but the protein will be deficient in one or more amino acids.

This occurs in several haemoglobin variants (mostly involving β-globin gene) and also in cystic fibrosis.

Duplications and insertions

These may result from unequal crossing over in meiosis. The effect depends on whether or not disruption of the reading frame occurs (if not there is little or no defect).

Fusion mutations

These arise from unequal crossing over between non-homologous genes resulting in the formation of fusion genes. The commonest example is red–green colour blindness.

Point mutations

The substitution of one base pair by another in double-stranded DNA: this may be purine substituted by purine or pyrimidine by pyrimidine (**transition**) or purine replaced by pyrimidine or vice versa (**transversion**).

About one third of all point mutations are not associated with alteration in coded amino acid because of degeneracy of genetic code. There are several different classes.

- **Mis-sense mutations**: base substitution leading to encoding of different amino acid. Not all have pathological consequences. Examples include sickle cell disease and α_1-antitrypsin deficiency.
- **Nonsense mutations**: converts a codon specifying an amino acid into a stop codon. The nearer to the 5' end the greater the truncation of the protein. Associated with the commonest cause of β-thalassaemia and with some cases of haemophilia A.
- **Stop codon mutations**: converts a stop codon into one encoding an amino acid.
- **Frameshift mutations**: occurs as a result of point mutation or via partial gene deletion. Results from either insertion or deletion of a single nucleotide which disturbs the reading frame so that a new set of codons is specified.
- **RNA splice mutations**: following transcription the original product must have introns removed for mRNA to be produced for translation. Most introns have GT sequence at 5' end of intron (**donor site**) and AG at 3' end (**acceptor site**). Mutations in either of these results in disturbance of splicing giving abnormal, non-functional mRNA.
- **Consensus sequence mutations**: splicing defects can occur due to mutations in consensus sequences.
- **Transcriptional mutations**: mutations in the blocks of DNA upstream from the 5' end which regulate transcription of the gene.

MITOCHONDRIAL DISORDERS

Each mitochondrion contains several copies of a circular chromosome consisting of a small amount of DNA which encodes some protein components of the respiratory chain and oxidative phosphorylation system as well as some special types of RNA.

Inheritance of mitochondrial genes in humans occurs entirely through the maternal line. Mitochondrial DNA has a high rate of mutations. **Examples** of disorders include:

- Leber's hereditary optic atrophy (late-onset bilateral loss of central vision; disturbances of heart rhythm)
- myoclonus with ragged red fibres
- mitochondrial myopathy with encephalopathy, lactic acidosis and stroke
- Kearns–Sayre syndrome (paralysis of external ocular muscles; complete heart block; pigmentary degeneration of the retina).

PART 2

Systemic pathology

The cardiovascular system

DISORDERS OF BLOOD VESSELS

THE ARTERIES: ATHEROSCLEROSIS

Altherosclerosis is the leading cause of death in Western countries. The term is derived from the Greek meaning 'porridge' (*athere*) and 'hardening' (*sclerosis*). The lesions, focal intimal thickenings, are seen in large elastic and muscular arteries, including the aorta, femoral, carotid and coronary arteries. Arteries smaller than 300 μm are not affected.

Mature atherosclerotic lesions show:

- a 'fibrous cap' made up of collagen-rich connective tissue
- intra-intimal collections of plasma-derived lipid
- a basal zone of necrosis, rich in lipid.

Clinical effects

- Increasing plaque volume: when > 75% of lumen cross-sectional area there is limitation of blood flow, potentially causing ischaemia (e.g. stable angina).
- Injury to plaque cap causes thrombosis (unstable angina, myocardial infarction or sudden death).
- Endothelial dysfunction: in areas of plaque there may be inadequate production of nitric oxide, or excess endothelin 1, causing disturbed vascular tone, e.g. inappropriate vasoconstriction on exercise.
- Medial atrophy beneath the plaque, causing aneurysm formation if severe.

Morphological appearances of atherosclerosis

Fatty streak

This is the first visible lesion, starting as a small yellow dot, 1–2 mm in size, above the adjacent intima. It is seen from early life onwards, appearing in the arch and upper ascending aorta, the dots forming parallel rows. They appear where there is a low blood flow shear rate, with thickening of the intima and a predilection for lipid deposition. Microscopic examination shows mild intimal thickening with intracellular accumulation of lipid within macrophages ('foam cells'), together with smooth muscle cells. There is evidence to suggest that there is a progression to the raised plaque, but this is not inevitable.

Gelatinous lesions

These are small blister-like intimal elevations, caused by focal oedema, which contain some extracellular fat. Some authorities believe these to be precursor lesions to mature plaques.

Fibrolipid plaque (raised lesion)

The archetypal lesion, responsible for occlusive arterial disease, such as ischaemic heart disease, stroke and limb ischaemia. Hypertension, hyperlipidaemia and diabetes mellitus are all associated with increased severity of raised lesions.

The lesions show:

- a sub-endothelial connective tissue cap
- 'atheromatous' basal pool.

If the cap is well developed the plaque is described as 'fibrous'; a large basal pool is present in a 'lipid' plaque. The basal pool can contain criss-crossed collagen strands from the cap to the base providing structure. If this is absent the pool is deformable, and more liable to rupture with consequent thrombosis. Dystrophic calcification is commonplace. Plaque instability is related to:

- large amounts of extracellular lipid
- a relative decrease in numbers of smooth muscle cells
- an increase in numbers of lipid-filled macrophages.

A plaque involving the entire circumference is concentric; the media is splinted and there is little change in calibre with changes in muscle tone. In eccentric plaques there still is potential for the media to respond to vasomotor signals.

Twelve per cent of the plaques involving the coronary arteries are eccentric and lipid rich and are most frequently associated with acute thrombosis. Large numbers of macrophages and relatively few smooth muscle cells within the cap are also risk factors for thrombosis.

PLAQUE GENESIS AND NATURAL HISTORY

The following phases are observed:

1. **Infiltration and retention of cholesterol-rich plasma-derived lipid within the intima.** It enters as intact low density lipoprotein (LDL), and is ingested by macrophages via the scavenger receptor after oxidation, possibly from free radicals generated by endothelial cells and macrophages. The LDL is a chemo-attractant for blood monocytes, and reduces their motility.

2. **Connective tissue (smooth muscle) cell proliferation, with collagen and matrix protein synthesis.** Smooth muscle cells show contractile and synthetic phenotypes, controlled by a number of chemical signals. There is strong evidence that this is a result of paracrine or autocrine growth factors from existing smooth muscle cells.

3. **Platelet derived growth factor (PGDF)**: Present in α granules of platelets, and also produced by endothelial cells, activated macrophages, and arterial smooth muscle cells. It is mitogenic for smooth muscle, and also has chemo-attractant properties. This would explain the migration of smooth muscle cells from the media to the intima in atherogenesis. Binding of PDGF to its receptor activates c-*fos* and c-*myc*, proto-oncogenes that initiate cell proliferation.

4. **Growth promoting potential of the macrophage**: As well as PDGF, macrophages produce fibroblast growth factor (FGF), transforming growth factor α and β.

5. **Necrosis of the cells, fibres and matrix at the plaque base, forming the lipid pool.**

PLAQUE INJURY AND THROMBOSIS

Life-threatening events (unstable angina and myocardial infarction) are related to plaque injury in 'unstable' plaques.

Superficial plaque injury

Denudation of the surface endothelium and superficial strands of collagen, leading to mural and occlusive thrombus deposition. This pattern accounts for 25% of thrombi related to damaged fibrolipid plaques.

Deep intimal injury

The development of a tear from the luminal surface through the connective tissue cap into the underlying lipid pool. Mixing of blood with the thrombogenic plaque contents activates platelets and the clotting cascade. The thrombus may remain confined within the plaque or extend into the lumen forming either mural or occlusive thrombus.

....

EPIDEMIOLOGY: RISK FACTORS

Age

There is strong and consistent association between age and atherosclerosis. Fatty streaks first appear in the aorta in the 1st decade, in the coronary arteries in the 2nd decade, and the cerebral vessels in the 3rd. Raised lesions appear in the 3rd decade and progress with age.

Sex

Clinical manifestation of atherosclerosis is far less frequent in women until middle age. After the menopause the difference is less marked. It is assumed female sex hormones are protective, and it is interesting that hormone replacement is associated with a reduced risk of ischaemic heart disease (IHD).

Race

There are striking geographic differences in prevalence, severity and extent of atherosclerosis. In the USA black people show less severe atherosclerotic disease than do whites.

Cigarette smoking

Smoking more than 15 cigarettes a day is strongly associated with IHD, stroke and peripheral arterial insufficiency.

The risk of IHD decreases quickly on giving up, and is thus thought to be related to changes in platelet function and clotting activity. Atherosclerosis, however, is more extensive and severe in smokers, and could be related to the free radicals in smoke.

Diabetes mellitus

Atherosclerosis is a major complication of diabetes in the West, accounting for 70% of deaths. The effect of diabetes is only seen in those predisposed to develop atherosclerosis. The increase in risk is marked in women who appear to lose the protection from sex hormones. Possible mechanisms include:

- type IV hyperplipidaemia (with ↓ HDL) is often seen in diabetes, with an increased IHD risk
- glycosylation of lysine residues of LDL, with a reduction in its catabolism
- glycosylation of fibrin, which is less susceptible to plasmin cleavage
- insulin resistance and high insulin levels appear to promote atherogenesis.

Systemic hypertension

An important risk factor for IHD where atherosclerotic clinical disease is common.

Hyperlipidaemia

- Athersclerotic lesions contain far more lipid (especially LDL,) than normal intima.
- Increased plasma LDL concentrations in animal models lead to increased formation of atherosclerotic lesions.
- Inherited hyperlipidaemias in man cause marked atherogenesis and an increase in IHD.
- High mean LDL levels are associated with an increased risk of IHD.
- The lipid profile is a result of genetic and environmental factors, diet being especially important. Raised plasma cholesterol is the most important modifiable risk factor.

ISCHAEMIC HEART DISEASE (IHD)

This description refers to a spectrum of clinico-pathological entities all resulting from atherosclerosis of the coronary arteries, with possible complication by thrombosis secondary to plaque injury:

- stable angina
- unstable angina
- variant (Prinzmetal's) angina
- syndromes associated with acute myocardial necrosis, or myocardial infarction (MI)
- sudden death
- chronic pump failure.

Epidemiology

- Commonest cause of death in the West, accounting for 140 000 deaths/year in the UK (27% of all deaths).
- It is a major drain on healthcare resources.

Risk factors

Most significant risk factors are related to lifestyle, but genetically determined factors are also involved (e.g. hyperlipidaemias, diabetes mellitus). For full details see under atherosclerosis.

Physiological factors influencing the expression of ischaemia

Energy requirements

By virtue of its constant contractile activity, cardiac muscle has high energy requirements. Contraction demands high energy phosphates. There are also considerable energy demands to maintain membrane integrity, and the concentration gradients of sodium, potassium and calcium.

Features of cardiac muscle:

- poor endogenous fuel reserves
- well vascularized
- aerobic metabolism.

Interruptions to blood supply are potentially catastrophic. At rest the heart extracts 80% of the oxygen in coronary blood; increased work demands an increase in blood flow. The heart is capable of using all fuels including glucose and fatty acids, the latter are oxidized preferentially – a feature of the glucose–fatty acid cycle.

Patterns of myocardial blood flow

Perfusion of the myocardium occurs in diastole; in systole the intramyocardial vessels are compressed by contraction. The flow depends on the difference between the pressure in the aortic root (above the closed aortic valve) and that in the left ventricular cavity. It is inversely related to the resistance of the vascular bed; in exercise the relaxing of small arteries and arterioles increases blood flow. Larger epicardial arteries in the **undiseased** state do not contribute to resistance. These larger arteries are regional, supplying an identifiable segment of myocardium. In humans and large animals sudden blockage of a major coronary artery branch results in necrosis of the segment supplied by that branch (functional end arteries).

General pathology of ischaemic myocardial injury

The time-related functional, biochemical and ultrastructural changes after coronary artery occlusion constitute a difficult area to study in humans; much of our knowledge has been derived from animal studies in dogs and pigs. The following have been observed:

- within minutes: cessation of contraction of ischaemic area
- coagulative necrosis over next 12 hours.

Necrosis may be inhibited if blood flow is re-established within 20–40 min.

Biochemical changes
- fall in oxygen tension
- loss of mitochondrial (aerobic) respiration
- anaerobic glycolysis of glycogen is sole source of energy; causing a rise in lactate which accumulates
- marked fall in intracellular ATP, to zero in 40–60 min

- creatine phosphate falls to zero within 15 min of ischaemia
- inhibition of myosin ATPase activity by H^+ ions leads to cessation of contraction.

The key to cell survival in ischaemia is **preservation of cell membrane integrity**. The generation of free radicals causes lipid peroxidation of unsaturated membrane lipids, which is highly damaging.

Generation of free radicals
- Superoxide anion is produced when electron carriers are highly reduced as in ischaemia.
- Release of endogenous catecholamines (a response to cardiogenic shock) causes oxidation of hypoxanthine and xanthine through xanthine peroxidase and produces superoxide and hydrogen peroxide.

If reperfusion occurs (spontaneously or as a result of therapeutic thrombolysis) the appearance of oxygen in hypoxic tissue with high concentrations of NADH and hypoxanthine causes much free radical generation with consequent membrane damage.

Structural changes occurring in ischaemic myocardium

Ultrastructural changes Mitochondrial and membrane damage is seen after 15–40 min. These changes are more severe upon reperfusion with swollen muscle cells, accumulation of hydrated calcium phosphate in mitochondria and sarcomere disturbance (shortened distance between Z bands). This latter change is thought to result from the myocyte being unable to relax because of the high concentration of intracellular calcium.

Light microscopic changes The first signs of damage appear at 4–8 h after occlusion, and the following sequence is seen:
- Appearance of neutrophils in the interstitium at 4 h.
- Appearance of macrophages in the ischaemic zone at around 4 days. Myocytes show coagulative necrosis (strong eosinophilic staining with loss of nuclei and cross-striations).
- Clearance of necrotic tissue by macrophages. Development of granulation tissue capillaries from

adjacent viable tissue for repair by scar formation at
4–5 days.
- Laying down of collagen fibres starts at day 9; repair
complete at 6 weeks.

THE SPECTRUM OF IHD IN HUMANS

Stable angina

Stable angina (reversible chest pain) is seen when increased
demands for oxygen cannot be met (e.g. exercise, cold,
sweating or emotion). It is predictable, occurring when
myocardial work exceeds a certain known level.

Coronary artery pathology in stable angina

The causative lesion is a fixed stenosis of the lumen of one
or more epicardial coronary arteries by more than 50%,
with a reduction of cross-sectional surface area of more than
75%. The reduction in flow is partly offset by a fall in the
vascular resistance beyond the obstruction.

Stenosis morphology: 76% of lesions are concentric, of
these more than 60% are fibrous plaques with small basal
lipid pools. The remaining 24% are eccentric, half with large
lipid pools, and half are fibrous. Some also may show plugs
of vascularized connective tissue, possibly representing
recanalization of occlusive thrombus.

Unstable angina

This is unpredictable chest pain, often at rest, varying in frequency, intensity and character. Over 3 months after onset,
4% of patients will die suddenly, 15% will undergo myocardial infarction, and the remainder will experience remission. Treatment with aspirin reduces these complications
suggesting thrombosis as a cause.

Stenosis morphology

Two patterns are seen:

- type I: smooth lumen outline
- type II: ragged lumen outline, overhanging edges.

Microscopic examination of type II lesions shows splitting and fissuring of the fibrous cap with thrombus deposition. At autopsy, platelet microthrombi are seen downstream of type II lesions.

Unstable angina with type I lesions is a result of localized muscle spasm; sometimes seen in lesion free coronary arteries-variant angina. It is regarded as an altered vasomotor response, possibly the result of:

- reduced production of nitric oxide (NO) – endothelium-derived relaxing factor (EDRF)
- reduced response to NO, possibly from the fibrous plaque acting as a barrier
- increased sensitivity of smooth muscle to vasoconstrictors
- adventitial inflammation affecting innervation
- neutralization of NO within the intima by plasma constituents, e.g. haemoglobin.

Acute myocardial necrosis (myocardial infarction)

Patterns of acute necrosis

Regional transmural infarction Large areas of coagulative necrosis confined to the territory of one major coronary artery branch.

Transmural: Extends from endocardial to epicardial surface (with sparing of the immediate myocardium beneath the ventricular surface). Total artery occlusion is seen within 1 h of onset of symptoms (pain and ECG changes). In 30% cases flow is restored from thrombolysis, leaving a type II lesion. A subsequent autopsy may not show the causal arterial pathology. Occlusive thrombus is largely associated with plaque fissuring.

Sub-endocardial: Less than 50% of the ventricular wall, involving the inner half. This is often seen at the margins of transmural infarcts. Pathogenesis is unclear, with a lower frequency of occlusive thrombus, and a possible greater degree of collateral flow.

Non-regional infarction Involves the whole circumference of the left ventricle, usually sub-endocardial. Seen with widespread coronary artery stenosis. At autopsy no occlusive thrombus is found in 15% of cases. It is caused by a global reduction in myocardial perfusion, brought about by a fall in perfusion pressure (fall in aortic root pressure or a rise in intraventricular diastolic pressure) or a shortened diastolic interval. Sub-endocardial muscle is affected.

Clinical situations:

- cardiogenic shock
- severe aortic valve disease
- end stage dilated cardiomyopathy
- grossly thickened ventricular wall.

The fall in cardiac output in a large regional infarct may compromise aortic root pressure and bring about superimposed diffuse sub-endocardial necrosis, thus setting up a vicious cycle with further fall in cardiac output.

Right ventricular infarction

Most cases of MI solely affect the left ventricle. Isolated right ventricular infarction is excessively rare, seen usually in marked right ventricular hypertrophy. Occlusion of the proximal right coronary artery can result in posterior left ventricular infarction with extension involving the right ventricle.

Complications of acute transmural infarction

Myocardial rupture

External cardiac rupture: third commonest cause of death after transmural infarction, often in older women. At autopsy may be confused with haemopericardium as a result of resuscitation. Typically seen as a tense bulging pericardium containing 300–500 ml blood.

Rupture through the interventricular septum: Complication of antero- and posteroseptal infarcts causes an additional haemodynamic burden on the heart, carrying a high mortality rate.

Rupture of papillary muscle: Ischaemic damage is common, and can lead to sudden catastrophic mitral valve incompetence.

Intraventricular thrombosis   After MI there is frequently an akinetic segment of myocardium, with overlying stasis of blood and resultant intraventricular thrombi, and possible systemic embolization.

Extension and expansion in myocardial infarcts Extension is seen with further episodes of ischaemia. Clinically there are further ECG changes and/or decreasing left ventricular function. Expansion is the stretching of the infarcted area with an increase in area but no new necrosis; it may result in a tear in the overlying endocardium.

Ventricular aneurysm formation A convex dilatation of the left ventricle with collagen making up the wall, as a result of full thickness infarction. There may be associated ventricular arrhythmias, cardiac failure mural thrombosis and systemic embolization. The fibrous tissue can undergo dystrophic calcification.

Sudden death Death occurring within 6 h in a previously symptom-free individual. IHD accounts for 60% of these fatalities. Half of these patients have no history of IHD.

Pathophysiology: Most deaths are due to fatal ventricular arrhythmias.

DISORDERS OF THE HEART VALVES

The heart valves are liable to damage from a number of differing disease process:

- acute rheumatic fever and chronic rheumatic valve disease
- non-rheumatic valve disease (aortic stenosis, aortic incompetence, mitral valve disease, pulmonary valve disease)
- infective endocarditis
- non-bacterial thrombotic endocarditis (NBTE).

ACUTE RHEUMATIC FEVER

A non-suppurative inflammatory disorder from an immune-mediated reaction to cell wall components of β-haemolytic streptococci. Many tissues are affected in the acute phase, but the heart valves are targeted in chronic disease.

The acute form is a disease of childhood, most commonly from 5–8 years, seen up to 20 years. There is a close association between acute rheumatic fever and subsequent chronic valve disease. The incidence of both have greatly declined in the West as a result of:

- improved socio-economic circumstances
- antibiotic treatment of streptococcal throat infections
- decreased incidence of such infections.

The disease is still common in the Third World.

Clinical features

A self-limiting sore throat caused by β-haemolytic streptococcus (Lancefield group A), followed by a combination of the following major and minor features (diagnosis depends on two major features or one major and two minor features):

Major: pancarditis, 'flitting' polyarthritis, chorea, subcutaneous nodules, erythema

Minor: fever, prolonged PR interval on ECG, elevated ESR.

Death from cardiac failure in the acute phase is occasionally seen. Subsequent episodes of streptococcal sore throat are associated with a high risk of recurrence and development of chronic valve disease.

Pathogenesis

The immune reaction to streptococcal antigens is idiosyncratic, seen in 3% patients with a streptococcal sore throat. The antibodies produced are directed against streptococcal cell wall components (fibrillary M protein), and cross-react with the following target tissues:

- heart muscle (sarcolemma and sub-sarcolemmal cytoplasm)
- heart valve connective tissue
- thymic cells
- human glomerular basement membrane
- neuronal cytoplasm in sub-thalamic and caudate nuclei in the brain
- skin
- lymphocytes.

These antibodies directed against self-antigens suggest that T-cell tolerance has been overcome, and indeed the tissue damage may be mediated by T cells, the antibodies reflecting an epiphenomenon.

Pathological features

The disease is characterized by a pancarditis.

Pericardial changes Fibrin-rich inflammatory exudate ('bread and butter heart'). The pericarditis completely resolves in most cases, with no scarring and no constriction of the heart.

Myocardial changes Where death occurs in the acute phase (1% cases), the heart is dilated with a flabby appearance. Two histological patterns are seen:

- A non-specific myocarditis (oedema, inflammatory cells and rarely a small-vessel arteritis).
- A specific granulomatous myocarditis present throughout the heart but most commonly in the interventricular septum: Aschoff nodules, composed of Aschoff giant cells (multi-nucleated macrophages), Anitschkow myocytes – cells with a characteristic bar of chromatin and 'owl's eye nucleus' (also macrophage in origin) – and lymphocytes, mostly T helper cells. With time the Aschoff nodule regresses to a small scar.

Endocardial changes

- Acute phase changes: thickening of valves from oedema, and a row of small, flat vegetations, 1–2 mm in size, composed of platelet-rich microthrombi, along the lines of closure. They arise from contact-related trauma and are not associated with embolism (unlike infective endocarditis).
- Neovascularization is then seen associated with fibroblast proliferation and laying down of collagen (as in wound healing).
- Subsequent fibrosis can be slight with little effect on valve function, or contraction and stiffening of cusps causing incompetence, and/or fusion of commissures causing stenosis.
- The mitral and then the aortic valve are most commonly affected.

- The chordae tendineae are also commonly affected contributing further to mitral valve incompetence.

....

CHRONIC RHEUMATIC VALVE DISEASE

All valves affected by:

- commissural fusion
- cusp scarring
- dystrophic calcification.

These changes are seen in any post-inflammatory valve disorder, and are not specific for rheumatic fever.

Mitral stenosis

Commoner in females (F:M 1:5–4:1). Largely caused by fusion of commissures, decreasing size of valve opening; increased cusp stiffness and chordal fusion are also factors. The commissural fusion is treatable by splitting the fused commissures, restoring normal function. Commissural fusion is also seen as a congenital cause of mitral stenosis.

Effects on the left atrium

The size varies from normal to gross dilatation, (when there almost always is thrombus formation). Thrombus develops in the left atrial appendage, often protruding into the atrial cavity and gives rise to systemic embolization. Thrombus is seen in up to 30% of cases. A sheet of thrombus covering the entire wall can form, which can calcify to be seen on X-ray. Rarely a spherical mass of thrombus forms, attached to the septum, and this can block the orifice in a ball valve fashion.

Pathophysiological effects

Significant mitral valve stenosis causes pulmonary venous hypertension, raised pulmonary wedge capillary pressure and pulmonary arterial hypertension. There is an increase in the right ventricle workload, with lipid deposition in the artery walls.

Morphological changes
- solid brown lungs with numerous haemosiderin-laden macrophages (recurrent bleeding from alveolar capillaries)
- fatty streaks and atheromatous plaques in pulmonary vessels
- right ventricular hypertrophy (from pressure overload).

Mitral incompetence

Pure MI is rarely seen in chronic rheumatic disease, but is often seen in association with stenosis. The incompetence is caused by cusp retraction from scarring, and thickening of the chordae tendineae. The incompetence causes left ventricular dilatation and hypertrophy from volume overload together with atrial enlargement.

Aortic valve changes in chronic rheumatic heart disease

Chronic rheumatic heart disease typically causes both stenosis and incompetence resulting from commissural fusion. Cusp scarring in the absence of fusion causes pure incompetence.

....

NON-RHEUMATIC VALVE DISEASE

Aortic valve

Normal anatomy and function

Three half moon-shaped cusps of equal size. These overlap in diastole, and the line of closure is below the free edge. The cusp area between the line of closure and the free edge is termed the 'lunula', which can become fenestrated in later life, without functional significance. Effective function requires overlapping and contact, so the cusp area must be greater than the aortic root (normal ratio 1.6:1). A decrease results in functional incompetence with regurgitation of blood back from the root area into the left ventricle in diastole. In systole the cusps fold into the aortic sinuses with no pressure gradient between the left ventricular cavity and the aortic root.

Age-related changes

Fibrous thickening occurs along the line of closure, and calcified nodules appear at the mid-point of each cusp (corpora Arantii), of no functional significance. Calcification develops with age, causing stenosis in the elderly. This results in rigid crescent-shaped masses of calcium, fixing the cusps in a semi-closed position. Abnormal closure patterns results in premature calcification.

Aortic stenosis (AS)

True congenital AS Failure of separation of valve cusps resulting in dome-shaped membrane with small central orifice. Five per cent of cases of congenital heart disease in UK result from AS. Requires early surgical intervention.

Bicuspid aortic valve Commonest single cause of AS in middle life (1–2% population); a small proportion of cases undergo sufficient calcification to cause stenosis. Clinically there is a short ejection systolic murmur. The valve shows a linear slit-like orifice.

The left ventricle shows a marked degree of concentric hypertrophy, typical of high pressure overload. There is a high risk of sudden death, related to arrhythmias. The high pressure gradient between the left ventricular cavity and the aortic root reduces myocardial perfusion, compromising sub-endocardial blood flow in the left ventricular wall. Furthermore 30–50% patients awaiting surgery also have coronary artery disease.

Aortic incompetence

Arises from a mismatch between the valve ring circumference and the cusp area.

Changes in cusp area
- Shrinkage/retraction of cusps: rheumatic disease, rheumatoid disease, ankylosing spondylitis.
- Perforation: infective endocarditis.

Changes in valve ring
- Inflammatory causes: autoimmune (HLAB27 associated) causes – rheumatoid disease, ankylosing spondylitis, non-specific urethritis, non-specific aortitis, syphilis.

There is destruction of elastic fibres and smooth muscle with a lymphoplasmacytic infiltrate. The intima is frequently irregular ('cobble-stoned') from medial scarring. The adventitia is often thickened.

- Non-inflammatory causes: aortic dissection (Marfan/ non-Marfan familial); idiopathic root dilatation.

Loss of both the elastic lamina, and smooth muscle, sometimes with mucin accumulation but no significant inflammation.

The valve ring circumference should be no more than 10.5 cm; beyond 12.5 cm there will be significant regurgitation. There may be secondary changes in the aortic cusps with widening of the commissures, and thickened rolled edges (especially seen in syphilis).

....

MITRAL VALVE DISEASE

Mitral valve incompetence

Normal function requires:

- **Active muscular narrowing of valve ring** Dystrophic calcification (commoner in women, diabetes and Paget's disease of bone) can splint the valve ring causing incompetence.
- **Normal mobility of valve leaflets** Restriction of movement from rheumatic post-inflammatory scarring (retraction of cusps and shortening or fusion of chordae tendineae) causing incompetence. Excessive cusp mobility, typically seen with 'floppy mitral valves' causes prolapse into the left atrium with incompetence. The increase in size is a result of accumulation of mucopolysaccharide within the valve matrix. It is associated with disruption of collagen fibres, either from breakdown or a failure of synthesis. Floppy mitral valves are subject to sub-endocardial injury with thrombus formation, emboli and infective endocarditis.
- **Normal area of leaflets** See under floppy mitral valve above.

- **Support from chordae tendineae**   Chordal rupture for whatever reason will lead to catastrophic regurgitation.
- **Contraction by papillary muscles**   Post-ischaemic scarring is a common cause of varying degrees of incompetence. Acute rupture with myocardial infarction is a rare cause of catastrophic incompetence.
- **Normal ventricular function and shape**   If the left ventricle is dilated there may be dilatation of the valve ring and disturbance of the 'line of pull' of the muscles causing incompetence.

··

PULMONARY VALVE DISEASE

- Rarely involved in chronic rheumatic disease.
- In carcinoid syndrome (50% cases) there is fibrosis of the ventricular aspect of the pulmonary valve cusps, giving a diffuse or plaque-like thickening. This results in stenosis and/or incompetence.

··

INFECTIVE ENDOCARDITIS

An inflammatory disorder of the endocardial surface of the heart from infection by a wide range of micro-organisms. It is characterized by masses of thrombus – vegetations – which contain the micro-organisms. In the past, two organisms were held responsible for most cases:

- *Staph. aureus:*   acute endocarditis
- *Strep. viridans:*   sub-acute endocarditis.

It is now recognized that many other organisms cause infective endocarditis and there is a wide clinical spectrum. Increasingly seen in older patients, fewer with pre-existing acquired valve disease, with more cases of staphylococcal infections, often associated with intravenous drug abuse.

Acute endocarditis

Acute onset, occurring without pre-existing cardiac haemodynamic abnormalities. Before antibiotics it followed a short course and was invariably fatal, with severe valve incompetence. Complicated by pyaemic abscesses from emboli.

Sub-acute endocarditis

Slow insidious onset, associated with haemodynamic abnormality, e.g. post-rheumatic heart disease, ventricular septal defect, prosthetic valves.

Pathogenesis

Haemodynamic injury   High-pressure jets/turbulent blood flow which damage endocardium.

Seen with congenital and acquired valve disease, as in mitral valve prolapse, congenital bicuspid valve, post-rheumatic valve disease, prosthetic valves. Also congenital valve defects, e.g. Tetralogy of Fallot, patent ductus arteriosus, coarctation.

The greater the virulence of the organism the greater the likelihood of endocarditis developing in the absence of a haemodynamic disturbance.

Bacteraemia
- 40–50% cases: α-haemolytic *Streptococcus viridans*
- 10–20% cases: Lancefield group D *Streptococci*
- 15–25% cases: *Staphylococci*, including *Staph. aureus*, and the less virulent *Staph. epidermidis* (especially prosthetic heart valves)
- Gram-negative organisms: frequently encountered in intravenous drug abuse. The tricuspid valve is a frequent target
- fungal infections (usually *Candida albicans*) typically seen in intravenous drug users, prosthetic heart valves, immunosuppressed patients.

Access to the bloodstream occurs with any minor invasive procedure, including dental work, cystoscopy, prostatectomy and gastrointestinal tract biopsy. Also important are *Staph.* infections of the skin, lungs or wounds. Colonization of the valve depends on the adhesive properties of the organism, with ligands for matrix proteins (e.g. fibronectin) and platelet receptor sites.

Cardiac lesions in infective endocarditis

Vegetations

The characteristic lesion is the vegetation, masses of thrombus adherent to the endocardial surface of the valve. Microscopically the luminal surface consists of platelets and fibrin with masses of organisms beneath. Adjacent to the valve is an inflammatory reaction with an associated granulation tissue response.

The vegetations can extend upwards to involve the posterior wall of the left atrium, into the interventricular septum, and into tissue adjacent to the valve causing deep paravalvular abscesses (making valve replacement particularly hazardous).

Release of proteolytic enzymes from neutrophils can cause destruction of valve tissue, causing perforations or chordal rupture.

Embolization, especially from the aortic valve, can cause myocardial abscesses and necrosis.

Complications

Embolic Embolization is common, potentially causing metastatic abscesses. Most lesions are bland. Cerebral infarcts are an important cause of death in infective endocarditis (20% cases); renal emboli are commoner with fewer consequences (50% cases).

Mycotic aneurysms are seen when the organisms invade the wall of the vessel in which the embolism is lodged, causing an inflammatory reaction, and weakening the wall (often seen in intracranial vessels).

Cardiac failure Rapidly developing volume overload, due to onset of valve regurgitation or worsening of pre-existing incompetence. Caused by valve cusp perforation or ulceration of the edge, or mitral valve chordal rupture.

Immune complex-mediated complications Any prolonged bacteraemia (as is seen in infective endocarditis) is associated with circulating immune complexes. Target organs:

Skin: purpuric haemorrhage from vasculitis.
Joints: arthralgia from localization of the complexes within the joints.

Kidneys: a focal mesangio-proliferative glomerulo-nephritis giving rise to 'nephritic' syndrome. Renal failure is a serious complication accounting for 25% of deaths from infective endocarditis.

NON-BACTERIAL THROMBOTIC ENDOCARDITIS (NBTE)

Small non-infected thrombotic vegetations found along the lines of the closure of the affected valve. By convention the vegetations seen in systemic lupus erythematosus and acute rheumatic fever are considered separately.

NBTE vegetations are seen in up to 10% of autopsy cases, and are composed of fibrin and platelets with no damage to the underlying valve. They are often seen in malignant disease (mucinous adenocarcinomas) and 50% of patients are hypercoaguable. Embolic complications are sometimes seen.

DISORDERS OF HEART MUSCLE: THE CARDIOMYOPATHIES

Cardiomyopathies are functional or structural abnormalities of the myocardium. They are *not* a result of volume or pressure overload from any cause (e.g. valve disease, congenital shunts, systemic or pulmonary hypertension, ischaemic heart disease).

They account for a significant proportion of heart disease especially in the Third World.

Classification

Aetiology and pathogenesis are poorly understood so rational classification is difficult (see Table 32.1). The WHO has moreover decreed that once the cause is known it is termed a 'specific muscle disorder'. Most cardiologists still follow the above definition with appropriate descriptive qualification, e.g. 'alcoholic-dilated cardiomyopathy'.

Table 32.1 Classification of cardiomyopathies

Type	Functional abnormality	Morphological abnormality
Dilated form	Loss of systolic contractile force with increased end-systolic volume, and an eventual increase in end-diastolic volume	Dilated thin-walled left ventricle with a large capacity
Restrictive form	Impaired diastolic relaxation, sometimes as a result of partial obliteration of left ventricular cavity	Various patterns

HYPERTROPHIC CARDIOMYOPATHY

Functional abnormality Decreased diastolic compliance, with enhanced abnormal early systolic contraction and impaired diastolic relaxation. There may be normal or increased contractility of the ventricle and a possible increased systolic ejection fraction.

Morphological abnormality Increased wall thickness (symmetric or asymmetric), with a disproportionate increase in thickness of the septum and a small cavity.

Defining features
- left ventricular hypertrophy
- no dilatation of left ventricular cavity.

The ratio of septal thickness to the free wall may be greater than 2:1 and the cut surface shows a whorled appearance rather like a uterine leiomyoma. The upper septum may bulge just below the aortic valve striking the anterior leaflet of the mitral valve thickening the endocardium to give a white patch.

Microscopically there is disarray of muscle fibres within cells (disorganization of myofibrils) and changes in tissue architecture giving whorling around a central focus of collagen. The extent of these changes varies from case to case, but are likely to account for at least 30% of the volume of the myocardium examined. As the hypertrophy increases there is scarring with focal myocyte loss and interstitial fibrosis.

Clinical presentation

Sudden death, syncope associated with exercise, anginal type chest pain, dyspnoea.

Outflow obstruction may appear to be present, but is more likely to reflect the high pressures late in systole when most of the blood has been ejected. Some patients also present with congestive cardiac failure.

Echocardiographic screening of families reveals more cases. The risk of death is greatest in adolescence.

Genetic abnormalities

Autosomal dominant with incomplete penetrance (15–35%). Although not sex-linked males are affected twice as commonly.

In 50% cases there is a change in the heavy chain of β cardiac myosin. More than 30 different point mutations have been described; those causing the greatest change in net molecular charge cause the greatest functional disturbance and hence symptomatic disease. Linkage studies have identified four other genes on different chromosomes all coding for proteins related to myofibrillary structure. Abnormalities of myosin-binding protein have also been found. The end result of these molecular abnormalities is the formation of abnormal contractile filaments disturbing the normal spatial arrangement. The heavy chain of β myosin is transcribed in lymphocytes thus providing a method of screening relatives.

....

DILATED CARDIOMYOPATHY

This is characterized by a decline in the ability of the ventricular myocardium to contract in systole and was formerly termed congestive cardiomyopathy (COCM). The left ventricular ejection fraction falls (< 0.4) so end-systolic and end-diastolic volumes both increase, causing gross ventricular dilatation.

Clinical features   Progressive cardiac failure, often rapidly progressive. Sudden death from ventricular arrhythmias is seen and there is often mural thrombus with embolic disease.

Morphological features Enlargement of the heart both in weight and volume (630 g in men and 550 g in women). Ventricular wall thickness may be normal. The myocardium is flabby and pale.

Microscopically the myocytes are hypertrophied with large hyperchromatic nuclei, showing square ends. Perinuclear vacuoles are seen containing glycogen or lipid. There may be loss of myofibrils and associated invasion by macrophages. Interstitial fibrosis is present sometimes with large areas of scarring. Focal collections of lymphocytes and macrophages can be seen resembling features of myocarditis. Similar changes with myocardial necrosis can result from viral infection, catecholamine-mediated damage and also cytotoxic chemotherapy e.g. anthracyclines.

Aetiology Dilated cardiomyopathy is best regarded as a common response to a wide range of insults rather than as a single disease. Table 32.2 lists its known associations.
In most cases the cause is unknown. Some of these cases may represent endstage viral myocarditis.

....

RESTRICTIVE CARDIOMYOPATHY

The least common cardiomyopathy, caused by a decrease in the ability of the myocardium to relax in diastole. Diastolic

Table 32.2 Known associations of dilated cardiomyopathy

Infective disorders	Bacterial, viral, protozoal
Familial neurological, neuromuscular or muscle disorders	Friedreich's ataxia, abetalipoproteinaemia, Duchenne's muscular dystrophy, mitochondrial myopathy
Inborn errors of metabolism	Wilson's disease, haemochromatosis, carnitine deficiency
Nutritional and metabolic disorders	Thiamine deficiency, protein malnutrition, diabetes mellitus, selenium deficiency
Autoimmune disease	Dermatomyositis, progressive systemic sclerosis, SLE
Cardiotoxic drugs and chemicals	Alcohol, cobalt, cocaine, anthracyclines, lead, lithium, mercury

filling is impeded with a rise in systolic pressure filling. Systolic function is normal and there is no significant hypertrophy (cf. HOCM). There may a reduction in the ventricular volume from mural thrombi or gross thickening of endocardium (endomyocardial fibrosis) – restrictive-obliterative cardiomyopathy.

The ventricular wall is stiffened, possibly from:

- generalized scarring
- infiltration of the myocardium (e.g. amyloid)
- scarring of the superficial myocardium or endocardium (splinting of ventricular wall).

Types of restrictive cardiomyopathy

Endomyocardial fibrosis

Commonest form worldwide, principally in the tropics but also elsewhere. It is associated with eosinophilia and affects young adults. The eosinophilia may be associated with leukaemias, polycythaemia rubra vera and parasitic infections. Patients present with CCF, mitral incompetence and pulmonary hypertension (left ventricle affected) or enlarged pulsatile liver, ascites and bilateral proptosis (right ventricle predominantly affected).

Macroscopic changes   Gross endomyocardial scarring with thick white fibrous tissue around the inflow tracts, immobilizing the posterior leaflet of the mitral valve to cause mitral incompetence. In the right ventricle the apex can be obliterated by the fibrosis.

Microscopic changes   Cellular hyaline fibrous tissue, with organizing fibrin on the luminal surface.

Amyloidosis

Restrictive cardiomyopathy from cardiac amyloid is most often seen with amyloid of immune origin (intact light chain or amino-terminal end of light chain). It is also seen in the inherited amyloidosis syndromes.

Macroscopic changes   Extreme thickening of ventricle wall, with sharp-cut edge of stiffened myocardium. The heart is pale brown.

Microscopic changes   Congo red positive hyaline deposits.

Excess iron storage

Seen with hereditary haemochromatosis, multiple blood tranfusions, thalassaemia and sickle cell disease.

Macroscopic changes Dilated heart, thickened myocardium with rusty red brown colour. Positive Perl's reaction.

Endocardial fibroelastosis (EFE)

Plaque-like thickening of ventricular endocardium associated with elastic fibres running tangentially to the surface.

Primary EFE Disease of infancy seen from 2 to 12 months with onset of CCF, 40% of cases showing features of mitral regurgitation (and tricuspid regurgitation if the right ventricle is involved).

Macroscopic features Dilatation of left ventricle, with thickened white endocardium, obliterating the papillary muscles.

Secondary EFE Endocardial thickening seen in association with cardiac malformations with obstruction to the left ventricular outflow tract, e.g. aortic stenosis, coarctation.

Miscellaneous associations with restrictive cardiomyopathy

- sarcoidosis
- inborn errors of metabolism, including storage diseases.

....

MYOCARDITIS

Heart muscle disorders where myocardial damage is associated with a significant inflammatory cell infiltrate.

Morphological classification

- acute non-specific myocarditis
- granulomatous myocarditis (TB, fungal, rheumatic, syphilitic, sarcoid, giant cell-idiopathic).

Pathogenetic mechanisms

Note that in many cases these are unknown.

- post-infectious
- drug related

- immune-mediated
- miscellaneous (according to histological appearances).

....

PERICARDIUM

A sac composed of two layers of thin fibrous connective tissue lined on the inside by mesothelial cells.

Pericardial effusions

An accumulation of fluid within the pericardial cavity resulting in acute or chronic tamponade.

- *Acute tamponade:* Typically seen in haemopericardium after rupture of either the myocardium (after full thickness myocardial infarction) or the intrapericardial portion of the aorta (after aortic dissection), where the sac is filled with blood. With rapid accumulation of fluid, the parietal pericardium cannot stretch and pressure rises within the sac preventing filling of the heart itself with just 200–400 ml blood. Cardiac output declines rapidly with death.
- *Chronic effusion:* A slow accumulation of fluid allows the pericardium to stretch to accommodate 1 litre fluid. This is seen in CCF, metastatic tumour and myxoedema. Symptoms of tamponade eventually appear with cardiac failure, pulsus paradoxus and muffled heart sounds.

Acute inflammation (pericarditis)

Characterized by fibrinous, serofibrinous, purulent or haemorrhagic inflammatory exudates.

- *Viral:* seen as an effusion, resolving in 1–2 weeks, caused by Coxsackie B, echoviruses, influenza, mumps and EBV.
- *Bacterial:* seen as a complication of septicaemia, pyemia, pneumonia, lung abscess, empyema and ulcerating tumours of bronchus and oesophagus. The causative organisms are usually pyogenic, e.g. *Staphylococcus aureus, Haemophilus influenzae* and streptococci.
- *Tuberculous:* arises by direct spread from a caseous node or by blood. The exudate is initially fibrinous or haemorrhagic and becomes chronic with scarring,

adhesion formation and a resultant constrictive pericarditis.

- *Non-infective causes:*

  — acute rheumatic fever
  — myocardial infarction
  — connective tissue disorders, including SLE and rheumatoid disease
  — uraemia
  — post-renal transplantation
  — post irradiation
  — post-cardiac trauma.

Chronic inflammation

Progressive scarring that obliterates the pericardial cavity, encasing the heart in thick fibrous tissue often with calcification, restricting atrial and ventricular filling. Tuberculosis is a common cause where there is a high prevalence of the disease. Patients present with features of congestive cardiac failure, with a raised JVP, ascites and hepatomegaly.

CONGENITAL CARDIAC DEFECTS

Defined as structural or functional disorders of the heart or great vessels, present at birth (see Table 32.3). Without treatment 60% cases would die in infancy, 25% in the neonatal period, and 15% would survive into early adulthood.

....

MAJOR FUNCTIONAL DISTURBANCES

Eighty per cent of cases are associated with abnormal communications between the right and left sides of the heart, with abnormal flows.

Left-to-right shunts

These cause volume overload of the right atrium, right ventricle and pulmonary vascular bed, initially with no pressure overload and no cyanosis. With time there is pulmonary intimal hyperplasia of small vessels causing

Table 32.3 Incidence of congenital cardiac defects

Frequency of defects	(%)
Ventricular septal defects (VSD)	32.5
Patent ductal arteriosus (PDA)	11.9
Pulmonary stenosis	7
Aortic coarctation	6.3
Fallot's tetralogy	5.9
Atrial septal defect	5.9
Aortic stenosis	5.1
Transposition of the great vessels	5
Hypoplastic left heart	2.8
Ebstein's anomaly	2.5
Atrioventricular septal defect	2.4
Double inlet atrioventricular connection	1.7
Persistent truncus arteriosus	1.1
Total anomalous pulmonary venous return	0.8

Classified according to:
- functional disturbance
- embryological developmental abnormality
- morphological abnormality.

irreversible pulmonary hypertension, with eventual reversal of flow, shunting deoxygenated blood into the left side of the heart (Eisenmenger's syndrome).

Ventricular septal defect

Commonest defect, after bicuspid aortic valve, (1 in 500 live births), and 60% cases are associated with other abnormalities e.g. Fallot's tetralogy. Most VSDs are peri-membranous. The pathophysiological effects depend on the defect size: small defects (< 0.5 mm) cause a high pressure, low volume shunt with an increased risk of infective endocarditis. With growth the defect becomes relatively smaller and may even close. A large VSD gives rise to a large volume overload, with raised pulmonary artery pressure, right ventricular hypertrophy and eventual flow reversal causing central cyanosis. Very large defects can cause serious heart failure early in life.

Patent ductus arteriosus

This is a normal channel passing from the pulmonary artery to the aorta in fetal life, allowing blood to bypass the unexpanded inactive lungs. After birth, with lung expansion, the pulmonary pressure falls and flow ceases in 1–2 days caused by spasm of the media. Failure of closure is poorly understood, but is mediated through decreased levels of prostaglandin E2, and can be related to the use of cyclo-oxygenase inhibitors such as indomethacin. The effects depend on the size of the patent ductus: a small defect results in a small flow throughout the entire cycle because of the constant pressure gradient between aorta and pulmonary artery (machinery murmur), a large defect causes a marked rise in pulmonary circulation with shunt reversal.

Atrial septal defect

Accounts for 30% of congenital heart defects in adult life. Most cases are a result of failure of the foramen ovale (a physiological valve allowing oxygenated blood to pass from the right atrium to the left in utero) to close after birth. Three patterns are described:

Ostium secundum defects   The commonest ASD, arising where there is mid-septal defect in the flap valve structure. Associated mitral valve prolapse is seen in 20–30% cases. Small defects are well tolerated; those in excess of 2 cm diameter cause left-to-right shunting and volume overload. ASD and acquired mitral stenosis (from rheumatic fever) precipitates pulmonary hypertension (Lutembacher syndrome).

Ostium primum defects   Accounts for 5% of cases of ASD, more correctly described as a defect in tissue bridging the two atria in the anterior leaflet of the mitral valve. There is associated mitral incompetence giving rise to a poorer prognosis than secundum defects.

Sinus venosus defects   These are rare.

Right-to-left shunts (with central cyanosis)

These are sub-divided into causes with diminished pulmonary blood flow, and normal or increased blood flow.

Diminished blood flow

Tetralogy of Fallot
- pulmonary stenosis (valve and/or infundibulum) to cause obstruction of the right ventricular outflow
- large high VSD beneath the aortic valve

- overriding aorta across the VSD
- right ventricular hypertrophy.

The functional abnormality is determined by the degree of narrowing of the pulmonary outflow, with a corresponding increase in right ventricular blood entering the aorta, causing a greater degree of cyanosis.

Clinical features   At birth there is often no cyanosis, which gradually develops as the child grows, together with poor exercise tolerance and failure to thrive. At around 4–6 months hypoxic episodes appear, related to spasm of the pulmonary outflow, preventing blood from the right ventricle entering the lungs. There can be deep cyanosis, breathlessness and loss of consciousness. These features can be reduced by the child squatting which helps to maintain blood flow through the lungs. There is also polycythaemia, clubbing and a right parasternal heave. Complications include cerebral thrombosis, cerebral abscess and infective endocarditis.

Pulmonary atresia with VSD   There is complete obstruction of blood flow from the right ventricle into the pulmonary artery from pulmonary atresia, together with a high VSD. Blood reaches the pulmonary circulation via the ductus or collateral vessels arising from the aorta, with early onset of cyanosis.

Cyanosis with increased pulmonary blood flow

Transposition of the great vessels   The second commonest cause of cyanosis, this describes the aorta arising from the right ventricle and the pulmonary artery from the left ventricle. The two circulations remain separate, with mixing taking place while the ductus remains open. With closure there is severe acidosis and cyanosis. Immediate management is to induce a defect in the atrial septum with a balloon, with follow-up definitive surgery at a later date. There can also be an associated VSD.

Common mixing of blood in the heart and great vessels

Persistent truncus arteriosus   A rare defect arising from failure of the truncus to divide into the aorta and the pulmonary artery, with an associated VSD. There is considerable overload of the pulmonary circulation which worsens as the pulmonary vascular resistance drops after birth.

Outflow obstruction without cyanosis

Coarctation of the aorta A stricture in the aorta at the point of insertion of the ductus arteriosus. It is a relatively common disorder, accounting for 6% congenital cardiac anomalies (M:F 3:1), and in women there is an association with Turner's syndrome. Coarctation is associated with bicuspid aortic valve, aortic stenosis, ASD, VSD, mitral valve anomalies and berry aneurysms of the circle of Willis. Pre-ductal narrowing is usually more severe, sometimes requiring surgery shortly after birth. Post-ductal narrowing may remain asymptomatic until adolescence.

CARDIAC FAILURE

Failure of the heart, despite normal venous pressure, to maintain output adequate to meet the body's needs. The clinical picture depends on which ventricle is predominantly failing.

....

RIGHT-SIDED FAILURE

Commonly results from:

- left-sided failure
- chronic lung disease (cor pulmonale)
- tricuspid/pulmonary valve disease
- left-to-right shunts (e.g. ventricular septal defects)
- mitral valve disease with secondary pulmonary hypertension
- isolated right-sided cardiomyopathy (rare)
- pulmonary embolism.

Clinical features Raised systemic venous pressure and distension characterized by:

- raised jugular venous pressure
- enlarged tender liver (nutmeg change)
- pleural transudates and ascites.

LEFT-SIDED FAILURE

Commonly caused by:

* ischaemic heart disease
* inadequately treated systemic hypertension
* aortic stenosis and incompetence
* mitral incompetence
* cardiomyopathies.

Clinical features Pulmonary vascular congestion from a raised left atrial pressure, transmitted back to the pulmonary capillaries. This causes intra-alveolar oedema with symptoms of fatigue, shortness of breath on exertion and at rest and paroxysmal nocturnal dyspnoea.

Mechanisms
* heart muscle dysfunction
* outflow obstruction
* volume overload
* obligatory high output e.g. severe anaemia, thyrotoxicosis, beri-beri, left-to-right shunts, Paget's disease of the bone
* restriction of ventricular filling, e.g. constrictive pericarditis, pericardial effusions, restrictive cardiomyopathy
* disturbances of rhythm.

ACUTE FAILURE

Seen in sudden onset of serious arrhythmias, severe myocardial infarction, pulmonary embolism, mechanical dysfunction (papillary muscle rupture, perforation of valve leaflet).

Pathophysiology: compensatory mechanisms

Ventricular dilatation

Decreased systolic ejection fraction results in an increase in blood in the ventricle after systole, causing a rise in end-diastolic volume. The resultant increased stretching of heart fibres causes increased contractility (Starling's law) to restore stroke volume. This effect flattens off with progressive failure and the stroke volume falls off significantly.

Neurohumoral activation

Sympathetic nervous system activation increases heart rate and contractility. Peripheral vein constriction is seen, increasing venous return to the heart and hence cardiac output; concomitant arteriolar constriction increases ventricular workload.

Renin-angiotensin system   The decreased cardiac output and arteriolar constriction reduces renal perfusion. The renin-angiotensin system is activated causing salt and water retention. The resultant increase in plasma volume initially maintains stroke volume (Starling's law) but progressive failure leads to pulmonary and systemic oedema.

Atrial natriuretic peptides (ANP)   The sodium retention from renal underperfusion causes release of ANP (short-chained peptides) which cause vasodilatation and loss of urinary sodium. ANP levels rise in cardiac failure to reduce the effects of pre-load and after-load.

SHOCK

This may be defined as systemic underperfusion of tissues because of prolonged and severe hypotension. The pathogenetic mechanisms are:

- hypovolaemic shock
- cardiogenic shock
- redistributive shock.

Morphological features of shock

There is evidence of ischaemia from underperfusion, and changes of disseminated intravascular coagulation (microthrombi and haemorrhage). Any tissue can be affected; organs most commonly damaged are lungs, heart, kidneys, liver, pancreas, gut, brain, pituitary and adrenals.

....

HYPOVOLAEMIC SHOCK

Characterized by a significant decrease in fluid volume, it is seen with severe haemorrhage, and excessive fluid loss as in diarrhoea, vomiting or extensive burns to the skin. To compensate the heart rate rises and there is marked peripheral vasoconstriction mediated by catecholamines, vasopressin and the angiotensin system.

CARDIOGENIC SHOCK

There is failure of the myocardial pump and this is commonly seen with acute myocardial infarction. Where there is loss of more than 35% of ventricular muscle there is a significant fall in cardiac output, leading to underperfusion of the sub-endocardium, with further necrosis and loss of function.

REDISTRIBUTIVE (SEPTIC) SHOCK

Here there is an excessive increase in capacity of the vasculature from vasodilatation.

- Associated with systemic infection with Gram-positive and -negative organisms, viruses (dengue fever) and fungi (candidiasis).
- The patient is hypotensive with a warm skin (unlike hypovolaemic and cardiogenic shock).
- There is tissue ischaemia (renal failure and ischaemic colitis), together with consumptive coagulopathy, adult respiratory failure (ARDS) and a reduced ventricular systolic ejection fraction.
- The complete picture of septic shock carries a mortality of 80–90%. This is preceded by the 'sepsis syndrome' (fever, tachycardia, oliguria and hypoxamia) with a lesser mortality rate of 10–20%, and is important to recognize clinically.

Pathogenesis

Most of the features can be explained by the action of bacterial endotoxin, a lipopolysaccharide found in the cell wall of many Gram-negative bacteria. It interacts with various cell types and plasma protein cascade systems causing the release of chemical signals, some of which are hypotensive, and others that contribute to disseminated intravascular coagulation. These include:

- Cytokines: tumour necrosis factor (TNF) 1α, interleukin (IL) 1, IL-6 and interferon (IFN) γ. In animal models TNF 1α alone produces most of the features of shock.
- Nitric oxide (NO). This is normally produced by vascular endothelium, and controls vascular tone. Endotoxin can induce NO production additionally from macrophages and vascular smooth muscle, causing inappropriate vasodilatation, and the vessels become refractory to vasopressor agents.
- Products of arachidonic acid metabolism: prostaglandins, leukotrienes, platelet activating factor.

Other bacterial toxins can cause redistributive shock – super-antigens. These bind to T cells, without requiring presentation with HLA class II proteins, and cause the release of large quantities of cytokines including TNF-1α and IFN-γ.

ANEURYSM

An abnormal permanent segmental dilatation in an artery, vein or the heart, involving the wall of the affected vessel. A false aneurysm is seen with rupture, and its wall is organizing connective tissue surrounding the haematoma.

Shape

- *Saccular* A bag-like dilatation involving just part of the wall circumference at the site of the wall weakness. The overlying blood flow is turbulent, with thrombus deposition within the cavity of the aneurysm.
- *Fusiform* An elliptical dilatation involving the entire circumference of the vessel, often lined by a sheath of poorly organized thrombus.

Cause

Most causes of vascular disease can cause aneurysm formation, and are related to atrophy or necrosis of the arterial media, and damage to the elastic lamina.

AORTIC ANEURYSMS

The aorta is the commonest site of aneurysm.

- **Syphilis**: a rare cause nowadays with the decline of tertiary syphilis.
- **Atherosclerosis**: the aorta is the commonest site of aneurysm. Most causes are now related to atherosclerosis, affecting the abdominal aorta. There is a prevalence of 1–4% of the population aged over 50 years.

Risk factors

- Age: strongly associated with increasing age, the frequency doubles from 50–80 years.
- Sex: marked male preponderance.
- Race: Caucasians more often affected than Blacks.
- Hypertension: Possibly related to incremental effect on atherogenesis.
- Cigarette smoking.
- Genetic factors: familial clustering around aortic aneurysm is well described: a first-degree relative with an aneurysm is associated with 12-fold risk of developing an aneurysm. There is a possible association with haptoglobin phenotype, types of cholesterol ester transfer protein and disorders of connective tissue.

Pathological features

The aorta distal to the origin of the renal arteries is most commonly affected, and may extend to involve the iliac arteries. Most cases are fusiform and the diameter ranges from 5–10 cm. Microscopic examination shows smooth muscle atrophy and loss of the elastic lamina.

Pathogenesis Atherosclerosis and proteolysis cause weakening of the wall, potentially resulting in localized dilatation, and so the distending force of systolic blood pressure increases, according to La Place's law.

Complications

- Rupture: This is related to wall tension and size. Aneurysms greater than 5 cm diameter at diagnosis have a risk of rupture of 25% over 5 years. Elective surgical repair carries a mortality of 5%, emergency repair carries a mortality of 40%.

- Bacterial infection: most commonly caused by blood-borne *salmonella* and *Staph. aureus*, patients complain of back pain, associated with fever and a tender pulsatile mass.
- Embolization: Distal emboli originating from thrombus associated with an aneurysm can cause areas of painful discolouration of the toes and ankles.

'INFLAMMATORY ANEURYSM'

An aortic aneurysm associated with fibrous thickening of the periaortic tissues, with a florid inflammatory cell infiltrate (T and B cells, and plasma cells). This closely resembles the changes of idiopathic retroperitoneal fibrosis, raising the possibility that both are a single disorder, consisting of a marked immune response, perhaps to oxidized lipid, causing fibrosis. The fibrosis can involve the ureters to cause hydronephrosis and renal failure.

THORACIC AORTIC ANEURYSMS

Sinus of Valsalva

- *Congenital*: defective insertion of aortic base with periaortic fibrosis, often associated with disorders of connective tissue matrix protein synthesis such as Marfan's and Ehlers–Danlos syndrome.
- *Acquired*: mycotic aneurysms associated with infective endocarditis, especially when the aortic valve is involved.

Aortic root

These aneurysms are associated with fragmentation of the elastic lamina, medial smooth muscle atrophy and accumulation of connective tissue mucin. These changes are collectively known as Erdheim's cystic medial necrosis and are seen in Marfan's syndrome (failure to produce fibrillin protein).

Ascending and descending thoracic aorta

- *Syphilis*: common before the introduction of antibiotics, with an autopsy incidence of 1% adults. As well as causing aneurysm, syphilitic aortitis can result in aortic root dilatation, with aortic incompetence and stenosis of the coronary artery ostia. The aorta shows a lymphoplasmacytic infiltrate in the media, focal smooth muscle necrosis and multi-nucleate giant cells (gummas), and an ingrowth of new blood vessels. The loss of muscle and elastin imparts a wrinkled appearance to the intima ('tree-bark' appearance).
- *Other causes*: tuberculosis, rheumatoid disease, giant cell arteritis and Takayasu (pulseless) disease are all causes of thoracic aneurysms.

....

AORTIC DISSECTION

Longitudinal splitting of the aortic wall by blood between the inner two-thirds and the outer third of the media. There is a tear of the intima, allowing blood to track into the media. This is related to haemodynamic stress and the resistance of the aortic wall. If untreated, dissection carries a high mortality rate, 75% dying within 2 weeks after presentation. The following are risk factors:

- Sex: 2–3 times commoner in males.
- Age: 50–70 years.
- Race: commoner in blacks in the US.
- Hypertension: 80% cases are hypertensive, often with left ventricular hypertrophy. Many are associated with accelerated hypertension.
- Connective tissue disorders: Marfan's syndrome – 44% patients with Marfan's syndrome have aortic dissection.
- Pregnancy: 49% dissections in patients under 40 occur in pregnant women, usually in the third trimester.
- Bicuspid aortic valve and coarctation.

- Miscellaneous: Turner's and Noonan's syndromes.
- Iatrogenic: dissection is associated with bypass cannulation.

Seventy-five per cent of cases are seen in the ascending aorta (type A). These tend to be more serious, and are seen in younger patients. Type B dissecting aneurysms occur in the descending aorta. The dissection may rupture into the pericardial cavity, the left pleural cavity, or back into the lumen affecting spontaneous repair.

INFLAMMATORY DISEASE AFFECTING BLOOD VESSELS: THE VASCULITIDES

These are inflammatory disorders of vessels with structural damage to the wall; necrotizing vasculitis is seen with a significant degree of acute necrosis (this includes hypersensitivity angiitis, allergic granulomatous angiitis, rheumatic arteritis, polyarteritis nodosa and temporal arteritis).

Classification is based on:

- size of vessels
- pathogenesis
- aetiology
- associated clinical features.

Pathogenesis

Immune mediated injury is involved in many cases.

- Lesions in animal models resemble some human vasculitis.
- Evidence of immune disturbance is seen in some vasculitides including; circulating immune complexes, plasma autoantibodies, changes in the complement system, changes in T cell and macrophage function.
- Immunosuppression improves condition.

Mechanisms

- Formation of pathogenic immune complexes, localizing in the vascular bed (Gell and Coombes type III reaction) – serum sickness model, with complement activation.

- Immediate hypersensitivity, mediated by IgE. Serum IgE levels are raised in polyarteritis nodosa and Churg–Strauss syndrome.
- Direct tissue damage from cytotoxic antibodies (Gell and Coombes type II reaction). This mechanism is well described in Goodpasture's syndrome and immune-mediated haemolysis, but there is less evidence for vasculitis.
- Tissue damage from activation of white cells by binding of antibody to white-cell antigens. Serum anti-neutrophilic cytoplasmic autoantibodies (ANCAs) are present in many necrotizing vasculitides including Wegener's granulomatosis, microscopic polyarteritis, crescentic glomerulonephritis and hypersensitivity angiitis. Two types of ANCA are described:

  — *c-ANCA* The entire cytoplasm is stained, the antibody reacting with primary lysosomes in neutrophils. c-ANCA is strongly associated with Wegener's granulomatosis, and some cases of polyarteritis.
  — *p-ANCA* This antibody stains the perinuclear region of neutrophils, binding to myeloperoxidase. p-ANCA is associated with polyarteritis, Churg–Strauss syndrome and crescentic glomerulonephritis.

- Tissue damage from cellular immune damage (often with granulomas).

Role of infectious agents

Any infectious agent can act via the above mechanisms. Relatively few infections are associated with a vasculitis. These include:

Herpes virus infections   These may directly affect endothelial cells, possibly exposing receptors for C3b and Fc.

Mycoplasma   This is associated with vasculitis at sites distant from the primary infection.

Rickettsial infections   The inflammatory process involves the arterioles. The organism grows within the endothelium, which becomes necrotic, with thrombosis. These changes are seen in the skin and other organs.

HTLV-I   The virus infects endothelial cells in culture, and vasculitis is well described in HIV infections.

Vasculitis in malignant disease

- hypersensitivity vasculitis is well described in malignant disease
- polyarteritis nodosa is associated with hairy cell leukaemia
- granulomatous vasculitis is associated with Hodgkin's disease.

The mechanism in some cases is due to pathogenic immune complex deposition. In others the blood vessel walls are invaded by tumour cells, typically in T-cell lymphoma (mycosis fungoides and lymphomatoid granulomatosis).

· ·

VASCULITIS INVOLVING LARGE AND MEDIUM SIZED BLOOD VESSELS

Takayasu's arteritis (pulseless disease)

A chronic inflammatory disease affecting both systemic and pulmonary circulations. The aorta is often involved, together with its major branches and coronary arteries.

Epidemiology and aetiology

Most commonly seen in the Far East, affecting young women from 15 to 45 years age. There is an association with HLA B5 sub-type and also autoimmune disorders including rheumatoid disease, ankylosing spondylitis, inflammatory bowel disease, retroperitoneal fibrosis and scleroderma. Manifestation of the disease depends on the site of affected vessels, e.g. absent pulses.

Clinical features

At the time of active vascular inflammation there are often systemic symptoms including fever, malaise, dizziness and arthralgia. The ESR is raised, along with raised acute phase proteins (C-reactive protein and α_2-globulin).

Pathological changes

There is an initial granulomatous panarteritis with patchy destruction of medial smooth muscle and the elastic lamina.

The inflammatory infiltrate includes lymphocytes, plasma cells and some giant cells. There is subsequent scarring of the artery wall with marked fibromuscular intimal proliferation, mural thrombosis, adventitial and periadventitial scarring. The artery can be left as a rigid stenotic tube or develop an aneurysm.

Giant cell arteritis (cranial and extracranial)

The commonest of the vasculitides, it is a granulomatous inflammatory process affecting any elastic and muscular artery. It is typically seen in the superficial temporal artery, often associated with polymyalgia rheumatica (pain and stiffness in the shoulder and pelvic girdles, raised ESR and malaise). There is a prompt response to steroids.

Cranial giant cell arteritis

Characterized by headache, scalp tenderness, blurring and loss of vision, musculoskeletal symptoms and general malaise. Classic changes show a focal inflammatory infiltrate in the media consisting of lymphocytes, plasma cells and macrophages. Giant cells may be present around the medial and intimal junction, associated with disrupted elastic lamina. Atypical giant cell arteritis lacks the presence of giant cells. Healed giant cell arteritis may just show prominent fibromuscular intimal thickening, with little inflammation. There may be collagenous replacement of the disrupted elastic lamina within the media. It is likely these changes are a result of release of macrophage-derived growth factors. Diagnosis is confirmed by tissue biopsy from a segment of superficial temporal artery, but may not be positive because of the focal nature of disease and its transient nature, particularly if steroids have been given.

Extracranial giant cell arteritis

Any large artery can be affected but only 10–15% patients present with clinical disturbances, usually intermittent claudication. Complications include myocardial ischaemia, aortic valve incompetence, aortic dissection and aneurysm.

Granulomatous angiitis of the central nervous system (isolated angiitis of the nervous system)

Rarely the intracranial vessels are exclusively involved by the inflammatory process. There is a severe headache, altered mental function and focal neurological deficits; systemic symptoms are absent. Angiography shows segmental changes including focal stenoses and dilatations. Biopsies show granulomatous inflammation, with necrosis of arteries, arterioles and venules. There is a strong association with malignant lymphoma or leukaemia, often accompanying herpes zoster infection.

Buerger's disease (thromboangiitis obliterans)

First described in young males in 1908 this is a syndrome of vascular insufficiency, progressing to gangrene.

- ischaemia usually seen in the lower limbs
- predominantly seen in males aged 20–45 years
- strongly associated with cigarette smoking
- absence of atherosclerosis and recognized risk factors for atherosclerosis
- associated migratory thrombophlebitis
- affects medium-sized arteries and veins.

Epidemiology and aetiology

Seen in all ethnic groups but commoner in Orientals and Ashkenazi Jews. There is an association with HLA A9 and B5 sub-types. Cigarette smoking is a major contributory factor; the disease worsens with continuing smoking and improves on stopping. Most patients show auto-antibodies against type III collagen.

Pathological changes

At amputation the diseased vessels resemble fibrous cords, with scarring around the vascular bundle. In the early stages there are cellular thrombi with microabscesses. The walls of both arteries and veins show transmural inflammation, with no disruption of the internal elastic lamina. Recanalization of the occlusive thrombi occurs with organization, with considerable narrowing of the lumen and further occlusion by thrombosis.

VASCULITIS INVOLVING MEDIUM AND SMALL SIZED VESSELS

Polyarteritis nodosa

A disease of early middle life; males are affected twice as commonly as females. If left untreated there is a high risk of death (5 year survival < 15%); there is a good response to immunosuppressive treatment.

Pathogenesis

No single pathogenetic mechanism explains the disease. Immune complex deposition is seen in many cases: Hepatitis B surface antigen, hairy cell leukaemia, and drugs are all described associations. Where there is no immune complex deposition ANCA is present in the serum.

Clinical features

The clinical picture is determined by which vascular bed is affected, together with systemic symptoms e.g. fever, headache, myalgia and weight loss. Dermal vessel involvement causes purpuric rashes, coronary artery involvement causes cardiac symptoms. Aneurysms are found in diseased medium-sized vessels.

Diagnosis and pathological changes

Any accessible tissue can be biopsied: skin changes do not always reflect systemic disease, and skeletal muscle carries a false negative rate of 65%. Arteries (and arterioles in microscopic polyarteritis) show fibrinoid necrosis, with a neutrophil infiltrate and thrombosis. With time the vessel wall undergoes fibrosis, both medial and intimal, with a lymphocytic and macrophage infiltrate. The artery acquires a nodular appearance.

Wegener's granulomatosis

Characterized by:

- necrotizing granulomas involving the upper and lower respiratory tracts
- systemic necrotizing vasculitis

- glomerulonephritis: ranging from focal segmental changes to rapidly progressive crescentic glomerulonephritis.

Clinical features

Seen from adolescence to old age, peak incidence is 40 years, more commonly in males, and associated with HLA–DR2 sub-type. Without treatment with immunosuppressives there is a poor outlook, with 82% cases dying within 1 year. Sixty per cent present with upper respiratory tract symptoms e.g. sinusitis, nasal obstruction, ulceration and severe otitis media and deafness; the remainder with lower respiratory tract symptoms including productive cough, haemoptysis and dyspnoea. There is renal involvement in 80% cases.

Diagnosis

ANCA is positive in most cases, but its specificity is low; biopsy is the most reliable means of diagnosis.

Pathological findings

Multiple well-circumscribed haemorrhagic necrotic lesions. Histology shows coagulative necrosis, surrounded by granulation tissue, sometimes with ghost outlines of vessels. Multi-nucleate giant cells may be seen, but well-formed granulomas are not usually present. The necrosis affects both arteries and veins, with thrombosis and distal infarction. Pathological changes can be sparse and absent on biopsy.

Churg–Strauss syndrome (allergic angiitis and granulomatosis)

Characterized by:

- asthma and eosinophilia
- pulmonary and systemic vasculitis
- extravascular granulomas.

There is usually an eosinophilia, and raised IgE in the vasculitic phase. Patients present with fever and weight loss.

Pathological findings

Eosinophilic vasculitis involving small arteries, veins and capillaries, with focal necrosis of vessel walls. The granulomas are poorly formed, with necrotic centres. Lesions are also found in the spleen, gastro-intestinal tract, and rarely in the heart and prostate.

Kawasaki's disease (muco-cutaneous lymph node syndrome)

An acute febrile disease in children under 5 years. There is a systemic vasculitis of medium sized arteries, including the coronaries. There can be aneurysm formation, in 5–10% patients. The aetiology remains unclear, although a tick-borne rickettsial infection has been postulated.

Clinical features

Fever, conjunctival congestion, dryness and inflammation of the oral cavity and lips, painful cervical lymphadenopathy, polymorphous skin rash and reddening of the skin of the palms and soles, with desquamation and oedema.

Pathological changes

In the acute stages there is a pancarditis, and dilatation/ aneurysm of the coronaries. This can then regress (seen when the diameter is < 4 mm) or result in stenosis or occlusion (when the diameter is > 8 mm), seen in 3–5% cases. The arteries show fibrinoid necrosis and thrombosis.

....

VASCULITIS CHIEFLY INVOLVING SMALL BLOOD VESSELS

Hypersensitivity vasculitis

Typical examples are serum sickness and drug induced vasculitis. The skin is commonly involved together with other sites. There is fibrinoid necrosis and a neutrophilic inflammatory reaction with nuclear fragmentation (leucocytoclastic vasculitis) and hypocomplementaemia. Immune complexes are frequently present in the lesions; the antigens are derived from micro-organisms, drugs and tumour antigens.

Clinical sub-types of hypersensitivity vasculitis include:

Henoch–Schönlein purpura

Seen in young adults and children, there is purpura, arthritis and abdominal pain, sometimes with intestinal bleeding. The kidney is involved in 30% patients, with proteinuria and haematuria from a focal mesangio-proliferative glomerulonephritis. The skin shows a necrotizing vasculitis with IgA deposition, and is probably the same condition as IgA nephropathy (Berger's disease).

Essential mixed cryoglobulinaemia

Characterized by small vessel vasculitis with glomerulonephritis, purpura and arthralgia. There is deposition of complement, IgG and IgM cryoglobulins.

Hypocomplementaemic urticarial vasculitis

Characterized by marked hypocomplementaemia, skin lesions, arthralgia, myositis and abdominal pain, and a possible glomerulonephritis. The skin lesions show a leucocytoclastic vasculitis, with IgG deposits in the vessel walls.

DISORDERS OF VEINS

NORMAL ANATOMY AND PHYSIOLOGY

- poorly defined internal elastic lamina
- little muscle in media, the amount depending on vessel calibre and intraluminal pressure.

Veins act as capacitance vessels, carrying two-thirds of the circulating blood volume. Via the autonomic nervous system there can be rapid redistribution of blood in various compartments of the vasculature controlled by changes in venous tone. In this way cardiac output can be maintained with haemorrhage.

Venous return from the lower limb is driven by pressure changes from the calf muscles in walking (muscle pump), together with changes in intra-abdominal and intrathoracic pressure. The action of the 'muscle pump' is facilitated by bicuspid valves in the communicating veins that join the superficial vein with the deep system. It ensures that blood returns from the lower limb in exercise and also reduces superficial vein pressure, so minimizing the effects of hydrostatic pressure on the skin.

It is the absence of exercise-induced venous hypotension that underlies much of venous pathology as in:

- Abnormalities of the 'muscle pump':
  calf-muscle weakness; decreased capacity of the deep vein after deep vein thrombosis; excessive dilatation and valve incompetence.
- Incompetence of the communicating veins.
- Incompetence of the superficial veins (giving rise to cosmetic problems).

DISORDERS OF VENOUS DRAINAGE

Varicose veins

These 'saccular dilatations' occur typically in the saphenous vein and superficial veins.

Epidemiology

Varicose veins are seen in 2% of the population, and are associated with increasing age, female sex (possibly as a result of increased venous pressure in pregnancy), obesity and long periods of standing. There is a hereditary component.

Secondary varicose veins are seen after deep vein thrombosis, and with pelvic tumours.

Pathophysiology

Tributaries of the long saphenous vein become dilated, elongated and tortuous. The media is disrupted by scar tissue and intimal fibrosis.

Complications
- Haemorrhage.
- Superficial thrombophlebitis: tender warm thickening along the course of the vein. There may be a systemic reaction with pyrexia, but embolization is not seen.
- Brown skin pigmentation: extravasation of red cells into surrounding connective tissue, often associated with skin ulceration.
- Lipodermatosis: progressive fibrosis of dermis and subcutis as a result of prolonged venous hypertension. It develops acutely as hot, red tense changes in the skin, which becomes stiff and shiny.

Venous ulceration

Seen in the lower limb, with associated vein abnormality and blood flow pattern. They are present in 0.2% of the population, and represent a significant drain on healthcare resources. There is often a history of preceding deep vein thrombosis, and incompetence of the communicating veins. The dermal capillaries become dilated and tortuous with leakage of fibrinogen. Increased deposition of fibrinogen and fibrin is seen in the pericapillary areas, which may lead to a 'diffusion block' to the skin with anoxic changes.

Deep vein thrombosis

This has already been discussed in Chapter 18.

NORMAL STRUCTURE AND FUNCTION

The nasopharynx is lined by squamous epithelium with a wide-ranging normal microbiological flora.

The paranasal sinuses, eustachian tubes and middle ear are lined by ciliated columnar epithelium (respiratory epithelium) with underlying submucous and serous glands.

Defence mechanisms

- **Mechanical**: sneezing, coughing and the gag reflex. Viscid mucus traps foreign particles, which are propelled up by cilia (muco-ciliary escalator). Viral infections depress ciliary function.
- **Local immunological defences**: there is abundant lymphoid tissue, with much secretion of IgA.
- **Abundant blood vessels**: rapid delivery of inflammatory cells.

INFLAMMATORY DISORDERS

These are infective or a result of type I (IgE mediated) hypersensitvity.

Acute nasopharyngitis (The common cold)

Caused by 200 different viruses – rhinoviruses (110 strains), adenoviruses (31 strains), parainfluenza (4 strains), enteroviruses (60 strains) and coronaviruses (3 strains). Although a trivial disorder it is of huge economic importance in terms of lost working days. The infections predispose to bacterial infections e.g. paranasal sinusitis.

Allergic rhinitis

IgE mediated hypersensitivity. Allergens include plant pollens, animal danders and house-dust mites. Exposure causes reddening and oedema of nasal mucosa with nasal obstruction. The resultant inflammatory infiltrate contains numerous eosinophils.

Nasal polyps

Islands of oedematous mucosa develop after repeated episodes of allergic rhinitis. There is associated hyperplasia of mucous glands and a mixed inflammatory infiltrate rich in plasma cells. Obstruction develops with resultant impaired drainage from the sinuses causing sinusitis.

Sinusitis

Characterized by nasal congestion, purulent nasal discharge and pain. Also related to deviation of nasal septum, trauma, foreign bodies, neoplasms, cystic fibrosis and Kartagener's syndrome (see page 294), immunosuppression and AIDS. Frontal and maxillary sinuses are involved in adults, the ethmoid in children. Causative organisms (isolated from direct puncture specimens) include *Haemophilus influenzae, Streptococcus pneumoniae* and *Moraxella catarrhalis*. Anaerobes are cultured in 25% of cases. Most cases respond to antibiotic treatment and decongestants. The inflammation can involve the orbit, the bony margins of the sinus and the skull itself, with a resulting thrombophlebitis.

Rhinoscleroma

A chronic inflammatory disorder affecting the nose, pharynx and larynx caused by *Klebsiella rhinoscleromatis*. The inflammatory infiltrate contains foamy macrophages which contain the organisms.

Mucormycosis

A fungal infection, typically seen in poorly controlled diabetes mellitus and immunosuppressed patients. The branching, wide, non-septate fungal hyphae invade blood vessels to cause thrombosis and necrosis. The infection can spread to the orbit and brain.

Wegener's granulomatosis

See vasculitis (page 276).

See vasculitis (page 276).

. . . .

NEOPLASMS

Papilloma

Affects males and presents as nasal stuffiness, obstruction or bleeding. Lesions arising on the lateral wall frequently show an invaginating proliferation into the fibrous stroma ('inverted papilloma'); not invasive, but tends to recur locally, to invade the orbit or skull. Three per cent of cases are malignant at presentation, and another 3% show subsequent malignant change. The prognosis for these is poor.

Juvenile angiofibroma

Seen in adolescent males aged 10–20 years. The lesions arise from erectile tissue in the posterior lateral wall of the nose, are androgen-dependent and show androgen receptors.

Macroscopy   Haemorrhagic polypoid masses.

Microscopy   Numerous blood vessels set in a fibrous stroma, with characteristic stellate fibroblasts and mast cells.

Natural history   May regress after puberty. Usually excised surgically (may recur); also treated with radiotherapy with a subsequent small risk of sarcomatous change.

Carcinoma of the paranasal sinuses

A rare tumour, usually seen in the maxillary sinus, typically squamous. Late presentation is common with invasion of the bony margin. Increased risk in nickel workers. Adenocarcinoma is seen in the ethmoid sinus and is associated with wood-workers.

Carcinoma of the nasopharynx

Geographic variation: frequently seen in adult males from South China, and children of both sexes from North Africa.

Aetiology Genetic factors, environmental factors and infection by the Epstein–Barr Virus (EBV). Patients show IgG antibodies to early EBV antigen and IgA to the capsid. Keratinizing nasopharyngeal carcinoma (NPC) is not associated with EBV and is seen in older patients.

Microscopy Non-keratinizing NPC can be undifferentiated (with an associated lymphoid infiltrate known as lymphoepitheliomas) or show some squamous features.

Natural history Clinically silent, often unresectable at presentation, with spread to regional lymph nodes. Undifferentiated NPC is radiosensitive, with a cure rate of 50%. Prognosis is better in younger patients if the ipsilateral lymph node involvement, and disease is confined to the upper neck.

Carcinoma of the minor salivary glands

Tumours are seen in the nose and paranasal sinuses, usually adenoid cystic carcinoma. Pleomorphic salivary adenoma is seen in the nose.

Olfactory neuroblastoma (aesthesioneuroblastoma)

Arises from the neuroepithelium of the olfactory membrane. Seen at any age, most often at 50 years. The tumour cells show an 11:22 chromosomal translocation, common to Ewing's sarcoma (see page 823) suggesting a common origin with other primitive neuroectodermal tumours (PNET).

Macroscopy Red-grey, vascular polypoid masses in the roof of the nasal fossa.

Microscopy A highly cellular tumour composed of small round cells, round nuclei, little cytoplasm, with rosettes. Immunocytochemistry is positive for chromogranin, neuron-specific enolase and catecholamines.

Natural history Local invasion of sinuses, orbit, palate, nasopharynx and base of skull. Distant metastasis to cervical nodes and lungs in 20% cases. The five-year survival is 50–60%.

LARYNX

STRUCTURE AND FUNCTION

Divided into three parts:

- **Supraglottis**: that part of the larynx above the vocal cords, and includes the epiglottis and the false cords.
- **Glottis**: the true vocal cords and the anterior commissure.
- **Infraglottic region**: the segment below the vocal cords.

Pathological processes are apparent as:

- abnormalities of phonation, e.g. hoarseness
- obstruction to normal airflow.

DISORDERS OF DEVELOPMENT

- **Laryngeal web**: a delicate membrane of connective tissue covered by epithelium arising between the anterior portions of the vocal cords.
- **Laryngeal stenosis**: caused by cysts or webs. Acquired stenosis is seen after trauma, such as exposure to caustic agents, and inflammation, e.g. TB.
- **Laryngocoele**: abnormal enlargement of laryngeal ventricle, aggravated by a rise in intralaryngeal pressure, as in coughing.

INFLAMMATORY DISORDERS

Acute infective laryngitis

Children are most commonly affected. The narrow airways are readily obstructed by oedema, which can be life threatening.

Acute epiglottitis

Affects also posterior tongue and larynx. Starts as sore throat, with stridor (airway obstruction) and septicaemia. The pharynx is inflamed and the epiglottis is swollen and hyperaemic (likened to a bright red cherry). Frequently caused by type B *Haemophilus influenzae*. This strain possesses a polyribose-ribitol-phosphate (PRP) capsular antigen and causes severe non-specific acute inflammation. Most individuals show antibodies to this antigen presumably from childhood infection. Non-encapsulated strains are found in 50% of healthy children.

Acute laryngotracheobronchitis

An uncommon complication of upper respiratory tract infections, often parainfluenza and influenza viruses. There is marked inflammatory oedema of the sub-glottis, with hoarseness, a barking cough and stridor. Children under 3 years are affected.

Diphtheria

Now extremely rare because of universal immunization. Caused by *Corynebacterium diphtheriae* which produces a toxin that disrupts elongation factor 2 – a translocase that controls protein synthesis. The inflammation causes the formation of a grey-white pseudomembrane in the pharynx and larynx, consisting of polymerized fibrin, necrotic epithelium and inflammatory cells and can cause respiratory obstruction.

Chronic infective disorders of the larynx

Tuberculosis

Complication of open active pulmonary TB, now seen less frequently. Presents with hoarseness, with nodular ulceration on the vocal cords that clinically can resemble squamous cancer. Microscopy shows granulomas ± caseation; diagnosis is confirmed by demonstrating *Mycobacteria* spp.

Fungal laryngitis

Hoarseness, with granulomatous lesions in which mycobacteria cannot be isolated. Common in US, caused usually by *Histoplasma* or *Blastomyces*. Often associated with marked pseudo-epitheliomatous hyperplasia.

Acute non-infective disorders of the larynx

Angioneurotic oedema

Acute attacks of laryngeal oedema, possibly causing laryngeal obstruction.

Hereditary Autosomal dominant deficiency of C1 esterase inhibition, which controls intravascular activation of complement with resultant low levels of plasma C1, C2 and C4. Can be triggered by trauma to skin or soft tissues, may be preceded by a rash.

Non-hereditary Associated with urticaria/atopy.

Chronic non-infective disorders of the larynx

Granulomatous reactions

Seen after intubation trauma and Teflon injections into paralysed vocal cords (used with recurrent laryngeal nerve damage).

Pyogenic granuloma

A florid nodular capillary overgrowth, seen after trauma, e.g. intubation or biopsy.

Vocal cord polyps

Arise from mechanical damage to the vocal cord connective tissue after persistent misuse of the voice (known for example as 'singer's nodule') to cause hoarseness. Seen when the cords are firmly pressed together with rapid vibration, to cause congestion, oedema and haemorrhage. The lesions are typically on the medial aspect of the mid-anterior portion of the cord. Microscopic examination shows fibrosis, new blood vessels, haemorrhage, haemosiderin deposition and hyaline change of collagen.

....

LARYNGEAL NEOPLASMS

Benign epithelial neoplasms

Juvenile papillomas

Seen in young children. Usually multiple and recur but regress after puberty. Fifty per cent show HPV types 6 and 11. The lesions are small, lobulated papillomas covered by well-differentiated non-keratinizing squamous epithelium. Rarely undergo malignant transformation.

Adult papillomas

Single lesion, composed of keratinizing squamous epithelium, with possible dysplasia. Malignant transformation is seen in 2–3% cases.

Malignant epithelial neoplasms

Intraepithelial neoplasia (carcinoma in situ)

Often seen at the margin of invasive squamous carcinoma, and may be the only lesion present on the vocal cord. Manifested by cytological atypia present within the epithelium; the greater the thickness involved, the higher the grade of intraepithelial neoplasia. The prognosis is difficult to predict and management is either excision, or stripping the epithelial covering of the cord.

Invasive squamous carcinoma

Ninety per cent or more malignant laryngeal neoplasms are squamous carcinoma.

Clinical features   Most cases are seen over 50 years; Males > females (24:1), and accounts for 2.2% of all male cancer cases, 0.4% female cancer cases. Tobacco smoking is a major risk factor, which is enhanced by heavy alcohol intake. They are classified according to location which affects pattern of spread (Table 33.1).

Table 33.1 Classification of invasive squamous carcinomas

Location	Cases (%)	Pattern of spread
Glottic	60	These arise from true vocal cords. Remain localized for a long time with late lymph node metastasis (few lymphatics, and tumour confined by cartilage). Good prognosis after irradiation or local resection of cord lesions (80% 5-year survival).
Supraglottic	30	Involves false cord, laryngeal ventricle or epiglottis. Spread to pre-epiglottic space is seen but not the cartilage; treated by local resection with preservation of the vocal cords. Treatment failure is from spread to the cervical lymph nodes (40% cases), (65% 5-year survival).
Transglottic	< 5	The tumour crosses the laryngeal ventricle; treated by total laryngectomy because of the risk of spread to cervical nodes (50%) 5-year survival).
Subglottic	< 5	May genuinely arise below the cord (very rare) or from the cord to extend into the subglottis. There is spread to the thyroid gland, cricoid cartilage and trachea. Lymph node metastasis is seen is 50% of cases (40% 5-year survival).

LUNGS

....

NORMAL ANATOMY

- Paired asymmetrical conical organs, combined weight 850 g (men) and 750 g (women).
- Attached at the hilum to move freely within the thoracic cavity. This can be lost with the formation of post-inflammatory adhesions which bridge the visceral and parietal pleura.
- The lungs are divided into lobes: three on the right, two on the left.
- Each lobe is sub-divided into bronchopulmonary segments; each is supplied by a first generation bronchus. These in turn give rise to lobules (polyhedral areas on the pleural surface) demarcated by connective tissue septa.

Classification of conducting airways

The conducting airways start with the trachea, which divides into the right and left main bronchi. The left bronchus divides at a greater angle, is longer and narrower giving a greater risk of obstruction from aspiration on the right side. The number of divisions from main bronchus to acinus varies from 8 to 25. The conducting airways are all lined by ciliated epithelium and have smooth muscle in the wall.

Bronchi   These possess cartilage in the walls, are lined with pseudo-stratified ciliated columnar epithelium and have smooth muscle arranged in spiral bundles in the wall. Mucous glands are present in the wall, providing the main source of bronchial mucus. Neuroendocrine cells that secrete peptide hormones (e.g. bombesin and calcitonin) are present.

Bronchioles   No cartilage in the wall, with a lining of simple ciliated columnar and non-ciliated secretory epithelial cells (Clara cells), reaching the terminal bronchiole which in turn supplies the acinus.

Acinus   Basic structural unit for gas exchange. Composed of subdividing respiratory bronchioles (muscular bronchioles carrying alveoli) which subdivide. The numbers of alveoli increases with each sub-division, and end with alveolar sacs – grape-like collections of spaces with a diameter of 250 μm. Each lobule supplies three to five acini, and there are around 300 million alveoli in each lung.

Alveolar septum and lining cells   Gas exchange takes place through the following structures:

- alveolar epithelium
- alveolar basement membrane
- interstitial space
- capillary basement membrane
- capillary endothelium.

Changes in the septum can greatly affect gas exchange. Mesenchymal cells are present in the interstitial space and can lay down collagen and elastin. The alveolar lining cells are of two types:

- *Type 1*: Thin cells with a diameter of 50 μm and thickness of 0.1 μm, 40% of alveolar cell population, covering 90% of alveolar basement membrane.

- *Type II*: Cuboidal cells with stubby microvilli, a prominent Golgi apparatus and secretory granules, which contain surfactant (seen on EM as close-packed layers of membrane-like material).

Surfactant is an acellular material lining the alveolar surface and containing lipids which lower surface tension. If absent (as in infantile respiratory distress syndrome) the alveoli cannot expand, causing collapse of the lungs.

....

NORMAL FUNCTION

- Gas exchange between air and blood: oxygen is added to and carbon dioxide is removed from pulmonary arterial blood (normal range O_2: 10.5–13.5 kPa, CO_2; 4.8–6.0 kPa).
- Occurs in acini: functional units defined as lung tissue distal to terminal bronchioles.
- Processes involved: ventilation, perfusion and diffusion.

Ventilation

The rhythmic movement of gases (inflation and deflation) in and out of the lungs. This depends on:

- natural elasticity of lung tissue
- lowering of surface tension by surfactant
- contraction of intercostal muscles and diaphragm lowering intrathoracic pressure
- elastic recoil of lung tissue and relaxation of the above muscles
- depth, rate and rhythm of respiration controlled by the respiratory centre in the medulla oblongata (monitors CSF CO_2 and arterial blood pO_2 levels in blood, sensed by carotid body).

Perfusion

- 5 litres of blood per minute pass through the pulmonary circulation
- arterial pressure: 15 mmHg with a corresponding low resistance

- the vascular resistance is raised by hypoxia: local ventilation falls with a reduction in local CO_2 levels. These two factors indicate a homeostatic mechanism to match ventilation with perfusion.

Increased vascular resistance

Occurs in chronic airflow obstruction, resection of large parts of the lung, inflammatory disorders of the pulmonary vasculature, pulmonary venous hypertension.

Diffusion of gases

The movement of gases within the alveolus is determined by diffusion through the alveolar lining epithelium, basement membranes, interstitial space and endothelium of the alveolar capillaries.

DEFENCE MECHANISMS IN THE RESPIRATORY TRACT

Some 10 000–20 000 litres of air pass through the respiratory tract each day, potentially carrying noxious gases, injurious dusts and infective micro-organisms.

The nose

The complex cross-sectional area of the nose promotes turbulent airflow encouraging deposition of air-borne particles on the nasal mucosa. They are trapped in surface mucus to be removed by ciliary action to the pharynx. The nose is also responsible for warming and humidifying the air.

Lower respiratory tract

The airways are covered in a superficial layer of mucus which is constantly swept upwards by ciliary action through the glottis for swallowing. This mechanism, the *muco-ciliary escalator*, removes foreign particles and excess secretions.

This mechanism is disrupted in Kartagener's syndrome (bronchiectasis, sinusitis and dextrocardia). There is an abnormality in dynein, the protein linking the microtubule sub-units in cilia.

Mechanical clearance: coughs and sneezes

Foreign particles and excessive tracheal and bronchial secretions are expelled from major airways. The reflex is reduced in the elderly and lost when unconscious, increasing the risk of aspiration and inhalation pneumonia.

Alveolar clearance: alveolar macrophage function

Particles deposited in alveoli are ingested by macrophages (covering 5% of the alveolar surface) which then move proximally via the terminal bronchioles on to the mucociliary escalator (cilia are not present beyond the terminal bronchiole). Macrophages also produce scar-promoting growth factors and present antigens to T-helper cells in the immune response.

CHRONIC AIRFLOW OBSTRUCTION

Chronic obstructive airway disease (COAD) is a set of disorders characterized by a diminished ability to expire air, manifested by reduced elastic recoil of lung tissue and/or reduced airway calibre. Lung function tests show a reduction in FEV_1/FVC.

Pathological causes

- chronic bronchitis
- emphysema
- chronic asthma
- bronchiectasis
- cystic fibrosis.

....

CHRONIC BRONCHITIS AND EMPHYSEMA

Chronic bronchitis The presence of chronic cough productive of mucus/mucopurulent sputum for at least three months over at least two consecutive years.

Emphysema A permanent over-distension of the airways distal to the terminal bronchioles, associated with the destruction of the walls.

The two conditions co-exist, and emphysema is seen twice as commonly as chronic bronchitics. Both are related to atmospheric pollution and especially to tobacco smoking.

Epidemiology

- International differences: related to differing degrees of atmospheric pollution. COAD is common in industrialized countries; in the UK it is the sixth commonest cause of death.
- Age and sex: deaths are commoner in males, as with other smoking-related illness.

Aetiology

- Cigarette smoking: cigarette smoke contains high concentrations of free radicals and nitric oxide. These cause direct damage to cell constituents, e.g. peroxidation of membrane lipids, and disrupt anti-proteolytic defences in the lung. They also cause release of injurious proteases from neutrophils and macrophages.
- Atmospheric pollution: the precise aetiological factors are not clearly understood.
- Infection: early childhood lung infections (e.g. respiratory syncytial virus) correlate with impaired respiratory function in adulthood.
- α_1-antitrypsin deficiency: an inherited disorder of anti-protease activity. Proteases, derived from neutrophils and macrophages (elastase and collagenase), can cause breakdown of the airspace wall connective tissue. This activity is counterbalanced by antiproteases e.g. α_1-antitrypsin, produced by the liver. There is a failure to transport the α_1-antitrypsin from the liver cell into the plasma, the anti-protease being seen as PAS positive globules in hepatocytes. Severe emphysema occurs when antiprotease activity is 40% normal, presenting as basal emphysema in patients under 40 years.

Pathological changes in chronic bronchitis

- Hyperplasia of tracheal and bronchial mucous glands. This can be studied quantitatively using the Reid Index (ratio of bronchial gland thickness to thickness of the bronchial wall). In non-bronchitics the ratio ranges from 0.14–0.36; in bronchitics it is 0.41–0.79. In chronic bronchitics the sputum contains more sulphated viscid mucins.
- Increased numbers of airway goblet cells. Goblet cell metaplasia in the small airways is responsible for excess intraluminal mucus that may cause obstruction, and also displace surfactant, altering their mechanical properties.
- Intraluminal mucus accumulation.
- Bronchiolar wall oedema.
- Increased tone and reactivity of smooth muscle.
- Peribronchiolar fibrosis: loss of tethering of the small airways to the adjacent interlobular septa. In expiration there is a greater degree of bronchial narrowing.

EMPHYSEMA

Four patterns are recognized depending on which region of the acinus is affected.

Proximal acinar (centriacinar) emphysema

Enlargement of the respiratory respiratory bronchioles. Two patterns are described:

Non-industrial centriacinar emphysema Dilatation and destruction of second- and third-order respiratory bronchioles. The upper lobes are more severely affected and the changes are typically seen at the centre of secondary lobules, with adjacent chronic inflammation and fibrosis. Associated with COAD.

Inhalation of dust (simple coalminers' pneumoconiosis) The changes parallel those seen in centriacinar emphysema, but without destruction of tissue, inflammation or scarring. There is carbon pigmentation at the centre of the secondary lobules with dust adjacent to the emphysematous spaces. The changes are seen throughout the whole lung. The prevalence has declined over the last 30 years.

Panacinar emphysema

The whole acinus is affected with destruction of tissue. There is total disorganization of the acini which are replaced by large irregular thin walled airspaces. This change is typical of α_1-antitrypsin deficiency.

Distal acinar emphysema

The least common form, present in the periphery of the acinus, often alongside septa (paraseptal emphysema). Usually seen in the sub-pleural posterior margins of the upper lobes, with scarring; it can cause spontaneous pneumothorax.

Irregular emphysema

The commonest and clinically least significant type, associated with scarring with no disturbance of lung function unless severe.

Effects of emphysema on lung function
- loss of elastic recoil decreases the force of expiration
- greater narrowing of small airways in expiration
- loss of surface area available for gas exchange.

....

CLINICOPATHOLOGICAL CORRELATES OF COAD

Obstruction to airflow can give rise to under-ventilation with resultant ventilation–perfusion mismatch causing hypoxaemia.

Effects of hypoxaemia on the pulmonary circulation

Constriction of pulmonary arterioles with a resultant rise in pulmonary artery pressure. If this is sustained there is right ventricular hypertrophy and eventual right-sided cardiac failure (cor pulmonale). The main pulmonary artery may resemble the aorta, with thickened walls and atheromatous change (fatty streaks and plaques). There is muscular hypertrophy of smaller vessels with fibrosis. The pulmonary veins also show arterialization (medial hypertrophy and the appearance of an internal and external elastic lamina).

The 'Blue Bloater' and the 'Pink Puffer'

In severe COAD the hypoxic stimulus to respiration can be reduced. Patients develop pulmonary hypertension, secondary polycythaemia and cor pulmonale, resulting in cyanosis, and CO_2 retention – the 'blue bloater'. Treatment with O_2 may reduce the hypoxic drive further and worsen the CO_2 retention to cause a respiratory acidosis. Where there is a predominance of emphysema the respiratory drive is maintained but dyspneoea is an early feature – the 'pink puffer'.

Other associations with COAD

- Weight loss: 25% patients with COAD show loss of lean body mass and fat. The underlying mechanism is unclear.
- Diaphragmatic changes: in emphysema the diaphragm area and mass are reduced, with flattening of the diaphragm seen on X-ray.
- Peptic ulceration: there is a prevalence of duodenal and gastric ulceration of around 15–43%. This is related possibly to high levels of CO_2 stimulating gastric acid secretion. Alternatively COAD patients are likely to smoke.
- CNS effects of hypercapnia: increased cerebral blood flow and raised CSF pressure have been reported, with drowsiness, and a 'flapping' hand tremor.

ASTHMA

Episodes of widespread airways narrowing (hyper-reactivity) associated with wheeze. There is muscle spasm, airway inflammation, oedema and increased mucus production.

Macroscopy Autopsy studies show over-inflated lungs that do not collapse on opening the chest, indicating air entrapment. The cut surface shows sticky plugs of mucus obstructing small and medium sized airways.

Microscopy The airways are blocked by non-sulphated mucins mixed with a proteinaceous serous inflammatory exudate, containing eosinophils and desquamated respiratory columnar cells. The mucosa is damaged with marked oedema and detachment of epithelial cells. Regenerating cells are frequently non-ciliated and the sub-epithelial basement membrane is thickened. The sub-mucosa is oedematous, congested with an inflammatory infiltrate of lymphocytes and eosinophils. There is hyperplasia of mucous glands and smooth muscle hypertrophy in the bronchial wall.

Examination of sputum
- Charcot–Leyden crystals – colourless hexagonal crystals derived from eosinophil granules, containing lysophospholipase
- Curschmann spirals (twisted casts of airways)
- Creola bodies (clusters of respiratory cells).

Clinical features
Increasing in prevalence especially in the 2nd decade of life; commoner in developed countries.

Extrinsic asthma

Associated with atopy and increased levels of IgE (bound to mast cells). Exposure to specific allergens causes an immediate reaction (muscle spasm) and a delayed reaction (mucosal inflammation and oedema). The former response is blocked by antihistamine, the latter reduced by corticosteroids and chromoglycate.

Intrinsic asthma

Patients are not atopic, and the asthma is provoked by widely disparate triggers ranging from exercise, cold air, emotion and certain drugs.

Triggering factors

Ninety per cent of asthmatic children are atopic with excessive levels of IgE. Exposure to the allergen (e.g. house dust, house-dust mite, pollens, fungal spores or, certain foods including milk, eggs, fish, cereals, nuts and, chocolate) causes release of mast cell contents by binding to specific IgE receptors. As well as bronchospasm sufferers frequently experience dermatitis, rhinitis and conjunctivitis.

BRONCHIECTASIS

The permanent abnormal dilatation of the bronchi. The prevalence was difficult to define before the introduction of modern imaging techniques and was estimated at 1.5 per 1000 population in the UK in the 1950s. It appears to have fallen markedly in the West because of effective vaccination against measles and whooping cough, effective treatment of childhood respiratory infections and a fall in fibrocaseous TB.

Aetiology and pathogenesis

1. Increased dragging forces on the bronchial wall. The lung is maintained in an expanded state from negative intrapleural pressure. This effect is far greater if adjacent lung parenchyma has collapsed, or is scarred, causing the bronchus to dilate. Collapse is seen:

   - in infection with airway obliteration (e.g. in non-specific bronchopneumonia and viral bronchiolitis)
   - compression by tumour or an enlarged lymph node
   - obstructing foreign bodies.

   Accumulation of secretions may contribute. Chronic lung infections may result in loss of lung parenchyma which also increases this effect.

2. Post-inflammatory weakening of the bronchial wall. In its most severe form there is damage and loss of cartilage in the bronchial wall. Severe infections are associated with this change, especially when there is disturbed mucociliary clearance as in Kartagener's syndrome and cystic fibrosis.

Structural changes

Third- and fourth-order airways are the most affected; larger airways being protected by thicker cartilage.

- infection typically affects basal segments. In cystic fibrosis the changes are generalized. The hilar regions are damaged in allergic bronchopulmonary aspergillosis.
- the bronchi can show a uniform cylindrical dilatation, fusiform or saccular changes. The appearances are unrelated to the cause or functional disturbance. The dilated bronchus continues to the pleural surface.
- the lumen contains pus with marked mucosal non-specific inflammatory changes, including extensive ulceration leaving a surface of fibrous or granulation tissue. Prominent lymphoid follicles may be present (follicular bronchiectasis).
- bronchial arteries show muscular hypertrophy and develop anastomotic connections with pulmonary arteries.
- infection and necrosis of the bronchi may extend into adjacent lung parenchyma causing an abscess cavity.

Complications

- infections with increased production of purulent sputum
- empyema
- colonization by fungi (e.g. *Aspergillus fumigatus*) within the cavity, to form a ball like mass – aspergilloma
- cor pulmonale
- massive haemoptysis, often from bronchial artery anastamoses
- metastatic abscess
- amyloidosis: reactive systemic type, sometimes causing the nephrotic syndrome and eventual renal failure.

RESTRICTIVE VENTILATORY IMPAIRMENT

Characterized by increased stiffness or loss of compliance of lung parenchyma; the ratio of FEV_1/FVC remains normal. The patient develops dyspnoea and a chronic cough. These changes are seen in:

- scarring (fibrosis)
- cellular infiltration
- interstitial oedema.

Localized scarring

At apex as in TB, rupture of emphysematous bullae or in relation to old infarcts.

Two patterns of widespread scarring are seen:

- involving the lung bases: diffuse alveolar damage, cryptogenic fibrosing alveolitis, chronic oedema, asbestosis
- sparing the lung bases: sarcoidosis, extrinsic allergic alveolitis, silicosis, berylliosis, Langerhans cell histiocytosis.

The scarring can be:

- intra-alveolar (fibroblasts migrating through basement membrane defects)
- interstitial
- obliterative (lumina of several adjacent airspaces are effaced, e.g. paraquat poisoning).

With extensive and advanced scarring these patterns are lost and the lung shows numerous cystic spaces – 'honeycomb lung'.

....

INTERSTITIAL LUNG DISEASES

Cryptogenic fibrosing alveolitis (idiopathic pulmonary fibrosis)

A chronic inflammatory disorder starting as an alveolitis and ending as severe interstitial fibrosis of unknown aetiology.

Clinical features

Prevalence 3–5 per 100 000 population, usually 50–60 years age, aggressive course with death 3–6 years from presentation. Physical examination shows clubbing and fine crackles are present over the lung bases on auscultation.

Pathological features

Two histological patterns are described:

- usual interstitial pneumonitis (UIP) – damage to alveolar walls
- desquamative interstitial pneumonitis (DIP) – accumulation of inflammatory cells in the alveolus.

Both now are regarded as variants of a single disease. DIP shows a good response to steroids and is less likely to progress to endstage fibrosis.

Microscopy

Increased numbers of inflammatory cells, especially neutrophils, are seen with damage to the alveolar wall. Loss of type 1 alveolar cells is seen with proliferation of type 2 cells, and expansion of the interstitial matrix with increased numbers of fibroblasts, myofibroblasts and smooth muscle. In its early stages the alveolar architecture is maintained; with time there is marked disturbance of airspaces with thickened distorted walls and the development of pulmonary hypertension.

Pathogenesis

The changes are a result of cellular damage and repair caused by secretory activity of activated macrophages. Neutrophils are recruited, with release of free radicals and proteolytic enzymes (e.g. elastase) causing damage, together with production of growth factors (e.g. fibronectin, PDGF) in the repair process.

Extrinsic allergic alveolitis

A chronic granulomatous disease caused by organic dusts (bacteria, fungi and animal proteins) acting as foreign antigens. Examples include farmer's lung, detergent packers' lung and birdfanciers' lung.

Clinical features

Presentation varies from sudden onset of symptoms (fever, rigor, cough, dyspnoea and haemoptysis) after exposure to the antigen, to an insidious history of increasing shortness of breath. Lung function shows a restrictive pattern, and an impaired diffusion capacity. Specific antibodies to the precipitating allergen are present in the serum.

Microscopy

Small non-caseating epithelioid granulomas, an interstitial pneumonitis (macrophages, lymphocytes and plasma cells), bronchiolar obstruction from mucosal ulceration and an ingrowth of granulation tissue. Foamy macrophages are present in the alveolar airspaces.

Natural history

In the absence of further allergen exposure the granulomas resolve after 6 months. The inflammation leads to scarring, predominantly affecting the upper lobes.

Sarcoidosis

A multi-system granulomatous disease of unknown aetiology. Lesions can be found at any site but the lungs are most often affected, with irreversible loss of lung function in 20–25% cases, and death in 5–10%. There is a decrease in lung volume and diffusing capacity, and often some airflow obstruction.

Epidemiology

Commonest in Sweden and black populations in the US.

Clinical features

Insidious onset with weight loss, fatigue, weakness, fever, erythema nodosum, dry cough and dyspnoea. Four patterns are seen according to chest X-ray findings:

Type 0: No obvious thoracic involvement.
Type 1: Bilateral hilar lymphadenopathy.
Type 2: Hilar lymphadenopathy with pulmonary parenchymal infiltrate.

Type 3: Parenchymal infiltrate without hilar lymph-adenopathy, seen typically in advanced cases with associated fibrosis.

Pathological features

Most cases show circumscribed, non-caseating granulomas, in alveolar walls, bronchioles and blood vessels. Interstitial fibrosis is seen in 25% cases. This rarely causes lung destruction and associated remodelling.

Studies of the alveolar cell population suggest there is activation of the T helper cell population. The blood however shows a lymphopaenia with a shift to T suppressor cells. Alveolar macrophages also appear to be activated with a resultant rise in serum angiotensin-converting enzyme ACE activity and hypercalcaemia from macrophage overexpression of 1α-hydroxylase. Although the increased ACE activity is not specific for sarcoid it provides a means of monitoring the disease activity.

Pulmonary histiocytosis X (eosinophilic granuloma)

One of a set of diseases characterized by the proliferation of Langerhans cells, which are involved with processing and presentation of antigens to lymphocytes. Ultrastructural studies show the presence of the Birbeck granule (X body) – a pentilaminar cytoplasmic inclusion.

Clinical features

A rare condition seen in young adults (20–40 years) associated with cigarette smoking. There is a non-productive cough, exertional dyspnoea and sometimes chest pain and fever. On chest X-ray small irregular nodules are seen in the upper and mid-zones. Lung function shows a mixed obstructive–restrictive pattern.

Pathological features

A cellular infiltrate is seen in the walls and lumina of alveoli, and around airways and vessels in the interlobular septa. There are collections of Langerhans cells admixed with eosinophils, and pigment-laden macrophages with scarring are seen in later lesions.

Natural history

The disease follows a variable course, some patients showing a rapid progression and others appearing to resolve spontaneously.

Pulmonary lymphangioleiomyomatosis

A rare disorder of females seen in reproductive life. There is a proliferation of immature smooth muscle throughout the lung derived from walls of lymphatic vessels. Patients show a progressive decline in respiratory function, spontaneous pneumothorax, chylous pleural effusions and pulmonary haemorrhage. May have a hormonal basis; progression is halted after the menopause.

....

PULMONARY OEDEMA (INCLUDING ADULT RESPIRATORY DISTRESS SYNDROME)

Oedema occurs with an increase in hydrostatic intra-capillary pressure and/or an increase in capillary permeability. Oedema is seen with more than 4–5 ml fluid/gm dry blood-free tissue.

High pressure pulmonary oedema

Cardiac causes

Left ventricular failure, ventricular and supra-ventricular tachycardias, pulmonary venous hypertension as in mitral valve disease, constrictive pericarditis.

Other causes

Severe anaemia, intravenous fluid overload, veno-occlusive disease, cerebral injury (related to raised intracranial pressure, sympathetic activity, release of catecholamines, pressure load on left ventricle), renal failure (related to sodium retention, hypertension), high altitude.

Cardiogenic pulmonary oedema

Clinical features

Shortness of breath, orthopnoea, cough with frothy pink sputum and paroxysmal nocturnal dyspnoea. Auscultation shows bilateral basal crepitations. The interstitial and intra-alveolar oedema reduces lung compliance and effective lung volume. There is hypoxaemia, and frequently a metabolic acidosis related to poor tissue perfusion.

Pathological features

At post-mortem the lungs are reddened, heavy and wet. Pink, granular fluid is seen within alveolar spaces, and in longstanding cases haemosiderin-laden macrophages are present from intra-alveoloar haemorrhage. There can also be interstitial fibrosis.

Increased capillary permeability: adult respiratory distress syndrome (diffuse alveolar damage, shock lung)

Seen after severe damage to alveolar capillary endothelium with a consequent rise in permeability.

Clinical features

- refractory hypoxaemia
- reduced lung compliance
- normal pulmonary capillary wedge pressure
- normal plasma oncotic pressure.

The syndrome resembles infantile respiratory distress syndrome. There is a 60–65% mortality. Conditions associated with ARDS include gastric aspiration, disseminated intravascular coagulation, pneumonia, trauma, multiple transfusions and bacteraemia.

Pre-clinical phase

Microvascular injury takes place, mediated by activation of neutrophils, platelets producing injurious free radicals and complement.

Acute phase

There is flooding of alveolar spaces with a protein-rich oedema fluid which disturbs gas exchange. The lungs become heavy, red and airless. Microscopy shows widening of alveolar septa from oedema, also present in alveoli, admixed with red cells. Endothelial and type I pneumocytes are swollen, indicative of injury. Hyaline membranes appear within the terminal airways 1–2 days after the oedema consisting of cellular debris, fibrin and glycoprotein.

Repair phase

Starts 2–3 days after the onset of acute phase. There is replacement of alveolar lining cells by proliferating type 2 pneumocytes, together with proliferation of fibroblasts within the interstitium and extending into and obliterating airspaces.

PNEUMONIA

Acute inflammation of lung parenchyma, caused by living micro-organisms, with filling of alveoli by inflammatory exudate: 'consolidation'.

Clinical features

- Commonest infective cause of death in the UK: 56 deaths/100 000 population.
- Predilection for the elderly.
- **Community acquired** cases seen in the elderly and the very young.
- *Nosocomial* infections in hospital: cause of death in 0.5–5% of hospital admissions. A special problem after surgery and in intensive care, related to intubation, immune suppression and changes in flora from antibiotic treatment.
- Considerable cause of morbidity and mortality in deprived Third World children (5×10^6 deaths worldwide/ year)

Classification

This takes account of:

Causal organism   Bacteria, *Mycoplasma*, viruses, protozoa.

Immune status   Healthy individuals susceptible to *Streptococcus pneumoniae*; post-viral infection: *Staphylococcus aureus* and *S. pneumoniae* in COAD: *Haemophilus influenzae*.

Opportunistic pneumonia is seen in the immune suppressed (cytotoxic agents, immunosuppressive drugs and

HIV infection): *Pneumocystis carinii, Toxoplasmosis*, fungi, mycobacteria and viruses.

Defects of neutrophils (numbers or function): infection from normal oral flora, Gram-negative bacilli (*Klebsiella*) and fungi.

Defects in antibody formation: *Strep. pneumoniae* and *Haemophilus* infections.

Anatomical distribution of inflammatory process

- *Lobar* one or more lobes involved by a **confluent** inflammatory process, spreading in infected oedema fluid through alveoli.
- *Broncho-pneumonia* Focal inflammation which remains localized on the airways. Affects the young and elderly. Many contributing factors including post-viral infections, COAD, cystic fibrosis, aspiration, suppression of cilia activity and a suppressed cough reflex from anaesthesia.

As both patterns can be seen with the same organism it is possible that rapid mobilization of neutrophils contains the infection in broncho-pneumonia and the production of infected oedema fluid favours lobar pneumonia.

....

SPECIFIC MICROBIOLOGICAL TYPES OF PNEUMONIA

Pneumococcal (lobar) pneumonia

Gram-positive diplococcus – *Streptococcus pneumoniae*; 82 different antigenic sub-types, based on the polysaccharide capsule. The capsule protects against phagocytosis, conferring pathogenicity (type III is the most virulent). Diagnosis is established from culture and identification of 'pneumococcal' antigen in serum by immunoelectrophoresis.

Clinical features

Commoner in males, and with increasing age.

Rapid onset with fever, unilateral sharp stabbing pain (pleuritic), rapid shallow breathing, prominent cough with 'rusty' sputum.

Pathological changes

Before the introduction of antibiotics four stages were typically seen:

Congestion   At post-mortem the cut surface of the lung is wet with frothy bloodstained fluid. Microscopy shows a marked increase in blood flow in alveolar capillaries with oedema fluid within alveolar airspaces. Gram-staining is positive for pneumococci.

Red hepatization   The lung is firm, 'meaty' and airless, with a pleural fibrinous exudate. The lung cut surface is dry. Microscopy shows a coagulative inflammatory exudate with fibrin and neutrophils within airspaces.

Grey hepatization   The lung becomes grey-red in colour: reduced blood flow, and continuing migration of inflammatory cells.

Resolution   Lysis of fibrin, restoring functional normality with a generalized inprovement in the clinical condition 8–9 days after onset of illness. If lysis is incomplete organization occurs with scarring.

Complications
* abscess formation
* empyema
* failure of resolution (scarring).

Legionella pneumonia

First recognized in 1976, lobar distribution, caused by a minute coccobacillus, staining poorly by Gram, but demonstrable by immunocytochemical techniques. Culture is difficult, but the organism can be recovered from bronchial washings, pleural fluid, lung biopsy and blood.

The organisms are ubiquitous in warm, moist conditions; outbreaks may be caused by infected aerosols from air-conditioner heat exchangers and shower heads. Debilitated and immunosuppressed patients are particularly susceptible.

Pathological changes
Closely parallel those seen in pneumococcal lobar pneumonia.

Staphylococcal pneumonia

Frequently seen as a post-viral complication. Spread to the lung occurs by inhalation or via the bloodstream (from skin abrasions, venepuncture sites and from bacterial endocarditis).

Pathological changes

The lungs are heavy and congested, with multiple centrilobular suppurative foci, often forming abscesses. Rupture of sub-pleural abscesses cause empyema.

Complications

Scarring, bronchiectasis, pneumatoceles (air-filled cysts).

Klebsiella pneumonia

A frequent commensal in the oral cavity, especially with poor oral hygiene. Diabetics and the elderly are susceptible. Increased frequency of infection may be related to wide-pread antibiotic use.

Pathological features

A confluent lobar pneumonia, often right-sided and uni-lateral. The organism has a mucoid capsule, and the consol-idated tissue is slimy, often with abscess and necrosis formation.

....

LUNG ABSCESS

A local area of suppuration walled off by a membrane com-posed of fibrin and granulation tissue. An abscess is likely to involve several airways, unlike bronchiectasis which is centred on a single airway.

- *Primary abscess* No preceding inflammatory conditions, a result of aspiration of infected oropharyngeal material, particularly with loss of consciousness, dysphagia and oesophageal dysfunction. Causative organisms include mixed anaerobes from the oral cavity, *Bacteroides* and *Strep. milleri*.

- *Secondary abscess* Related to obstruction, foreign objects, bronchiectasis, pneumonias and bronchial carcinoma.

Natural history

Spontaneous rupture into a bronchus can result in improvement or spread throughout the bronchial tree. The cavity may become walled off to form a cyst or develop into a pneumatocoele.

NEOPLASMS OF THE LUNG

PRIMARY MALIGNANT NEOPLASMS

Epidemiology
- rare 30–40 years ago
- largest cancer cause of death in the UK: 35 000 deaths/year
- 30% of all male cancer deaths
- male: female ratio: previously 7:1, now 2:1
- rise in incidence in women parallels increase in numbers of female smokers.

Aetiological factors

Cigarette smoking
- Case-control studies: Mortality is related to duration of smoking and number of cigarettes smoked. Greater risk with cigarette smoking compared with pipe smoking. No difference between urban and rural dwellers.
- On stopping smoking lung cancer death rate falls, taking 10–15 years for the risk to equate with non-smokers.
- Increased risk in passive smokers.
- Autopsy studies show a high prevalence of squamous metaplasia, with dysplasia. The latter is thought to be a precursor lesion.
- Analysis of cigarette smoke:

Tar phase components:

- polycyclic hydrocarbons – known to induce skin tumours experimentally

— nitrosamines, cadmium, nickel and polonium-210, all believed to be carcinogenic.

Gas phase components: large numbers of free radicals, including nitric oxide, hydrazine, nickel carbonyl, vinyl chloride and nitrosodiethylamine – all are carcinogenic.

Environmental and occupational factors

- Risk is greater in industrialized urban areas.
- Asbestos exposure amplifies the effects of smoking.
- Petrochemicals (polycyclic hydrocarbons).
- Organic compounds: mustard gas, vinyl chloride, chloromethyl ether. The risk is related to the total dose, and most tumours are small cell.
- Metal refining/smelting: nickel, chromium and cadmium.
- Arsenic: vineyard workers exposed to arsenical insecticides.
- Ionizing radiation: radon exposure in miners.
- Diet: low intake of vitamin E and β-carotene (antioxidants) may increase the risk of lung cancer.

Molecular changes

ras oncogenes (H-*ras*, K-*ras*, N-*ras*) are activated in human lung cancer. They code for G proteins, a cell membrane protein which transduces growth signals. Thirty per cent of lung adenocarcinomas show a point mutation of K-*ras*, which appears to correlate with a poorer prognosis. Amplification of c-*myc* has been described in small cell carcinoma.

Chromosomal deletions

Small cell carcinoma shows deletion of the short arm of chromosome 3 – possibly a tumour suppressor gene.

Classification of lung cancer

The purpose of classification is to define sub-types with better or worse prognosis, and establish appropriate treatment protocols (see Table 33.2). A crucial distinction is between small cell (a greater propensity for early spread) and non-small cell carcinoma.

Table 33.2 WHO classification of lung cancer

25–40%	Squamous carcinoma

15–25%	Small cell carcinoma
	    a) oat cell
	    b) intermediate cell type
	    c) combined

30–50%	Adenocarcinoma
	    a) acinar adenocarcinoma
	    b) papillary adenocarcioma
	    c) bronchioloalveolar adenocarcinoma
	    d) solid carcinoma with mucin

10–20%	Large cell carcinoma
	    a) giant cell
	    b) clear cell
	Adenosquamous carcinoma
	Carcinoid
	Bronchial gland carcinoma
	    a) adenoid cystic
	    b) mucoepidermoid
	Others

Staging

Staging is essential for defining treatment and giving a prognosis. Surgical resection offers the best option for survival but 66% cases are inoperable at diagnosis.

Intrathoracic staging

- Assessment of history and clinical findings, e.g. superior vena caval obstruction indicates mediastinal spread.
- Imaging techniques: mediastinal nodal disease indicates inoperable disease. CT scanning has a sensitivity of 80–94% compared with mediastinoscopy and lymph node sampling. A negative CT scan has a predictive value of 90–95%. Mediastinoscopy is performed less frequently now because of imaging.
- Any pleural effusion should be drained for cytological examination.

Extrathoracic staging

- Clinical examination may show obvious extrathoracic spread from organ enlargement, or clinical signs. Metastatic deposits in palpable lymph nodes can be confirmed by fine needle aspiration for cytology.

- Biochemical screening may produce evidence of likely spread, e.g. a low serum albumin is suggestive of disseminated disease. Hypercalcaemia can indicate bony metastatic disease (or secretion of parathyroid hormone-related peptide by squamous carcinoma).

Pathological staging

The most accurate assessment of intrathoracic spread comes from careful examination of resected specimens. Mediastinal lymph node involvement carries a poor prognosis.

....

CLINICAL FEATURES OF LUNG CANCER

Local spread

Intrapulmonary spread

Can cause cough (irritation of bronchial receptors), haemoptysis (erosion of blood vessels), airway obstruction (wheeze/ stridor, pneumonia and bronchiectasis), chest pain.

Spread to adjacent structures

- Pleura (pleural effusion).
- Invasion of nerves:

  - recurrent laryngeal nerve: hoarseness
  - phrenic nerve: diaphragmatic paralysis
  - brachial plexus: shoulder and arm pain and weakness
  - involvement of the sympathetic plexus: Horner's syndrome – unilateral constriction of pupil, ptosis, enophthalmos and loss of sweating)
  - Pancoast's syndrome encompasses brachial plexus involvement and Horner's syndrome.

- Mediastinum: compression of the superior vena cava causes facial congestion, oedema and distended veins of the neck and chest.
- Chest wall: chest pain.
- Pericardium: pericardial effusion and cardiac tamponade.

Distant spread

The clinical effects depend on the sites of secondary deposits.

Paraneoplastic syndromes

These are systemic abnormalities unrelated to tumour spread, mediated by tumour derived chemical signals (see Table 33.3). Small cell carcinoma is most frequently associated with ectopic hormone production, and cases show a shorter survival period.

Pathology of lung cancers

Squamous carcinoma

Bronchoscopy may show an exophytic, cauliflower-like mass. The right lung and the upper lobes are more often affected, except with asbestosis-related cases, where the lower lobes are involved. Growth into the airway causes obstruction with collapse of the distal segment, associated with infection, bronchiectasis and endogenous lipoid pneumonia (accumulation of intra-alveolar lipid laden macrophages). Central cavitation is seen in large tumours, sometimes mistaken for an abscess on chest X-ray. Extension to the pericardium or pleura is seen, and mediastinal metastasis is present in 50% cases.

They arise centrally in the larger airways, often grossly visible with a friable grey cut surface

Table 33.3 Paraneoplastic syndromes

Syndromes	
Non-endocrine	Weight loss, fever, loss of appetite
Dermatolgical	Acanthosis nigricans, dermatomyositis, tylosis (hyperkeratos of palms and soles)
Vascular	Thrombophlebitis migrans, non-infective thrombotic endocarditis, disseminated intravascular coagulation
Skeletal	Clubbing, hypertrophic osteoarthropathy
CNS	Cerebellar syndrome, peripheral neuropathies, myaesthenia gravis and encephalopathy
Endocrine and neuro-endocrine	Cushing's syndrome, inappropriate ADH secretion, hypercalcaemia, gynaecomastia.

Microscopic examination reveals islands of cells, sometimes showing keratinization. Squamous differentiation can be confirmed with immunocytochemical staining for cytokeratins 4, 10 and 13, as well as involucrin (a precursor protein of the protein envelope).

Small cell carcinoma

Aggressive behaviour with early dissemination. Often associated with paraneoplastic syndrome. Small to medium-sized cells (3–5 times the size of a lymphocyte) with little cytoplasm. The nuclei appear packed together (nuclear moulding). Immunocytochemical investigation reveals evidence of neuroendocrine differentiation – neuron-specific enolase (NSE) and neural protein PGP 9.5 positive. Antibodies to low molecular weight cytokeratins also positive.

Electron microscopy   Small cytoplasmic granules with a dense core and clear halo.

Combined small cell carcinoma   Seen in resected material, the small cells are seen together with squamous cell carcinoma or adenocarcinoma.

Adenocarcinoma

These arise peripherally, sometimes seen in association with central scarring and dust pigment.

Microscopy shows mucin production or the presence of tubular/papillary structures.

The possibility of metastatic deposits from e.g. pancreas, ovary and kidney must be considered and excluded. Multiple tumours favour metastasis; hilar lymph nodes and significant scarring associated with a single tumour favour primary lung origin.

Bronchioloalveolar carcinoma

A highly differentiated adenocarcinoma arising in the peripheral lung beyond the bronchi, with growth upon the walls of pre-existing alveoli.

Microscopy shows 'alveolar colonization' – mucin-secreting carcinoma cells along alveolar septa with no stromal reaction to spread throughout the lung.

Large cell carcinoma

Applied to those cases where neither squamous nor glandular differentiation is apparent on light microscopy. The tumour cells are frequently large, with much cytoplasm, and large irregular nuclei, sometimes with giant cell forms.

....

OTHER PRIMARY EPITHELIAL TUMOURS OF THE LUNG

Carcinoid tumours

These are derived from cells from the diffuse neuroendocrine system, found in the surface epithelium and bronchial glands characterized by neurosecretory granules containing steroid and peptide hormones (e.g. 5-HT, bombesin, calcitonin and ACTH). They account for 1–2% of primary lung neoplasms, seen at a younger age, with no sex difference and no relation to smoking or environmental pollution.

Macroscopic features   Central or peripheral location, with a well-defined edge, growing into the lumen (sometimes causing obstruction) and into adjacent lung. The cut surface is yellow.

Microscopic features   A monotonous cell population with regular nuclei, small nucleoli, and clear or granular cytoplasm. The growth pattern can be 'packeted', or show intertwining cords and ribbons of cells, separated by intervening fibrous tissue septa carrying delicate blood vessels. Lung carcinoids derived from the embryological foregut show *argyrophilia*, and are positive to neuro-endocrine immunocytochemical markers (NSE, PGP 9.5 and chromogranin).

Clinical behaviour   Carcinoids are potentially malignant but rarely metastasize. Atypical carcinoids (characterized by pleomorphic nuclei, coarse chromatin, prominent nucleoli, tumour necrosis and a high mitotic rate) are more aggressive, 70% showing metastasis.

Adenochondroma (chondroid hamartoma)

A well-defined mass composed of cartilage and containing clefts lined by bland cuboidal epithelial cells. Formerly regarded as hamartomas, classified now as benign tumours of connective tissue, with entrapped epithelial structures.

THE PNEUMOCONIOSES

Legally defined as permanent alteration of lung structure from inhalation of mineral dusts and subsequent tissue reactions.

Mechanisms of injury

Changes in the lung range from:

- focal collection of dust-laden macrophages
- massive local fibrosis
- diffuse fibrosis with and without cavitation.

The reaction depends on:

- intrinsic properties of the dust
- amount and duration of dust exposure
- individual idiosyncratic and immune responsiveness.

The dust particle is engulfed by resident macrophages. In large numbers the clearance mechanism may be overwhelmed with accumulation of macrophages. Proliferating type I pneumocytes grow over the nodule separating it from the lumen which can be partially occluded. A fine reticulin network appears between the macrophages, which can progress to broad bands of collagen.

....

ASBESTOS-RELATED DISEASE

Asbestos may be defined as fibrous silicates with fire-resisting properties used in a wide range of products including asbestos cement, floor tiles, brake linings, wicks and lagging. It exists in two forms: serpentine (curly fibres) and amphibole (straight). Serpentine fibres (chrysotile) tend to break into smaller fragments whereas the amphiboles (crocidolite, amosite, tremolite) remain intact.

Inhalation of asbestos fibres

The ultimate destination within the lung is the parietal pleura. Penetration of the fibre depends on the cross-sectional surface area; the curly serpentine fibres penetrate less than amphiboles and appear to cause less damage. Straight fibres of 50–100 μm reach the alveoli; longer fibres are deposited in respiratory bronchioles and alveolar ducts.

Once deposited the fibres are ingested by macrophages and cleared via the lymphatics or the muco-ciliary escalator (chrysotile more so than the amphiboles).

Asbestos bodies Amphibole fibres coated in yellow/brown iron-containing protein, highlighted by Perl's stain for iron. Many more uncoated asbestos fibres are present in the lung but cannot be seen on conventional light microscopy. Up to 100 000 000 amphibole fibres are present per gram of dried lung tissue.

Pathological changes after exposure

- asbestosis – a type of interstitial fibrosis
- benign pleural disease – pleural plaques and diffuse thickening
- mesothelioma
- lung carcinoma.

Asbestosis

Fibrosis affecting the lower lobes, with associated fibrous thickening of the pleura. It can develop up to 20 years after exposure, or as little as 5 years after substantial continuous exposure. As with other interstitial lung diseases there is reduced compliance and ventilation–perfusion mismatch.

Pathogenesis Like other interstitial lung disease there is activation of pulmonary macrophages, release of cytokines, free radicals and growth factors causing cell damage and scarring.

Pathological changes The earliest change is septal scarring of alveolar walls with increased numbers of septal and intra-alveolar macrophages, and type 2 pneumocytes. Sub-pleural areas show severe changes of disturbance of lung architecture with honeycombing.

Grading This depends on the amount of lung involved (A – none, B – < 25%, C – 25–50%, D – > 50%) and the severity of distortion of lung architecture (0 – none to 4 – severe).

Benign pleural disease

Pleural plaques are markers of asbestos exposure. They appear as shiny white thickened plaques on the parietal pleura. Histological examination shows an increase in dense collagen fibres. Diffuse thickening is also seen which involves the visceral pleura, encasing the lung.

Malignant mesothelioma

A malignant neoplasm arising from the mesothelium, first recognized in the 1950s, closely associated with asbestos exposure. Males are more commonly affected, possibly related to occupational exposure. It is seen from 50–70 years of age, after a long latent period following exposure.

Amphiboles are more dangerous than serpentine fibres, and crocidolite is the most dangerous amphibole. Mesothelioma is also associated with exposure to another fibrous silicate: zeolite.

Pathological features The tumour arises from either visceral or parietal pleura, forming a thick white layer. The lung is encased by the tumour causing a restrictive ventilatory defect. The prognosis is poor and metastasis to lymph nodes, kidney, liver and CNS is well recognized.

Four histological patterns are recognized:

- tubulopapillary (epithelial)
- sarcomatous (spindle cells, producing collagen)
- undifferentiated (polygonal cells)
- mixed patterns.

The epithelial type resembles adenocarcinoma, but may be distinguished by immunocytochemical techniques (absence of epithelial markers) and demonstrating long slender microvilli by EM.

COAL MINERS' PNEUMOCONIOSIS

Formerly a significant problem with up to 3000 miners diagnosed each year with occupationally related lung disease. Following introduction of preventative measures this has fallen to around 400 cases in the UK.

Development of pneumoconiosis depends on the length and intensity of exposure, and the nature of the coal dust. High-rank coal contains more carbon and less mineral than low-rank coal; it is more toxic to macrophages and appears to carry a greater risk of pneumoconiosis. The risk from low-rank coal depends on its mineral content.

Simple pneumoconiosis

Usually does not cause symptoms; it is recognized from small black macules, 2–5 mm in size on the pleural surface and in the lung cut surface. Microscopically there are aggregates of dust-laden macrophages at the centre of the acinus, sometimes with associated mild centriacinar emphysema. Fibrogenic dusts cause the development of collagen-containing nodules that become palpable (typically from low-rank coals with a high mineral content).

Complicated pneumoconiosis (progressive massive fibrosis)

Characterized by well-demarcated, hard, rubbery black collagen-rich nodules greater than 10 mm in size. The lesions are single or multiple, often in the upper lobes towards the posterior aspect. If close to the periphery there is marked puckering and scarring. Some lesions show central necrosis with cavitation. Microscopically there is a haphazard proliferation of fibrous connective tissue with dust-filled macrophages and inflammatory cells at the periphery. The lesions may develop from fusion of small individual nodules (low-rank coal) or enlargement of a single nodule (high-rank coal).

Caplans' syndrome

First described in coalminers with rheumatoid disease, exposed to a relatively low dust burden, showing nodular lung lesions. The nodules are sub-pleural, up to 50 mm diameter and contain concentric layers of dust. They otherwise resemble large rheumatoid nodules. These changes are also seen in rheumatoid patients exposed to silica dusts other than coal.

....

SILICOSIS

A severe disabling chronic disease from inhalation of crystalline silica (silicon dioxide); amorphous silica is harmless. Following engulfment in the macrophage there is disruption of lysosomes, release of enzymes and cellular breakdown with release of the silica particle, and so the process repeats itself. The lung develops numerous nodules, 2–6 mm in diameter, which become hyalinized with time. There is scarring and thickening of the pleura. Exposure to silica is a predisposing factor for tuberculosis. Clinical features include worsening exertional dyspnoea, with cough and weight loss in late stages.

DISORDERS OF THE PULMONARY CIRCULATION

....

PULMONARY EMBOLISM (PE)

- 50 000 deaths/annum in the US
- autopsy studies show pulmonary embolism in at least 10% unselected cases.

Source of emboli

Venous thrombi in the lower limbs (80% in calf veins). Emboli from larger thigh veins and pelvic veins account for most clinically significant episodes.

Clinical features

1. **Massive PE** causing death or severe right ventricular strain, typically seen with at least obstruction of 50% of the pulmonary circulation. Occlusion of either the main pulmonary arteries or the pulmonary trunk can occur, with coiling of a long length of worm-like thrombus seen at autopsy. Sudden death occurs, often with the patient apparently straining at stool. Alternatively there may be severe dyspnoea and a rapid feeble pulse, or cardiovascular collapse. The underlying pathogenesis is not fully understood. As well as the effects of mechanical obstruction release of vasoactive humoral factors e.g. thromboxane A_2, leukotrienes, from platelets that accumulate at the site of impaction may be involved. Blood gas analysis shows a lowered pO_2 with a normal or reduced pCO_2, from ventilation–perfusion mismatch.

2. **Silent embolism** with no clinical effect.

3. **Medium-sized embolism** causing pulmonary infarction, typically seen with obstruction of peripheral arteries. The likelihood of infarction is greater with underlying venous congestion, as in left ventricular failure and mitral valve disease. At autopsy the lung shows a wedge-shaped area deep to the pleura, with the apex at the point of occlusion. The cut surface is firm, and blue–red in colour. Histology may show complete necrosis (complete infarcts), or more usually blood filled airspaces, and viable alveolar walls (incomplete infarcts). Complete infarcts are converted to fibrous scars, incomplete infarcts may resolve completely. Complete infarction is rare, probably because of the dual blood supply that the lung receives via the bronchial vasculature.

4. **Recurrent embolism**: raised pulmonary artery pressure and eventual congestive cardiac failure (cor pulmonale). This manifestation is rare and may be explained by repetitive thrombi causing multiple foci of intimal hyperplasia with eventual small-vessel obstruction, pulmonary hypertension and congestive heart failure.

PULMONARY HYPERTENSION (PH)

Defined as a systolic/diastolic pressure consistently exceeding 30/15 mmHg.

Pathogenetic causes

- hyperkinetic: increased blood flow, e.g. left-to-right shunts in congenital heart disease
- pulmonary venous causes: left-sided heart disease, e.g. left ventricular failure, mitral valve disease, pulmonary veno-occlusive disease
- embolic: thrombo-embolic, parasitic (e.g. schistosomes), tumour emboli
- pulmonary fibrosis
- hypoxia
- plexogenic pulmonary arteriopathy: primary PH and PH with associated liver cirrhosis.

Vascular lesions of pulmonary hypertension
(see Table 33.4)

Pulmonary trunk

Before birth the aorta and pulmonary trunk are identical; by 9 months of age the intima is thinned, with an irregular media and incomplete elastic laminae.

- Congenital PH: retention of 'fetal aorta-like' appearance.
- Later onset PH: smooth muscle hypertrophy with thickening of the media; atherosclerosis seen in the intima.

Table 33.4 Grading of pulmonary vascular lesions

Grade	Pathological features
1	Medial hypertrophy
2	Grade 1 + cellular intimal proliferation
3	Grade 2 + intimal fibrosis
4	Grade 3 + plexiform lesions
5	Grade 4 + dilatation (angiomatoid) lesions
6	Grade 5 + necrotizing arteritis

Conducting arteries

These extend from the pulmonary trunk to vessels of 1 mm diameter, accompanying airways. They show an increase in medial elastic tissue, with numerous elastic laminae. In PH there are lesions of atherosclerosis and medial smooth-muscle hypertrophy.

Muscular arteries

These lie adjacent to the terminal and respiratory bronchioles, and control the pulmonary vascular resistance. The ratio of the medial thickness to the overall vessel diameter should be less than 7%. The following changes are seen:

- Medial hypertrophy – the commonest finding and may be the only change apparent. It is particularly marked with hyperkinetic causes (congenital heart disease) and is less so with thromboembolic causes. Venous medial hypertrophy is also seen with raised pulmonary venous pressure. The ratio of media to external diameter may reach 0.25%.
- Cellular intimal proliferation can be a frequent and prominent finding. Significant amounts of collagen are associated with severe PH.
- Dilatation lesions: typically seen are hyperkinetic PH, primary PH and PH associated with chronic liver disease (cirrhosis). Three patterns are described, all proximal to an occlusive lesion:

  Plexiform: aneurysmal dilatations contained within an elastic lamina layer and filled with cellular connective tissue in which endothelial-lined channels are seen (possible organization of thrombus).
  Simple dilatation lesions: simple aneurysmal sacs.
  Angiomatoid lesions: multiple dilated thin-walled vessels joining a hypertrophied muscular artery with its capillary bed.

- Fibrinoid necrosis/necrotizing angiitis: a rare finding seen with a very high and rapidly rising pulmonary artery pressure. There is necrosis of smooth muscle and accumulation of fibrin with an inflammatory reaction.

Pulmonary arterioles

Normally there is no media, but in PH a muscular media may develop. Table 33.4 gives a grading of pulmonary vascular lesions.

Specific types of pulmonary hypertension

Primary PH

A diagnosis of exclusion, possibly requiring open lung biopsy, which shows changes of severe PH discussed above. A rare condition, more often seen in young females. Thirty per cent of cases have positive serology to anti-nuclear factor, and 10% have Raynaud's disease. Right-heart failure develops with oedema and ascites. Effective treatment is by heart-lung transplantation. A similar picture is seen with liver cirrhosis, sometimes with portal vein thrombosis.

Hypoxic pulmonary vascular disease

Hypoxia causes pulmonary vasoconstriction of the muscular arteries as in:

- COAD
- diseases affecting thoracic movement (e.g. kyphoscoliosis, obesity)
- high altitude hypoxia.

Primary venous hypertension

Mild hypertension is seen with a raised left atrial pressure. The following changes are seen in mitral stenosis:

- arteries: dilatation of pulmonary trunk with atherosclerosis
- muscular arteries: medial hypertrophy and intimal fibrosis, sometimes with thrombosis
- pulmonary arterioles: prominent media
- capillaries: gross dilatation and congestion
- pulmonary veins: medial hypertrophy
- lymphatics: gross dilatation, especially in oedematous interlobar septa at the bases causing Kerley B lines on chest X-ray.

Pulmonary veno-occlusive disease

A rare condition of unknown aetiology affecting children and young adults. There is obliteration of the lumina of pulmonary veins by scarring, associated with marked medial hypertrophy. The vein may no longer be apparent. There is resulting severe interstitial oedema, fibrosis and haemosiderosis (collections of iron-laden macrophages within the alveoli, with encrusted capillary basement membrane material and calcification).

DISORDERS OF THE PLEURA

- Infections in the absence of underlying lung disease.
- Primary neoplasia: malignant mesothelioma.
- Changes secondary to:

  — local inflammatory disease of the lung
  — lung neoplasia
  — systemic disorders, e.g. systemic lupus erythematosus.

PLEURAL EFFUSION

Most pleural disorders are associated with a pleural effusion (> 15 ml), amounting to more than 1 litre. Underlying mechanisms are:

- increased intravascular hydrostatic pressure (e.g. congestive cardiac failure)
- increased vascular permeability (inflammation, leaky vessels associated with tumours)
- decreased plasma oncotic pressure (nephrotic syndrome)
- decreased lymphatic drainage (obstruction/trauma to the thoracic duct, or hilar vessels by tumour).

The effusions are all transudates, except with increased vascular permeability. The type of fluid depends on the relative concentrations of water and protein:

- serous: large amounts of water present, usually non-inflammatory, may be seen in TB, often bilateral
- fibrinous: polymerized fibrin is present on serosal surfaces

- serofibrinous
- purulent
- haemorrhagic: seen with tumour involvement, bleeding diathesis, infection (rickettsial).

Inflammatory effusions are seen with disease in underlying lung, for example tuberculosis, pneumonia, abscess and bronchiectasis. Bacterial seeding can cause an empyema. Pleural infection arises from direct extension, after penetrating injury, sub-phrenic abscess, bacteraemia, oesophageal rupture and after thoracic surgery.

Non-infective causes include pulmonary infarction, rheumatoid disease and systemic lupus erythematosus.

ANATOMY

The oral cavity is lined by stratified squamous epithelium. There is variable keratinization.

CONGENITAL DISORDERS

Major developmental disorders

Hare-lip and cleft palate

Epidemiology   More than 200 types of facial clefts are described. Frequency of 1/800 live births. Commonest is clefting of upper lip (hare-lip) which is unilateral in 80% (left:right 2:1). M:F 3:2. Hare lip may be isolated but in 50% cases is associated with cleft palate. Cleft palate occurs in 1/2500 live births, is more common in females and in 40% is associated with Pierre–Robin syndrome (abnormally small mandible, backward displacement of chin and small tongue which is displaced posteriorly and downwards).

Mechanism   Failure of fusion of facial processes at about the 7th gestational week. Some may be related to lack of TGF-α (tumour necrosis factor-α) gene. Some forms of hare-lip may be inherited in X-linked recessive pattern. Some cases of cleft palate are associated with trisomies 13 and 18.

Hemifacial hypertrophy

Mechanism: Hard and soft tissues (may include teeth and tongue) on one side of face grow more rapidly than on the contralateral side.

Focal abnormalities

Fordyce's granules

Epidemiology   Seen in 50% normal adults.

Macroscopy   Small yellow-white granules on lateral part of vermilion of upper lip or buccal mucosa.

Microscopy   Ectopic sebaceous gland.

Clinical features   Of no clinical significance.

Congenital lip pits

Epidemiology   May be associated with hare-lip, cleft palate and agenesis of second premolars in autosomal dominant fashion or as isolated phenomenon.

Macroscopy   Usually bilateral on lower lip.

Microscopy   Small fistulae connecting mucous gland to overlying epithelium.

Endogenous pigmentation

Melanin pigmentation of lips, oral mucosa and circumoral skin.

Associations   Neurofibromatosis, fibrous dyasplasia of bone, Addison's disease, haemochromatosis and Peutz–Jeghers syndrome.

Congenital epulis

Epidemiology   Occurs almost exclusively in females.

Macroscopy   Masses on gum present at birth.

Microscopy   Aggregates of large granular cells (similar to cells of granular tumour) covered by squamous epithelium. Electron microscope suggests these are fibroblasts or perivascular pericytes. S100 protein is not seen.

White sponge naevus

Epidemiology   Autosomal dominant inherited disorder.

Macroscopy   Shaggy white patches on oral mucosa. Buccal areas most frequent.

Microscopy   Patches composed of hyperplastic well differentiated squamous epithelium with marked intra- and intercellular oedema.

INFLAMMATORY LESIONS OF MOUTH, LIPS AND TONGUE

These may be infective or non-infective.

Bacterial infections

Acute ulcerative gingivitis

Cause Mixture of spirochetes and fusiform bacilli. Risk increased by malnutrition.

Macroscopy Ulceration of gum usually between the teeth.

Actinomycosis

Cause Actinomyces, which form part of normal oral flora, invade oral tissues through mucosal defects.

Macroscopy Firm mucosa swelling from which pus containing 'sulphur granules' exudes.

Microscopy Abscesses with zones of central necrosis surrounded by granulation and fibrous tissue. Granules are colonies of Gram +ve filamentous bacteria surrounded by eosinophilic club-shaped bodies.

Tuberculosis

Epidemiology Rare in West. Usually spread from pulmonary lesion.

Macroscopy Tongue most frequent site with irregular ulcers.

Microscopy Typical caseating granulomas.

Syphilis

Epidemiology Rare.

Macroscopy May see all three stages of chancre (usually lips or tongue), snail-track ulcers in secondary stage and gummatous lesions of tertiary stage (usually on tongue or palate).

Microscopy Similar to lesions seen elsewhere.

Viral infections

Herpes simplex virus (HSV)

Two inflammatory lesions:

1. **Acute herpetic gingivo-stomatitis**

Epidemiology Most frequent in children (1–3 years).

Macroscopy Blisters and ulcers of the oral mucosa.

Clinical features Associated with fever and enlargement of draining lymph nodes. Lesions usually heal in 2–3 weeks.

2. **Herpes labialis** (cold sores)

Epidemiology Common recurrent disease due to latency of the virus.

Clinical features Lesions can recur repeatedly at the same site.

Pathogenesis Virus becomes latent in neurones because of the presence of a repressor for the viral IE (Intermediate Early) gene. Latency is interrupted for instance by fever or sunlight exposure triggering virus formation in neurones. The virus travels down the neurone to the skin where the lesions occur.

Macroscopy Clusters of vesicles usually at junction between skin and lip vermilion. Vesicles rupture to become ulcers and heal without scarring.

Herpes zoster

Epidemiology Varicella zoster usually involves the skin but may affect oral mucosa. Usually unilateral.

Clinical features Usually unilateral. Painful.

Macroscopy Vesicles on reddened mucosa.

Coxsackie virus type A (herpangina)

Virology Caused by strains 2, 4, 5, 6, 8 and 10 of the type A Coxsackie virus (an enterovirus).

Clinical features Abrupt onset of fever, sore throat, anorexia, dysphagia and vomiting or abdominal pain.

Macroscopy Reddened oropharynx with discrete vesicles on the anterior pillars of the fauces, on the palate, uvula and tongue. Self-limiting.

Human papilloma virus (HPV)

Macroscopy   Warty lesions.

Microscopy   Some lesions show typical features of HPV infection such a koilocytosis but others do not.

Human immunodeficiency virus (HIV)

Pathogenesis   Pathological manifestations of HIV infection in the mouth are related to decline in cell-mediated immunity resulting in infections and neoplasms.

Clinical features   Oral infections may be bacterial, viral or fungal. Of the fungal infections oral candidiasis is the commonest (50–70% infected individuals). Epstein–Barr virus-related oral leukoplakia is also seen. The commonest neoplasm in the oral cavity is Kaposi's sarcoma, most commonly affecting the palate.

Fungal infections

The most important fungus affecting the oral cavity is *Candida albicans* which may present in a number of ways.

Oral candidiasis (thrush)

Epidemiology   Most common in neonates, young infants and immunosuppressed adults. In neonates 5–10% are affected, infection being acquired during vaginal delivery.

Macroscopy   Discrete white patches which may involve any part of the oral mucosa or tongue.

Microscopy   Pseudomembrane might be present containing keratinous debris as well as many yeasts and which covers a denuded base.

Acute atrophic candidiasis

Macroscopy   Red tongue associated with atrophy of the filiform papillae.

Clinical features   Tongue is painful. May occur as a result of prolonged antibiotic therapy or local immunosuppression due to steroids (inhalers or topical within mouth).

Treatment   Removal of predisposing factor.

Candida cheilitis

Clinical features   Affects angles of the mouth or lip vermilion. Associated with excessive licking of the lips or
topical steroids.

Candida leukoplakia

Clinical features   Lesions appear anywhere on oral or
lingual mucosa with pain or burning sensation.

Macroscopy   Discrete area of epithelial hyperplasia.

Microscopy   Hyperplastic epithelium with candida in the
superficial layers. Cellular atypia may be present. Carcinoma
has been reported as late complication. Candida infection is
also seen in up to 90% of cases of hairy leukoplakia.

··

NON-INFECTIVE INFLAMMATORY LESIONS

Aphthous ulcers

Epidemiology   Commonest inflammatory lesion in the
mouth affecting up to 40% of the population. Most frequent
in the first two decades.

Cause   Unknown. Some associated with Behçet's syndrome, trauma, endocrine disturbances (including menstruation and pregnancy), stress and allergy.

Clinical features   Abrupt onset of localized discomfort or
burning sensation. When ulcerated they are painful. Self-
limiting disorder which heals without scarring. Recurrence
common.

Macroscopy   Intense red mucosa with dilation of sub-
epithelial vessels. Well-demarcated ulcers 1–2 mm in diameter.

··

LEUCOPLAKIA

The term is descriptive and is not a single disease entity.

Aetiology   Frequently no specific cause. Some cases associated with tobacco use (particularly chewing), trauma (e.g.
poorly fitting dentures) and dietary irritants.

Macroscopy White patches on oral mucosa. Occasionally patches appear red (erythroplakia).

Microscopy Epithelial hyperplasia and increased surface keratin. There is a spectrum in the presence and severity of abnormal keratinocyte proliferation, maturation and the presence of dyaplasia (nuclear enlargement, increased nuclear-cytoplasmic ratio, mitoses that are abnormal in morphology or location). Erythroplakia is associated with increased blood flow due to vascular dilation in the lamina propria.

Clinical features Severe dysplasia is more common in erythroplakia which carries a higher risk of malignant transformation (about 50%) compared to 1–30% (risk in the order of 5–6% is more likely) for ordinary leukoplakia.

Hairy leukoplakia

Epidemiology Almost exclusively seen in patients with HIV infection.

Aetiology Epstein–Barr virus.

Macroscopy White patches usually on lateral border of tongue with corrugated or hairy surface.

Microscopy Epithelial thickening and hyperkeratosis. Presence of herpes-type intranuclear inclusions and cytoplasmic ballooning in deeper epithelium. Frequently associated with candida infection.

....

MALIGNANT TUMOURS OF THE ORAL CAVITY

Epidemiology

Malignant tumours of the oral cavity account for 4% cancer deaths in male and 2% in females. There are marked geographical differences being most common in the Indian subcontinent and with a mean incidence (male and female combined) of 4/100 000 in the West.

Males are more frequently affected than females particularly for carcinomas of the lip (M:F 10:1). Carcinoma of the oral cavity usually affects middle-aged and elderly individuals with a steep increase in incidence after 70 years. The commonest type of malignant oral tumour is squamous cell carcinoma (95% cases).

Squamous cell carcinoma

Aetiology
Several aetiological agents are thought to be important.

- smoking: 2–4 times increased risk of oral carcinoma. Particularly associated with holding tobacco in mouth (snuff-dipping) or tobacco chewing (e.g. as part of 'pan', chewed in south-east Asia)
- alcohol: If this is associated with smoking the increased relative risk becomes 6–15-fold
- human papilloma virus infection: HPV type 16 is identified in up to 50% cases
- sunlight: particularly for carcinomas of the lip.

Genetics
In cell-line studies loss of multiple chromosome regions appears important including 18q (100%), 19p (80%), 8p (70%) and 3p (60%). Also deletion of short arms of acrocentric chromosomes is seen in 70% and additional copies of 7p in 90% of cell lines. Amplification and over-expression of epidermal growth factor receptor, bcl-2, int-1, and cyclin D-1 has been seen.

Sites
The tongue (mostly the ventrolateral surface) and floor of mouth are the most frequent sites (50%). Rarest sites are dorsum of tongue and hard palate.

Macroscopy
Early lesions appear as opaque plaques or warty areas. Later lesions ulcerate with a firm rolled edge and indurated bed.

Microscopy
Most are well-differentiated keratinizing squamous cell carcinomas. Keratin pearls are commonly present. The margins are marked by islands and strands of neoplastic cells which may infiltrate deeply into connective tissue, muscle and

underlying bone. Some are poorly differentiated (particularly those at tongue base). Well-differentiated tumours express involucrin and cytokeratins 1 and 10 (or 4 and 13 if non-keratinizing) while poorly differentiated tumours are involucrin negative and express cytokeratins 8 and 18.

Spread

Local invasion is often pronounced. Lymph node metastasis follows the pattern of lymph drainage and is frequently present at diagnosis. Distant spread may involve mediastinal nodes lungs, liver and bone.

Natural history

Depends on location (lower lip 90% 5-year survival; anterior tongue 60%; posterior tongue, floor of mouth, tonsil, gum, hard palate all 40% and soft palate 20%), stage and histological grade (poor prognosis associated with less differentiated tumours).

Verrucous carcinoma

This is a variant of squamous carcinoma.

Epidemiology Mostly in elderly men.

Site Buccal mucosa and gum of lower jaw most frequent.

Macroscopy Bulky soft cauliflower-like lesions which frequently become infected and therefore smell unpleasant.

Microscopy Extremely well-differentiated squamous carcinoma. Rete pegs are thick with a bulbous pattern. Stromal invasion only in late stages. Increase in size of the squamous cells is a useful diagnostic indicator. Differential diagnosis from hyperplastic lesion can be difficult.

Other oral tumours

Granular cell tumour (granular cell myoblastoma)

This is a benign tumour of uncertain histogenesis but thought to be derived from Schwann cells.

Site Any site but tongue is commonest.

Microscopy Sheets of large pink-staining cells with small nucleus and granular cytoplasm containing periodic-acid-Schiff (PAS) positive material. Perineural tumour may be seen. Often associated with pseudoepitheliomatous hyperplasia of overlying epithelium.

THE SALIVARY GLANDS

....

ANATOMY

The glands are classified as being either major or minor. The minor glands are situated in the sub-mucosa of the mouth, pharynx and upper respiratory tract. The major glands consist of three paired glands named in accordance with their location.

Parotid glands

Location   Below and anterior to the external ear.
Divided into two parts (superficial and deep) by the facial nerve. Drain via main (Stensen's) duct into floor of mouth.

Submandibular glands

Location   In groove between lower jaw and tongue.
Drain via Wharton's duct through small caruncles on either side of the frenulum of the tongue into the floor of the mouth.

Sublingual glands

Location   In the sublingual fossae of the mandible.
Drain via Bartholin's duct into a series of small openings on either side of the groove below the tongue. Occasionally the main excretory duct joins the submandibular gland duct.

Histology

The microanatomy of all the glands is similar.

Secretory apparatus

Lobular gland containing many acini of wedge-shaped cells with a central lumen. In the parotid all the cells are serous cells with a basally situated nucleus and granular basophilic cytoplasm. These granules contain amylase and stain magenta with PAS stains. The submandibular contains a mixture of serous and mucinous acini and the sublingual gland contains mucinous cells only. Between the epithelium and the basement membrane there are myoepithelial cells which are contractile and exhibit epithelial and mesenchymal characteristics.

Intercalated ducts

The acini drain into intercalated ducts lined by flattened or cuboidal epithelium. These blend into the striated ducts also lined by cuboidal epithelium with striations on the basal aspect due to invaginations of the basement membrane and mitochondria. Myoepithelial cells are also seen.

Interlobular ducts

The striated ducts emerge from the lobules and drain into the interlobular ducts running in the interlobular connective tissue being lined by pseudostratified columnar epithelium. These drain into the principal excretory duct, the lining of which becomes squamous near its orifice.

Function

Lubrication   Allows swallowing due to the high water content of saliva.

Digestion   Amylase in saliva digests complex carbohydrates.

Protection   Secretory IgA in the saliva and non-specific antibacterial compounds (muramidase and lactoferrin) protect against infection. Saliva protects the teeth against decay by the low pH produced by acid-producing bacteria.

....

DISORDERS OF SECRETION
Xerostomia

Definition   Decreased or absent secretion of saliva.
Cause   May be functional or structural.

- Functional xerostomia: Usually drug related due to anti-histamines, tricyclic anti-depressants, phenothiazines, certain hypotensive agents and some anti-emetic drugs.
- Structural xerostomia: Due to loss of secretory tissue as a result of irradiation of the head and neck or autoimmune destruction as seen in Sjögren's syndrome.

Mumps and sarcoidosis cause a decrease but not cessation of saliva flow. In the case of mumps complete return to normal occurs after resolution of the inflammation.

Sialorrhoea (ptyalism)

Definition   Increased flow of saliva.

Cause   Seen in association with inflammation of mouth or gum and linked to aphthous or herpetic ulcers and teething in infants; is occasionally seen in mercury poisoning, pemphigus, epilepsy, Parkinson's disease and myasthenia gravis.

....

INFLAMMATORY DISORDERS
Acute inflammatory disorders

Causes   Most are bacterial or viral. Bacterial infections usually result from ascending infection from the mouth in the context of reduced saliva flow.

Clinical features   Most present with painful enlargement of the gland with pus discharging into the mouth from the duct orifice.

Salivary calculi

Epidemiology   Submandibular duct affected 2–3 times more often than parotid. Calculi are the commonest cause of unilateral parotid swelling.

Clinical features   Submandibular calculi are found mostly in the main duct and can be palpated in the floor of the mouth. Complete obstruction causes pain and swelling (particularly associated with meals). In the parotid complete obstruction of a duct is associated with decreased secretion of the drained acinar units so the association of pain and swelling to meals is absent. In these glands the swelling is associated with inflammation.

Chemistry Salivary calculi are mostly calcium phosphate with calcium carbonate the second most abundant component.

Chronic obstructive sialadenitis

Epidemiology Most commonly in the submandibular glands.

Macroscopy Dilated ducts. Firm glandular tissue.

Microscopy Dilated ducts contain eosinophilic glycoprotein and may be lined by metaplastic squamous epithelium. There is expansion of the interlobular connective tissue with associated intralobular fibrosis and acinar loss. A mild to moderate chronic inflammatory infiltrate is frequently seen.

Chronic recurrent parotitis

Epidemiology Mostly children 5–15 years. Males > females.

Clinical features Recurrent episodes of parotid swelling and tenderness lasting 7–10 days and associated with fever and malaise. Intervals between attacks may be weeks or months.

Microscopy Acinar atropy with dilation of smallest ductules (sialectasis).

Sjögren's syndrome

Definition Autoimmune disease characterized by the appearance in the serum of organ-specific (e.g. anti-thyroid) and non-organ-specific antibodies.

Clinical features Affects salivary and lacrimal glands resulting in dry mouth (xerostomia) and dry eyes (conjunctivitis sicca). May be isolated (primary) or associated with other autoimmune diseases of which the commonest is rheumatoid arthritis but includes primary biliary cirrhosis, scleroderma, polymyositis and systemic lupus erythematosus. The eyes and mouth are more severely affected in primary Sjögren's syndrome which also shows salivary gland swelling and systemic manifestations such as Raynaud's phenomenon, lymphadenopathy and lung and renal involvement.

Immunology Primary Sjögren's syndrome is associated with HLA-DR3 and positive finding of anti-SS-A 0(Ro; 75%), anti-SS-B (La; 40%), rheumatoid factors (95%), anti-salivary gland antibodies and rheumatoid arthritis precipitin (5%), while secondary Sjögren's syndrome is strongly associated with rheumatoid arthritis precipitin (85%), rheumatoid factors (100%) and anti-salivary gland antibodies (70%) but not with anti-SS-A (10%) or anti-SS-B (5%) (25%).

Epidemiology Peak incidence in 4th–5th decades; M:F 1:9. Possibly associated with viral infection such as Epstein–Barr virus or HTLV-1. HIV p24 protein more commonly seen in patients with Sjögren's syndrome (30%) than normal population (1–4%).

Microscopy Focal chronic inflammatory infiltrates adjacent or replacing acinar tissue consisting of at least 50 lymphocytes, plasma cells and macrophages in both major and minor salivary gland. Epimyoepithelial islands ('benign lymphoepithelial lesions') consisting of lymphocytes infiltrating islands of epithelial and myoepithelial cells are seen but are not specific to Sjögren's syndrome and may be seen as an isolated finding in females in their 5th–6th decade.

··

TUMOURS OF THE SALIVARY GLANDS

Epidemiology Any gland can be affected but the parotids are the most frequent. Ratio parotid:submandibular:sublingual: minor salivary gland 100:10:1:10. Benign tumours account for 90% of the tumours but a greater proportion of the tumours arising in the minor salivary glands are malignant. Salivary gland tumours are rare, accounting for only 1–2% of all tumours. Aetiology: salivary gland tumours are associated with irradiation.

BENIGN EPITHELIAL TUMOURS

Adenomas

Pleomorphic salivary adenoma (mixed salivary tumour)

Epidemiology Commonest salivary gland tumour. Occurs at any age with peak in 4th and 5th decades. Slight female preponderance.

Site Most arise in superficial parotid (above facial nerve), 10% occur in deep part of the parotid gland.

Macroscopy Rounded masses with well-defined edge and connective tissue capsule. Frequently shelled out from their bed at surgery but with risk of leaving small projections behind. Most tumours are firm. Cut surface may show foci resembling cartilage.

Microscopy Highly variable both between and within single tumours. Epithelial component (thought to arise from intercalated ducts) show well-formed duct structures and/or compact masses of myoepithelial cells. Squamous metaplasia of the myoepithelial islands may occur. The stroma shows accumulation of basophilic material rich in connective tissue mucins which can resemble cartilage. The stroma may be very bulky with only a few strands of myoepithelial cells in some cases.

Natural history Benign. Tendency to recur if not completely removed at surgery. Small proportion (1–5%) show malignant change if untreated for long periods.

Treatment wide excision with rim of normal tissue which in the parotid usually entails a superficial parotidectomy.

Adenolymphoma (Warthin's tumour)

Definition A monomorphic adenoma with heavy lymphocytic infiltrate.

Epidemiology Accounts for 8% of all tumours in the parotid. M:F 3–4:1. Peak incidence 6th and 7th decades.

Site Almost exclusively seen in the parotid gland with most in the superficial part. About 10% are bilateral and multiple tumours in a single gland can be seen.

Macroscopy Soft well-defined brown mass. Cut surface is polycystic with papillary ingrowths of epithelium into cyst cavities and clefts.

Microscopy The cysts and clefts are lined by a double layer of pink epithelial cells. The inner layer is of tall columnar cells with eosinophilic granular cytoplasm and the outer layer is composed of smaller cuboidal/pyramidal cells. Electron microscopy shows the cells contain numerous mitochondria (a feature of so-called oncocytes). The stroma contains a florid lymphocytic infiltrate with lymphoid follicles containing germinal centres.

Origin Thought to arise from striated ducts.

Natural history Virtually always benign. If malignant transformation occurs this is in the epithelial component. Slow growing. May become infected with abscesses within the tumour.

Oxyphilic adenoma (oncocytoma)

Epidemiology Rare. Accounts for less than 1% of all parotid tumours, less common in other glands.

Macroscopy Well-defined round or oval masses with pinkish cut surface.

Microscopy By definition the tumour is composed of oncocytes – large granular eosinophilic epithelial cells which may be in solid clumps or with obvious tubule formation. Electron microscopy shows the cells to contain many mitochondria.

....

MALIGNANT EPITHELIAL TUMOURS

Adenoid cystic carcinoma

Site About 15% of submandibular gland tumours are adenoid cystic carcinomas compared with 2% of parotid tumours and 15–20% of tumours in the minor salivary glands (majority in palate).

Macroscopy Appears well-circumscribed. Uniform cut surface with no areas of haemorrhage or cystic change.

Microscopy Epithelial cells are believed to originate from the intercalated ducts. Myoepithelial cells are the greater proportion of these cells and may form compact masses within which mucoid material accumulates (adenoid areas). If the cystic spaces are large and numerous the term cribriform carcinoma can be applied. In some parts the cells may be in solid clumps or a tubular pattern. The cellular islands are surrounded by a sheath containing either hyaline connective tissue or mucoid material derived from basement membrane material. The tumour has infiltrative margins with a marked predilection for perineural invasion.

Natural history   Slow-growing but highly malignant. The tumour can infiltrate widely and insidiously into nose and antrum. This insidious invasion makes complete resection difficult and local recurrence is common. Distant metastasis occurs at late stage with lungs as most common site.

Prognosis   Related to histological pattern. Predominantly solid pattern has worst prognosis (50% 5-year survival) and a tubular pattern the best (more that 90% 5-year survival); the cribriform carries an intermediate prognosis.

Acinic cell tumour

Epidemiology   Rare, 2–3% of parotid tumours. Occurs at any age with peak incidence in the 5th decade. Slight female preponderance.

Site   Most occur in the parotid.

Macroscopy   Solid well-circumscribed tumours, slightly firmer than surrounding gland. Cut surface is grey with occasional yellow flecks.

Microscopy   Cells closely resemble secretory cells of parotid. The cytoplasm is basophilic and granular showing positive staining with periodic-acid-Schiff (PAS). Areas with ductular epithelium may be seen but some areas of acinic cells are mandatory for the diagnosis. Tumour cells may be arranged in a solid acinar pattern or in compact sheets. Fluid can accumulate between cells bestowing a lattice-like appearance. Overt features of malignancy (cellular pleomorphism and increased mitotic rate) are rare.

Origin   Thought to arise from stem cells of the intercalated duct.

Natural history In the majority growth is slow and presentation is with a painless enlargement of the parotid. Rarely growth may be accelerated and the lesion painful. Local recurrence occurs in 12–20% and distant metastasis in 8–10%.

Mucoepidermoid carcinoma

Definition A tumour composed of both mucin-secreting and epidermoid epithelial cells.

Epidemiology Occurs at any age with a peak in 3rd and 4th decades.

Site Accounts for 3–5% of tumours in the parotid and submandibular gland. Commoner in minor salivary glands where it accounts for up to 15% of tumours. Palate a frequent site.

Macroscopy Appears well circumscribed. Cut surface depends on the relative proportion of mucin-secreting and epidermoid elements. If the former predominate the tumour may show numerous cysts.

Microscopy Variable mixture of mucin-secreting and epidermoid cells, the latter showing typical intercellular bridges. The mucin-secreting cells can occur in solid clumps or lining small cystic spaces. Frequently infiltrative growth pattern at the edge with irregular extension into surrounding tissue.

Natural history Usually slow-growing painless mass. Local recurrence frequent if not adequately excised. All mucoepidermoid tumours have malignant potential but only about 10% show metastasis and these tend to be high grade with overt evidence of malignancy on microscopic examination. Five-year survival rate in the order of 90%.

OTHER TUMOURS OF THE SALIVARY GLANDS

These include non-epithelial tumours, principally haemangiomas, lymphomas that mostly arise from mucosa-associated lymphoid tissue (MALT) acquired in Sjögren's syndrome, and secondary tumours.

ANATOMY

Length   25 cm.

Position   Cricopharyngeus muscle (6th cervical vertebra) to gastro-oesophageal junction (10/11th thoracic vertibra). All but distal 1.5 cm intrathoracic.

Histology

Intrathoracic portion lined by stratified squamous epithelium with basal layer amounting to 15% thickness. Wide submucosa containing oesophageal glands secreting sulphated acid mucins. Thick muscularis mucosae – inner circular and outer longditudinal layers. Upper third contains voluntary muscle fibres. No serosa on intrathoracic part.

Nerve supply

Extrinsic   From autonomic nervous system including sympathetic (thoracic spinal nerves) and parasympathetic (vagus).

Intrinsic   From myenteric plexus (between layers of muscularis mucosae) exerting stimulatory and inhibitory stimuli.

FUNCTION

1. Propulsion of food from mouth to stomach (swallowing)

Requires:

- freedom from obstruction such as foreign bodies, webs, abnormal contraction rings (usually at cardia), neoplasms
- normal motor function including propulsion (peristalsis) and relaxation of functional gastro-oesophageal sphincter

- absence of narrowing from scarring from e.g. caustic chemicals, radiation, sclerosis surrounding tumour.

2. Prevention of reflux

Achieved by lower oesophageal sphincter (segment of smooth muscle 2–4 cm long situated just above gastro-oesophageal junction with pressure 10–30 mmHg above intragastric pressure.

....

DISORDERS OF FUNCTION (DYSPHAGIA)

Obstructive disorders

Congenital oesophageal atresia/stenosis

Most often combined with tracheo-oesophageal fistula (1:800/1500 live births). May be part of VATER syndrome: **V**ertebral defects, **A**nal atresia, **T**racheo-(o)**E**sophageal fistula, **R**enal dysplasia. Associated with maternal hydramnios. Several anatomical variants.

Oesophageal webs

Most common at level of cricoid cartilage. Fibrous tissue layer covered by normal epithelium nearly obstructing lumen. May be part of Paterson–Brown–Kelly syndrome (syn. Plummer–Vinson syndrome, sideropaenic dysphagia) – iron deficiency anaemia, oesophageal web, achlorhydria, atrophy of mucosa of tongue, pharynx and stomach. Almost exclusively affects females. May predispose to upper (post-cricoid) oesophageal carcinoma.

Oesophageal rings (Schatzki's rings)

Constrictive rings at level of gastro-oesophageal junction. Projection of epithelial connective tissue covered by either squamous or columnar epithelium or both.

Foreign bodies

Food (fish/meat bones; fruit stones) or non-food material (coins; broken toys; dentures) inappropriately or deliberately swallowed.

Neoplasms

Motor disorders

Achalasia (failure of relaxation)

Increased basal tone of lower oesophageal sphincter, failure of sphincteric relaxation and reduced peristaltic contractions.

Morphological correlate Loss of ganglion cells from myenteric plexus. May be congenital (5%) or acquired (95%) usually after 40 years. M=F. Similar changes seen in Chagas' disease as a result of infection by *Trypanasoma cruzi*. May lead to marked dilation of oesophagus.

Symptoms Dyspepsia and regurgition of food which can be aspirated into the airways May get secondary oesophagitis with ulceration and bleeding. Possible increased risk of carcinoma.

Diffuse muscular spasm

Occurs either at rest or after swallowing very hot or cold liquids. Caused by irregular contractions of the lower two-thirds of the oesophagus.

Morphological correlate Focal of diffuse hypertrophy of smooth muscle up to 1 cm in thickness.

Neuropathies associated with systemic disorders

Autoimmune neuropathies associated with diabetes mellitus or amyloidosis. Impaired primary peristalsis associated with long-term alcohol over-ingestion.

Connective tissue disorders

Most associated with systemic sclerosis (progressive systemic sclerosis) – 75% of patients with this condition. Also in dermatomyositis, systemic lupus erythematosus and other connective tissue diseases.

Morphological correlates Progressive atrophy of smooth muscle, loss of peristalsis and dysfunction of lower oesophageal sphincter.

Pharyngeal/oesophageal diverticula

Pharyngeal pouch

Commonest upper GI diverticula. Posterior aspect of oesophagus. Herniation of mucosa through fibres of inferior constrictor and the oblique thyropharyngeal muscles. Enlarge and put pressure on oesophagus. M:F 3:1. Most over 50 years.

Traction diverticula

Middle and lower third. Associated with inflammation of mediastinal lymph nodes (mostly TB) due to fibrous adhesions between nodes and oesophagus.

Epiphrenic diverticula

Just above the diaphragm. Due to raised luminal pressure.

Diffuse intramural oesophageal diverticulosis

Small (1–3 mm) diverticulae within the wall. Mostly upper third. Possibly cystically dilated submucosal gland ducts.

Gastro-oesophageal reflux

Aetiology   Pressure of lower sphincter falls below critical level.

Causes   Hormones (oestrogen/progesterone, glucagon, seratonin, cholecystokinin, prostaglandin E2), drugs (atropine, theophylline, meperidine) and dietary factors (low fat intake, smoking, alcohol, chocolate).

Symptoms   Usually episodic. heartburn (burning substernal pain) and water brash (awareness of acid juice in oesophagus).

Morphological correlates   Acute inflammation (neutrophils and eosinophils) and epithelial proliferation (papillomatosis and basal cell hyperplasia). May lead to ulceration.

Barrett's oesophagus

Definiton   Columnar epithelium lining distal oesophagus.

Morphological features   Epithelium can be intestinal (usually small intestinal) or mucosa of gastric fundus or cardia-type.

Associations Associated with dysplasia and 30–40-fold risk of developing carcinoma (mostly adenocarcinoma).

Hiatus hernia

Definition Presence of intrathoracic gastro-oesophageal junction and/or part of stomach.

- Two types: sliding (90%) – herniation through hiatus through which oeophagus passes. May be congenital (occasionally familial) or acquired.
- Rolling (paraoesophageal 10%) – stomach herniates through diaphragm alongside oesophagus.

Oesophagitis not related to reflux

1. Infective

Most are seen in the immunosuppressed as a result of drugs or associated with lymphoma/leukaemia or AIDS. Viral (herpes simplex, cytomegalovirus) or fungal (candida).

Herpes simplex – lesions start as small vesicles becoming ulcerated. See multi-nucleated giant cells with intranuclear viral inclusions.

2. Non-infective

Seen due to ingestion of chemical irritants (strong acid/alkali), irradiation, graft-versus-host disease, physical trauma (nasogastric tubes) or systemic disease (pemphigoid, epidermolysis bullosa, uraemia).

....

NEOPLASMS

Benign tumours

Rare. Most involve connective tissue. Commonest is leiomyoma. Also haemangioma, lipoma, nerve sheath tumours. Squamous papillomas (small warty lesions) occur rarely.

Malignant tumours

Carcinoma

Type Squamous (90%), adenocarcinoma (10%).

Incidence 5.2–10.4/100 000 population per year. 2–5% deaths from malignant disease per year.

Geography Wide variation worldwide and within populations (high = China, Japan, Finland, France, parts of Iran and South Africa) suggestive of environmental factors.

Aetiological factors Tobacco (all types), alcohol (spirits > wine and beer), low trace metals (particularly molybdenum), hot beverages, pickled vegetables (nitrosamine-containing), low intake of fresh fruit and vegetables. Chronic oesophagitis.

Site Middle third (50%), lower third (30%) and upper third (20%).

Macroscopy Crateriform, polypoid/fungating or stenosing.

Microscopy Squamous carcinoma – all grades of differentiation from keratinizing with well-formed nests to anaplastic. May extend laterally under mucosa. Adenocarcinoma – most arise from metaplastic epithelium (Barrett's). Some may arise from oesophageal glands.

Spread Direct – conspicuous spread through wall. Once through muscularis propria frequently involves trachea, main bronchi, lung and mediastinum; less commonly the aorta, pericardium, heart and recurrent laryngeal nerves. Metastatic – through lymphatics. Has usually occurred at time of diagnosis.

STOMACH

Size J-shaped, capacity 1.2–1.5 l.
Location Left hypochondrium.

....

ANATOMY

Four zones:

- cardia (small area 0.5–3.5 cm distal to gastro-oesophageal junction)
- fundus (above horizontal line drawn though gastro-oesophageal junction)

- body (main region, two-thirds of the remaining stomach)
- pyloric antrum (remaining third leading into the pyloric sphincter).

Histology

Mucosa

Glands of varying types in loose meshwork of vascular connnective tissue leading to straight-sided crypts. Surface covered by single layer of tall mucin-secreting epithelial cells with basal nuclei. Crypt and gland morphology differ between regions. All crypt and gland-lining cells are derived from pluripotent stem cells in the neck region.

Cardia

Crypts occupy 50% mucosal thickness. Glands lined by mucin-secreting cells. Occasional acid and pepsin-secreting cells. Endocrine cells common.

Body

Responsible for acid and pepsin secretion. Crypts one-quarter of mucosal thickness. Remainder is glands with two main secretory cell types – **parietal cells** (upper part of glands, secrete acid, intrinsic factor and blood group substances) and **chief cells** (deeper parts of gland, secrete pepsinogen and other proteolytic enzymes).

Antrum

Gastric pits occupy 50% mucosal thickness. Fewer glands than body, lined with mucus-secreting cells.
Neuroendocrine cells can be found in all areas of the stomach and secrete a large number of products including gastrin, somatostatin, serotonin, vasoactive intestinal peptide and pancreatic polypeptide.

Acid secretion

From parietal cells. Secretion of H+ by action of H+K+ ATPase proton pump exchanging with K+ in gastric lumen.

Control

Endocrine Stimulatory – gastrin from G cells in antral mucosa under control of:

- gastrin-releasing peptide (homologous to bombesin) from mucosal nerve endings
- intraluminal breakdown products of proteins.

Inhibitory – somatostatin acting on parietal and G cells in paracrine fashion. Release is mediated by B-adrenergic stimuli, cholecystokinin, luminal acid, locally synthesized prostaglandins and weakly by gastrin.

Nervous Release of acetylcholine by mucosal nerve endings.

Paracrine Histamine from mucosal mast cells.

Pepsin secretion

Produced from the inactive precursors pepsinogens I and II from chief and neck cells of fundus and body (types I and II) and glands in the cardia antrum and duoneum (Brunner's glands) (type II only).

Control

Stimulation Vagal cholinergic pathway. Secretin and vasoactive intestinal polypeptide.

Protection of gastric and duodenal mucosa

Mucus and bicarbonate production Surface layer of mucus and bicarbonate acts as barrier to back-diffusion of acid allowing maintenance of alkaline pH at mucosal surface. Dependent on rates of mucus secretion and break-down, rate of bicarbonate secretion and degree of penetration of mucus layer by acid.

Prevention of back-diffusion of H+ ions Glandular epithelial cells form high resistance intercellular junctions at the apical cell membranes. This can be disrupted by aspirin.

Local production of prostaglandins (chiefly E-type) Decrease in local prostaglandins decreases bicarbonate production (possible mechanism of aspirin-induced ulcergenesis as aspirin blocks prostaglandin production by inhibiting cyclo-oxygenase.

......

DEVELOPMENTAL ABNORMALITIES

Congenital hypertrophic pyloric stenosis

Incidence   1:400 live births, commoner in first born. M:F 4:1.

Genetics   Polygenic inheritance. Increased risk in siblings and offspring of affected individuals.

Associations   Rarely associated with other gut abnormalities such as imperforate anus and oeophageal atresia.

Clinical presentation   Projectile vomiting usually at 2–4 weeks. Failure to thrive. Hypochloraemic alkalosis. Hypertrophied pyloris can be felt on palpation after feeding.

Pathology   Hypertrophy of the circular layer of muscuris propria by factor of 2–4 from pyloris proximally for about 2 cm.

Treatment   Surgical incision through hypertrophied muscle.

......

GASTRITIS AND PEPTIC ULCERATION

A set of disorders of the gastric and duodenal mucosa ranging from acute mild inflammation to chronic deeply penetrating ulcers. Represents an imbalance between factors that damage the mucosa (e.g. acid and pepsin) and factors that are protective (e.g. bicarbonate and mucus).

Helicobacter pylori and gastroduodenal disease

Helicobacter pylori (H. pylori)

Gram-negative microaerophilic curved spiral and flagellate bacillus. First cultured in 1983. Initially termed *Campylobacter pylori*, but was later found to be different from true campylobacters and renamed (1989). Produces a powerful urease which increases local pH. Also produces catalase, lipase, proteolytic enzymes and cellular toxins.

A non-invasive organism lying on the surface only of gastric epithelium (including gastric metaplasia in duodenum, rectum and Meckel's diverticulum).

Detection

- Can be directly visualized in gastric biopsies on H&E stained sections or by using histochemical stains employing silver deposition on the organism (Warthin Starry) or other tincturial stains (toluidine blue, Giemsa, crysal violet, Gram stain). Can be stained with specific immunocytochemical antisera.
- Detection of antibodies in the blood implies current or previous infection.
- Urea breath tests: patient ingests C14 or C13 labelled urea which is converted to CO_2 in the stomach by *H. pylori* derived urease, absorbed into blood and expired in breath.

Infection

Lifelong infection thought to occur mostly in childhood. Dependent on both host (transient hypochlorhydria) and organism (urease, flagella, adhesion properties) factors. Probably faeco-oral or oro-oral route. Infection related to poor and crowded living conditions. Autoeradication is rare. Infection rates vary in different populations but is approximately 10% by 30 years and 60% in 60-year-olds in developed countries representing cohorts of individuals infected in childhood. In developing countries infection rates are about 80% by 2 years.

Disease

H. pylori is associated with the generation of chronic gastritis, gastric and duodenal ulceration, gastric carcinoma and gastric lymphoma.

Eradication

Much debate still surrounds the best treatment regimens, their doses and duration. All are multi-agent and most contain an acid suppressor (anti-histamine or proton pump inhibitor) with antibiotics (usually metronidazole, clari-

thromycin, ampicillin or tetracycline in some combination).
Antibiotic resistance (particularly to metronidazole) is
already emerging.

Acute gastritis (acute erosive gastropathy)

Definition   Hyperaemic mucosa with evidence of bleeding
or mucosal erosions in severe cases.

Causes   Direct mucosal damage caused by alcohol and cigarettes, corticosteroids, aspirin and non-steroidal anti-
inflammatory drugs, strong acids and alkalis, bile reflux.
Can be associated with systemic infections and 'stress' (e.g.
trauma, burns, sepsis, hypothermia) possibly via mucosal
ischaemia.

Microscopy   Hyperaemia, oedema and focal haemorrhage.
Erosions are focal necrosis of the surface epithelium.

Chronic gastritis

Set of mucosal inflammatory disorders that can be classified
on the basis of histological or aetiologial features.

Histological features
This involves assessment of four characteristics and leads
to a recognition of two patterns (Table 34.1).

Aetiological features
Two major types.

Type A
- mainly body region
- low acid secretion, high plasma gastrin levels and
  decreased secretion of pepsinogen
- often associated with anti-parietal cell antibodies
  (50–90% in patients with pernicious anaemia, 20–40%
  patients without).

Thought to be organ-specific autoimmune disease. IgG antibodies bind to parietal cell gastrin receptor.
    Other antibodies react with intrinsic factor.

Type B
- mainly antrum. Patchy in body
- high or normal acid secretion. Normal pepsinogen

Table 34.1 Patterns of chronic gastritis

Disorder	Type of mucosa	Level of involvement	Inflammatory infiltrate	Intestinal metaplasia
Chronic superficial gastritis	Any area	Superficial, glands spared	Neutrophils (may invade epithelium), plasma cells and lymphocytes. Lymphoid follicles are seen in association with *H. pylori*	None
Atrophic gastritis	Body and antrum	All layers with atrophy and loss of specialized cells	Similar to superficial gastritis but more severe	Present in two forms • complete: mucin-secreting goblet cells and specialized absorptive cells with brush border • incomplete: mucin producing cells only. Either sialomucins (88%) or sulphated mucins (12%). Sulphated mucin production associated with risk of carcinoma (90% of sulphated mucin producers)
Gastric atrophy (most severe form)	Thin mucosa	Few specialized cells	Less conspicuous but lymphoid aggregates may survive.	Prominent. Long-term cancer risk 2–4%.

- high frequency of *H. pylori* infection
- not associated with anti-parietal cell antibodies.

There are two further subdivisions:

1. Hypersecretory gastritis – increased secretion of acid and pepsin leading to gastritis and ulceration. Metaplasia not a feature. No increased risk for carcinoma development.
2. Environmental gastritis – no increase in acid or pepsin. Inflammation starts at antral–body junction in multiple foci. Intestinal metaplasia common. Wide geographical variation – found where gastric carcinoma is common, e.g. Japan.

Associations with gastritis

Gastric ulcer.   Usually type B variety. Associated with *H. pylori* infection, the use of non-steroidal anti-inflammatory drugs or biliary reflux.

Iron deficiency anaemia.   May be the result of occult chronic bleeding or to failure to absorb non-haem iron for which gastric acid is necessary.

Gastric carcinoma.   Greater risk of carcinoma in association with chronic atrophic gastritis possibly linked to sulphated mucin producing incomplete intestinal metaplasia.

Peptic ulceration

Definition   Well-circumscribed area of mucosal defect found only in areas exposed to acid and pepsin.

Location   Most are found in the stomach and first part of the duodenum; also in oesophagus (due to reflux), at gastrojejunal anastamosis sites, in or adjacent to Meckel's diverticula (if ectopic gastric mucosa present) and in lower parts of the small intestine (second part of duodenum to upper jejunum) in patients with gastrin-secreting tumours (Zollinger–Ellison syndrome).

Types
- Erosions: focal loss not amounting to full mucosal thickness
- acute ulcer: involving full thickness of mucosa; may penetrate deeper layers but with no scarring at the base

- chronic ulcers: always through the muscularis mucosae but to a variable depth through the wall and always with scarring of the ulcer base.

Epidemiology Gastric and duodenal ulcers have different prevalence.
- duodenal ulcer: incidence 1–3.5/1000 population/year. M:F 4:1, peak age 4th decade
- gastric ulcer: incidence 0.5/1000 population/year. M:F 1.5:1, peak age 6th decade.

Sites
- duodenal ulcer: most 1 cm distal to the pylorus, anterior or posterior aspect of bulb
- gastric ulcer: most on lesser curve just distal to body–antrum junction.

Pathogenesis Disruption of balance of defensive and injurious factors.

Genetic factors Duodenal and prepyloric ulcers more common in individuals with blood group O and HLA B5. High concordance in monozygotic twins. High risk of duodenal ulcer in some genetically determined syndromes e.g. Zollinger–Ellison; systemic mastocytosis (30% have duodenal ulcer); a familial syndrome including tremor nystagmus and narcolepsy (50% with duodenal ulcer); familial hyperpepsinogenaemia I.

Pathophysiology of duodenal ulcer
- Increased maximal gastric ulcer secretion in one-third of patients; higher than normal basal acid secretion in one-third, caused by increased parietal cell mass and increased parietal cell sensitivity.
- Maximal pepsinogen and intragastric proteolytic activity higher. Most marked for pepsinogen I.
- Gastrin secretion. Basal gastrin secrtion is normal but post-feeding plasma gastrin levels are increased.
- Gastric emptying. This is abnormally fast in many duodenal ulcer patients with acid unbuffered by food entering the duodenum.

Diseases associated with duodenal ulcer
Chronic obstructive airways disease, hyperparathyroidism, liver cirrhosis, chronic renal failure and α-1-antitrypsin deficiency.

Macroscopic features

Round to oval with well-demarcated margins, usually single (multiple in 5% cases). Most less than 3 cm diameter. Proximal margin frequently overhanging, distal margin usually sloping. Active ulcer bases are covered by grey–white exudate and are firm due to scar formation. In the stomach the surrounding mucosa is flattened close to the ulcer with mucosal folds radiating out from the ulcer.

Microscopic features

All active chronic peptic ulcers have similar features with four areas distinguishable (Askanazy's zones).

1. On the mucosal aspect a layer of exudate containing fibrin, acute inflammatory cells and dead cell debris.
2. A layer of necrotic tissue appearing as an amorphous eosinophilic layer with moderate number of leucocytes.
3. A layer of inflammatory granulation tissue with large capillaries and mixed inflammatory infiltrate.
4. A layer of dense fibrous tissue replacing the muscularis propria which contains blood vessels with fibromuscular thickening.

At the edge of the ulcer fusion of the muscularis mucosae and muscularis propria is common. When healing has commenced regenerating epithelium is present at the ulcer edge.

Complications

- Haemorrhage – occurs in 15–20% ulcer patients (most common in stomal and post-bulbar duodenal ulcers. Mortality from acute large bleed is about 5%.
- Perforation – occurs in less than 10% ulcer patients. Most frequent in ulcers located in anterior gastric antral wall. Gastric/duodenal contents lead to sudden onset of severe abdominal pain because of peritoneal irritation but these symptoms may be absent in the elderly.
- Penetration – inflammatory reaction on the serosa deep to an ulcer may lead to adhesion between this area and adjacent structures – most frequently the pancreas. Localized inflammation in the pancreas leads to severe back pain. Occasionally anterior gastric ulcers penetrate into the transverse colon to give a gastrocolic fistula.

- Obstruction – due to scarring. In ulcers in the middle of the stomach this can lead to a curious malformation termed 'hourglass stomach'.
- Malignant transformation – less than 1% ulcers.

....

NEOPLASMS OF THE STOMACH

Gastric carcinoma

Epidemiology

The leading cause of death from malignancy at the beginning of the twentieth century. Now has a decreasing incidence (mainly of intestinal type). It is still the third most common malignancy of the gastrointestinal tract in US. Marked geographical variation with high-risk areas in Japan (8 × prevalance of risk for both sexes), China, Chile, Brazil, Colombia, Iceland and Spain. Also variation within countries (in the US blacks and American Indians have a higher incidence than whites). Migrant adult populations from high- to low-risk areas maintain the high risk of the area of origin but their children adopt the low risk of the country of destination. This suggests an environmental factor acting early in life.

Aetiology and pathogenesis

Genetic factors:

- familial clustering – in San Marino 25% gastric carcinoma sufferers have a first-degree relative with disease (5.6% in control population) and in China the cancer risk in relatives of carcinoma patients is 8 times that for controls
- blood group A associated with development of diffuse cancers (50% belong to this group)
- phenotype for secretion of one type of pepsinogen.

Environmental factors

- nitrosamines – possible relationship between high levels of nitrates in the diet and carcinoma. These nitrates are converted to nitrites in the stomach which combine with

amines and amides to form potentially carcinogenic N-nitroso compounds
- cigarette smoking
- high salt diet
- low vegetable content in diet – these contain anti-oxidants such as vitamin C and E
- low intake of animal protein and fat
- high intake of complex carbohydrates.

Pre-cancerous conditions
- pernicious anaemia – risk of cancer development increased by 3–4 times
- presence of gastric stump – risk increased by 3–6 times with peak at 20–30 years after surgery
- intestinal metaplasia
- epithelial dysplasia – where this is present there must be a careful search for co-existing carcinoma. Dysplasia is characterized by the presence of cellular atypia (increased nuclear cytoplasmic ratio, nuclear pleomorphism and hyperchromasia, irregular nuclear arrangement giving pseudostratification appearance), abnormal differentiation (loss of secretory granules, intestinal metaplasia, loss of Paneth cells) and disorganized mucosal architecture. Classified as mild, moderate or severe.

Early gastric carcinoma

Definition Carcinoma limited to mucosa alone or mucosa and submucosa.

Frequency Increase in last few years as a result of advances in endoscopy and introduction of screening in Japan where the number of cases of early cancer has increased from 4% to 30%.

Macroscopy Three main types:
- I protruded
- II superficial (a) elevated (b) flat or (c) depressed
- III excavated.

Combinations can be seen. In these cases the dominant pattern is cited first (e.g. I + II(c))

Microscopy Most early carcinomas remain intramucosal until they exceed 3 mm. Invasion of the submucosa is through breaches in the muscularis mucosae associated with lymphoid aggregates. The submucosal diameter then grows to exceed the mucosal diameter. Lymph node metastasis is not incompatible with the diagnosis and occurs in up to 4.2% with mucosal and 16.8% with submucosal tumour.

Prognosis Much better than lesions involving muscularis propria at diagnosis (80–100% 5-year survival compared with 12% 5-year survival for deeper lesions).

Advanced gastric cancer

Definition Cancer extending beyond muscularis propria.

Incidence More than 80% gastric carcinoma patients are in this category in US and UK.

Location Mainly in the pre-pyloric region, pyloric antrum and lesser curve.

Macroscopy Three types:
- Ulcerating – commonest. Irregular margins with raised everted edges. Thick mucosal folds radiating away are thicker with loss of pattern seen around benign ulcer. Malignant ulcers tend to be bigger than benign ulcers.
- Nodular or fungating – found most often in body or fundus. Protruding friable tissue on broad base. Often large at time of diagnosis.
- Infiltrating – may have plaque-like appearance. More often involves the whole stomach wall causing increased thickness and lack of distensibility called 'linitis plastica' or 'leather-bottle stomach'. This type carries the worst prognosis.

Microscopy The most widely used classification is that of Lauren (Table 34.2).

Any typical adenocarcinoma may also show areas with neuroendocrine differentiation without effecting behaviour or prognosis.

Clinical features Onset often insidious with non-specific symptoms including abdominal pain (66%), wieght loss (50%), nausea and vomiting (32%), anorexia (25%), dysphagia (23%) or bleeding (23%).

Spread Spread can occur by:
- direct invasion
- lymphatic permeation: common, 85% have lymph node deposits at post-mortem (90% for intestinal, 71% for

Table 34.2 Lauren classification of advanced gastric cancer

	Description	M:F	Mean age (years)
Intestinal type	• Most frequent in countries with high cancer risk • Related to environmental factors • Tumour has glandular structure but frequently with some solid or papillary areas	2:1	55.4
Diffuse type	• Separated single cells or malignant cells in small aggregates • Glandular structures uncommon • Cells are small, uniform and have small dark nuclei • Mitoses are infrequent • Mucin production is prominent with intracellular accumulation giving signet ring appearance • Intramucosal spread is more common and the cells elicit a desmoplastic stromal response	1:1	47.7

diffuse if the serosa has been reached). Metastases can be seen in mediastinal nodes and occasionally in cervical nodes

- blood vessels: to give distant metastases in liver, lungs, adrenals and ovaries
- transperitoneal: about 25% cases with involvement of serosa. Metastases are embedded in peritoneum. May get bilateral ovarian metastases (Krukenberg tumour).

Other types of gastric carcinoma

Neuroendocrine differentiation

1. Typical carcinoid tumours
Well-differentiated slow growing tumours of the endocrine cell, normally found in the stomach.

Macroscopy May be small polyps.

Microscopy Small uniform cells with granular eosino-philic cytoplasm arranged in trabeculae, ribbons or small islands. Cells express neuroendocrine markers including neuron-specific enolase and chromogranin. May secrete gastrin (tumours usually single in antrum) or made up of enterochromaffin cells (usually associated with atrophic gastritis and intestinal metaplasia). May be associated with pernicious anaemia enterochromaffin. Good prognosis.

2. Atypical carcinoids
Invasive neuroendocrine tumours with increased mitotic activity and necrosis. Better prognosis than adenocarcinoma but not as good as typical carcinoids.

3. Small cell carcinoma
Similar to those seen in lung. Very aggressive.

Mucoid adenocarcinoma
Macroscopy Glistening colloid appearance.

Microscopy Associated with abundant extracellular mucin production which accumulates in large pools containing islands of tumour cells.

Behaviour Indolent with mean survival up to 9 years.

Hepatoid adenocarcinoma
Microscopy Admixture of cells of glandular type and those resembling liver cells (large, esinophilic and polygonal). Cells synthesize α-fetoprotein and α-l-antitrypsin.

Choriocarcinoma
Macroscopy Large, fleshy and frequently haemorrhagic, with areas of necrosis.

Microscopy Presence of large bizzare cells resembling syncytiotrophoblast. Secrete β subunit of human chorionic gonadotrophin.

Connective tissue neoplasms
These are uncommon tumours. Most are smooth muscle, remainder are nerve sheath but many show structural and immunohistochemical features of both and all of

these tumours are best considered as gastric stromal tumours.

Presentation Gastric bleeding due to ulceration of overlying mucosa.

Macroscopic Firm, well-circumscribed with tan, grey or pink colour. Arise within stomach wall. May project either into stomach lumen or from serosa.

Microscopic Most have bundles of spindle shaped cells. Occasionally tumour cells have a more epithelioid appearance with abundant cytoplasm which may appear vacuolated in fixed tissue. Features that are associated with malignancy include large tumour size (> 5 cm diameter), high mitotic rate (> 5 mitoses per 10 high powered fields) and marked pleomorphism or areas of necrosis. Express CD117 (c-kit) which can be detected immunocytochemically.

Lymphoma

This accounts for 2–5% of all gastric malignancies. The majority are high-grade diffuse B cell lymphomas. The majority of low-grade lymphomas belong to the group of tumours known as lymphomas of mucosa associated lymphoid tissue (MALT).

Macroscopy May have minimal changes with gastritis-type picture and thickened mucosal folds, or present as polypoid lesion or ulcer.

Microscopy Similar to MALT lymphomas elsewhere. Diffuse infiltrate of atypical lymphoid, centrocyte-like cells around and over-running reactive lymphoid follicle centres. Almost all (92–98%) associated with *H. pylori* infection.

Clinical features Present with non-specific abdominal symptoms. Mass or bleeding is rare.

Treatment These tumours can be successfully treated by surgery, radiotherapy and chemotherapy either alone or in combination. More recently 70% of early low-grade tumours have been shown to regress with eradication of *H. pylori* alone.

Prognosis Good. Dissemination is rare and occurs late in the course of the disease. Prognosis most dependent on stage and slightly less so on grade.

ANATOMY

Location   Pylorus to ileocaecal valve. Constituted by duodenum, jejunum and ileum. No sharp distinction between jejunum and ileum.

Length   3.5 m. First 20–25 cm is duodenum (most fixed and widest part). Jejunum makes up 40% and ileum 60% of the remainder.

Blood supply   Coeliac artery supplies stomach, duodenum, pancreas and liver. Superior mesenteric artery supplies jejunum and ileum with extensive collateral circulation through arcades between the mesentery and intestinal wall.

Macroscopy   The mucosa of the small intestine is thrown into numerous folds (valvulae conniventes) most prominent in the jejunum. The surface of the mucosa is arranged in villous processes.

HISTOLOGY

Villi are about 320–570 μm high and 85–140 μm wide. Covered by columnar epithelial cells with microvillous brush border, occasional mucin-secreting and neuroendocrine cell.

Crypts lie between each pair of villi. Depth is about one-third villous height. New epithelial cells derive from stem cells in the crypt bases which migrate up villi and shed into the lumen (cycle = 2–4 days). Crypts also contain Paneth and neuroendocrine cells.

Within the mucosa there is abundant lymphoid tissue constituting the normal gut associated lymphoid tissue (GALT) involved in the generation of mucosal immunity. Highest concentration is in Peyer's patches of terminal ileum. Within the dome epithelium there are adapted epithelial cells, so-called M-cells, which transport antigens from the lumen for presentation to the lymphoid tissue. GALT is composed of lymphoid follicles (follicle centre, mantle zone and a well-developed marginal zone), lamina propria plasma cells, and lamina-propria and intraepithelial T cells. Once activated the B cells are thought to leave the follicles into the bloodstream via efferent lymphatics and home back to the mucosa as IgA-secreting plasma cells.

....

FUNCTIONS

- Completion of digestion.
- Food breakdown by pancreatic enzymes, fat solubilized by bile salts.
- Absorption of food components:

  — large absorptive area
  — specific transport mechanisms.

- Transport of non-absorbed materials. This requires normal motility and normal balance of water and electrolyte transport across mucosa.
- Immunological surveillance of dietary organisms and micro-organisms (commensals and pathogenic).

....

CONGENITAL ABNORMALITIES
Meckel's diverticulum

Definition   Remnant of vitello-intestinal duct.

Epidemiology   Occurs in 2% of the population.

Macroscopy   Blind-ending diverticulum on anti-mesenteric border approximately 1 m from ileocaecal valve with same diameter as small intestine and 2–12 cm in length. Mostly the blind end is free, occasionally attached to umbilicus by fibrous cord. All layers of normal bowel are present.

Microscopy   Lined by gastric epithelium in 50%. Peptic ulceration may occur. There may be acute inflammation in patients presenting with appendicitis-like symptoms. Heterotopic pancreas may also be seen.

Clinical features Most asymptomatic. Some present with symtoms related to ulceration or sequelae such as haemorrhage or perforation.

Atresia or stenosis of small intestine

Position Usually in second part of duodenum.

Aetiology May be due to local vascular insufficiency during fetal life.

Macroscopy Blind segments may be linked by fibrous cord.

Failure of physiological rotation (exomphalos)

Pathogenesis Adherence or failure of return of midgut into the abdominal cavity following normal rotation in fifth week of fetal life.

....

DISORDERS OF FUNCTION

Malabsorption syndromes

Causes Reduction of absorptive area (pathological or iatrogenic e.g. following extensive surgery), disturbance of a specific transport mechanism or failure of adequate digestion of food. Many diseases may cause malabsorption.

Consequences Failure to absorb fat, fat-soluble vatamins and other nutrients.

Coeliac disease

Synonyms Coeliac sprue, gluten sensitive enteropathy.

Definition Chronic disease associated with variable degree of malabsorption caused by abnormal reaction to dietary wheat gliadin (alcohol-soluble portion of wheat gluten) or homologues (prolamins) in barley rye and oats.

Associations Can be associated with insulin-dependent diabetes mellitus, selective IgA defficiency and dermatitis herpetiformis.

Epidemiology Mostly seen in whites (1:1000–1200), highest in West Ireland (1:300), seen occasionally in Indians and rarely in Chinese, Japanese and indigenous Africans. First presentation at any age.

Pathogenesis Unclear. Several mechanisms have been proposed including:
- enzyme deficiency (unlikely as changes are usually reversed by gluten withdrawal)
- abnormal glycosylation of cell membrane glycoprotein leading to lectin-like binding between gluten and absorbtive cells
- genetic component (most likely – 70% concordance in identical twins and high familial association with 8–12% prevalence in first-degree relatives of sufferers) Associated with HLA class II antigens HLA-DR3 (70–90% N Europeans), HLA-DQw2 (> 90%) and HLA-B8
- immune mechanisms resulting in increased anti-gliadin antibodies. Other antibodies that have been found include anti-endomysium and antibodies to human jejunum
- cell-mediated immunity. There is an increase in intraepithelial T cells most of which are CD8+ and express the gamma/delta T cell receptor.

Macroscopy Surface of the mucosa has a flattened feature-less appearance.

Microscopy The features are not specific. Total/sub-total villous atrophy and crypt hyperplasia. Increased intraepithelial lymphocytes with clear halos (feature of T lymphocytes) and lamina propria plasma cells. Neutrophils, eosinophils and mast cells may be seen in the lamina propria. The diagnosis is formally confirmed by improvement following gluten withdrawal and relapse after reintroduction of dietary gluten (although the latter step is often omitted).

Prognosis Patients with coeliac disease are at increased risk of the development of malignant disease, predominantly lymphoma arising from intraepithelial T lymphocytes but also for carcinoma of the oropharynx, breast, oesophagus and small intestine.

Tropical sprue

Definition Coeliac-like syndrome occuring in inhabitants or visitors to certain areas of the tropics.

Epidemiology Endemic in Caribbean (excluding Jamaica), northern part of South America, Puerto Rico, India, parts of South East Asia and the Philippines.

Aetiology Thought to be infective, particularly associated with certain toxin-producing *Escherichia coli*.

Microscopy In some patients small intestinal biopsies are normal. In others there is villous atrophy with an inflammatory cell infiltrate that is rich in eosinophils.

Whipple's disease

Definition Rare multi-system disease usually presenting with steatorrhoea, abdominal cramps and fever. Can present with flitting polyarthritis, skin pigmentation, lymphadenopathy, CNS involvement and amyloidosis.

Epidemiology Chiefly white males (M:F 10:1).

Aetiology Intracellular organisms which have not yet been cultured.

Microscopy Large numbers of macrophages in the lamina propria distended by PAS positive material which on electron microscopy appear to be bacilli.

Bacterial overgrowth and malabsorption

Definition Malabsorption characterized by steatorrhoea, diarrhoea and protein malnutrition caused by abnormal flora.

Aetiology Increased bacterial flora caused by:
- decreased mechanical clearing of small gut by peristalsis (e.g. blind loop autonomic neuropathy)
- decreased gastric acidity or bile salts that normally destroy or inhibit proliferation of organisms before they reach the gut
- loss of secretion of immunoglobulins into intestine
- segmental stasis
- gastro-colic/enterocolic fistula.

Effects Inhibition of brush border enzymes. Damage to mucosa by secondary bile acids (formed by bacterial hydroxylation of primary bile acids). Deconjugation of bile acids inhibiting micelle formation.

Diagnostic test Culture of aspirated small intestinal juice. Breath test following ingestion of C 14-labelled glycine ingestion (false negative rate = 30%).

Abetalipoproteinaemia

Definition Autosomal recessive disorder caused by failure of synthesis of apoprotein B48 within enterocyte.

Clinical features Steatorrhoea in infancy with failure to thrive. Atypical retinitis pigmentosa involving the macula and ataxic neuropathy (degeneration of posterior columns of spinal cord).

Pathogenesis Inability to assemble chylomicrons within small intestinal wall with accumulation of dietary fat as intracytoplasmic triglyceride. Lack of lipids for cell membrane synthesis causes CNS abnormalities.

Congenital lymphangiectasia

Definition Abnormal development of intestinal and frequently limb lymphatics.

Pathogenesis Protein loss from gut leads to hypoproteinaemia. Failure to absorb fat.

Clinical features If lower limb involved the striking presentation is lower limb oedema. Pleural and peritoneal effusions may be seen.

Microscopy Thickened villi. Gross dilation of lymphatics in villi. Frequently fat droplets in lamina propria.

Ischaemic small intestinal disease

Epidemiology Acute transmural infarction occurs most often in the middle-aged and elderly.

Aetiology Severe underperfusion as a result of occlusion of superior mesenteric artery or one or more of its major branches or severe vasoconstriction of substantial mesenteric bed. Occasionally caused by obstruction of the mesenteric vein, usually thrombotic.

Pathogenesis   May be acute or chronic that will determine pathophysiology, resulting in pain after eating (intestinal angina) localized fibrosis resulting from chronic ischaemia or ischaemic necrosis confined to mucosa and submucosa or of full thickness (usually associated with severe lack of perfusion due to superior mesenteric artery occlusion either thrombotic or embolic).

Clinical features   Presentation with abrupt onset of severe abdominal pain, vomiting, fever and abdominal distention. Failure of peristalsis results in loss of bowel sounds.

Macroscopy   Infarcted bowel is dark reddish-purple in colour. Non-viable segments have dull (rather than shiny) serosa. On opening there may be a pseudomembrane, ischaemic ulceration or perforation.

Microscopy   Necrosis of the cells lining the villous tips is the earliest morphological change. The necrosis may extend into the mucosa or submucosa. A pseudomembrane composed of inflammatory exudate and necrotic tissue may be seen. Regeneration of ulcerated areas is associated with pseudo-pyloric metaplasia. There may be granulation tissue in the submucosa.

Prognosis   Associated with high mortality (50–75% treated, 100% if untreated).

Acquired diverticula

Position   Most in duodenum.

Epidemiology   Mostly in elderly people.

Macroscopy   Herniations of mucosa through the muscularis propria at vascular points of entry.

....

OBSTRUCTION OF THE SMALL INTESTINE

This may be complete or incomplete with the onset sudden or gradual. The cause can be **neural, vascular** or **mechanical**. The latter can be caused by lesions within the lumen (foreign bodies, gallstones, food; tumour or meconium in neonatal period), within the gut wall (fibrosis secondary to inflammation due to e.g. Crohn's disease or enteric coated tablet ingestion, congenital atresia/stenosis, strictures following ischaemia) or to lesions outside the wall causing external compression.

....

HAMARTOMAS OF THE SMALL INTESTINE

Peutz–Jeghers syndrome

(Hamartomatous gastrointestinal polyposis associated with mucosal and cutaneous pigmentation)

Definition Autosomal dominant syndrome with excessive melanin pigmentation in perioral mucosa and occasionally of skin of fingers and toes.

Macroscopy Polyps of variable size from a few mm to 5 cm most commonly found in jejunum, ileum and stomach, less frequently in colon.

Microscopy Branching muscularis mucosae covered by native-type epithelium and glands. Occasionally glands are misplaced into the deeper layers of the wall.

Prognosis Most common complication is recurrent bouts of intussusception. Carcinoma very rarely develops. Positive correlation with risk for ovarian sex cord neoplasms and breast carcinoma.

Cronkhite–Canada syndrome

Definition Polypoid changes in the stomach, small intestine and colon.

Clinical features Functional abnormality leads to protein loss.

Associations Hyperpigmentation of skin, baldness and nail atrophy.

Brunner's gland hamartoma

Location First and second parts of the duodenum in relation to the Brunner's glands.

Microscopy Abnormally branched muscularis mucosae similar to Peutz–Jeghers syndrome.

Clinical features Bleeding and occasionally obstruction.

....

NEOPLASMS OF THE SMALL INTESTINE
Adenomas

Very rare (with the exception of the ampulla of Vater). Tubular, tubulovillous or villous. May undergo malignant transformation.

Adenocarcinoma

Epidemiology Less frequent (40–60 times) than in the large intestine. May arise as complication of Crohn's disease or very rarely Peutz–Jeghers syndrome.

Location Most common in the upper part with 40% in duodenum mostly at ampulla of Vater.

Macroscopy Those at the ampulla of Vater have a papillary appearance. Others have stenosing 'napkin-ring' appearance.

Microscopy Most are well differentiated adenocarcinomas producing mucin. Many express CEA, some express murmidase. Other histological variants include small cell carcinomas.

Carcinoid tumours

Definition Tumours with wide spectrum of behaviour arising from neuroendocrine system. Most are argentaffin (secretory granules deposit silver salts in the absence of reducing agents) the remainder are argyrophil (silver salt deposition requires reducing agents).

Origin In gut either from Kulchitsky (enterochromaffin) cells found within crypts or from sub-epithelial neuroendocrine cells.

Location Anywhere in gut, 60–80% in appendix and ileum (mid-gut origin), 10–20% in large gut (hind-gut origin) and the remainder in the rest of the small intestine, stomach and oesophagus (foregut origin). Apart from the appendix the commonest site for mid-gut carcinoids is the ileum.

Macroscopy   Usually the nodule is covered by intact mucosa. Following formalin fixation cut surface is usually yellow.

Microscopy   Classic carcinoids have solid cellular islands (insular pattern). The cells are uniform, with scanty, pale-pink granular cytoplasm, round to oval nuclei with inconspicuous nucleoli and stippled chromatin. The cells at the periphery of the islands are palisaded. The mitotic index is low. Variants include goblet cell (crypt cell) carcinomas characterized by signet ring cells. The cells show evidence of epithelial and neuroendocrine differentiation expressing both low molecular weight cytokeratins and endocrine related antigens such as chromogranin, neurone-specific enolase, serotonin and synaptophysin.

Prognosis   Influenced by site of origin (appendix and rectum rarely aggressive while ileal, colonic and gastric carcinoids are often malignant). Around 15–35% of small intestinal carcinoids are multiple.

Clinical features   Slow growth rate but highly invasive with metastatic potential (with the exception of appendix carcinoids). Secondary tumours in lymph nodes and liver most frequently. Metastases are associated with the carcinoid syndrome. This is the result of pharmacologically active compounds and is characterized by flushing and cynosis, asthma-like wheezing, watery diarrhoea, episodic hypertension and palpitations, and right-sided cardiac failure.

....

CONNECTIVE TISSUE NEOPLASMS
Gastrointestinal stromal tumours

Definition   Term applied to connective tissue neoplasms of the gastrointestinal tract that show evidence of smooth muscle and nerve sheath differentiation.

Macroscopy   Can be well-defined nodular lesions in the bowel wall.

Microscopy   Spindle-cell tumours.

Prognosis Depends on the size and features of malignancy such as mitotic rate and presence of necrosis.

LYMPHOMA

Immunoproliferative small intestinal disease (IPSID, mediterranean lymphoma, α-chain disease)

Definition Variant of B-cell lymphoma of mucosa associated lymphoid tissue frequently associated with abnormal α-chain synthesis.

Microscopy Infiltration of the lamina propria by monoclonal plasma cells with few B cellls and occasional lymphoepithelial lesions. In the later stages blast cells become more frequent.

Clinical features In the very early stages IPSID will respond to antibiotic therapy.

Enteropathy associated T-cell lymphoma

Definition Malignant lymphoma of intraepithelial T cells mostly associated with coeliac disease.

Epidemiology Mostly in middle-aged patients with a history of coeliac disease which may be of adult onset or poorly controlled.

Macroscopy Can be shallow ulcers without obvious tumour within the spectrum of ulcerative jejunitis, or as tumour masses.

Microscopy Variable. Frequently large cells with variable number of smaller cells. Eosinophils may be present.

Burkitt's lymphoma

Common in Middle East. Chiefly at ileo-caecal valve.

Multiple lymphomatous polyposis

Definition Mantle cell lymphoma presenting with intestinal polyps.
Location Usually in ileo-caecal region.

ANATOMY

Length   40–20 cm (mean 7 cm).

Position   Diverticulum of caecum which may lie in a variety of sites around the caecum/terminal ileum region.

HISTOLOGY

Lining similar to that of the large bowel. Non-branching crypts lined by absorptive and mucin-secreting cells. Neuroendocrine cells at crypt bases and in the lamina propria.

ACUTE APPENDICITIS

Epidemiology   Common in Western Europe and North America but rare in non-white communities in Africa and Asia. Uncommon in children less than 5 years, with peak incidence in second and third decades.

Pathogenesis   Obstruction of lumen thought to be important and may be due to lumenal block by inspissated faecal material (faecolith; seen in 9–90% cases), lymphoid hyper-plasia in the wall or may be functional due to muscle contraction in the appendix wall. The obstruction results in increased lumenal pressure leading to mucosal ischaemia, loss of the mucosal lining and invasion of the wall by micro-organisms. Many types of organism may be involved including yersinial infection and actinomycosis. Viral infections such as measles and adenovirus may precipitate appendicitis probably due to lymphoid hyperplasia. The appendix can also be involved in specific inflammatory conditions such as tuberculosis, Crohn's disease and schisto-somiasis.

Macroscopy   In the early stages there may be mild to moderate swelling with serosal hyperaemia. As inflammation advances the serosa becomes opaque with fibinous/fibropurulent exudate. With further progression the appendix becomes soft.

Microscopy There is acute inflammation of the appendix wall with focal ulceration of the surface. In advanced cases (gangrenous appendicitis) there will be abscesses with destruction of the wall as a prelude to rupture. In yersinial infections there is characteristically micro-abscess formation in the lymphoid follicle centres.

Consequences
- perforation: associated with peritoneal soiling and either generalized peritonitis and risk of septic shock or, if the process remains localized, the development of an appendix abscess
- thrombosis of small veins of mesoappendix: infective thrombi which may extend to larger vessels, spread to portal circulation and cause multiple liver abscesses (suppurative pylephlebitis)
- formation of adhesions: may lead to intestinal obstruction
- fibrous occlusion of appendix: following healing there may be fibrous obliteration of the appendiceal tip. If fibrosis is more proximal there may be accumulation of mucinous secretions in the tip leading to a mucocele.

....

NEOPLASMS OF THE APPENDIX

Carcinoid tumours

Epidemiology Commonest appendicular tumour (80%) present in up to 0.3% of appendices as an incidental finding.

Pathogenesis The majority are of midgut type but hindgut carcinoids do occur.

Macroscopy Frequently seen as a small yellowish nodule in the tip of the appendix.

Microscopy Similar to those seen in the small intestine.

Behaviour See small gut carcinoids.

Polyps

Types Metaplastic, hamartomatous (Peutz–Jeghers and juvenile types) and adenomatous polyps are seen.

Macroscopy The adenomas are different from other large bowel adenomas being predominantly diffuse papillary lesions with a sessile base. May be associated with copious mucin formation and dilation of lumen (cystadenoma).

Microscopy Similar to large bowel lesions with a variable degree of dysplasia.

Clinical features Cystadenomas may rupture to give pseudomyxoma peritonei.

Adenocarcinoma

Epidemiology Rare.

Pathogenesis Arise on basis of pre-existing adenomas.

Microscopy Requires the identification of true invasion of the appendix wall.

Spread Lymph node metastasis present in up to 25% patients at diagnosis.

Treatment Right hemicolectomy.

Prognosis Overall 5-year survival in region of 65%.

INFECTIOUS AND INFLAMMATORY BOWEL DISEASE

....

ACUTE INFECTIOUS ENTEROCOLITIS

General considerations

Epidemiology A leading cause of death in the Third World, the incidence is profoundly affected by adverse socioeconomic conditions. It is estimated that 4.5–6 million children in Africa, Asia and South Americal die of these disorders. In the USA the mean incidence of infective enterocolitis is 1.5–1.9 attacks per person per year causing considerable morbidity.

Pathogenesis   There are several mechanisms.
- release of toxins within lumen without tissue invasion. Toxins may be ingested without the presence of bacteria.
- invading the bowel wall, damaging the lining epithelium and causing an inflammatory response
- invading the bowel wall and localizing to Peyer's patches.

The occurrence and severity of the infection depends on an interaction between the dose and virulence of the infecting organism and the host defences. Host defences include normal gastric acid, gastrointestinal mobility, the normal bacterial flora and the immune status.

Cholera

Aetiology   *Vibrio cholerae*.

Bacteriology   Comma-shaped toxin-producing bacillus.

Pathogenesis   There is no invasion of the wall. The toxin results in prolonged activation of adenylate cyclase with consequent sustained production of cAMP. The result is that villious cells are prevented from absorbing sodium, chloride and water and the crypt cells pump out sodium, chloride and bicarbonate with associated water loss.

Source   One of the commonest water contaminants in the Third World.

Clinical features   Profuse watery diarrhoea (up to 20 litres per day) with tiny flecks of mucus (rice-water stool).

Treatment   As the transport of glucose (which is coupled with sodium) is unaffected, oral rehydrating solutions of glucose or rice with sodium chloride are effective.

Toxin-producing *Escherichia coli* enteritis (traveller's diarrhoea)

Aetiology   Some types of *Escherichia coli*.

Pathogenesis   The heat-labile toxin produced by these organisms are similar in effect as those of *Vibrio cholerae*.

Shigella dysentery

Aetiology *Shigella dysenteriae, S. flexneri, S. boydii* and *S. sonnei*.

Bacteriology Slender Gram-negative bacilli. Natural habitat is the primate gut. Minimal infective dose is less than 1000 organisms. As well as endotoxin (lipopolysaccharide) derived from the cell wall there is an exotoxin that affects the bowel and CNS.

Source 'Food, fingers, faeces and flies'.

Pathogenesis Invasion of the mucosal epithelium is followed by the formation of small abscesses in the wall of the colon and terminal ileum.

Clinical features Sudden onset of abdominal pain, fever and watery diarrhoea. Within a few days the stool becomes more solid with mucus and blood.

Microscopy there is stippling of the normal lining, bleeding and the formation of a pseudomembrane of fibrin cell debris, necrotic mucosa, acute inflammatory cells and bacteria. Ulcers are usually shallow but deep ulcers may occur, healing of which results in mucus retention cysts.

Campylobacter infections

Aetiology *Campylobacter jejuni* is commonest.

Bacteriology Motile Gram-negative comma-shaped bacilli.

Source Food, drink and infected animals.

Pathogenesis Organisms multiply in the small intestine, invade the bowel wall and produce acute inflammation. In addition to the small bowel the appendix, colon and rectum can be involved.

Clinical features Fever, abdominal pain and bloody diarrhoea.

Clostridium difficile and pseudomembranous colitis

Aetiology *Clostridium difficile.*

Pathogenesis Following suppression of normal gut flora by some antibiotic therapy the organism (present as normal flora in 2–10% normal individuals) multiplies to excess. The bacterium produces two toxins: one is cytotoxic, the other is cytotoxic but also has features similar to those of cholera-toxin.

Laboratory findings Diagnosis is established by identifying toxin in stool.

Site In severe cases the rectum is often involved.

Macroscopy Pale yellowish-grey plaques of membrane adhere to the surface varying in size from a few millimetres to 15–20 cm.

Microscopy Initial focal mucosal necrosis is covered by mushroom-shaped tufts of fibrin, mucus and acute inflammatory cells.

Yersinia enterocolitis

Aetiology *Yersinia enterocolitica* and *Yersinia pseudotuberculosis*.

Bacteriology Short Gram-negative bacilli. Various animals are the natural host. Minimal infective dose is large (10^8–10^9).

Source Food or drink contaminated by faeces of infected animals.

Pathogenesis Organisms multiply intramucosally.

Clinical features In infants symtoms of acute gastroenteritis but in older children symtoms are of acute appendicitis.

Microscopy Acute inflammation, ulceration and microabscesses in the mucosa but also affecting lymphoid tissue including mesenteric lymph nodes. Macrophages cluster around abscesses. True granulomas are rare with *Y. enterocolitica* but common with *Y. pseudotuberculosis*.

Natural history and prognosis Usually self-limiting but can be associated with pneumonia and meningitis.

Salmonella infections

Aetiology There are many *Salmonella* species.

Bacteriology Motile Gram-negative bacilli. Mean infective dose is 10^5–10^8, except for *S. typhi* which may be as low as 10^3.

Source Inoculation is via the mouth. *Salmonella typhi*, *Paratyphi A*. and *Schottmulleri* (formally paratyphi B) come from another human. Other species come from a wide variety of animal sources.

Pathogenesis Typhoid fever follows invasion of the bowel wall and localization of organisms in the Peyer's patches. Organisms multiply in macrophages in the gut, associated lymphoid tissue and in the regional lymph nodes. There is bacteraemia and organisms are ingested by tissue macrophages in liver sinusoids and the spleen. Some organisms are excreted in the bile, reach the gallbladder and make a second appearance in the gut lumen.

Clinical features *Salmonella* infection may cause enterocolitis (many types, mostly *S. typhimurium*), bacteraemia or typhoid fever (enteric fever, caused by *S.typhi*, *Paratyphi* A and *Schottmulleri*). *Salmonella* enterocolitis follows 8–48 h after inoculation with nausea, vomiting, fever, headache and watery diarrhoea. Typhoid fever presents during the bacteraemic phase with fever, malaise, headache, myalgia and mental clouding. There may be bradycardia and there is often constipation. Fever plateaus in the second week decreasing in the third and fourth weeks. In the second week a maculopapular rash (rose spots) appears, lasting a few days.

Laboratory features Organisms can be cultured from stool and urine.

Macroscopy There may be oval ulcers with their long axis along the length of the bowel.

Microscopy Ulcers show large numbers of rounded macrophages. Neutrophils are scarce. The macrophage response can be seen in lesions outside the bowel.

Complications Common in weeks 3 and 4 of illness with the most important being haemorrage and perforation but also acute cholecystitis, paralytic ileus, myocarditis, focal necrosis in liver and kidneys and Zenker's degeneration of abdominal muscle.

Intestinal tuberculosis

Aetiology *Mycobacterium tuberculosis* and *Mycobacterium bovis*.

Source Primarily from drinking infected milk (*M.bovis*); secondary source is the swallowing of infected sputum in patients with pulmonary disease.

Site Most commonly the jejunum and ileum; may occur in the following sites (in order of frequency): appendix, colon, rectum and duodenum. Very rare in oesophagus, stomach or anus.

Macroscopy Ulceration is usually circumferential. There may be an inflammatory process extending through the thickness of the bowel forming a mass of inflamed fibrous tissue.

Intestinal *Mycobacterium avium intracellulare* infection

Pathogenesis Seen in patients with AIDS in whom cell-mediated immunity is disturbed.

Microscopy Lamina propria infiltrated by many large granular macrophages.

Intestinal spirochaetosis

Aetiology Organisms of genus *Borrelia*.

Clinical features Probably non-pathogenic.

Chlamydial infections

Site Rectum.

Clinical features Anal pain, tenesmus and passage of blood and mucus per rectum.

Macroscopy Reddened, friable and ulcerated mucosa.

Microscopy Florid non-specific inflammation with much fibrosis.

Rotavirus

Epidemiology Commonest cause of severe diarrhoea in infants and young children accounting for about 34% of hospitalizations of children under 2 years. There are 3.5 million cases per year in the USA and 125 million cases of diarrhoea per year in developing countries, 18 million of which are severe; 800 000–900 000 are fatal.

Virology A Reovirus with double stranded RNA and a non-enveloped icosahedral structure.

Source Transmitted by faecal–oral route.

Norwalk virus

Epidemiology Causes diarrhoea in adults and school-aged children. Important cause of epidemic gastroenteritis in institutions.

Source Infected water or poorly cooked shellfish from infected waters.

Adenovirus

Epidemiology Mainly children under 2 years accounting for up to 20% of cases in this age group.

Aetiology Adenovirus group F, serotypes 40,41.

Clinical features Watery diarrhoea which may be followed by vomiting.

Astrovirus

Epidemiology Probably very common as 70% British children have antibodies by 4 years old. Mostly children 1–7 years.

Clinical features Watery diarrhoea.

Giardiasis

Aetiology Giardia lamblia.

Epidemiology Greatest in areas with poor hygiene and sanitation.

Source Drinking contaminated water.

Site Duodenum and jejunum.

Clinical features In areas where *Giardia* is prevalent many of the indigenous population are asymptomatic carriers while people newly infected (e.g. travellers) develop diarrhoea, abdominal pain and occasionally steatorrhoea.

Microscopy In some there may be no abnormality while in others there is an increase in intraepithelial and lamina propria lymphocytes. There may be villous atrophy particularly in those with malabsorption.

Cryptosporidiosis

Epidemiology Found in 14–26% AIDS patients with diarrhoea.

Parasitology Oocysts release sporozoites in small intestine which become attached to the brush border. These enter the cells and undergo asexual development releasing merozoites that invade other cells in the vicinity.

Clinical features Depends on immune competence of the individual. In competent individuals there is watery diarrhoea, cramping abdominal pain and loss of appetite lasting 5–14 days. In immunosuppressed individuals the illness can be more severe and prolonged.

Microscopy In the small intestine the appearances range from normal to markedly inflamed with crypt abscesses, villous shortening/destruction. The parasites can be seen on the brush border as basophilic bodies 3–4 μm diameter and can be highlighted by Ziehl–Neelsen stains.

Isospora belli

Epidemiology Found in 2–6% AIDS patients with diarrhoea.

Parasitology Oocysts release sporozoites which enter the epithelium.

Source Contaminated water or food.

Site Small bowel epithelium.

Clinical features Diarrhoea and malabsorption. In immune suppressed individuals *I. belli* causes a chronic illness with cramping abdominal pain, nausea and weight loss.

Microscopy Variable degree of villous atrophy and a moderately intense inflammatory response with lymphocytes and plasma cells. Parasites may be seen in epithelial cells.

Amoebic dysentery

Aetiology   *Entamoeba histolytica.*

Epidemiology   Worldwide distribution but more common in the tropics.

Parasitology   Exists either in a mobile vegetative form (found in stool of patients with active illness) or in cystic form (passed in stool). The cyst wall dissolves in the intestinal lumen following ingestion. The amoeba produces proteolytic enzymes which are ulcerogenic and phagoctose red blood cells.

Site   Most common in caecum and rectum but can be seen anywhere in the large bowel.

Clinical features   Moderately severe diarrhoea with blood and mucus.

Macroscopy   Ulcers tend to be circumferential.

Microscopy   Ulcers have a narrow neck and broad base (flask shape). Amoebae can usually be found on or just below the ulcer surface. Can be highlighted by periodic acid-Schiff stain.

Complications   Perforation is rare but frequently fatal. Amoebae may penetrate the bowel wall and travel to the liver in the portal circulation to form single or multiple amoebic abscesses which may subsequently rupture through the diaphragm into lung/pleural cavity, into the pericardial cavity or into the peritoneum. More distant spread via small hepatic venules may also occur.

....

NON-INFECTIOUS CHRONIC INFLAMMATORY BOWEL DISEASE

Crohn's disease

Definition   Characterized by inflammation that is granulomatous in 60% and can occur anywhere in the gastrointestinal tract from mouth to anus (small bowel 66%, large bowel 17%, both in 17%) and most often in a discontinuous pattern, with involvement of the full thickness of the bowel wall and involvement of extraintestinal sites (e.g. skin, vulva and bone/joints).

Epidemiology   Most common in temperate climates and among those of Euopean origin. Jews are more often affected than non-Jews (Ashkenazy > Sephardic). Annual incidence of 2–5/100,000 and prevalence of 30–75/100,000. There appear to be three age peaks 20–29 (highest), 50–59 and 70–79.

Aetiology   Unknown but suggested factors include microorganisms (*Mycobacteria* and viruses, particularly measles virus), genetic factors, environmental factors (including cigarette smoking and intake of refined sugars) and other immune-mediated factors (including increased concentrations of antigen-presenting cells, and altered activities of natural killer cells and activated lymphocytes).

Site   Although Crohn's can occur anywhere in the gastrointestinal tract involvement of the terminal ileum is common (terminal ileitis).

Clinical features   Variable. Diarrhoea is present in 80% (associated with blood if the colon is involved). There may be fever and lower abdominal pain which is abrupt in onset, severe and localized in 20%, suggesting a surgical emergency. In others presentation is related to changes such as stricture formation (symptoms related to chronic or sub-acute obstruction), fistula formation or malabsorption (if terminal ileum involved and including pernicious anaemia).

Macroscopy   In the early phases there are small superficial ulcers. These coalesce to become serpiginous and the combination of the ulcers and intervening oedema and lymphoid hyperplasia gives the characteristic **cobble-stone** appearance. The submucosa and muscularis becomes oedematous and inflammation may involve the serosa. Multiple **skip lesions** may be seen. With disease progression there is formation of deep fissures penetrating the wall which may form the basis for fistulae between bowel loops, with the skin or other hollow viscera (e.g. bladder). Anal fistulae are seen in up to one-third of patients. Oedema and fibrosis at this time confers a rigid **hose-pipe** appearance to the affected segments.

Microscopy   There are several features of Crohn's disease that are characteristic:

• transmural inflammation from mucosa to serosa
• marked oedema of the submucosa

- the presence of lymphoid aggregates and follicles
- patchy mucosal ulceration and fissuring ulceration
- presence of non-caseating tuberculoid granulomas (only seen in 60%) at any level of the bowel wall and also seen in lymph nodes.

Other features that may be present include pseudo-pyloric metaplasia in mucosa glands, thickening of nerve fibres and thickening of the muscularis mucosae.

Natural history and prognosis There is an increased risk of developing carcinoma as a late complication (3% patients).

Extraintestinal complications can affect:

- eyes – 4% experience inflammatory conditions of the eye e.g. conjunctivitis, episcleritis or uveitis
- joints – 15% suffer sacro-ileitis or mono-articular arthritis. Ankylosing spondylitis is seen in 1–6%
- liver – fatty change is common. Sclerosing cholangitis is rare (< 1%)
- skin – erythema nodosum is seen in 5–10% and pyoderma gangrenosum occurs in about 1%.

Ulcerative colitis

Definition Inflammatory condition of unknown cause affecting primarily large bowel mucosa starting in the rectum and spreading proximally in continuity.

Epidemiology Commoner than Crohn's disease with an annual incidence in Europe and the USA of 8–11/100 000 and a prevalence of 80–120/100 000. Whites are more commonly affected than blacks and Jews more than non-Jews.

Aetiology No infectious agent has been seriously implicated. There is some evidence that genetic factors may play a role. There is a negative correlation with smoking. There is no clear data implicating abnormal immune-mediated mechanisms although there is an increase in antibody-producing cells in the affected mucosa and type 1 hypersensitivity is increased in frequency in ulcerative colitis patients.

Clinical features Diarrhoea with blood and mucus. Attacks last for a variable time from days to months.

Site Confined to the colon although some involvement of the terminal ileum may occur (backwash ileitis). Tends to affect the rectum and spread proximally in continuity.

Macroscopy The bowel appears shortened which is most appreciated in relation to the rectum and distal colon and is not due to fibrous scarring. The affected mucosa is reddened with a roughened friable velvety appearance. Later small ulcers appear which may coalesce to form irregular ulcerated areas. Intervening non-ulcerated mucosa may be oedematous and polypoid in appearance. Occasionally ulcers extend laterally tunnelling under non-ulcerated mucosa.

Microscopy In actively inflamed mucosa there is marked hyperaemia and an inflammatory infiltrate in the lamina propria in which plasma eosinophils and neutrophils are prominent. Neutrophils infiltrate the crypts and destroy part of the crypt wall (**crypt abscess**). The mucosal surface shows loss of suface epithelium and pus. The inflammatory process is confined to the mucosa with little spill-over into the superficial submucosa. However if fulminating colitis supervenes the inflammation becomes transmural. Active inflammation is accompanied by loss of goblet cells. In the course of resolution there is restoration of lost crypts with the new crypts showing irregularity and branching. If there has been severe mucosal loss the new crypts will not regrow to reach the muscularis mucosae and there will be persistent shortening. Longstanding diease is associated with the appearance of Paneth-cell metaplasia, endocrine cell hyperplasia and adipose tissue in the mucosa.

Natural history and prognosis Disease pursues a chronic course punctuated by episodes of relapse and remission. In a proportion of cases (5–10%) a fulminating diarrhoeal illness can develop in which a part of the bowel (mostly the transverse colon) becomes dilated to greater than 5 cm diameter and the wall becomes markedly thinned (toxic megacolon). Perforation may occur in which case there is a high mortality.

Long-standing extensive ulcerative colitis carries an increased risk for carcinoma with some studies showing 7.2% of patients with total/extensive colitis developing carcinoma after 20 years rising to 16.5% at 30 years. These tumours are often multiple, flat and diffusely infiltrative and are preceded by epithelial dysplasia. Mucinous carcinomas are relatively over-represented as a group in these patients.

Extraintestinal manifestations include:

- cirrhosis of the liver
- sclerosing cholangitis (12% patients).

Collagenous colitis

Definition Abnormally thick layers of collagen present beneath the basement membrane.

Epidemiology Most are middle-aged females.

Clinical features Watery diarrhoea.

Site Most obvious in the rectum and left side of colon. May be patchy.

Microscopy in addition to the thickened collagenous layer there is a mild to moderate non-specific inflammatory infiltrate in the laminal propria.

Colitis in graft-versus-host disease

Epidemiology Patients who have received allogenic bone marrow transplantation.

Microscopy There is focal apoptosis in the crypt epithelium which may be associated with crypt abscess formation. Neuroendocrine cells survive while other epithelial cells in the crypts are lost.

Radiation colitis

Epidemiology Following irradiation particularly seen following pelvic irradiation.

Clinical features Acute damage is associated with diarrhoea, colicky abdominal pain and tenesmus. Chronic damage may lead to obstruction.

Microscopy Acute changes include loss of surface epithelium and damage to crypt epithelium with an infiltration of the lamina propria and epithelium by eosinophils. Chronic damage is associated with scarring, oedema, homogenization of the collagen, the presence of atypical fibroblasts and vascular changes (e.g. fibrinoid necrosis of small vessels, endothelial cell swelling, thrombosis and sub-epithelial accumulations of lipid-laden macrophages).

The solitary rectal ulcer syndrome (mucosal prolapse)

Epidemiology   Mostly young adults.

Site   Usually ulcer on anterior or anterolateral rectal wall.

Pathogenesis   Associated with faulty motility of the affected bowel segment resulting in straining at stool. Ischaemia of the mucosa may be the cause of the histological changes.

Clinical features   Rectal bleeding, pain and passage of mucus in stools.

Macroscopy   There may be ulceration.

Microscopy   Scarring in the lamina propria associated with splitting and arborization of the muscularis mucosae with fibres arranged vertically in the mucosa. The crypts are hyperplastic, have a characteristic diamond shape and show depletion of the goblet-cell population.

THE COLON AND RECTUM

....

ANATOMY

Size   Approximately 1.5m long.

Regions   Divided into caecum, ascending colon, transverse colon, descending colon, sigmoid colon and rectum.

Site   The large bowel extends from the ileocaecal valve to the anus. The caecum and transverse colon are completely surrounded by peritoneum apart from the mesenteric attachments. The ascending and descending colon are covered by peritoneum on their anterior aspects only. The upper third of the rectum is covered by peritoneum on anterior and lateral aspects, the middle third on the anterior aspect only and the lower third is below the peritoneal reflection.

Blood supply   The right side of the colon and half the transverse colon are supplied by branches of the superior mesenteric artery and the left side and rectum is supplied by the inferior mesenteric artery with the 'watershed' area being the splenic flexure. The arterial branches are accompanied by veins with a well-formed plexus in the submucosa and a less well-developed one in the serosa.

Lymphatic drainage Lymph either drains into nodes lying close to the gut wall or via lymph nodes adjacent to blood vessels. Lymphatics draining the lowest part of the rectum drain into internal iliac and to some extent inguinal nodes.

Nerve supply Parasympathetic fibres are derived from the vagus and sacral spinal nerves with their pre-ganglionic fibres terminating in the myenteric (Auerbach's) plexus between the layers of the muscularis propria. The sympathetic supply is from the lower thoracic and lumber spinal nerves with the pre-ganglionic fibres terminating in the superior and inferior mesenteric ganglia. The postganglionic sympathetic fibres terminate either in the myenteric plexus or in Meissner's plexus in the sub-mucosa.

HISTOLOGY

The mucosa

There are no villi. The epithelium is arranged in non-branching crypts perpendicular to the surface. There are four principal cell types (Table 34.3).

Table 34.3 Principal cell types of the mucosa

Mature columnar cells	Majority cell component. Absorb water and electrolytes. Secrete brush-border enzymes. Transport IgA to the lumen
Goblet cells	Secrete acid mucins
Endocrine cells	Most on left side of colon, in lower part of crypts. Secrete peptides e.g. somatostatin, 5-hydroxytryptamine, glucagon and a VIP-like product
Undifferentiated stem cells	Give rise to all other types. Situated in lowest part of crypts. Daughter cells move up crypts to surface over period of 3–7 days

The crypts are separated from the surrounding well-vascularized lamina propria by a basement membrane and thin (7 μm) collagenous plate. The lamina propria contains IgA secreting plasma cells, fibroblasts, mast cells, eosinophils, macrophages and occasional lymphoid follicles.

Sub-mucosa and muscularis propria

The sub-mucosa is similar to that of the rest of the intestine. The muscularis propria is arranged in an inner circular layer forming a continuous sheath while the outer longitudinal layer, while also a continuous layer, is concentrated into three linear bands (taeniae coli). These muscle bands are slightly shorter than the overall length of the large bowel with resulting outpouchings (haustra).

HIRSCHSPRUNG'S DISEASE (CONGENITAL MEGACOLON)

Definition Megacolon is a gross dilation of the colon usually associated with severe constipation.

Epidemiology Present from birth. Affects 1/5000 live births. M:F 4:1. Seen 10 × more often in patients with Down's syndrome (2% Down's syndrome infants) compared with normal.

Pathogenesis Defective migration of cells from the neural crest results in absence of ganglion cells in the submucosal and myenteric plexuses. This leads to defective peristalsis and functional obstruction. In most cases (82%) the involved segment is short and does not extend above the descending–sigmoid colon junction but in 13% the whole colon is involved.

Clinical features Severe constipation with onset any time from a few days after birth to adulthood. In some cases this can be associated with a severe enterocolitis.

Macroscopy The segment lacking the ganglion cells is narrowed. The gut proximal to this shows gross dilation with muscle hypertrophy (due to increased workload).

Microscopy Diagnosis is established by demonstrating the absence of ganglion cells. There is a marked degree of nerve fibre hyperplasia which contains large amounts of acetyl-cholinesterase (an abnormal finding in the gut). The dilated portion proximal to the obstruction has normal numbers of ganglion cells.

Neuronal intestinal dysplasia

This is a condition related to Hirschsprung's disease with identical clinical and radiological features but normal ganglion cells. It is characterized by abnormalities of the parasympathetic innervation of the large intestine including hyperplasia of nerve fibres of myenteric plexus, increases acetyl cholinesterase activity and presence of giant ganglion cells. These features are either localized or diffuse.

Adynamic bowel syndrome

Another related condition with deficiencies in cholinergic fibres.

Acquired megacolon

Aetiology May be associated with obstruction (e.g. due to tumour or post-inflammatory scarring), and endocrine disorder (e.g. hypothyroidism), drugs, central nervous system disorders (e.g. Parkinson's disease), psychogenic disorders or to destruction of ganglion cells (e.g. Chagas' disease caused by *Trypanosoma cruzi*, common in South America and in particular Brazil).

DIVERTICULAR DISEASE

Definition Includes the presence of diverticula (diverticulosis) and the condition when one or more diverticula become inflamed (diverticulitis).

Epidemiology Prevalence increases with age with two-thirds of those over 80 years affected in Western communities. There is a marked geographic variation with the condition being rare in communities that are predominantly vegetarian with a high fibre diet, (e.g. rural Africa).

Site Sigmoid colon predominantly. Rectum never involved.

Pathogenesis These are pulsion diverticula thought to be related to exaggeration of normal peristalsis and high intra-luminal pressure although direct evidence for this is lacking. Diverticulitis develops when the surface is eroded by hard faecal material allowing the entry of infected material into the underlying tissues.

Clinical features Diverticulosis is frequently an incidental finding at autopsy. In the living, it presents with left-sided abdominal pain, tenderness in the left lower quadrant, fever and occasionally signs of peritoneal irritation.

Macroscopy The diverticula are seen as rounded sacs protruding through potential defects in the circular muscle associated with blood vessel penetration. They lie in rows between the mesenteric taenia and the two anti-mesenteric taeniae either within the serosa or pericolic adipose tissue.

Microscopy Outpouchings of mucosa extend through the muscle coat to the serosa. Once diverticulitis supervenes there are small abscesses in the pericolic tissue and there may be a foreign body giant cell reaction to faecal material.

Natural history and prognosis Characteristically inter-mittent course with remissions and exacerbations. Complications include perforation, haemorrhage, fistula formation and low colonic obstruction.

....

VASCULAR DISORDERS OF THE COLON AND RECTUM

Ischaemia

Aetiology May result from defective perfusion (e.g. hypo-tension or hypovolaemia), vascular stenosis (athero-sclerosis, thrombosis, embolism), arterial spasm or vasculitis.

Pathogenesis Damage is due to underperfusion. Free radical mediated reperfusion injury may aggravate the damage.

Macroscopy There may be full thickness, gangrenous, necrosis or ischaemic enterocolitis (when the changes are confined to the mucosa).

Natural history and prognosis Ischaemic stricture may occur with fibrous tissue repair of necrotic segments. Iscaemic enterocolitis may result in complete resolution.

Necrotizing enterocolitis of the newborn

Epidemiology Rare. Affects premature infants.

Site Both small and large bowel may be affected.

Clinical features Abdominal distension, bloody diarrhoea and vomiting.

Macroscopy Patchy necrosis of the mucosa and submucosa. Full thickness necrosis with perforation may occur. Submucosal gas-filled cysts (pneumatosis intestinalis) are common.

Angiodysplasia (angioectasia)

Epidemiology Chiefly elderly patients. May occur in association with von Willebrand's disease, hereditary haemorrhagic telangectasia (Rendu–Osler–Weber disease).

Site More common on right side, frequently opposite the ileo-caecal valve.

Clinical features Often presents with iron-deficiency anaemia due to blood loss. More rarely there may be acute massive haemorrhage. Diagnosed by angiography or colonoscopy.

Microscopy Groups of thin-walled blood vessels in the mucosa and submucosa.

Cavernous haemangioma

Site Most often sigmoid colon or rectum.

Clinical features Usual presentation is with rectal bleeding.

Macroscopy Mucosa appears plum-coloured but usually no mass is visible.

Microscopy Many tortuous vessels are seen. Some contain thrombus.

NON-NEOPLASTIC POLYPS OF THE COLON AND RECTUM

Hyperplastic polyp

Epidemiology   Seen in 30–50% of adults.

Site   Anywhere in colon and appendix.

Macroscopy   Small (up to 5 mm diameter) usually sessile and may be multiple.

Microscopy   No increase in crypt number but the lower third is lined predominently by goblet cells. The upper part has a saw-tooth outline with hyperplastic mucin-secreting columnar cells. Natural history and prognosis: these are **not** pre-malignant.

Juvenile (retention) polyp

Epidemiology   Commonest polyps in children with two-thirds of all cases occurring in childhood.

Site   Commonly sigmoid.

Clinical features   Causes rectal bleeding. Occasionally there are multiple polyps (multiple juvenile polyposis). May be seen as part of the Cronkhite–Canada syndrome associated with baldness, nail atrophy and hyperpigmentation.

Macroscopic   Often single but may be multiple. The surface is red and granular and the cut surface shows mucin-filled cysts.

Microscopy   The cysts are dilated crypts distended by mucus. The lamina propria is inflamed. Natural history and prognosis: no malignant potential.

Hamartomatous polyps

Seen in Peutz–Jehger's syndrome or in Cowden's syndrome (autosomal dominant inherited disease) in association with tumours and tumour-like lesions of skin and mucosae together with an increased incidence of malignancy.

....

TUMOURS OF THE COLON AND RECTUM

Adenoma

Definition   A lesion, usually polypoid, representing a focus of intraepithelial neoplasia in the gut mucosa.

Epidemiology   Found in approximately 30% adult postmortems. Frequency increases with age.

Site   May be single or multiple. Seen in right side (40%), left side (40%) and rectum (20%).

Clinical features   Most are asymptomatic but can present with rectal bleeding. Villous adenomas may be associated with fluid and electrolyte, particularly potassium, loss.

Macroscopy   In the early stages may be sessile but most become pedunculated as a knob-like lesion projecting into the lumen on a stalk lined on each side by normal mucosa. In some adenomas the surface is thrown into velvety folds (villous adenomas).

Microscopy   Crowded mass of branched tubules lined by epithelium showing differing degrees of severity (tubular adenomas). One third of lesions show a papillary configuration alone (villous adenoma) or in combination (tubulovillous adenoma).

Natural history and prognosis   All adenomas have malignant potential but carcinoma occurs more commonly in villous adenomas (30–79%).

Adenocarcinoma

Epidemiology   One of the commonest tumours in the West causing 19 000 deaths annually in the UK. There is considerable geographic variation, the disease being commonest in the developed world (Europe, North America, and Australia) and rarest in developing countries (Africa, South America and Asia).

Aetiology   May be associated with meat consumption.

Pathogenesis   Most are thought to arise from pre-existing adenoma.

Genetics   Well-defined inherited syndromes are associated with the development of carcinoma.

Multiple familial polyposis syndromes

- inherited as autosomal dominant or recessive
- include familial adenomatous polyposis coli (dominant), Gardner's syndrome (dominant, associated with fibromatoses, osteomas of skull and mandible, cysts in skin and other extracolonic manifestations) and Turcot's syndrome (recessive, associated with malignant tumours of the CNS)
- account for 1% colon cancers
- polyps not present at birth, appearing any time 4–70 years
- two patterns: either carpet (numerous tiny polyps) or multiple discrete larger polyps
- development of carcinoma inevitable unless prophylactic colectomy undertaken.

Familial adenomatous polyposis coli (FAPC)

- occurs in 1/8000–1/29 000 individuals with a quarter to one-third of these new mutations
- mean age of presentation 39 years
- life expectancy without colectomy is 42 years
- also associated with gastric hyperplastic polyps (30–50%), duodenal adenomas (around ampulla of Vater, 90%), papillary carcinoma of thyroid, ileal carcinoid tumours, brain tumours.

Hereditary non-polyposis colorectal cancer

Two types:

- Lynch syndrome I – excess of cancer affecting colon/ rectum only.
- Lynch syndrome II – excess of cancer affecting colon/ rectum as well as endometrium, ovary and pancreas.

In both cases the proximal (right side) colon is affected most.

Molecular genetics

There is thought to be a sequential progression from normal mucosa through adenoma to carcinoma.

Activation of ras oncogene

Only somatic mutation commonly occurring in colorectal neoplasms. *Ki-ras* is affected in 80%. About 50% of colorectal carcinomas show *ras* mutations as do a similar proportion of adenomas >1 cm, but it is present in only 10% of those <1 cm.

Abnormalities of long arm of chromosome 5

Deletions in region 5q15–22 (*fap* gene) are associated with FAPC and allelic losses in this region resulting in inactivation of this tumour suppressor gene is seen in 20–50% colorectal carcinomas and 30% of adenomas.

Deletions on long arm of chromosome 18

Loss of material from region 18q21–22 (DCC [deleted in colon cancer] gene) is seen in 70% of carcinomas and 50% of large adenomas.

Deletions on short arm of chromosome 17

Loss of material resulting in inactivation of *p53* has been reported in up to 75% colorectal carcinomas but few adenomas.

Site

About 50% occur in the rectum or recto-sigmoid, about 15% occur in the caecum and lower ascending colon and the rest are evenly distributed along the remaining bowel.

Clinical features

Tumours arising in the caecum, where the lumen is wide, frequently remain asymptomatic until late in the course of the disease but may present with symptoms of anaemia from chronic blood loss. Carcinomas lower down the colon (e.g. sigmoid and rectum) present with passage of fresh blood per rectum. Constricting lesions, particularly if in the lower colon where the faeces are solid may present with altered bowel habit due to obstruction (less noticeable more proximally where the faeces are liquid).

Laboratory findings

Colonic carcinomas produce a variety of proteins the most studied of which is carcino-embryonic antigen (CEA).

Although this is produced by too many tumours to be diagnostic measurements of serum CEA can be used in follow up with the reappearance of this marker suggesting recurrence.

Macroscopy

Four main types are seen:

- protuberant masses – most common in the caecum and ascending colon they affect only part of the circumference and are not associated with proximal obstructive changes
- plaque-like lesions that undergo ulceration – commonly seen in the rectum and recto-sigmoid regions these tumours have a rolled and everted edge
- deeply infiltrative tumours affecting whole circumference – if there is an associated sclerotic (desmoplastic) tissue response these tumours can produce a tight constriction with features of obstruction in the proximal bowel including marked dilation of the lumen
- tumours producing large amounts of mucin – on naked-eye examination these have a gelatinous appearance.

Microscopy

Most are clearly adenocarcinomas with tubule formation and in some, mucin secretion. Mucin dominates the picture in 10–15% (mucinous carcinomas either with intracellular mucin [signet ring carcinoma] or extracellular mucin lakes [colloid carcinoma]). Tumours are graded as well (20%), moderately (60%) or poorly differentiated (20%) on the basis of tubule formation and nuclear appearances. There are numerous stategies for staging colorectal carcinoma, most of which depend to a greater or lesser extent on depth of penetration through the wall and extent of extracolonic spread. One of the most widely used was originally described by Dukes (Table 34.4).

Colorectal carcinoma spreads by direct invasion, via lymphatics (50% have lymph node involvement at the time of resection) or via the blood stream.

Table 34.4 Dukes classification of tumours

Dukes stage A	Tumour not penetrated the muscularis propria. No lymph node involvement
Dukes stage B	Tumour extends through muscularis propria and into pericolic/perirectal tissue No lymph node involvement
Dukes stage C	Lymph node deposits present

Natural history and prognosis

Prognosis is dependent on tumour type (mucinous has poorer prognosis), grade and stage. Dukes A tumours should be cured by resection, stage B tumours have a 70% chance of cure but stage C has a 5-year survival of only 30–35%. Invasion of veins outside the colonic wall reduces survival but invasion of small veins within the wall does not affect survival.

THE ANUS

ANATOMY

Site Connects the lower end of the rectum to the perianal skin. Demarcated by the proximal and distal margins of the internal sphincter.

Size Approximately 3–4 cm long.

HISTOLOGY

The junction of the anus with the skin is marked by the appearance of skin adnexal structures. Above this the anus is lined for about half its length by stratified squamous epithelium with the remainder covered by mucosa indistinguishable from that of the rectum. The junction between these two epithelia is marked by the anal valves which form the inner boundary of the anal crypts (branching ducts passing into the submucosa). The valves collectively form the pectinate line. Immediately above the pectinate line is a narrow zone 0.3–1.0cm long, the transitional or cloacogenic zone lined by epithelium similar to the transitional epithelium of the bladder.

CONGENITAL DISORDERS
Atresia or stenosis of the anus

Epidemiology   One or the other affects about 1/5000 live born infants. Atresia is 9 times more common.

Macroscopy   Atresia is characterized by a gap between a blind-ending rectum and the external surface. In some cases the anus is marked by a dimple on the surface while in others (10%) the anal canal is formed but ends short of the rectum.

Natural history and prognosis   Those atresias in which the rectum ends above puborectalis component of the levator ani muscle (40% of cases) are associated with severe degree of obstruction, other congenital abnormalities and defective innervation of the muscles of the pelvic floor. In this variety a fistula tract to the urinary bladder, urethra or vagina is commonly seen. In those with a more distal atresia the obstruction is rarely severe and the pelvic floor innervation is normal. Simple surgery is curative in these cases.

INFLAMMATORY DISORDERS
Anal fissure

Site   Commonest on posterior aspect of lower anal canal.
Clinical features   Pain on defaecation.
Macroscopy   Triangular mucosal lesion.
Microscopy   Non-specific chronic inflammation.

Anal fistula

Definition   Abnormal track opening into the anal canal.
Site   Usually at level of the pectinate line.

Macroscopy Track may open on to perianal skin surface or may end blindly in perianal soft tissue.

Microscopy Begin with sepsis in perianal crypts. Multinucleated giant cells of foreign body type are present. The track is frequently lined by epithelium.

Crohn's disease

Epidemiology The anus is involved in 25% of cases of small intestinal Crohn's disease and 75% of cases involving the large bowel.

Clinical features Chronic anal fissure, anal fistula or perianal oedema may be present.

Microscopy Diagnosis depends on the identification of typical granulomatous lesions in anal/perianal biopsies. The features must be distinguished from anal tuberculosis.

Pilonidal sinus

Epidemiology More common in males. Associated with hirsutism and obesity.

Pathogenesis Penetration of skin of the natal cleft by hair shafts.

Microscopy Sinus track from skin into soft tissues which has a complex branching pattern and is lined partly by squamous epithelium and partly by inflamed granulation tissue. Foreign body giant cell reactions to hair material are common.

Haemorrhoids

Definition Prolapse of one or more anal vascular cushions (complexes of arterioles, arteriovenous communications and venules).

Aetiology Thought to be related to straining at stool.

Pathogenesis Prolapse of the cushions interferes with vascular return resulting in further engorgement.

Clinical features Most frequently bleeding (usually mild and chronic but may be massive). Thrombosis or strangulation may occur.

Microscopy Dilated vessels with thick muscular layer.

TUMOURS OF THE ANUS

Perianal Paget's disease

Epidemiology   Rare most often found in elderly.

Macroscopy   Red scaly area.

Microscopy   Epidermis is infiltrated by large vacuolated cells containing mucin.

Natural history and prognosis   Most are associated with low grade adenocarcinoma of the apocrine gland ducts which may have a long pre-invasive course. Very occasionally Paget's disease is associated with an adenocarcinoma arising in the anal canal.

Squamous carcinoma

Epidemiology   Commonest malignant tumour of the anus, but still rare. Associated with passive male homosexuals.

Aetiology   Association with human papilloma virus particularly type 16 in some tumours. Also associated with poverty and poor hygiene.

Clinical features   Presents with bleeding and/or pain most commonly but some present with a mass or local pruritis. About 25% are assymptomatic.

Site   Carcinoma in the anal canal is 3 × as common as those on the anal skin.

Microscopy   Variable degree of differentiation. One varient, the basiloid cloacogenic carcinoma, shows cellular nests with peripheral pallisaded cells.

Natural history and prognosis   This is dependent on grade. Carcinomas proximal to the pectinate line tend to spread proximally to the rectum or laterally to the perianal tissues. Inguinal node involvement can be seen late in tumours of the anal canal but is the principal route of spread for tumours of the anal margin.

The liver, biliary system and exocrine pancreas

35

THE LIVER

ANATOMY

Weight   Male 1.4–1.8 kg; female 1.2–1.4 kg.

Site   Right hypochondrium extending to epigastrium. The greater part is under the ribs and the superior surface is in contact with the diaphragm.

Organization   Divided into right and left lobes by the falciform ligament. The quadrate and caudate lobes are conventionally considered part of the right lobe but are functionally part of the left lobe of liver.

STRUCTURE AND HISTOLOGY

Parenchyma

The acinus

Basic functional unit of the liver. That part of the liver perfused by the vessels of a single portal tract. Portal vein and hepatic artery branches in the portal tract divide into sinusoids and drain into terminal hepatic venules (central veins) which therefore receive blood from more than one acinus.

The zones

Each acinus is divided into three zones on the basis of distance from portal tract with zone 1 the nearest and zone 3 the furthest.

The liver cell plates

Liver cells radiate out from the triads in columns one cell thick (liver cell plates) separated by sinusoids. The portal tract is surrounded by a concentric layer of liver cells which is breached by the sinusoids. The portal tract/hepatic parenchyma interface is the limiting plate.

The liver cell

Hepatocytes are large (long axis 20–30 nm) with single round nuclei. Most are diploid but there may be increased ploidy during regeneration. 'Intranuclear' vacuoles can be seen particularly in patients with diabetes and Wilson's disease. The hepatocyte plasma membrane on both sinusoidal and bile canalicular borders show multiple microvilli liver cells containing microfilaments which are important in transport of bile into the canaliculus, well-developed smooth endoplasmic reticulum, up to 800 mitochodria and primary and secondary lysosomes.

Blood supply

Portal vein
Formed by splenic and superior mesenteric veins this supplies about 75% of the blood *reaching* the liver. Normal pressure is 5–10 mm Hg.

Hepatic artery
Carries remaining 25% of liver's blood but furnishes about 50% of the oxygen.

Sinusoids
Wide endothelial lined spaces between liver cell plates. There are no tight junctions, some of the cells contain holes (fenestrae) and there is no subendothelial basement membrane. This allows the free access of plasma from sinusoidal blood to liver cell. The endothelium is separated from the underlying liver cells by the **space of Disse**. On the luminal aspect of the sinusoids are **Kupffer cells** which function as tissue macrophages and **pit cells** which are large granular lymphocytes and are thought to function as natural killer cells. Within the sinusoids are **perisinusoidal (Ito) cells** which are believed to be derived from myofibroblasts and secrete the extacellular matrix of the space of Disse.

Hepatic vein: drains blood from the liver.

Bile

The bile ducts

Liver cells secrete bile into canaliculi in which the bile flows in the opposite direction to blood (towards the portal tract). From the canaliculi bile flows into pre-ductules (canals of Hering) then into bile ductules at the periphery of the portal tracts, interlobular bile ducts and segmental ducts.

Bilirubin

This is the catabolic product of haem, mostly from effete red cells at the end of their 120-day life but also from cytochrome P450, catalase and other oxidizing enzymes. About 250–300 mg bilirubin is excreted daily. Formation of bilirubin begins with removal of the haem group from haemoglobin which is oxidized to biliverdin and subsequently reduced to bilirubin. These events occur in fixed-tissue macrophages in splenic and hepatic sinusoids. Bilirubin has a hydrophobic surface and is insoluble in water; this is therefore transported to the liver bound to albumin. Bilirubin is taken up into liver cells from the space of Disse and binds in the cell to proteins known as ligandin and protein Z. Conjugation occurs with the addition of glucuronic acid which renders the bilirubin soluble in aqueous solution.

Secretion of bile

Bile formation is the route for excretion of conjugated bilirubin, some detoxified chemicals, cholesterol and bile salts. Bile is secreted either by a bile-acid dependent or bile-acid independent pathway.

Disorders of bilirubin

Gilbert's syndrome

Epidemiology May affect 3–7% of population. Male preponderance. Usually presents initially in 2nd or 3rd decades.

Biochemistry Reduced activity of glucuronyl transferase. Late presentation might be due to hormone related changes in glucuronyl transferase at puberty.

Clinical features   Mild intermittent episodes of jaundice in about one third while the remainder have vague symptoms such as abdominal discomfort or excessive fatigue.

Crigler–Najjar syndrome type 1

Genetics   Autosomal recessive inheritance.

Biochemistry   Absent or reduced glucuronyl transferase activity leads to increased plasma unconjugated bilirubin.

Clinical features   Recognized in first few days of life.

Microscopy   Canalicular cholestasis.

Natural history and prognosis   Deposition of free bilirubin causes severe brain damage, usually apparent within first 18 months of life.

Crigler–Najjar syndrome type 2

Genetics Autosomal   dominant inheritance with variable penetrance.

Biochemistry   Degree of reduction of glucuronyl transferase not so severe.

Microscopy   Unremarkable.

Natural history and prognosis   Brain damage not as severe. Life expectancy may be normal.

Dubin–Johnson syndrome

Genetics   Autosomal recessive inheritance.

Biochemistry   Failure of transport of conjugated bilirubin from liver cell to canaliculus.

Clinical features   Conjugated hyperbilirubinaemia usually presents in early adult life.

Macroscopy   Darkly pigmented liver.

Microscopy   Liver cells contain granular coarse brown pigment (thought to be lipofuscin).

Rotor syndrome

Genetics   Autosomal recessive inheritance.

Biochemistry   Failure of transport of conjugated bilirubin from liver cell to canaliculus.

Macroscopy   Unpigmented liver.

Cholestasis

Failure to drain bile may lead to the appearance of increased concentrations of all bile constituents in the plasma.

Aetiology

Extrahepatic   Gallstones, neoplasms obstructing flow, sclerosing cholangitis, bile duct atresia, pancreatitis and pancreatic tumours.

Intrahepatic   Associated with obstruction – granulomas, metastatic neoplasms, cystic fibrosis and intrahepatic bile duct atresia.

Not associated with obstruction – some infections, α-1-antitrypsin deficiency, pregnancy, viral hepatitis, some drugs, idiopathic recurrent cholestasis, familial progessive cholestasis (Byler's disease) early stages of primary biliary cirrhosis and cirrosis of other types.

....

DISORDERS AFFECTING THE PARENCHYMA

Acute viral hepatitis

Pathogenesis

Viruses may be directly cytopathic or the virally infected cells may express viral neo-antigens in association with MHC class I proteins leading to attack by cytotoxic T cells.

Macroscopy

This is only undertaken in cases of fulminant hepatitis which has led to fatal liver failure. The liver is usually reduced in weight, with wrinkling of the liver capsule. The cut surface may have a uniformly red cut surface but in cases in which regeneration is commencing yellowish areas may exist on the red background of necrotic liver.

Microscopy

There is evidence of liver cell damage which is most severe in zone 3 which is seen in one of two forms. There is either **ballooning degeneration** with cells swollen to twice normal size with empty-looking cytoplasm or **acidophilic degeneration** which indicates irreversible cell damage with increased eosinophilia and condensation of the cytoplasm which in the extreme results in the formation of balls of eosinophilic material representing the result of apoptosis (**Councilman bodies**). There is a diffuse infiltrate of lymphocytes, plasma cells and macrophages which is most severe in zone 3 around the central veins. The portal tract is also the site of inflammation with lymphocytes, plasma cells and macrophages and not uncommonly neutrophils and eosinophils. In severe cases there is extensive liver cell death with loss of a confluent area bridging the area between portal tract and central vein (**bridging necrosis**) associated with collapse of the reticulin network.

Hepatitis A

Epidemiology   Infection is relatively common, with antibodies detectable in 29% Swiss blood donors and 90% in Israel and Yugoslavia.

Virology   RNA enterovirus of *Picornaviridae* group. A small non-enveloped single stranded RNA virus approximately 27 nm diameter.

Mode of infection   Via attachment of virus to receptors on target cell. Viral replication only occurs in liver cells.

Mode of transmission   Faecal–oral route. Some edible shellfish appear to concentrate the virus.

Incubation period   3–7 weeks.

Clinical features   Abrupt onset of malaise, nausea and anorexia, sometimes associated with fever. After 10 days there is jaundice.

Laboratory findings   There are raised plasma concentrations of liver enzymes (alanine aminotransferase) at the onset of symptoms, which decline at 10 days.

Microscopy   Cholestasis is more prominent than in other types.

Natural history and prognosis   Chronic hepatitis does not occur and there is no carrier state. Infection confers lifelong immunity. Mortality is less than 0.1%.

Hepatitis B

Epidemiology   Occurs worldwide with marked geographic distribution. High-risk areas (SE Asia, China, Philippines, Indonesia, Middle East [excluding Israel] Africa, Pacific Islands, Eskimo and Amazon basin) with 8–15% of the population showing HbsAg in serum and 60% with some marker of HBV infection. An intermediate group (eastern and southern Europe, the former USSR, Central Asia, Japan, Israel and the northern part of South America) with 2–7% showing HbsAg and 20–60% showing some marker of infection. The low-risk group (North America, Western Europe, New Zealand, Australia and the southern part of South America) shows less than 2% with HbsAG in their serum and less than 20% with serological markers of infection. Overall about 300–400 miilion people worldwide have chronic hepatitis B infection with 250 000 deaths annually attributable to acute or chronic HBV infection.

Virology   A member of the hepadnavirus group (hepatotropic DNA viruses). Spherical and 42 nm diameter Dane particle.

Mode of infection   Replication follows entry of the virion into the host cell where it uncoats. The viral DNA forms covalently closed circular DNA which acts as a template for the formation of RNA which itself forms a template for DNA formation using virus derived reverse transcriptase. The negative strand of DNA so generated then replicates to form a positive strand of DNA.

Mode of transmission   Perinatal (vertical) transmission from mother to infant via infected blood or liquor amnii at or shortly after birth, or horizontally by exposue to infected blood or blood products (e.g. infected needles used by drug abusers, in the course of tattooing or from infected blood transfusions. The last accounts for less than 1% hepatitis B infections in the UK. Sexual transmission is important in areas where there is low prevalence and may be acquired either by homosexual or heterosexual intercourse.

Laboratory findings   The first marker to appear is hepatitis surface antigen (HbsAg) detectable 1 week to 2 months after exposure and anywhere from 2 weeks to 2 months before onset of symptoms. The second marker is hepatitis E antigen which is correlated with maximum infectivity. With the onset of symptoms there is anti-hepatitis B core antibody (IgG and IgM). The last marker to appear is anti-hepatitis surface antibody. Failure to clear HbsAg after 6 months indicates chronicity.

Laboratory findings are summarized in Table 35.1.

Clinical features Incubation period 4–26 weeks, but typically 6–8 weeks.

Hepatitis C

Virology A small single stranded RNA virus distantly related to the flavivirus and pestivirus family.

Transmission In about 5–10% transmission is via blood transfusion; about 40% have a history of parental drug abuse, in less than 5% there has been occupational exposure to blood and in about 10% the only identifiable source is heterosexual contact. In the remainder there is no history of possible parenteral infection.

Clinical features Most infections are sub-clinical with only about 25% of patients becoming jaundiced.

Microscopy In addition to those features common to all viral hepatitis there are cytopathic liver cell changes, the presence of lymphocytes and macrophages in the sinusoids, a portal tract chronic inflammatory cell infiltrate which may include the presence of lymphoid follicles, evidence of intrahepatic bile duct damage and small droplet fatty change.

Natural history and prognosis Half the patients show evidence of chronicity and 20% of these will develop cirrhosis. Carriers have an increased risk for the development of liver cell carcinoma.

Hepatitis D

Epidemiology Worldwide distribution but with high-risk areas such as southern Italy, Venezuela, Colombia, the Amazon basin and western parts of Asia.

Virology This is a defective RNA virus which needs to be encapsulated by pre-surface and surface antigens of hepatitis B virus for infectivity.

Table 35.1 Laboratory findings in hepatitis B

Significance	HBsAg	HBeAg	Anti-HBe	Anti-HBc	Anti-HBc IgM	Anti-HBs
Acute HBV infection	+	+/-	+/-	+	+	-
HBV carrier (high infectivity)	+	+	-	+	- or weak +	-
HBV carrier (low infectivity)	+	-	+	+	-	-
Past HBV infection	-	-	+/-	+	-	+
Past HBV immunization	-	-	-	-	-	+

Mode of transmission There is either co-infection with hepatitis B or super-infection of a hepatitis B carrier by hepatitis D.

Natural history and prognosis There is a greater risk of developing fulminant liver failure if there is co-infection than for hepatitis B but the risk for chronic hepatitis is very small. When there is superinfection there is also greater risk of fulminant hepatitis but also a much greater risk of developing chronic liver disease.

Hepatitis E

Epidemiology Endemic in areas with low standards of sanitation and an undernourished population.

Virology Single stranded non-enveloped RNA virus related to the calicivirus group.

Mode of transmission Faecal–oral route.

Clinical features Incubation period of 3–9 weeks (average 6 weeks).

Natural history and prognosis Usually self-limiting. Fulminant liver failue occurs in 0.5–3%. However, in pregnant females infected in the third trimester 20% develop fulminant hepatitis and die of liver failure.

....

OTHER VIRAL INFECTIONS AFFECTING THE LIVER

Yellow fever

Virology An RNA virus transmitted by mosquito bites (*Haemogogus* variety in the jungle, *Aedes aegyptii* in urban areas). Endemic in primates in Central Africa and Central and South America. Replicates in host and vector.

Clinical features Many are clinically inapparent. Others show fever, headache, nausea and vomiting. Jaundice is present in severe cases.

Microscopy Liver cell abnormalities are most apparent in zone 2 with acidophil change and Councilman bodies (apoptosis). Ballooning degeneration and fatty change may be seen. Kupffer cells show acidophil change associated with the presence of virus in those cells.

Herpes virus infections

Epstein–Barr virus

Epidemiology   Usually young adults.

Virology   A herpes virus.

Clinical features   The commonest consequence is infectious mononucleosis (glandular fever) presenting with fever, malaise, sore throat and lymph node swelling. Hepatitis is seen in approximately 15%.

Microscopy   Little evidence of liver-cell damage or death. There is usually a marked degree of regenerative activity and a florid lymphocytic infiltrate.

Cytomegalovirus

Epidemiology   Infection is common with a peak prevalence in early adult life. Immunosuppressed patients are at increased risk.

Virology   A herpes virus.

Clinical features   Adult infection is usually associated with fever often with hepatitis and occasionally a polyneuropathy of Guillain–Barré type.

Microscopy   Similar to that seen in other types of viral hepatitis. Occasionally granulomas are seen and characteristic viral inclusions may be present (in about 20%) either in the liver cells or vascular endothelial cells.

Herpes simplex

Epidemiology   Disseminated infection is seen in neonatal life or immunosuppressed adults.

Virology   A herpes virus.

Microscopy   Haemorrhagic necrosis with the surrounding liver cells showing viral inclusions. There is a mononuclear cell reaction.

Arenavirus infection

Lassa fever

Epidemiology   Endemic in parts of West Africa.

Virology   Caused by an arenavirus.

Mode of transmission   From a rodent host *Mastomys natalensis*.

Clinical features   Multi-system disease with myocarditis, encephalitis, myositis and an abnormal bleeding tendency.

Microscopy   Liver shows focal necrosis with extensive acidophil change. This is particularly marked in zone 3 and there is a macrophage response.

Filovirus infections

Marburg virus

Virology   A filovirus.

Mode of trasmission   From African green monkeys.

Clinical features   Fever, conjunctivitis, hepatitis, diarrhoea, disordered renal fuction and an abnormal bleeding tendency.

Microscopy   Focal necrosis, beginning with acidophil change with only a mild inflammatory reaction.

Ebola virus

Epidemiology   Antibodies are present in 12.4% of the population of of six African countries including Sudan and Zaire.

Virology   A filovirus.

Clinical features   Severe haemorrhagic fever.

Microscopy   Similar to Marburg virus with numerous foci of necrosis.

Natural history and prognosis   Mortality of 70%.

Chronic hepatitis

Definition   Chronic inflammatory process which may be associated with liver cell necrosis and which lasts more than 6 months.

Epidemiology In Western Europe and North America chronic hepatitis due to hepatitis B infection is uncommon but this association exists in China and the Far East.

Aetiology May follow an attack of acute hepatitis or have an insidious onset without an antecedent attack of acute hepatitis. It can also be seen in association with reaction to certain drugs (including α-methyldopa, oxpheniatin, halothane, isoniazid and nitrofurantoin), in autoimmune disorders, Wilson's disease and α$_1$-antitrypsin deficiency.

Microscopy Most people now believe that there is a spectrum of changes ranging from chronic persistent hepatitis to chronic acive hepatitis rather than these two being distinct entities.

Chronic persistent hepatitis

Microscopy There is a brisk mononuclear cell infiltrate of the portal tract connective tissue which does not transgress the limiting plate, preservation of normal acinar architecture and and absence of patchy hepatocyte death in the area of the acinus abutting on the portal tract (piecemeal necrosis).

Chronic lobular hepatitis

Definition Variant of chronic persistant hepatitis.

Microscopy Preservation of the acinar architecture associated with patchy liver cell damage with ballooning degeneration and acidophil change. There may be collapse of the reticulin framework in the region of the terminal hepatic veins and some clustering of Kupffer cells containing ceroid pigment.

Chronic active hepatitis

Microscopy The hallmark is the presence of piecemeal necrosis (destruction of hepatocytes at the acinus/portal tract border by immunologically competent cells) which if severe may lead to bridging necrosis. There is portal tract inflammation with activation of Kupffer cells and connective tissue producing cells. Avoidance of regeneration is a prominent feature. Segmental bile duct lesions may be present (both small and large ducts) with epithelial hyperplasia leading to narrowing or occlusion.

Natural history and prognosis May progress to cirrhosis.

Chronic autoimmune hepatitis (lupoid hepatitis)

Epidemiology Chiefly in young women.

Pathogenesis Immune-mediated mechanisms are suggested by the findings of a positive LE phenomenon in 10%, plasma anti-nuclear antibodies in 50% of patients and anti-smooth muscle antibodies in 40–60%. There may be antibodies to a receptor on the liver cell membrane and/or microsomes. There is a heavy plasma cell infiltrate in the liver and there is a rapid response to immunosupressive agents.

Clinical features Jaundice, acne, amenorrhoea, liver and splenic enlargement and high plasma immunoglobulin concentrations. Evidence of multi-system disease such as Sjögren's syndrome, ulcerative colitis, arthritis, thyroid disease and fibrosing alveolitis may be present in 14% patients.

Natural history and prognosis If untreated it is associated with poor prognosis, death being associated with liver failure.

CIRRHOSIS

Definition Final stage of several pathogenetic mechanisms characterized by fibrosis **and** formation of structurally abnormal parenchymal nodules.

Aetiology The main pathways to cirrhosis are through chronic active hepatitis, steatohepatitis (fatty change with evidence of liver cell damage and inflammation), portal fibrosis or fibrosis occurring in acinar zone 3. The first two account for most cases with alcohol-induced steatohepatits accounting for more than 60% of cases of cirrhosis in the Western world.

Chronic active hepatitis

Aetiology Viral, Wilson's disease, chronic autoimmune hepatitis, α_1-antitrypsin deficiency and certain drug-related conditions.

Pathogenesis The cirrhosis occurs on the basis of regeneration occurring on a substrate of continuing necrosis of liver cells and with inflammation both in the portal tracts and liver acini. Bridging necrosis and intra-acinar necrosis are thought to be the most important features determining cirrhosis development.

Steatohepatitis

Aetiology   Particularly associated with alcohol abuse but also in the very obese and occasionally following amiodarone treatment.

Microscopy   There is large droplet fatty change, ballooning degeneration of liver cells most severe in acinar zone 3, an inflammatory infiltrate composed of lymphocytes as well as lymphocytes, new collagen around liver cells and in some instances Mallory bodies.

Portal fibrosis

Aetiology   Seen in genetically determined haemochromatosis and in those with chronic biliary obstruction.

Pathogenesis   Begins with scarring of the portal tracts that eventually link up and eventually cirrhosis develops.

Microscopy   The nodule outlines tend to be irregular.

Fibrosis in acinar zone 3 (centrilobular fibrosis)

Aetiology   Hepatic outflow obstruction at any level from small hepatic venules (e.g. in alkaloid induced venoocclusive disease) to chronic cardiac tamponade (e.g. constrictive pericarditis).

Pathogenesis   There is scarring around the terminal hepatic venules with linkage to zone 3.

Pathogenesis of fibrosis in cirrhosis

Active growth of the connective tissue matrix occurs in relation to the liver cell plates and the space of Disse with production of matrix proteins by the Ito cells which line the abluminal aspect of the sinusoidal basement membrane.

Morphological classification of cirrhosis

Determined by the size and uniformity of the nodules, the width of the fibrous septa and special histological features suggesting a specific cause.

Micronodular Nodules uniform in size and small (< 3 mm diameter). Fibrous septa uniform in thickness. See Table 35.2.

Macronodular Nodules vary in size and are larger (3 mm–1 cm diameter). Fibrous septa vary in thickness (up to several mm thick).

Mixed Range of nodule sizes from small to large.

Microscopy

Fibrous septa often contain blood vessels (venous radicles and small arteries), small bile ducts and bile ductules. The regenerative nodules are surrounded by fibrous tissue septa and do not contain normally situated hepatic venules. The liver cell columns in the nodules are more than one cell thick (NB: in a six-year-old child liver cell columns are normally two cells thick). There may be evidence of continuing liver cell damage with piecemeal necrosis. Other features may suggest a specific cause.

....

MICRONODULAR CIRRHOSIS (Table 35.2)

Alcoholic liver disease

Epidemiology

The majority of heavy drinkers develop fatty change; more severe damage is seen in 20–30% of such drinkers while biopsy-confirmed cirrhosis develops in 17–30% of heavy drinkers. Average daily intake for cirrhotics has been calculated to be 180 g over a period of 25 years but there is a continuum in risk with increasing intake (for males intake of 0.2 g gives relative risk of cirrhosis of 1, 40–60 g relative risk of 6, 60–80 g gives relative risk of 14). Threshold intake level is lower in females than in males but the pattern of intake (bingeing vs. soaking) has no effect.

Metabolism of alcohol

Normal metabolism of alcohol involves three pathways:

- oxidation of alcohol to acetaldehyde (by alcohol dehydrogenase in liver cytosol)
- coversion of acetaldehyde to acetate (in mitochodria)
- release of acetate into the blood.

Table 35.2 Micronodular cirrhosis

Frequency	Aetiology	Typical microscopic appearance
60–70%	Alcohol	Fatty change and/or ballooning degeneration of liver cells. Mallory bodies may be haemosiderin in liver cells. Neutrophils in inflammatory infiltrate.
5%	Primary biliary cirrhosis	Heavy lymphoid infiltrate in portal tracts in early stages. Epithelioid granulomas in portal tracts. Destruction of medium sized bile ducts. Cholestasis in zone 1. High level of copper in liver cells. Mallory bodies in some.
< 5%	Large bile duct obstruction	Severe degree of cholestasis. Marked bile ductule proliferation. Irregular nodule outline.
5%	Haemochromatosis	Large amounts of haemosiderin in liver cells, Kupffer cells and ductular epithelium.
Rare	Intestinal bypass	Marked fatty change in liver cells. Mallory bodies in some cases.
Rare	Cystic fibrosis	PAS positive material in proliferated ductules in portal tracts.
Rare	Indian childhood cirrhosis	Mallory bodies.

The oxidation of alcohol to acetaldehyde uses one of two pathways:

1. The first requires NAD, which is reduced to NADH resulting in an increase in the NADH/NAD ratio in the liver cells and a reduction in the redox state of the cells. This change is associated with most of the acute metabolic effects of alcohol including:

   • inhibition of gluconeogenesis leading to hypoglycaemia
   • impairment of fatty acid oxidation leading to increased fat accumulating in the liver cells.
   • decrease in the activity of the citric acid cycle.

Acetaldehyde itself has several deleterious effects on the liver:

- form adducts with protein with the potential to form new antigens which can result in a cell-damaging antibody response
- inactivates certain enzymes
- produces alterations in microtubules, mitochondria and plasma membranes
- causes depletion of the major intracellular scavenger systems based on reduced glutathione and therefore promotes free radical mediated damage.

2. The second pathway occurs within the microsomes and is termed the microsomal ethanol oxidizing system (MEOS). Increased activation of this produces increased acetaldehyde but also results in the formation of oxygen free radicals which may cause damage to hepatocytes via a number of pathways.

Pathological features

Three sets of pathological changes can occur in alcohol abusers either in isolation or in combination.

1. Alcoholic fatty liver

Epidemiology Most frequent and earliest change.

Pathogenesis Direct toxic effect rather than malnutrition.

Macroscopy Liver is grossly enlarged (1.5–2.5kg), pale yellow and feels greasy. In extreme cases the liver may float in water.

Microscopy Hepatocytes usually contain large fat droplets which compress the nucleus and other organelles against the plasma membrane. Occasionally there may be several smaller fat droplets rather than a single large one. The membranes of adjacent fat laden hepatocytes may rupture to form fat cysts. The development of fibrosis around terminal hepatic venules and pericellular scarring in zone 3 is a marker of increased risk of cirrhosis.

Natural history and prognosis Expected to resolve if alcohol intake is stopped.

2. Alcoholic hepatitis (steatohepatitis)

Epidemiology Less common than alcoholic fatty liver.

Clinical features May be symptom free. Vague abdominal discomfort may be present or presentation with a frankly hepatitic illness can occur in a few with jaundice, fever nausea, abdominal pain and a neutrophil leucocytosis.

Microscopy There is ballooning degeneration of hepatocytes particularly in zone 3. Large droplet fatty change is present in many hepatocytes. There is focal hepatocyte death with a neutrophil response. **Mallory's hyaline** (irregular clumped material staining reddish-blue with H&E, representing deranged cytoskeleton) is seen in liver cells which show ballooning. Grossly enlarged mitochondria may be seen (stain red with trichrome stains) usually indicating recent heavy drinking and disappearing after several weeks' abstinence. There may be cholestasis. Some degree of fibrosis around terminal hepatic venules and around hepatocytes in zone 3 is almost always present. There may be linkages of the fibrous tissue in zone 3 to the portal tract associated with hepatocyte loss in that area of the acini (**central hyaline sclerosis**).

Natural history and prognosis Incidence of full blown cirrhosis is 9 × higher than for alcoholic fatty liver. In those who persist with alcohol abuse one third will develop cirrhosis in 2 years. Resolution of the pathological changes occurs in those who stop drinking alcohol.

3. Alcoholic cirrhosis

Macroscopy In early cases the liver is enlarged, mostly due to intracellular fat, and the liver is pale yellow. The cut surface has a fine uniform nodularity. With increased duration there is loss of the uniform pattern with the development of some large nodules, fat is less conspicuous, the colour of the liver becomes brown and the size decreases.

Microscopy In the early stages the fine nodularity is due to fibrous septa connecting portal tract connective tissue to the terminal hepatic venules. These septa either enclose individual lobules or, more frequently, subdivide the lobules so that the normal vascular relationships are lost. The portal tracts may contain chronic inflammatory cells and there may be bile ductule proliferation. Stainable iron may be increased.

Complications The combination of fibrosis and regeneration has a major effect on the blood flow within the liver. The perivenular fibrosis and intimal thickening in the terminal venules leads to outflow obstruction and additional compression of hepatic veins by regenerating nodules may result in **post-sinusoidal portal hypertension**.

Natural history and prognosis Survival depends on whether diagnosis is followed by abstinence from alcohol and whether jaundice, ascites or haematemesis have supervened. In those in whom none of these complications has occurred and who abstain the 5-year survival is 88.9% falling to 62.8% if drinking continues. There is a fall in survival in those who susequently abstain but have developed jaundice (57.5%), ascites (52.4%) or haematemesis (35%) which again falls if alcohol consumption continues to 33.3% for those with jaundice, 32.7% with ascites and 21% following haematemesis.

Primary biliary cirrhosis (PBC)

Definition More accurately described as a chronic non-suppurative destructive cholangitis in which cirrhosis is a relatively late development. Usually considered to be an autoimmune disease.

Epidemiology Most are middle-aged females (M:F 1:9) and 75% are aged 40–59. Rare disease with prevalence estimated as 3.7–14.4 cases /100 000 population and estimated incidence of 5.8–15/million population per annum. Accounts for 0.6–2% of deaths due to cirrhosis.

Aetiology Disturbance of immune regulation is suggested by the finding of increased levels of serum immunoglobulins (particularly IgM), the presence of auto-antibodies (apart from anti-mitochondrial antibodies others are found reacting to nuclear membrane, thyroid, lymphocytes, acetylcholine receptors and RNA), skin anergy, the presence of granulomas, decreased suppressor T-cell function, association with other auto-immune disorders (non-hepatic disorders are seen in up to 70% patients including Sjögren's syndrome, CREST syndrome, autoimmune thyroiditis and interstitial lung disease) and chronic activation of the complement system.

Pathogenesis Starts with inflammation and destruction of small septal and interlobular bile ducts (35–75 μm diameter) only later proceeding to fibrosis and the formation of abnormal parenchymal nodules. Damage is mediated by cytotoxic T cells.

Clinical features Patients may be asymptomatic and identified following the finding of unexplained enlargement of the liver or abnormal liver function tests (raised serum alkaline phosphatase and γ-glutamyl transpeptidase). Symptomatic patients present with pruritis (itch) and slowly progressive jaundice.

Laboratory findings High titres of anti-mitochondrial in the plasma are found in 95% of cases.

Macroscopy In long-standing cases the liver is large with a green colour due to prolonged and severe cholestasis.

Microscopy In the early stages there is inflammatory destruction of interlobular or septal bile ducts. There is a florid lymphocyte and plasma cell infiltrate in the portal tracts where no bile ducts are seen. Damaged bile ducts show epithelial swelling and breaks in the basement membrane. There may be epithelioid granulomas in affected portal tracts. With progression there is cholestasis with bile plugs in canaliculi in acinar zone 1 and widening of portal tracts due to fibrosis and bile ductule proliferation. Extension of the inflammatory process to involve parenchyma of zone 1 of the acinus is often seen (piecemeal necrosis). The distinction between PBC and chronic active hepatitis is helped by the identification of changes in zone 1 hepatocytes associated with chronic cholestasis (swelling and pallor of the liver cells, the accumulation of coarse granules due to the accumulation of copper and copper-binding protein by lysosomes and the occasional appearance of Mallory bodies. Continuing damage results in nodular regeneration and the development of true cirrhosis.

Complications In addition to the complications of cirrhosis there may be special features associated with prolonged cholestasis including the development of xanthomata (as a result of increased serum lipid concentrations), an increased risk for developing duodenal ulcer and a risk of developing the disorders of bone remodelling – osteomalacia and osteoporosis.

Natural history and prognosis Variable. The duration of the disease may be very long. The level of serum bilirubin level is the best indicator of prognosis with a steep rise suggesting that death may occur within two years. Signs of liver failure (ascites, oedema, decreased serum albumin levels, increased prothrombin time) carry a poor prognosis. Other indicators of poor prognosis include the presence of other autoimmune disorders and the presence in liver biopsies of bridging necrosis, cholestasis and piecemeal necrosis.

Sclerosing cholangitis

Definition Progressive and incurable disorder characterized by irregular periductal fibrosis affecting intra- and extrahepatic bile ducts.

Epidemiology Male predominance (M:F 2:1). Most present in 3rd–5th decade.

Aetiology Unknown but well-known association with chronic inflammatory bowel disease (50–70% patients with sclerosing cholangitis) mainly ulcerative colitis but occasionally retroperitoneal fibrosis, mediastinal fibrosis and chronic pancreatitis. There may be a genetic association with HLA-B8 and DR3.

Clinical features May be asymptomatic (with raised serum alkaline phosphatase) or patients can present with jaundice, fatigue and pruritis. In long established cases examination reveals hepatomegaly, splenomegaly and jaundice. The diagnosis is made on the basis of a combination of biochemical, radiological and histological criteria.

Laboratory findings Increased serum alkaline phosphatase. There may be abnormalities in copper metabolism (common to all varieties of biliary cirrhosis and possibly the result of long-term cholestasis).

Radiological finding Retrograde cholangiography shows diffusely distributed annular strictures which appear multifocal with intervening normal bile ducts, short band-like strictures and sac-like outpouchings which together give a beaded appearance to the intrahepatic bile ducts.

Macroscopy Involved extrahepatic ducts have the appearance of fibrous cords with obliteration of the lumen by scar tissue.

Microscopy May not be visible on core biopsies but can be seen on wedge biopsies. There is concentric layering of fibrous tissue around the ducts with atrophy of the epithelium. The duct lumena become filled with fibrous tissue and eventually the smaller ducts within portal tracts disappear leaving fibrous scars. In the early stages there is a brisk inflammatory reaction in the portal tracts. In the later stages there is cholestasis, portal fibrosis and eventually true cirrhosis.

Natural history and prognosis Complications are similar to those for primary biliary cirrhosis but in addition there is an increased risk of developing gallstones, recurrent episodes of cholangitis (acute duct inflammation) and carcinoma of the gallbladder.

Secondary biliary cirrhosis

Definition Consequence of long-standing unrelieved extra-hepatic biliary obstruction.

Aetiology Post-inflammatory stricture of the common bile duct (e.g. post-operative), congenital biliary atresia, neoplasms of the bile duct, head of the pancreas and ampulla of Vater, and impaction of gallstones in the extra-hepatic biliary system.

Microscopy Bile stasis is an early finding with bile in the lumina of the interlobular bile ducts as well as the canaliculi, liver cells and Kupffer cells. There are associated neutrophils in and around the duct lumina. There may be associated liver cell necrosis associated with bile staining (**bile infarcts**) in which central liquefaction sometimes develops producing **bile lakes**. Eventually the adjacent portal tracts become linked by fibrosis and cirrhosis develops.

....

IRON STORAGE DISORDERS AFFECTING THE LIVER (HAEMOCROMATOSIS AND HAEMOSIDEROSIS)

Aetiology Certain red cell disorders can be associated with increased iron absorption such as thalassaemia major and hereditary sideroblastic anaemia. Liver disease such as alcohol related cirrhosis may be complicated by iron overload with the excess iron present in Kupffer cells. Iron overload can occur in people taking parenteral iron but there is debate as to whether overload can occur in metabolically normal people taking large amounts of oral iron (e.g. in alcoholic beverages).

Pathogenesis Where plasma iron levels are high and the degree of transferrin saturation is greater than 60% iron tends to be deposited in hepatocytes with associated cell damage. The degree of parenchymal iron overload rather than total body iron determines the severity of the disease. In iron overload states in which the plasma iron concentrations are not high (e.g. following repeated blood transfusions) the iron is principally stored in the reticulo-endothelial system and this is associated with little tissue injury or scarring (**haemosiderosis**).

Normal iron metabolism

Normal total body iron 4–5 g in males.

Iron in tissues Half is accounted for by haemoglobin, about a quarter is stored (mainly in the cells of the reticulo-endothelial system) and the remainder is located in other body cells. Most stored iron is bound to **apoferritin**. A small amount of ferritin circulates in the plasma and an increase in this indicates an excess of stored iron.

Iron in plasma Transported bound to **transferrin**. Circulating transferrin is usually about a third saturated and there is sufficient transferrin in the plasma to transport 300 µg of iron per 100 ml blood.

Iron absorbtion from the gut Regulated in the small gut wall by a mechanism that is poorly understood but depletion of total iron stores results in increased absorption and when iron stores are increased absorption is decreased.

Iron excretion In males daily loss of iron is about 1 mg with about 65% lost across the gut and the remainder in urine and sweat. In females there is 15–30 mg lost in each menstrual cycle. Pregnancy also increases needs.

Haemochromatosis

Definition Inherited disorder of iron metabolism characterized by defective regulation of iron absorption across the small intestinal epithelium.

Epidemiology One of the commonest genetic disorders. Autosomal recessive inheritance. Linked to the type A genes of the MHC on the short arm of chromosome 6. HLA-A6 is seen in haemachromatosis patients with a frequency in the order of 70%. M:F 5:1.

Pathogenesis Deposition of excess iron in the parenchymal cells of the liver and other organs leading to cell damage, scarring and eventually to organ dysfunction. There is also an increase in total body iron due to an inappropriately high level of iron absorption. Over a period of 25–50 years as much as 15–50 mg iron may be stored in tissues. Toxicity of intracellular iron is thought to be due to the generation of reactive oxygen free radicals resulting in depletion of anti-oxidant defences and eventual membrane damage as a result of lipid peroxidation.

Macroscopy and microscopy are outlined in Table 35.3.

Table 35.3 Macroscopy and microscopy of haemochromatosis in venous organs

Macroscopy

Liver	Greatly enlarged, often > 2 kg with reddish-brown colour that can be demonstrated by the development of blue colouration if a slice of liver is immersed in a mixture of potassium ferrocyanide and dilute hydrochloric acid: Prussian blue or Perl's reaction
Pancreas	Often deep brown colour
Skin	May have a metallic grey colour

Microscopy

Liver	Fibrous septa extend out from portal triads and surround groups of liver cell acini. In the early stages iron is seen in liver cells but with increased duration there is deposition in bile duct epithelium and in Kupffer cells. The full picture of cirrhosis develops late in the disease
Pancreas	Haemosiderin seen in acinar and ductal epithelium, islets of Langerhans and interstitial connective tissue
Heart	Most cases show haemosiderin in cardiac fibres and AV node involvement is quite common
Skin	There is an increase in melanin in the basal layers of the epidermis. Haemosiderin deposition does occur but is mostly in the fibrous tissue surrounding sweat glands
Joints	There is deposition of iron and calcium pyrophosphate in the synovium (chondrocalcinosis)

Natural history and prognosis In patients in whom advanced cirrhosis has developed there is a high risk (8–22%) for development of hepatocellular carcinoma. Carbohydrate intolerance occurs in 80% with overt diabetes mellitus in 60% with the intensity of the haemosiderin deposition mirroring the severity of the diabetes. About 15% of patients show some abnormality of cardiac function, the commonest being dysrrhythmias or progressive cardiac failure (which may have a rapid onset). About 25–50% have an arthropathy.

MACRONODULAR CIRRHOSIS
Wilson's disease

Definition   Inherited defect in copper metabolism.

Epidemiology   Rare with a worldwide prevalence of 1/30 000. Autosomal recessive inheritance with the genetic defect in one of a pair of genes on the long arm of chromosome 13.

Pathogenesis   Small net positive copper balance from birth onwards (normal net balance is zero throughout life) leading to accumulation of large amounts of copper and deposition in liver, brain, kidney, eye, skeleton and a number of other organs. In Wilson's disease there is a deficiency of the copper transporting protein **caeruloplasmin** and an abnormally high copper content in the liver. The handling of the copper in the liver is abnormal and the lysosymes contain 40 times the amount of copper as normal.

Laboratory findings   Low total serum copper, excess urinary copper and low amounts of copper in the bile.

Clinical features   The disease rarely presents before 5 years old. Neurological disturbances, mostly associated with basal ganglia disease often appear in adolescence and deposits of copper in Descemet's membrane of the cornea (Kayser–Fleischer rings) occurs later than liver disease.

Microscopy   In the early stages the liver shows large droplet fatty change. The nuclei are large and appear empty because of the presence of glycogen. With progression there is a mild focal mononuclear cell infiltrate in some, which may be followed by fibrosis. In others there is the picture of

435

chronic active hepatitis which in a few cases can be complicated by fulminant hepatitis and sub-acute necrosis of the liver. Untimately macronodular cirrhosis develops.

Natural history and prognosis   The use of chelating agents increases copper excretion in the urine and can reverse the clinical abnormalities in most cases.

α-1-antitrypsin deficiency

Definition   Genetic disorder which causes pan-acinar pulmonary emphysema or chronic liver disease or both in adults or children.

Genetics   α-1-antitrypsin is coded for on the long arm of chromosome 14. The gene locus shows marked pleomorphism with over 70 alleles identified. The various different protein products that arise from this number of alleles have been separated on the basis of their electrophoretic mobility. The commonest (80% of the normal population) is the M variant and the genotype of an individual homozygous for an allele producing this form is termed PiMM (Pi=protein inhibitor). A variant associated with abnormal function is the Z form which may be inherited as heterozygous or hemizygous (PiZ-).

Pathogenesis   α-1-antitrypsin is a powerful anti-protease with a role in the inhibition of the tissue-damaging effects of neutrophil derived elastase.

Clinical features   In infancy there may be neonatal hepatitis presenting with cholestatic jaundice. Later childhood cirrhosis may develop if jaundice lasts for more than 6 months and there is chronic hepatitis. In adulthood there may be macronodular cirrhosis which may not be associated with lung disease and usually develops in the 6th and 7th decades.

Microscopy   The neonatal hepatitis is characterized by marked cholestasis, liver cell necrosis, a mononuclear cell infiltrate, portal fibrosis and proliferation of bile ductules, Globules of α-1-antitrypsin (AAT) are not easily demonstrable before 6 months using conventional histological techniques but can be seen by staining with antibodies to AAT with immunohistochemistry or by using an electron microscope. In macronodular cirrhosis in adults AAT can usually be demonstrated.

Natural history and prognosis There is a considerably increased risk of developing hepatocellular and intrahepatic bile duct cholangiocarcinoma but this is only in males and is not seen in females.

Other causes of macronodular cirrhosis

- chronic viral hepatitis
- various drugs and toxins
- hereditary haemorrhagic telangectasia
- cryptogenic cirrhosis.

The commonest causes of macronodular cirrhosis are chronic viral hepatitis and cryptogenic.

HEPATIC TUMOURS

TUMOUR-LIKE CONDITIONS OF THE LIVER

Focal nodular hyperplasia

Epidemiology Lesions occur at any age, F > M. Not associated with oral contraceptives.

Pathogenesis Unknown but thought to be related to preexisting vascular anomalies.

Clinical features Most are asymptomatic and discovered incidentally. Must be distinguished from hepatic adenoma which usually necessitates resection.

Macroscopy Well-demarcated tan-coloured nodule but with irregular margin. Only partly (if at all) encapsulated. Firmer and paler than normal liver. Cut surface shows fibrous septa radiating from central scar dividing lesion into lobules.

Microscopy Liver cells are arranged in columns which are thicker than normal and are separated by sinusoids. The normal vascular relations are lost. The scarred areas show thick-walled blood vessels and possible duct-like structures.

Nodular transformation

Aetiology Associated with systemic disorders including SLE and rheumatoid disease.

Clinical features Presentation is usually due to complications of portal hypertension induced by this disorder.

Macroscopy Multiple nodules in the hepatic parenchyma.

Microscopy Combination of liver plates that are more than one cell thick but with preserved vascular relationships and small rounded hepatocyte nodules in which no hepatic radicles are seen. There is no fibrosis between the nodules (distinguishing it from micronodular cirrhosis).

....

TUMOURS OF THE LIVER
Hepatic adenoma

Epidemiology About 90% occur in women of childbearing age. Associated with oral contraceptive use.

Clinical features Most present with acute abdominal pain associated with intra-tumoural haemorrhage or rupture of tumour into peritoneal cavity with intraperitoneal haemorrhage.

Macroscopy Usually single. Diameter exceeds 10 cm in almost half. Tumour is not always encapsulated but is pale on cut surface.

Microscopy Absence of normal acinar structure, portal tracts and bile ducts.

Natural history and prognosis Some undergo malignant transformation (possibly up to 10%).

Hepatocellular carcinoma (HCC)

Epidemiology One of the commonest malignant tumours worldwide (annual incidence about 250 000). There is a marked geographical variation with a high incidence in south-east Asia and sub-Saharan Africa with a peak in Mozambique (104/100 00 males and 31/100 000 females) but lower in the UK (1–2/100 000). Typically middle to old age. M:F 3–4:1.

Aetiology The likeliest candidate as an environmental aetiologic agent is hepatitis B virus. The evidence for is:

- high degree of correlation between frequency of HBV infection and frequency of HCC. Patients who develop chronic hepatitis related to HBV infection have a 40–59% lifetime risk of developing HCC. Patients can also develop HCC associated with HBV infection in the absence of hepatitis (particularly in cases of vertical transmission)

- positive correlation between HBV infection and presence of liver cell dysplasia
- finding of HB viral antigens in cells of HCC
- finding of part of the HBV genome in the cells of some HCC
- a similar hepadna virus causes hepatitis in woodchucks with some animals developing cirrhosis and liver cell carcinoma.

Other possible aetiological factors include cirrhosis, haemochromatosis, homozygous α-1-antitrypsin deficiency, tyrosinaemia, glycogen storage disease type 1 (von Gierke's disease), aflatoxins (produced by *Aspergillus flavus*), certain drugs and toxins (e.g. thorotrast, a radiological contrast agent used in the 1930s and 1940s) and cigarette smoking.

Clinical features   The most frequent complaint is abdominal pain and discomfort. Loss of appetite, weight loss, fever and jaundice are also common. The commonest finding on examination is hepatomegaly and smaller lesions (less than 3 cm diameter) can be seen on ultrasound.

Laboratory findings   Many patients with HCC show elevated serum levels of α-fetoprotein (500 µg/l) – sustained rises in the serum are also seen in malignant liver cell tumours of childhood (hepatoblastoma), and malignant gonadal and extra-gonadal teratomas. Lower levels can be found in patients with chronic liver disease but without tumour. Also some variants of HCC (fibrolamellar, minute and pedunculated HCCs) produce lower levels resulting in a low sensitivity as a screening test. Some patients also show raised levels of β-sub-unit of human chorionic gonadotrophin.

Macroscopy   Many macroscopic variants exist. Some are large, apparently single and expansile while others are infiltrative or multi-focal. There may be large tumour nodules within the portal vein or hepatic artery. If the main hepatic veins are obstructed there may be acute congestion and necrosis of the liver (Budd–Chiari syndrome). HCC is rather soft and may have a green colour if well differentiated and bile secreting. Necrosis and haemorrhage can be seen.

Microscopy Depends on the differentiation and architectural organization of the tumour. In well-differentiated tumours the cells resemble non-neoplastic hepatocytes and bile secretion can be found. In other cases with less differentiation there are tumour giant cells and in some cases spindle cells. Mallory's hyaline may be occasionally seen and α-1-antitrypsin and α-fetoprotein can be demonstrated in 60–80% of tumours. The commonest architectural pattern is a trabecular pattern with cords 2–5 cells thick bordered by a sinusoidal type blood supply.

Variants of hepatocellular carcinoma

Minute carcinoma

Epidemiology Most frequently seen in Japanese.

Macroscopy Small tumour nodules seen against a background of cirrhosis. Firmer and paler than surrounding liver tissue.

Microscopy Similar to classic HCC.

Pedunculated carcinoma

Macroscopy These protrude from the capsular surface of the liver with little or no invasion of the underlying liver.

Natural history and prognosis Relatively easy to surgically resect and have a better prognosis than classic HCC.

Fibrolamellar carcinoma

Epidemiology Occurs at a much younger age with more than 90% in patients under 25 years and is seen in populations where HBV carrier rate is low. Females are quite often affected.

Site Unusual, in that about 65% arise in left lobe.

Macroscopy Usually a single multi-nodular mass which is sometimes encapsulated.

Microscopy There are islands and columns of cells with eosinophilic rather than granular cytoplasm which are separated from each other by broad collagen bands. Hyaline globules and PAS-positive inclusions may be seen in the cytoplasm of some cells. α-fetoprotein is usually absent but the neural antigen protein gene product (PGA) 9.5 is seen in all cases.

Natural history and prognosis This type is often resectable and has a better prognosis than classic HCC with 5-year survival of 60%.

Cholangiocarcinoma

Definition Tumour arising from extrahepatic bile ducts or bile ductules within the liver.

Epidemiology Tumours arising from intrahepatic bile ductule comprise 6–7% of primary liver carcinomas. Peak incidence in 6th decade.

Aetiology No correlation with HBV or cirrhosis. Rare cases are associated with sclerosing cholangitis. In the Far East cases are associated with liver flukes. Thorotrast has also been implicated in cholangiocarcinoma but less frequently than for hepatocellular carcinoma.

Microscopy Most intrahepatic cholangiocarcinomas are well differentiated mucin secreting adenocarcinomas with marked stromal fibrous reaction. Intravascular spread is rare but tumours can grow within vessel walls.

Natural history and prognosis Blood-borne metastases to the skeleton, brain, adrenals and lung occur.

Hepatoblastoma

Definition Embryonal tumour of liver.

Epidemiology Most common in infants up to 3 years in which age group it is the commonest liver tumour. Males > females.

Clinical features There are usually constitutional symptoms including anorexia, nausea, abdominal pain and vomiting.

Laboratory findings Serum α-fetoprotein is usually raised.

Microscopy Two types are described:
• an epithelioid type with cells resembling fetal liver which in well-differentiated tumours are arranged in columns separated by sinusoids with a second

embryonal (small and darkly staining) population arranged in nests and primitive acini

* a mixed type in which primitive mesenchymal stroma with focal evidence of differentiation into various forms of connective tissue (cartilage, osteoid or muscle) separates fetal and embryonal cells.

Benign cavernous haemangioma

Epidemiology   Commonest benign neoplasm of liver. Found in up to 1% of all autopsies. Peak incidence in 3rd and 5th decades.

Clinical features   Most are asymptomatic but in larger cases there may be a consumptive coagulopathy.

Macroscopy   Most are single and small but larger lesions (> 4 cm) occur.

Infantile haemangioendothelioma

Epidemiology   Exclusively in children under 6 months old.

Clinical features   Often associated with vascular lesions at other sites.

Macroscopy   May be single or multicentric. Lesions appear reddish-brown with spongy areas and focal calcification.

Microscopy   Vascular spaces lined by plump endothelial cells which may form solid masses within vascular channels.

Natural history and prognosis   Associated with a high mortality due to liver failure or high output cardiac failure.

Angiosarcoma

Epidemiology   Adult males most affected.

Aetiology   Cirrhosis, exposure to vinyl chloride (plastics manufacturing), thorotrast (with latent period 20–40 years) and arsenic (prolonged ingestion of therapeutic doses).

Macroscopy   Usually enlarged liver with numerous dark reddish-brown nodules. Occasionally cystic spaces filled with blood.

Microscopy   Spindle-shaped tumour cells either lining vascular channals or in solid masses. Extramedullary haemopoiesis may be present.

Natural history and prognosis Spread is usually rapid and may involve lymph nodes at the porta hepatis, the spleen or the lungs. Prognosis is poor with survival usually about 1 year after presentation.

Secondary malignant tumours in the liver

Epidemiology Commonest tumour found in the liver. Up to 40% patients with malignant tumours will have liver metastases. The finding of secondaries confined to the liver suggests the primary is drained by the portal system.

Site Usually visible on capsular surface. Nodules of variable size with central umbilication (due to central necrosis).

Natural history and prognosis Median survival with hepatic metastases is 4–15 months. A 3-year survival of 40% can be achieved in a highly selected group undergoing resection of metastases.

LIVER DISEASE SPECIFIC TO INFANCY AND CHILDHOOD

JAUNDICE

Aetiology In addition to physiological jaundice causes of unconjugated hyperbilirubinaemia include haemolytic disease of the newborn (usually rhesus incompatability) bacterial infections, hypoglycaemia, galactosaemia and fructosaemia.

Conjugated hyperbilirubinaemia is never physiological and may be due to:

- infections
- inherited metabolic diorders
- toxic or deficiency disorders
- endocrine disorders (some cases of hypothyroidism, hypoadrenalism and hypopituitarism)
- bile duct anomalies
- vascular disorders (veno-occlusive disease, lymphatic defects).

Natural history and prognosis   Unconjugated hyperbilirubinaemia must be treated promptly to avoid irreversible damage associated with kernicterus.

Galactosaemia

Genetics   Autosomal recessive inheritance.

Biochemistry   Low levels of enzyme galactose-1-phosphate uridyl transferase in liver and blood cells leading to accumulation of galactose, galactose-1-phosphate and galactitol.

Epidemiology   Liver is affected within 2 weeks of birth.

Microscopy   Fat accumulates in liver cells and there is bile ductule proliferation. There is pseudo-acinar transformation of liver plates and iron deposition. Cirrhosis may develop in months.

Natural history and prognosis   Cataract formation is characteristic and mental retardation develops.

Fructosaemia

Biochemistry   Absence of fructose-1-phosphate aldolase or fructose-1-6-diphosphatase.

Clinical features   Symptoms appear as fructose is introduced into the diet at weaning. The child eats poorly, fails to thrive and vomits frequently. Drowsiness and coma may supervene. On examination the liver is enlarged.

Microscopy   There is marked fatty change. Liver cell necrosis and multi-nucleated liver cells may be present and fibrosis of portal tracts is seen. Cirrhosis will ultimately develop if untreated.

Alagille's syndrome

Genetics   Autosomal dominant inherited disorder.

Clinical features   The facial appearances are characteristic – prominence of the forehead, straight nose and deep-set eyes. Cardiovascular anomalies are frequently present. Itching may be prominent and the degree of jaundice is variable.

Microscopy   Hypoplasia of intrahepatic bile ducts is present by the age of 1 year.

Natural history and prognosis   Jaundice clears within a year or two and death from liver disease is uncommon.

Changes associated with total parenteral nutrition

Pathogenesis   Prolonged intravenous feeding without oral nutrition in early infancy leads to bile stasis and liver cell damage.

Clinical features   Jaundice.

Microscopy   Expansion of portal tract connective tissue and bile ductule proliferation.

Natural history and prognosis   If untreated can lead to cirrhosis and hepatocellular carcinoma. Withdrawal of intravenous nutrition and institution of oral feeds causes jaundice to disappear and liver changes to resolve.

Extrahepatic biliary atresia

Definition   Post-inflammatory obliteration of segment of extrahepatic biliary system.

Epidemiology   One of the commonest causes of prolonged cholestatic jaundice in infants. Incidence of 1/14 000 live births.

Microscopy   There is oedema and fibrosis of portal tracts, bile duct reduplication and in 50% giant cells.

Natural history and prognosis   Surgically correctable. If obstruction not relieved then secondary biliary cirrhosis develops and death occurs by 1–2 years.

Choledochal cyst

Definition   Cystic dilation of bile duct.

Epidemiology   More common in females.

Site   May involve intra- and extrahepatic bile ducts.

Clinical features   Depends on age at which symptoms appear. In infants there may be prolongation of physiological jaundice, in older children there is recurrent upper abdominal pain and jaundice.

Microscopy   Similar to biliary atresia.

Natural history and prognosis   The cyst readily becomes infected leading to ascending inflammation in the biliary system (ascending cholangitis). The cyst may rupture leading to biliary peritonitis. Gallstones may form and there may be subsequent episodes of pancreatitis. Malignant transformation of the epithelium is rare.

Reye's syndrome

Epidemiology   Affects children in over 90% of cases.

Aetiology   Characteristically there is a recent history of viral illness. About 95% of children have been given aspirin.

Clinical features   Severe vomiting, irritability and disturbances of consciousness.

Laboratory findings   Increase in serum transaminase and increased plasma ammonia concentrations.

Microscopy   Small droplet fatty change but no necrosis. Electron microscopy shows mitochondrial abnormalities.

Natural history and prognosis   Mortality is high (40–50%) and survivors show evidence of brain damage.

Indian childhood cirrhosis

Epidemiology   Confined to Indian sub-continent, Sri Lanka and Malaysia. In certain areas of India it is the 4th commonest cause of death in young children. Presentation is usually between 6 months and 4 years.

Aetiology   Unknown. Possibly due to accumulation of copper in liver which may be associated with drinking boiled buffalo's milk which has been stored in copper containers.

Clinical features   Two main forms are seen. Initially there is anorexia, nausea and irritability followed by abdominal distension and hepatomegaly. Over the next few months signs of portal hypertension appear. In about 25% of cases the picture is dominated by a hepatitis-like syndrome.

Microscopy   In the earliest phase there is patchy liver cell necrosis with a focal inflammatory response. Mallory's hyaline appears. Fibrous septa divide liver into small nodules but there is little regenerative activity. The liver content of copper is high (10–60 × normal).

Congenital hepatic fibrosis

Genetics   Autosomal recessive inherited disorder.

Pathogenesis   Possibly due to failure of normal involution of embryonal ductal plates (earliest forms of bile ducts).

Clinical features   Affected children have enlarged firm livers and may show signs of portal hypertension.

Microscopy   Linkage of portal tracts by fibrous bands in which cystic spaces lined by bile-duct epithelium are seen. No evidence of hepatocellular damage.

Natural history and prognosis   In patients with the hepatitis-like presentation, death occurs 3–4 months after onset. Treatment with copper-chelating agents at a stage before ascites or jaundice have appeared gives a 50% survival.

VASCULAR DISORDERS OF THE LIVER

IMPAIRMENT OF HEPATIC VENOUS DRAINAGE
Chronic venous congestion

Epidemiology   Common finding in the liver at post-mortem.

Aetiology   Severe chronic congestion is seen in chronic heart failure, especially if the right side is involved.

Pathogenesis   Dilated and congested venous radicles in zone 3 together with hypoperfusion leads initially to fatty change and then atrophy of zone 3 hepatocytes.

Macroscopy   A variegated red and yellow appearance likened to the surface of a nutmeg.

Microscopy   The dark areas correspond to dilated and congested venous radicles and zone 3 sinusoids and the yellow areas are represented by fatty and atrophic hepatocytes. In some severe cases there is necrosis in zone 3. In chronic congestion (e.g. patients with tricuspid valve incompetence) fibrous tissue may be laid down in the perivenular area which eventually may form bridges with adjacent scarred areas. In these patients the acinar pattern may become exaggerated with reverse lobulation (false impression that veins lie at the centre of acini) with the liver appearing finely nodular (cardiac cirrhosis).

Hepatic vein occlusion (Budd–Chiari syndrome)

Definition Occlusion of the hepatic veins at their ostia or of the vena cava distal to its junction with the hepatic veins.

Aetiology Usually either thrombosis (e.g. in primary myeloproliferative disorders, paroxysmal nocturnal haemoglobinuria, clotting disorders such as presence of lupus anti-coagulant, Behçet's syndrome, oral contraceptive use, vasculitides and during or following pregnancy) or infiltration of veins by carcinoma (particularly hepatocellular or renal cell). About 10% have no predisposing factor.

Clinical features Ascites (96%), enlargement of the liver (90%) and spleen (64%), abdominal pain (80%), oedema (46%), jaundice (44%), fever (40%) and occasionally hepatic encephalopathy (22%) and gastrointesinal bleeding (14%).

Microscopy Most of acinus is replaced by blood with a rim of zone 1 hepatocytes.

Occlusion of intrahepatic venous radicles (veno-occlusive disease)

Definition Non-thrombotic lumenal narrowing of hepatic vein radicles and sub-lobular veins.

Aetiology Poisoning with pyrrolizidine alkaloids, irradiation of the liver, treatment with anti-tumour drugs, conditioning for bone marrow transplantation with cyclophosphamide and irradiation (within 4 weeks of transplant, 13–20% of patients) and graft-versus-host disease.

Pathogenesis Growth of new layer of sub-endothelial connective tissue.

Clinical features Similar to Budd–Chiari syndrome.

Arterial underperfusion

Aetiology May be functional (low output cardiac failure and shock) or structural (atherosclerosis, polyarteritis nodosa, embolus or invasion by tumour).

Microscopy In functional underperfusion zone 3 is the target. In some cases of shock there is cholestasis in the canaliculi adjacent to portal tracts. Infarction of the liver is rare (due to double blood supply from hepatic artery and portal vein).

Peliosis hepatitis

Aetiology Originally seen in patients with wasting diseases (tuberculosis and cachexia of malignant disease) but also seen in patients taking oral contraceptives and anabolic steroids.

Clinical features The liver is usually enlarged and there is jaundice.

Microscopy Blood-filled cystic spaces in continuity with sinusoids which are partly lined by endothelium within the liver parenchyma.

EFFECTS OF LIVER DISEASE

Portal hypertension

Aetiology Generally due to increased resistance to blood flow anywhere in the portal system, increased portal blood flow or both. The majority are due to increased resistance in the pre-hepatic, hepatic or post-hepatic vascular tree.

Physiology and consequences Normal portal blood flow is 1–1.2 l/min with a pressure of 7 mm Hg. In portal hypertension there is a significant diversion of blood from the portal to the systemic circulation. Collateral vessels open up in the oesophagus and gastric fundus becoming tortuous and dilated (varices). In the oesophagus this is associated with atrophy of the mucularis mucosae. The severity of oesophageal varices is graded 1–3. Other dilated collateral vessels form on the anterior abdominal wall (caput medusae) and in the rectal submucosa. There may be shunting into the left renal vein and there may also be portal–portal shunting around obstructions in the extrahepatic part of the portal vein. Congestive splenomegaly is the other main consequence of portal hypertension.

Classification At a functional level portal hypertension can be divided into three main groups:

- post-sinusoidal: either extrahepatic due to pathology in the heart (increased atrial pressure e.g. constrictive pericarditis), the inferior vena cava or large hepatic veins or intrahepatic due to pathology in the small hepatic veins

- sinusoidal: intrahepatic and the commonest cause of hypertension in Europe and North America. It is due to cirrhosis, non-cirrhotic nodules, acute alcoholic hepatitis, drugs and vitamin A intoxication
- pre-sinusoidal: may be intrahepatic due to portal tract lesions (e.g. schistosomiasis, early primary biliary cirrhosis, congenital hepatic fibrosis, chronic active hepatitis, some toxins, sarcoidosis and idiopathic causes) or extrahepatic due to lesions in the portal vein (mainly thrombosis, sometimes associated with tumour infiltration but also post surgery and associated with Crohn's disease), splenic vein or due to increased portal blood flow. Extrahepatic pre-sinusoidal portal hypertension in the absence of portal vein obstruction is sometimes termed non-cirrhotic portal hypertension.

Ascites

Definition   Accumulation of free fluid in the peritoneal cavity.

Physiology   Mostly transudate with protein of 1–2 g/100 ml.

Aetiology   Lesions leading to raised pressure in the venous end of the splanchnic capillaries, sinusoidal portal hypertension with increased formation of hepatic lymph, hepatic decompensation with decreased plasma albumin (lowering plasma oncotic pressure) or lesions leading to retention of sodium and as a consequence water.

Hepatic encephalopathy

Definition   Spectrum of neuropsychiatric disturbances caused by liver disease.

Aetiology   Either in association with acute liver failure or against a background of chronic liver disease such as cirrhosis. In those with chronic liver disease encephalopathy may be precipitated by infection, haemorrhage in the upper gastrointestinal tract, electrolyte disturbances and certain drugs/toxins (e.g. morphia, benzodiazepines, barbiturates and alcohol).

Pathogenesis The central development is the presence of portal blood in the systemic circulation without being first exposed to the metabolic functions of the liver. The main culprits appear to be nitrogenous compounds such as ammonia, derivatives of aromatic amino-acids, false neuro-transmitters (e.g. octopamine) and neuro-inhibitors (e.g. γ-aminobutyric acid and endogenous benzodiazepines).

Clinical features In acute cases there is a rapid onset with drowsiness which may be associated with delirium and fits. In some cases there is decerebrate rigidity. The patient may become unresponsive and comatose. In cases associated with chronic liver disease the encephalopathy may be episodic and associated with specific clinical events such as gastrointestinal haemorrhage. The onset is usually gradual with mood changes (either euphoria or depression) followed by confusion often accompanied by deterioration in handwriting (constructional apraxia) and a flapping tremor (asterixis). There may be characteristic delta-type slow waves on EEG.

Biochemistry There is usually elevation of blood ammonia and increased glutamine in the cerebrospinal fluid.

Macroscopy The brain may appear entirely normal but in about half there is cerebral oedema.

Microscopy In the early stages there is increased number and size of protoplasmic astrocytes in the deeper layers of the cortex, basal ganglia, in the dentate nucleus and cerebellum. In late stages in patients in whom there have been many episodes of encephalopathy the cortex is thinned with loss of neurones and fibres. Rarely there may be demyelination.

....

OTHER MANIFESTATIONS OF LIVER FAILURE

Effect of liver failure on the cardiovascular system

Patients may have a hyperkinetic circulation with high cardiac output and decreased peripheral resistance associated with vasodilation (of unknown cause).

Effect of liver disease on the lungs

A number of changes may occur, including reduced arterial saturation due to a shift in oxygen desaturation, curve of haemoglobin to the right and microscopic arteriovenous shunts in the lungs. There may be vasodilation that fails to respond to hypoxia leading to ventilation perfusion mismatch. Pulmonary hypertension may develop.

Effect of liver disease on endocrine function

The chief endocrine effects are on gonadal function with hypogonadism and gynaecomastia.

Effect of liver disease on blood cells and clotting

Red cells   There may be anaemia due to increased destruction in the spleen (hypersplenism), increased plasma volume, recurrent bleeding or failure of marrow responses. The red cells may be normocytic, macrocytic (associated with disordered vitamin B_{12} and folate metabolism) or microcytic. Abnormalities in red cell shape include presence of target cells, echinocytes (spiky appearances on wet film) or acanthocytes. About 3–12% of patients with hepatocellular carcinoma have increased red cell counts associated with raised erythropoietin levels.

Leucocytes   There may be leucopaenia (especially with cirrhosis and associated with marrow suppression and hypersplenism) or leucocytosis (associated with fulminant hepatitis, malignancy, ascending cholangitis and alcoholic hepatitis).

Platelets   There may be a mild thrombocytopaenia caused by pooling in the spleen, decreased survival and marrow failure. Platelet function may also be impaired.

Clotting   There may be decreased synthesis of clotting factors, naturally occurring anticoagulants (e.g. proteins C, S and antithrombin III), profibrinolytic and anti-fibrinolytic proteins. Some proteins may be abnormally formed (e.g. fibrinogen, Factor VIII and von Willebrand factor and the vitamin K dependent factors). There may also be decreased clearance of activated clotting factors, plasminogen activators and thrombin/antithrombin III complexes. The net effect of these is determined by the balance of all the abnormalities but patients mostly have prolonged one-stage prothrombin time and accelerated fibrinolysis. Disseminated intravascular coagulation occurs in some patients.

Effect of liver disease on the skin

There may be the development of spider naevi and palmar erythema (liver palms).

DRUGS AND THE LIVER

Epidemiology   Drug-related liver injury is responsible for 2% of all cases of jaundice and 25% of cases of fulminant acute liver failure. More than 600 drugs have been implicated in the causation of liver disease.

Definition   Damage may be **predictable** (related to dose) or **unpredictable** (inadequate intracellular defences or unusual immune response).

Normal biochemistry   Most drugs reaching the liver are lipid-soluble and are converted to water-soluble metabolites before excretion in urine or bile is possible. In most instances this requires two steps involving:

- oxidation of the compound by cytochrome P-450
- conjugation of the compound with a polar water soluble group (e.g. glucuronic acid).

Activation of cytochrome P-450 leads to the formation of highly reactive electrophilic compounds, semiquinone free radicals (from which reactive free radicals can form) and free radicals which are derived from haloalkanes. The cell damage results from covalent binding of electrophilic compounds to DNA, lipid peroxidation of unsaturated fatty acids in plasma membranes and depletion of antioxidants such as reduced glutathione.

Halothane-induced hepatitis

Definition   Immune-mediated reaction to the anaesthetic agent halothane. Similar reactions are thought to operate with imipramine, erythromycin and α-methyldopa.

Pathogenesis Liver cell plasma membranes are trifluoro-acetylated by a reactive product of halothane. These act as new antigens and cause the formation of cytotoxic antibody. Genetic factors are thought to determine which individuals will become immunized by these products.

MICROSCOPY OF DRUG-RELATED LIVER DAMAGE

There may be changes in:

1. Liver cells

   - coagulative necrosis – paracetamol, carbon tetrachloride
   - cytolyic necrosis – halothane, erythromycin isoniazid, α-methyl DOPA
   - Acute hepatitis-like picture – phenothiazines, sulphonylureas, tricyclic antidepressants
   - chronic hepatitis-like picture–nitrofurantoin, oxyphenisatin, methotrexate, α-methyldopa
   - large droplet fatty change – alcohol, methotrexate
   - small droplet fatty change – tetracyclines, valproic acid
   - phospholipidosis – amiodarone, perhexiline maleate, 4, 4′ diethylaminoethoxhexestrol
   - granulomatous hepatitis – sulphonamides, allopurinol, carbamazepine, phenylbutazone, quinine
   - neoplasm – oestrogens, thorotrast, anabolic steroids.

2. Bile ducts

   - acute bland cholestasis (no inflammation or necrosis) – oral contraceptives, anabolic and androgenic steroids
   - prolonged cholestasis – chlorpromazine, paraquat, some arsenical derivatives
   - lesions resembling sclerosing cholangitis – floxuridine infusion into hepatic artery.

3. Blood vessels.
4. Mononuclear phagocytes.

Anatomy

Location Pear-shaped sac in the gallbladder fossa between the quadrate and right lobe of the liver.

Size About 7–10 cm long with capacity of about 50 ml.

Histology

The mucosa is thrown into folds and lined by tall columnar epithelium. No muscularis mucosae. Muscularis propria or longitudinal fibres with collagen and elastic tissue.

Function

The liver secretes 0.5–1 l of watery bile per day. The gallbladder concentrates this by a factor of 5–10 and stores the bile prior to release. Release of bile is associated with eating fatty food mediated by plasma cholecystokinin.

....

GALLSTONES (CHOLELITHIASIS)

Epidemiology Common, affects 10–20% adults in UK and USA. F:M 2:1.

Risk factors Obesity, diabetes mellitus and high oestrogen levels (female gender, oral contraceptive).

Chemistry There are two main types of gallstone:

1. **Cholesterol stones**

   In Western countries more than 75% gallstones contain significant amounts of cholesterol either as pure cholesterol stones (90% content cholesterol) which are usually single, large (> 2.5 cm), white/yellow, easy to cut with radiating crystalline cut surface or mixed stones (50% cholesterol, rest mucoprotein, calcium and bilirubin) which are smaller (0.5–2.5cm), multiple and have a faceted appearance.

2. **Pigment stones**

   In Western countries these account for 10% of gallstones but are more common in Asia. They may be either black pigment stones (Commonest, found worldwide, associated with haemolysis and cirrhosis) composed of polymerized degradation products of oxidized bilirubin or brown pigment stones (found in Far East, associated with bile duct infections and helminth infestations) which are soft with laminated cut surface and are composed mainly of calcium bilirubinate.

Pathogenesis Normal hepatic bile is composed of 97% water with 3% solutes – (bile salts – 67%; phospholipids 22%; protein – 4.5%; cholesterol – 4% and bilirubin – 0.3%) – the composition of which is crucial to gallstone formation. Cholesterol is insoluble in aqueous solutions but is made soluble in bile by the bile salts and phospholipids. If the relative concentrations of these components is altered by an increase in cholesterol output (associated with increasing age, obesity, oestrogens, lipid-lowering drugs), decrease in bile salts (associated with decreased resorption in gut or impaired synthesis in liver) or a combination of these, then the bile becomes supersaturated with cholesterol (lithogenic). Stone formation begins with tiny crystals of cholesterol (nucleation) resulting in bile sludge which is promoted by pregnancy, prolonged total parenteral nutrition, starvation, rapid weight loss and the antibiotic ceftriaxone. Calcium stone formation is enhanced by impaired acidification of bile. Cholestasis is another risk factor and may be associated with pregnancy, oral contraceptive use and total parenteral nutrition.

Clinical features Most patients are asymptomatic. Symptoms are usually precipitated by impaction and the site of this (usually cystic duct) determines the symptoms and pathology. Most symptoms relate to right upper quadrant or epigastric abdominal pain.

Consequences Stones may pass into the common bile duct to cause obstruction and jaundice, ascending infection (cholangitis; may result in hepatic abscess formation), secondary biliary cirrhosis and pruritis. Stones passing through the common bile duct may cause acute pancreatitis due to obstruction of the pancreatic duct or the ampulla of Vater leading to bile reflux into the pancreatic duct which activates pancreatic enzymes. Occasionally inflammation of the gallbladder results in adhesion between that organ and the bowel (most frequently small intestine). The walls of each may erode to form a fistula through which a large stone can pass causing small intestinal obstruction at a more distal point (gallstone ileus).

....

INFLAMMATORY DISORDERS
Ascending cholangitis

Clinical features Presentation consists of fever and chills, pain and jaundice (Charcot's triad). Fever is absent in 20%. There may be dark urine. Septicaemia may supervene.

Acute cholecystitis

Definition Acute inflammation of the gallbladder. May be associated with suppuration and necrotizing inflammation.

Epidemiology Most associated with stones but 10% have no stones (more commonly males, M:F 2:1).

Pathogenesis Most due to cholestasis caused by gallstone impaction. Around 10% in absence of stone may be associated with defective filling/emptying of gallbladder (associated with immobilization) or rarely due to infections (notably *Salmonella*) or ischaemia in cases of vasculitis.

Macroscopy Gallbladder is enlarged with hyperaemic and oedematous wall. The lumen may contain pus (empyema of gallbladder) or mucous gland secretions which may be watery (hydrops of gallbladder) or sticky (mucocele of gallbladder). A stone may be present in the cystic duct.

Microscopy Features of acute inflammation with vasodilation and oedema with a neutrophil infiltrate varying from mild to florid with suppuration and necrosis of the wall. In the latter case (more common in the absence of stones) there may be perforation and peritonitis.

Clinical features Patients present with a severe abdominal pain, nausea, vomiting and fever, and they have a raised neutrophil count. Generalized peritonitis is rare but has a 30% mortality.

Chronic cholecystitis

Epidemiology More common than acute form. M:F 1:3.

Pathogenesis Poorly understood, a minority follow recurrent episodes of acute cholecysitis. Strongly associated with gallstones.

Clinical features Presents with vague upper abdominal pain, dyspesia, flatulence and intolerance of fatty food.

Macroscopy Gallbladder may be enlarged or shrunken and fibrosed. Wall may be thickened or atrophic. Stones (usually mixed type and multiple) present in 95% cases.

Microscopy Variable. If the wall is thick this is due to scarring and muscle hypertrophy. Out-pouchings of mucosa extending through the muscularis (Rokitansky–Aschoff sinuses) are frequent. A chronic inflammatory infiltrate is usually present and may include lymphoid follicles.

Cholesterolosis of gallbladder

Epidemiology Predilection for middle-aged females. Present in 25% gallbladders removed surgically and 12% at autopsy.

Macroscopy Bright yellow flecks project slightly above mucosal surface – 'strawberry gallbladder'. A localized variant of this may include cholesterol polyps.

Microscopy Aggregates of foamy macrophages in mucosa.

....

TUMOURS OF THE GALLBLADDER

Adenoma

Resemble adenomas of the large intestine.

Macroscopy May be pedunculated or sessile.

Microscopy May be tubular, tubulovillous or villous. Some degree of dysplasia may be found.

Carcinoma of the gallbladder

Epidemiology Rare. Majority (> 90%) in people over 50 years with peak incidence in 7th and 8th decades, M:F 3–4:1. In USA incidence is commonest in native American

Indians and Hispanics, rare in whites of European origin and very rare in blacks.

Aetiology Associated with gallstones (75% patients with carcinoma have stones) but occurs in only 0.5% patients with stones. Also associated with fistulae between gallbladder and gut, with extensively calcified gallbladder (porcelain gallbladder), sclerosing cholangitis, ulcerative colitis and hereditary intestinal polyposis syndromes.

Macroscopy May be diffuse (70%) with marked fibrosis of the wall which is gritty to cut or polypoid (30%) with a cauliflower-like pattern protruding into the lumen.

Microscopy Most are adenocarcinomas with variable differentiation. The glands are lined by one or more layers of cuboidal cells with cellular atypia and are surrounded by abundant cellular stroma. Evidence of spread is seen in 90% of cases at diagnosis which commonly involves direct invasion into liver, stomach or duodenum.

Prognosis Determined by stage. Stage I (intramucosal) and II (mucosa and muscularis involved) tumours are cured by cholecystectomy. Stage III (all three layers of wall involved) and IV (all layers and cystic lymph node) tumours have 11% 5-year survival while stage V (liver or other organs involved) are uniformly fatal.

Carcinoma of the extra-hepatic bile ducts

Epidemiology M=F.

Associations Weak association with gallstones. Associated with ulcerative colitis, sclerosing cholangitis, *Clonorchis sinensis* (liver fluke) infestation, and a variety of congenital bile duct anatomical abnormalities.

Site Occurs at any site excluding the ampulla of Vater but most common in upper third.

Macroscopy Three variants – a diffuse sclerosing variant with ill-defined thickening of the wall, nodular variant (most often middle third) and papillary variant (most distal third).

Microscopy Adenocarcinomas. The sclerosing variant may spread proximally to involve intrahepatic bile ducts. Perineural invasion may be prominent.

Prognosis Poor, overall 10% 5-year survival rising to 25% for tumours of distal third.

Other tumours of the gallbladder

Rarely tumours may arise from the connective tissues and these include paraganglioma, leiomyoma, lipoma and granular cell tumour.

THE EXOCRINE PANCREAS

Anatomy

Site Retroperitoneal on posterior wall of abdomen.

Size Approximately 12–15 cm long weighing 60–70 g.

Organization Normally divided in to head (disc shaped, lies in concavity of duodenum), neck, body and tail (in lienorenal ligament and in contact with splenic hilum. The uncinate process is that part of the head extending to the left behind the superior mesenteric vessels. The main duct of the pancreas begins at the tail and runs the length of the gland, opening into the ampulla of Vater with the bile duct (60% individuals) or drains separately into the duodenum. The accessory duct drains the upper part of the head and drains into the duodenum a short distance above the main duct.

Blood supply Splenic and superior and inferior pancreatoduodenal vessels. Each lobule is supplied by a single artery.

Histology

The pancreas is a lobulated gland in which the secretory cells are arranged in tubular or flask-shaped groups. A narrow intercalated duct is at the centre of these groups lined by centroacinar cells. The secretory cells have deeply basophilic cytoplasm with the apical portions containing eosinophilic zymogen granules. The more distal ducts are lined by columnar cells.

Development

From two gut-derived buds, one ventral and one dorsal. The ventral bud rotates to the left to fuse with the dorsal bud which ultimately forms most of the body and tail. The original ducts of the dorsal and ventral sections anastamose to form the main duct while the accessory duct is formed by part of the dorsal duct.

······

ABNORMALITIES OF DEVELOPMENT

Pancreas divisum

Epidemiology   In 5% of the population.

Pathogenesis   Failure of the two duct systems to anastamose.

Natural history and prognosis   Some patients develop segmental chronic pancreatitis in later life.

Annular pancreas

Definition   Ring of pancreatic tissue encircling the duodenum.

Epidemiology   M:F 3:1. About one-third associated with trisomy 21.

Pathogenesis   Probably failure of migration of ventral bud.

Clinical presentation   Most present as infants with vomiting probably related to duodenal narrowing.

Ectopic pancreas

Epidemiology   Found in up to 2% autopsies.

Pathogenesis   Displacement of pancreas along intestine before or during rotation.

Site   Commonly duodenum (28%), stomach (25%), jejunum (16%) or Meckel's diverticulum (6%).

Macroscopy   Small firm rounded mass in the submucosa (50%), muscularis (25%) or serosa (10%).

Microscopy   May be well formed with acini, ducts and islets of Langerhans, mainly ducts with few acini or proliferating ducts only.

....

INFLAMMATORY DISORDERS

Acute pancreatitis

Definition Expression of sudden enzymatic destruction of pancreatic parenchyma.

Epidemiology Usually adults 30–70 years but may be seen in children with type I hyperlipidaemia.

Aetiology Four main groups of causes:
- biliary disease and gallstones causing obstruction of the pancreatic duct (about 53% of cases in Europe)
- chronic alcoholism (mechanism unknown, about 6% of cases in Europe)
- idiopathic
- variety of other factors including duct stenosis, infections (e.g. mumps, Coxsackie virus and hepatitis), toxins (e.g. diuretics, α-methyldopa), endocrine disorders (e.g. hyperparathyroidism, steroids) metabolic disorders (hyperlipidaemias types I and V), vascular disorders/ ischaemia (e.g. shock), hypothermia and trauma.

Pathogenesis The pivotal event is thought to be the activation of trypsinogen to trypsin. In patients with gallstones this activation may be due to reflux of bile.

Site The distribution of ischaemia-related pancreatitis is different to those associated with ductal disease being located at the periphery of the lobe (furthest from the arterial inflow).

Macroscopy There is fat necrosis appearing as chalky white patches within and around the pancreas. In more severe cases there may be coagulative necrosis of acinar tissue with areas of haemorrhage. There may be thrombosis in adjacent blood vesels or frank haemorrhage if these vessels are disrupted.

Microscopy Initially there is a mild white-cell reaction. In some cases infection supervenes with abscess formation. There is perilobular fat necrosis.

Natural history and prognosis In some patients reparative fibrosis of areas of liquefactive necrosis results in these areas being walled off as a pseudocyst. Up to 40% patients develop shock associated with acute pancreatitis, 33%

develop transient hypocalcaemia and 15–25% develop transient hyperglycaemia associated with high glucagon and low insulin levels. There may be impaired lung fuction (a few will develop adult respiratory distress syndrome, ARDS) or renal function.

Chronic pancreatitis

Epidemiology   Males more often affected than females.

Aetiology   In Western countries more often associated with chronic alcoholism (60–85%) than biliary tract disease.

Pathogenesis   In alcohol-related cases thought to result from serotonin-mediated secretion of high protein fluid that blocks pancreatic ductules. In other cases related to gallstones and developmental abnormalities the pathogenesis is related to obstruction.

Clinical features   Pain is a major symptom and may be chronic or associated with episodes of superimposed acute pancreatitis.

Microscopy   Loss of acinar tissue and replacement by inflamed scar tissue. The endocrine tissue is less affected and appears more prominent. Inspissated protein-rich material and calcification are commonly seen in alcohol-related cases.

Natural history and prognosis   Patients may develop malabsorption (after 90% of gland destroyed), diabetes mellitus (30–40% of cases) or extra-hepatic biliary obstruction (5–10% of cases).

Cystic fibrosis (mucoviscidosis) and the pancreas

Epidemiology   Occurs in about 1 in 2500 live births as an autosomal recessive inherited disorder.

Aetiology   Mutation of the gene encoding cystic fibrosis transmembrane conductance regulator gene on chromosome 7 (region 7q31).

Pathogenesis   Viscid secretions in the pancreas lead to obstruction of the duct system, dilation of the ducts, post-obstructive atrophy and fibrosis.

Laboratory findings High concentration of chloride and sodium in sweat.

Macroscopy At birth the pancreas is macroscopically normal but by two years the pancreas appears lobulated and is much firmer than usual. The cut surface has cystic spaces containing cloudy fluid.

Microscopy Dilation of pancreatic ducts and ductules containing inspissated proteinaceous secretions together with acinar atrophy which is very marked in advanced cases.

....

TUMOURS OF THE PANCREAS

Benign

Papillary adenoma

Epidemiology Uncommon. M:F 1:1 with peak age 50–70 years.

Microscopy Resemble colonic tubulovillous adenomas. Cellular atypia may be marked.

Serous cystadenoma

Epidemiology Uncommon. Tends to occur in elderly females. Some cases may be associated with von Hippel–Lindau syndrome.

Macroscopy Quite large (6–10 cm diameter) with cut surface showing multiple small cysts.

Microscopy Cysts are lined by cuboidal epithelium.

Solid and cystic tumour

Epidemiology Chiefly in young females (10–35 years).

Macroscopy Large rounded masses (9–10 cm) with partly solid, partly cystic cut surface.

Microscopy Solid sheets of small regular cells with tumour breakdown resulting in small cysts and a pseudo-papillary pattern.

Malignant

Carcinoma

Epidemiology   Incidence increasing. Fourth most common cause of cancer-related death in males and fifth in females.

Pathogenesis   Associated with mutations of *Ki-ras* proto-oncogene in 90%.

Site   About two-thirds arise in head of pancreas.

Clinical features   Carcinomas of the head of the pancreas may present with obstructive rather painless jaundice and the gallbladder may become distended and palpable. Some patients may have an associated migratory thrombophlebitis. Carcinomas of the tail present later with symptoms related to invasion of local organs (e.g. vertebral column, stomach and colon).

Macroscopy   Carcinomas of the head of the pancreas tend to be small while those in the tail are larger.

Microscopy   The majority are fairly well differentiated adenocarcinomas of ductal type with fibrous stromas response. Other variants include acinar, adenosquamous, giant cell and mixed cell types. Squamous and small cell carcinomas, cystadenocarcinoma, pancreatoblastomas and osteoclast-like tumours are also described.

Natural history and prognosis   Very poor prognosis with 5-year survival of 2%.

The kidney

DISORDERS OF THE KIDNEY

ANATOMY

Size Approximately 11 cm long, 6 cm in breadth and 3 cm antero-posteriorly.

Weight About 150 g in males and 135 g in females.

Organization

There is a medial hilums where the renal artery enters and the renal vein and ureter leave. The cut surface shows an outer **cortex** 4–6 mm thick and an inner **medulla**. The medulla consists of 12 wedge-shaped **pyramids** with their base on the cortico-medullary junction and their apices draining into the minor calyces via the **papillae**. The prolongation of cortex between the pyramids is the **column of Bertin**. The cortex consists of both glomeruli and tubules; the medulla contains no glomeruli and is the site of the collecting tubules.

Blood supply

Arterial supply is via the main renal artery arising from the abdominal aorta which divides at the hilus to anterior and posterior branches. These further divide into five segmental arteries (with no collaterals). These branch at the cortico-medullary junction to form a series of arcuate arteries which curve around the medullary pyramids and give rise to the interlobular arteries. From these are derived the afferent arterioles which divide into glomerular capillaries which then fuse to form the efferent arteriole (smaller than the afferent vessel). Efferent arterioles branch into a capillary network running close to the renal tubules. The renal papillae are supplied by arteriolae rectae spuriae derived from efferent arterioles. The medulla also receives blood from arteriolae rectae verae directly from the interlobular arteries and these two systems constitute the vasa recta.

Venous drainage mirrors the arterial supply. Peritubular capillaries drain into interlobular veins which empty into arcuate veins, then segmental veins and eventually the renal vein. The vasa recta drain back into the arcuate veins.

The glomerulus

Glomerular capillary tuft

Lined by a single layer of fenestrated endothelium which lies on an incomplete basement membrane. The part of the tuft facing the mesangium has no basement membrane and here the lumen is separated from mesangial cells by endothelial cytoplasm.

Glomerular basement membrane (GBM)

About 300 nm thick. Consists of three layers; the lamina rara interna (in places in contact with the capillary lumen), lamina densa (thickest) and lamina rara externa. The GBM is the site of two antigens – amyloid P component and the Goodpasture antigen. The outer surface is covered by epithelial cells which have 'foot processes' (visible by EM) separated from each other by a gap of 20–50 nm (filtration slit). The epithelial cells are important for protein synthesis and signal reception but also synthesize and secrete basement membrane components (type IV collagen, laminin and heparan sulphate).

Glomerular polyanion

The GBM and the sides of the epithelial cell foot processes are covered by a negatively charged polyanion important in regulating clearance of molecules from the glomerular capillary blood (preventing leak of the major plasma proteins which are negatively charged and promoting separation of foot processes by mutual repulsion).

Glomerular clearance

About 150 litres of blood are filtered per day. Clearance of molecules depends on molecular size and charge, the presence of the glomerular polyanion and glomerular blood flow.

The mesangium

Matrix

Connective tissue containing collagen, fibronectin, laminin and entactin surround the mesangial cells. Some plasma reaches the mesangium through endothelial fenestrations and large molecules can become trapped between matrix fibrils where they are endocytosed by mesangial cells or engulfed by phagocytes. Plasma leaves by a number of routes including through epithelial cells into the urinary space. Macromolecules can potentially be trapped against the basement membrane at this point.

Intrinsic mesangial cell

Capable of contractile activity. Has receptors for angiotensin II and atrial natriuretic peptide and synthesizing functions (interleukin-1 which acts as an autocrine growth factor).

Mesangial mononuclear phagocytes

Normally present in very small numbers.

The juxtaglomerular apparatus (JGA)

Granular cells   Modified smooth muscle cells found in terminal part of afferent arteriole. Granules contain active renin and angiotensin II.

Lacis cells   Lie in the V formed at the glomerular hilum by afferent and efferent arterioles. Resemble intrinsic mesangial cells.

Macula densa   Part of the wall of the distal convoluted tubule lying nearest to the glomerular hilum in close apposition to lacis cells.

Function of JGA

Chief source of renin. Renin release is stimulated by fall in blood pressure, decreased concentration of sodium and chloride in macula densa, sympathetic discharge in small nerve endings. Renin is released into the interstitium and gains access to the blood via peritubular capillaries initiating the sequence.

- angiotensinogen–angiotensin I
- angiotensin I–angiotensin II (angiotensin converting enzyme, ACE)
- angiotensin II acts as potent vasoconstrictor and stimulus for aldosterone secretion
- aldosterone triggers sodium resorption from distal nephron.

Therefore the JGA is important for sodium/water regulation and control of arterial blood pressure.

DEVELOPMENT OF THE KIDNEY

The **pronephros** originates from mesodermal cells on the ventral surface (nephrogenic cord). This starts to degenerate as soon as it is formed but gives rise to the mesonephros (second primitive kidney). The mesonephros (Wolffian duct) rises from the caudal end of the pronephros and shows some differentiation into glomeruli and tubules (secretes urine until fourth gestational month). A ureteric bud arises from the postero-medial aspect of the mesonephric duct near the cloaca after degeneration of the mesonephros. From this and from primitive cells of the metanephric blastema arises the metanephros from which the mature kidney is formed. The ureteric bud gives rise to the ureter, renal pelvis, calyses and collecting tubules. The anterior growing end (ampulla) is responsible for outward extension of the bud, cell division, induction of nephron formation by blastema and establishment of communication between the bud and proximal portions of the nephron.

ABNORMALITIES OF DEVELOPMENT
Bilateral agenesis

Epidemiology   M:F 2:1.

Aetiology   Either absence of lower half of mesonephric duct or failure of the duct to give rise to the bud.

Clinical features Failure or fetal urinary secretion causes oligohydramnios.

Associations Pulmonary hypoplasia, absence or deformity of lower limbs, Potter facies (low set ears, receding chin, widened flattened and beaked nose and wide-set eyes with prominent inner canthus).

Natural history and prognosis Incompatible with more than a few hours of life and many are stillborn.

Unilateral agenesis

Epidemiology Found in 1/500 post-mortems of neonates and stillborn infants. Males more than females.

Macroscopy Single kidney is hypertrophied.

Natural history and prognosis Although a single kidney is compatible with normal life there are frequently other associated congenital abnormalities.

Renal aplasia

Definition Ureter is present but no functioning renal tissue.

Aetiology Defect in renal blastema or stimulatory effect of ureteric bud.

Horseshoe kidney

Aetiology Fusion of lower poles of metanephric duct in early embryonic life.

Associations When found in stillborn infants or neonates it is associated with other abnormalities. Sometimes occurs with trisomy 18.

Renal dysplasia

Definition Developmental abnormality covering a spectrum of abnormalities ranging from massive polycystic kidney to a small, irregularly shaped organ.

Aetiology Anomalous differentiation of metanephric blastema. May occur as part of various autosomal recessively inherited familial syndromes.

Associations Almost always associated with other renal tract abnormalities such as duplication of ureters, ureteric ectopia and posterior urethral valves.

Microscopy Expressions of maldifferentiation include primitive ducts (surrounded by mantle of primitive mesenchymal cells), metaplastic cartilage, immature glomeruli and multiple fibrous walled cysts.

Renal cystic disease

Aetiology of renal cysts

- Polycystic kidney   Autosomal dominant
  Autosomal recessive.
- Medullary cysts   Medullary cystic disease
  Juvenile nephronophthisis
  Medullary sponge kidney.
- Acquired cystic disease associated with chronic renal failure.
- Associated with hereditary syndromes.
- Renal dysplasia.

Mechanism of cyst development   Three possible mechanisms are suggested including intratubular obstruction, increased basement membrane and hyperplasia of tubular epithelium of which the latter seems more likely.

Polycystic renal disease

Autosomal dominant type (ADPKD-1)

Epidemiology   Mostly presents in adult life. In USA 6000 new cases each year.

Aetiology   Some are spontaneous mutations. In 80% there is a mutant gene on the short arm of chromosome 16. Penetrance is virtually complete but expression is variable. Other cases are associated with an abnormality on the long arm of chromosome 4, at 4q13–q23 (less severely affected).

Pathogenesis   Cysts originate from small groups of cells which proliferate abnormally and extend the wall of the affected tubule with undifferentiated epithelium.

Clinical features Flank pain is present and haematuria each occurring in 60%, hypertension in 50% and stone formation in 10–20%. Nocturia and urinary tract infections also occur.

Associations Aortic aneurysm, colonic diverticula, ovarian cysts and heart valve defects (including floppy valves). Liver cysts are found in 30–40%. Cerebral aneuysms affecting the circle of Willis are present in 10–20%.

Macroscopy Both kidneys are grossly enlarged and diffusely cystic with marked irregularity of the sub-capsular surface. Cysts are present in cortex and medulla. Some cysts communicate with renal tubules.

Natural history and prognosis Progressive renal failure develops in 50%. Accounts for 10% of all cases of chronic renal failure.

Autosomal recessive type

Epidemiology Rare. Found in 1/16 000 live births. Most present in infancy but a few present in adult life.

Clinical features Most have bilateral loin masses.

Associations Hepatic fibrosis is present in all cases.

Macroscopy Capsular surface is smooth. The cut surface has many small cysts (1–2 mm diameter) in the cortex which connect with radially orientated dilated channels derived from collecting duct epithelium.

Natural history and prognosis If fully developed at birth then death is usual in early infancy due to renal failure. If the disease is mild the hepatic changes may predominate.

Cystic disease affecting the renal medulla

Juvenile nephronophthisis

Epidemiology Presentation in childhood or adolescence.

Genetics Autosomal recessive inheritance.

Clinical features Anaemia, growth retardation and chronic azotaemia associated with polyuria and salt wasting.

Natural history and prognosis Usually progresses to end-stage renal failure by age 20.

Medullary cystic disease

Epidemiology   Usually presents in adult life.

Genetics   Autosomal dominant inheritance.

Macroscopy   Both kidneys are small and fibrotic. The cut surfaces show numerous small cysts in cortico-medullary region.

Microscopy   Often associated with glomerular scarring and interstitial fibrosis.

Medullary sponge kidney

Epidemiology   Usually presents in adult life. Affects about 1/5000 people.

Clinical features   Haematuria and renal stone formation.

Macroscopy   Diffuse and bilateral irregular dilatations of the medullary and papillary collecting ducts but may be restricted to only a few papillae.

Simple renal cysts

Epidemiology   Incidence increases with age – 50% of people over 50 years have at least one simple cyst.

Pathogenesis   Outpouchings of distal tubules or collecting ducts.

Clinical features   Most are asymptomatic but there may be flank pain, haematuria, urinary tract infections or hypertension.

Macroscopy   Cysts may be single or multiple, unilateral or bilateral. Occur typically in the cortex but deeper portion of the medulla may also be affected. Most are less than 1 cm diameter but may be 3–4 cm diameter.

Acquired renal cystic disease

Epidemiology   Confined to patients with advanced chronic renal failure, particularly those on dialysis for end-stage renal disease, occurring in 30–50% patients in this group with risk increasing from third year of dialysis.

Macroscopy   Multiple small cysts (5 mm diameter) distributed throughout shrunken endstage kidney. Found in cortex and medulla. Cysts may contain haemorrhagic fluid.

Microscopy Cysts are lined by flattened cuboidal epithelium. Atypical hyperplasia is common and may explain high prevalence of neoplasms.

Natural history and prognosis Neoplastic lesions are found in 25%. Most are adenomas but about 15% are renal cell carcinomas.

....

GLOMERULAR DISEASE

Epidemiology Accounts for more than one third of cases of chronic renal failure. At any time there are about 7000 patients with renal failure of this type in Britain.

Pathophysiology Disturbance of sieving function leads to **proteinuria**, disturbance of regulatory functions leads to **oedema** and **hypertension**, inability to keep red cells in the capillary lumen gives **haematuria** and there is a decline in glomerular filtration rate.

Clinical features These functional abnormalities give a number of different clinical presentations (Table 36.1).

May be complicated by thrombosis (particularly renal veins) and infections (particularly with *Streptococcus pneumoniae*).

May be associated with minimal change disease, membranous glomerulonephritis, focal segmental glomerulonephritis, reactive systemic amyloidosis, diabetes mellitus, some cases of mesangio-capillary (membranoproliferative) glomerulonephritis and some cases of systemic lupus erythematosus.

Table 36.1 Clinical features of nephritic and nephrotic syndrome

Nephritic syndrome	some reduction of urine volume
	mild to moderate proteinuria
	hypertension
	retention of sodium and water
	some expansion of intravascular volume
	haematuria (macroscopic or microscopic)
Nephrotic syndrome	massive protein loss in urine (> 3.5 g/day)
	hypoalbuminaemia
	oedema

Rapidly progressive renal failure (over period of weeks or months and usually not accompanied by hypertension).

Chronic renal failure

Proteinuria

Protein loss greater than 150 mg/day is abnormal and proteinuria of > 1 g/day usually indicates glomerular as well as tubular damage. Loss may be selective (implies clearance of proteins of lower molecular weight such as albumin and transferrin) or non-selective (involves high molecular weight proteins such as IgG and IgM as well). Protein loss of >3.5 g/day exceeds the liver's capacity for protein synthesis and leads to hypo-albuminaemia.

Haematuria

May be gross or detectable only by microscopy. Presence of red cell casts in the urine strongly suggests glomerular disease.

Correlations

There is no correlation either between syndromes and microscopic patterns or between pathological entities and clinical syndromes.

....

MECHANISMS OF GLOMERULAR INJURY

Immunological glomerular injury may occur as a result of:

- deposition of pre-formed immune complexes (about 45% of human glomerulonephritis)
- formation of immune complexes in situ
- activation of alternate pathway of complement
- nephrotoxic antibody binding to glomerular basement membrane (5%).

Non-immune mechanisms may be associated with hyperfiltration.

PRIMARY GLOMERULAR DISORDERS

Morphological classification rests on three criteria:

1. Distribution of abnormal glomeruli.
   If more than 70% of the glomeruli in a given section is involved then the disease is **diffuse** otherwise the disease is **focal**.
2. The distribution of abnormalities in the glomerulus.
   If the whole glomerulus is involved the disease is **global.**
   If only a part of the glomerulus is affected the disease is **segmental**.
3. The nature of the disease.

Cell proliferation Endothelial cells, mesangial cells or inflammatory cells.

Basement membrane appearances Normal, diffuse or focal thickening, splitting or abnormally thin.

Presence or absence of immune complexes or binding of antibody to glomerular structures Identified by EM or immunohistochemistry as being sub-epithelial, sub-endothelial, intramesangial or intrabasement membrane.

Minimal change glomerular disease (MCD, epithelial cell disease)

Epidemiology Commonest cause of nephrotic syndrome in childhood. Most cases before 6 years. More than 75% of cases of nephrotic syndrome under 16 years are due to MCD. Accounts for 15–25% nephrotic syndrome in adults. In children M:F 2:1 but this is abolished at 15 years.

Aetiology Unknown. No immune complexes although non-complement binding complexes can be found in plasma. An association is seen with atopy and Hodgkin's disease and there is some evidence for T cell dysfunction.

Laboratory findings Heavy proteinuria which is highly selective.

Clinical features Dramatic response to steroids.

Morphological features
- cell proliferation – absent
- basement membrane alteration – absent
- immune complex deposition – absent.

Macroscopy   In fatal cases the kidneys are enlarged and have pale cortex very clearly demarcated from the medulla.

Microscopy   Glomeruli appear normal. Tubular epithelium may show increased lipid. Immunohistology: absence of localized immunoglobulins, complement or fibrin.

Electron microscopy   There is fusion or withdrawal of epithelial foot processes.

Natural history and prognosis   Some cases are complicated by focal glomerular sclerosis which in 50% of cases may go on to chronic renal failure.

Membranous glomerulonephritis

Epidemiology   Accounts for 30% cases of nephrotic syndrome in adults. In the West most are idiopathic (70%).

Associations   Neoplasms (approximately 10% cases, strongest with carcinomas of the bronchus and large bowel), heavy metal toxicity (e.g. gold and mercury), penicillamine, persistent hepatitis B infection, quartan malaria, some cases of systemic lupus erythematosus and syphilis (congenital and acquired).

Clinical features   Insidious onset. Presents with nephrotic syndrome or asymptomatic proteinuria (non-selective).

Morphological features
- cell proliferation – absent
- basement membrane alterations – uniform thickening. Spikes of new basement membrane material protrude from epithelial aspect between sub-epithelial immune complexes eventually enclosing the complexes
- immune complex deposition – sub-epithelial.

Microscopy   Diffuse thickening of the capillary basement membrane in the glomerular tuft.

Immunohistology   Granular deposits of IgG (virtually all cases) and C3 (about one-third of cases) along the basement membrane.

Electron microscopy   See Table 36.2.

Natural history and prognosis   Spontaneous remission in 25%. Another 25% continue to show proteinuria over many years without renal impairment. The remainder ultimately develop renal failure.

Table 36.2 Electron microscopy of membranous glomerulonephritis

Stage 1	The earliest event is accumulation of sub-epithelial electron-dense deposits. There is fusion of foot processes. At this stage the light microscopy is normal.
Stage 2	Basement membrane substance increases and protrudes between immune complexes seen as **spikes** by light microscopy on sections stained with methenamine silver.
Stage 3	Spikes of basement membrane fuse to enclose complexes (some of which appear less electron-dense).
Stage 4	Glomeruli are collapsed and fibrosed on light microscopy. Complex densitiy is similar to basement membrane making them difficult to see on EM.

Focal segmental glomerulonephritis

Epidemiology Accounts for 10–20% of cases of nephrotic syndrome in adults and about 10% in children (mostly before 6 years).

Clinical features In most there is no history of preceding illness and presentation is usually with nephrotic syndrome. Proteinuria is usually non-selective. Haematuria is present in 50–75% (usually microscopic).

Morphological features
- cell proliferation – very mild increase in number of mesangial cells
- basement membrane alterations – thickening and wrinkling.
- immune complex deposition – absent.

Microscopy Affects mainly the juxta-medullary glomeruli. Segmental and non-proliferative sclerosis or hyalinization often accompanied by adhesions between glomerular tuft and Bowman's capsule. Eosinophilic hyaline droplets may be seen in glomerulus and large lipid-laden macrophages may be present in mesangium. PAS-positive material may accumulate within the lesions.

Immunohistology Segmental IgM or C3 has been seen but is not thought to be pathogenetic.

Electron microscopy Thickening and wrinkling of the basement membrane with splitting. Fusion of foot processes is characteristic and may be seen in cortical glomeruli which appear otherwise normal.

Natural history and prognosis Hypertension and renal failure tend to occur late (mostly in adults) and ultimate prognosis is poor.

....

PROLIFERATIVE GLOMERULONEPHRITIDES
Anti-glomerular basement membrane disease

Definition There is focal segmental necrotizing glomerulonephritis, circulating anti-basement membrane antibodies and linear deposition of IgG on the glomerular basement membrane.

Epidemiology Accounts for about 5% of cases of glomerulonephritis. Commonest in young adults, especially males. There is a major genetic component with 90% possessing HLA-DR2 antigen.

Clinical features There may be severe and rapid progressive glomerulonephritis with or without pulmonary haemorrhage. Patients present with acute renal failure or rapidly progressive renal failure associated with heavy proteinuria. Haematuria is invariably present at least at the microscopic level.

Laboratory findings Plasma contains IgG antibodies to the globular non-collagen domain of pro-collagen (Goodpasture antigen) which bind to basement membrane of the glomerulus, lung alveolus and choroid of the eye. Fifty per cent have antibodies to tubular basement membrane. Other antibodies may be found including anti-neutrophilic cytoplasmic antibodies (ANCA, 30%).

Morphological features
- cell proliferation – some increase in mesangial cells and in infiltrate of neurophils in affected glomerular segments
- basement membrane alterations – some irregularity and thickening (not a characteristic feature)
- immune complex deposition – linear IgG along basement membrane.

Microscopy Crescents (proliferations of cells partly or totally obliterating the space between the glomerular tuft and Bowman's capsule – thought to be linked to escape of fibrin from damaged glomerulus into Bowman's space) are present and usually extensive. Some glomeruli show focal necrosis of part of the tuft. There may be some increase in mesangial cells.

Immunohistology Linear IgG (less often IgM or IgA) in a non-granular fashion. C3 is also present in 50%.

Natural history and prognosis Patients with glomerular disease often develop rapidly progressive renal failure with dialysis needed in 70% of sufferers and in whom the outlook is bleak.

Goodpasture's syndrome

Definition Nephritic syndrome associated with pulmonary haemorrhage.

Pathogenesis The initiator of the antibody response is unknown, but candidates include a cross-reacting anti-viral antibody, an alteration of the patient's own tissues, or other environmental events that may expose sequestered basement membrane antigen.

Clinical features Haemoptysis of varying severity commonly associated with haematuria (> 90%). Granular casts are seen in the urine in more than 50%.

Macroscopy At autopsy the lungs are bulky, firm and congested due to intra-alveolar haemorrhage.

Microscopy The renal histology is the same as for cases unaccompanied by lung haemorrhage. The lungs show thickening of the alveolar septa with some showing disintegration or rupture.

Immunohistology Linear IgG and complement is also seen along pulmonary basement membranes.

Other causes of crescentic glomerulonephritis

Multi-system diseases SLE, mixed cryoglobulinaemia, Henoch–Schönlein purpura, polyarteritis nodosa, Wegener's granulomatosis, malignant hypertension and the haemolytic uraemic syndrome.

- Post-infectious glomerulonephritis.
- Membrano-proliferative (mesangio-capillary) glomerulonephritis.

Acute diffuse proliferative glomerulonephritis (acute diffuse endocapillary glomerulonephritis, post-infectious glomerulonephritis)

Pathogenesis Glomerular lesions are thought to be initiated by by immune complexes formed in situ in the glomeruli as a result of localized streptococcal antigen on glomerular basement membrane.

Clinical features Renal symptoms appear 10–18 days after infection. This used to be exclusive to group A β-haemolytic streptococcus but may be associated with other bacteria as well as viral and parasitic diseases. Most present with acute nephritic syndrome with oedema of the face, hypertension and decline in urine output.

Laboratory features Urine shows moderate proteinuria, haematuria, neutrophils and a variety of casts. There is usually a decline in plasma C3 and circulating antibodies reacting with several glomerular basement membrane antigens. Immune complexes may be found.

Morphological features
- cellular proliferation – all glomeruli are hypercellular due to proliferation of mesangial cells with neutrophils and monocytes both in the mesangium and capillary lumen. Endothelial cells are swollen
- basement membrane alterations – not thickened
- immune complex deposition – large sub-epithelial deposits with dome shape. Some smaller deposits at other locations may be present.

Macroscopy In the rare cases coming to autopsy the kidneys are slightly enlarged with smooth greyish surface which may show petechial haemorrhages. Swollen glomeruli may be seen as grey dots.

Microscopy There is diffuse involvement of the glomeruli with increased cellularity of the tufts which contain neutrophils. There may be fibrin in Bowman's space, capsular crescents and there is occasional glomerular necrosis.

Immunohistology Granular IgG and C3 (lumpy-bumpy pattern) along basement membrane.

Electron microscopy Large dome shaped sub-epithelial electron-dense depositis (humps) which are often related to

481

fused foot processes. Some deposits may be present in the mesangium and beneath the epithelium (usually smaller and of variable shape).

Natural history and prognosis Good prognosis but up to half show morphological evidence of chronicity. Poor prognostic indicators in biopsies include tubular atrophy, interstitial fibrosis and large confluent electron-dense deposits, particularly if associated with a marked degree of cellular proliferation.

Mesangio-capillary (membrano-proliferative) glomerulonephritis

Definition Proliferation of both mesangial cells and glomerular capillary basement membrane.

Associations SLE, malaria, ventriculo-atrial shunts, persistent hepatitis B infection, chronic renal allograft rejection, some cases of liver cirrhosis associated with α-1-antitrypsin deficiency, infective endocarditis, deficiencies in the complement system and epithelial and lymphoreticular malignancies. In the majority there is no identified cause.

Type I disease

Epidemiology Usually found in the 8–16 age group. Females are more frequently affected.

Clinical features Variable including nephrotic syndrome, nephritic syndrome and recurrent haematuria. Most patients have at least microscopic haematuria and about one in three have hypertension.

Laboratory findings Hypocomplementaemia is characteristic but not universal, with about 50% having reduced C_3 at diagnosis. C_3 nephritic factor (C3nef, an immunoglobulin which stabilizes C3bBb convertase of the alternate pathway of complement activation promoting alternate pathway complement activation) may be present in 30%.

Morphological features
- cellular proliferation – increased mesangial cell numbers and bulk of mesangial matrix. Small numbers of neutrophils may be present

- basement membrane alterations – basement membrane appears thickened on H&E stained sections but split (tramline) when stained with silver stains
- immune complex deposition – electron-dense deposits are seen in the sub-endothelial layer of the mesangium. Sub-epithelial deposits are also seen in 15–20%.

Microscopy Glomeruli are enlarged, hypercellular and tend to be lobulated. There is an increase in mesangial matrix. Mesangial cells are increased in number. The capillary wall is thickened with a tramline appearance on inpregnation with silver.

Immunohistology Irregular granular deposition of C3 in the periphery of the lobules and in the mesangium. C1q and C4 may be found and IgM and IgG may be found on the same distribution but IgA is not found.

Electron microscopy Mesangial cell cytoplasm is interposed between the capillary basement membrane and the endothelial cells. There is loss of epithelial cell-foot processes. Sub-endothelial electron dense deposits are characteristically found.

Natural history and prognosis Chronic renal failure develops in most but this may be delayed. Overall 10-year survival is about 49%.

Type II disease (linear dense-deposit disease)

Epidemiology Equal sex incidence but with a younger age of onset.

Pathogenesis Inappropriate activation of complement plays an important though probably not exclusive role in the pathogenesis.

Clinical features Essentially similar to type I. Some patients show a partial lipodystrophy with absence of sub-cutaneous fat over the trunk.

Microscopy In many cases it is impossible to distinguish type I from type II disease by light microscopy. Crescents are not unusual. In later stages there is tubular atrophy and interstitial fibrosis.

Immunohistology Usually C3 alone in the glomeruli.

Electron microscopy Extremely electron-dense deposits are present within the lamina densa causing marked thickening of the capillary wall. Dense deposits may also be seen around the tubular basement membranes. Epithelial foot processes are fused. There is an increase in mesangial cells and matrix.

Mesangial proliferative glomerulonephritis

Definition An inflammatory disorder of the glomeruli in which there is increase in mesangial cell number and increase in mesangial matrix.

Associations IgA nephropathy, Henoch–Schönlein purpura, infective endocarditis, SLE, some instances of Goodpasture's disease and Alport's syndrome.

IgA nephropathy (Berger's disease, recurrent haematuria syndrome)

Definition Haematuria (gross, mild or microscopic) and deposits of IgA and usually C3 in the mesangium of most glomeruli.

Epidemiology Striking geographical variations with high prevalence in France (accounting for 20% of nephritis), Italy, Japan, Singapore, South Korea and Australia. In Japan IgA nephropathy is present in 40% of renal biopsies for primary glomerular disease compared with 10% in Britain.

Clinical features Patients are commonly children or young adults (only 15% over 40 years) who present with haematuria which may be associated with acute infections (e.g. respiratory tract infections) but may be associated with trauma or periods of vigorous exercise. There may be mild proteinuria, but no hypertension or other stigmata of renal disease.

Microscopy The changes may be subtle. There is localized crowding of nuclei in the glomerular tuft associated with absence of visible capillary lumena. Tuft necrosis may be seen but is not common. The lesion progresses to segmental hyaline scarring. A small number of crescents may be seen but diffuse crescentic disease is rare.

Immunohistology There is IgA in the glomeruli and some IgG and C3 may be seen.

Electron microscopy Mild mesangial cell proliferation is seen. Electron-dense deposits are localized within the mesangium most of which are located in the region related to the capillary wall furthest from the urinary space. Sometimes the deposits extend to sub-endothelial or sub-epithelial locations.

Natural history and prognosis Only 50% of patients are alive with good renal function 20 years after diagnosis.

Thin basement membrane nephropathy with persistent haematuria of renal origin

Epidemiology Can occur sporadically or be inherited with autosomal dominant pattern.

Microscopy Normal.

Electron microscopy Abnormally thin basement membrane (mean 191nm ±28 [normal 350nm ±43]).

CHRONIC GLOMERULONEPHRITIS

Aetiology This is the common destination of many types of renal disease. The proportion of various conditions progressing to end-stage renal disease is shown in Table 36.3.

Macroscopy Size is usually reduced by one-third. The capsules strip with difficulty and the surfaces have a finely granular appearance. The cut surface shows cortical thinning and blurring of the distinction between cortex and medulla. Peri-pelvic adipose tissue is usually increased.

Table 36.3 Proportion of conditions progressing to end-stage renal disease

Diffuse crescentic GN	90%
Membranous GN	50%
Mesangio-capillary GN	50%
Focal glomerulosclerosis	50–80%
IgA nephropathy	30–50%
Acute diffuse endocapillary GN	1–2%

Microscopy Many glomeruli show partial or complete obliteration of the capillary tuft and mesangium by acellular connective tissue which stains positive with PAS. Concentric fibrosis around Bowman's capsule of affected glomeruli (periglomerular fibrosis) may be seen. The remainder of the nephron undergoes ischaemic atrophy. In those nephrons where the glomeruli are unaffected there is tubular hypertrophy. There is an increase in interstitial connective tissue and a moderate interstitial lymphocytic infiltrate can be seen in some cases. Changes associated with hypertension can be seen in the renal vasculature.

Chronic renal failure

Pathophysiology There is a decreased ability to excrete nitrogenous waste (e.g. urea and creatinine), changes in the regulation of water and electrolytes, changes in acid–base regulation leading to metabolic acidosis, changes in the renal handling of calcium and phosphate and changes in the production of renal hormones (erythropoietin, renin and prostaglandins).

The first stages on the path to chronic renal failure are shown in Table 36.4.

Table 36.4 The path to chronic renal failure

Stages	Abnormalities
Diminished renal reserve	
Renal insufficiency	Some retention of nitrogenous waste products. Impaired concentration of urine. Some degree of normochromic normocytic anaemia may be present
Renal failure	Increasingly severe anaemia, increased phosphate and decreased calcium, metabolic acidosis, fixed urinary specific gravity
Uraemia	Additional abnormalities involving the cardiovascular, gastrointestinal, nervous and locomotor systems and the skin

TUBULOINTERSTITIAL DISEASE

Definition Disease localized to the renal interstitial tissues and tubules usually associated with interstitial oedema, scarring and inflammatory infiltrate with atrophy or necrosis of some tubules.

Aetiology In 30% of patients with acute and a smaller percentage of those with chronic tubulointerstitial disease no cause is found but known causes include infection, drugs, immune reactions, urinary tract obstruction, renal papillary necrosis, heavy metal poisoning, acute toxic injury, metabolic disorders (hereditary and acquired), hereditary tubular disorders, neoplasms and glomerular disorders.

Clinical features In the acute form there is sudden onset (commonest types are acute bacterial pyelonephritis and acute hypersensitivity caused by drugs) but in the chronic form (commonest types are chronic pyelonephritis, analgesic nephropathy, chronic potassium deficiency and ischaemia) there may be no symptoms until late in the natural history, when patients present with chronic renal failure.

Microscopy The acute form is characterized by interstitial oedema and an inflammatory infiltrate dominated by lymphocytes, plasma cells and macrophages but usually accompanied by neutrophils and eosinophils. The chronic form is characterized by interstitial fibrosis, tubule atrophy and an interstitial lymphocyte/macrophage infiltrate.

Functional effects The medulla is the chief physiological target, resulting in inability to concentrate urine (causing polyuria and nocturia) which is termed **nephrogenic diabetes insipidus** if severe. There is reduced ability to secrete hydrogen ions leading to a **metabolic acidosis** and a decrease in tubular resorption of sodium and other solutes (salt losing nephropathy) resulting in hypotension and vascular collapse. In acute diffuse tubulo-interstitial disease the pathophysiological picture is dominated by reduction in glomerular filtration rate causing oliguria, proteinuria, haematuria and hypertension. The general pattern of tubular dysfunction is modified, depending on the principal target of the damaging agent.

Proximal tubule damage

Leading to proximal tubular acidosis (loss of bicarbonate leading to acidaemia, reduction in extracellular volume and consequent stimulation to aldosterone production leading to potassium loss and hypokalaemia).

- heavy metal poisoning
- multiple myeloma
- paroxysmal nocturnal haemoglobinuria.

Distal tubule damage

Leading to distal tubular acidosis (defect in hydrogen ion secretion so urine cannot be maximally acidified, associated with salt wasting, hyperkalaemia and decreased ability to concentrate urine).

- methicillin nephritis
- hypercalcaemia
- chronic urine outflow obstruction
- renal transplantation
- granulomatous inflammation
- Balkan nephropathy.

Medullary damage

Leading to inability to concentrate urine.

- analgesic nephropathy
- acute pyelonephritis
- sickle cell disease
- hyperuricaemia
- hyperoxalaemia
- polycystic disease of the kidney
- sarcoidosis.

Chemical injury and tubulointerstitial disease

Pathogenesis   Kidney is susceptible to chemical injury due the large blood supply to the metabolically active cortex, concentration of certain chemicals and precipitation of certain compounds at acid pH in the distal tubules. Pathways include direct effects, hypersensitivity and a cumulative effect of recurrent mild injury.

ACUTE TUBULOINTERSTITIAL DISEASE

Acute drug-induced hypersensitivity: interstitial nephritis

Aetiology   Methicillin, ampicillin, rifampicin, cephaloxin, allopurinol, phenytoin, non-steroidal anti-inflammatory drugs and possibly frusemide and thaizide diuretics.

Pathogenesis   Possible mechanisms include development of anti-tubular basement membrane antibodies, a cell-mediated immune response or an IgE mediated reaction.

Clinical features   Mostly acute renal failure with or without oliguria with an acute decline accompanied by fever, maculo-papular skin rash, high blood eosinophil count and arthralgia.

Microscopy   Glomeruli appear normal. There may be a florid interstitial infiltrate of lymphocytes, plasma cells, eosinophils and less frequently neutrophils. There is focal epithelial necrosis and hyaline droplet change in the distal tubules. Multi-nucleate epithelial cells are sometimes seen. On EM fusion of epithelial foot processes may be seen in some (10–20%) glomeruli.

Acute pyelonephritis

Epidemiology   Women are more susceptible to urinary tract infections than men (M:F 1:20).

Aetiology   Infection may reach the kidney via the bloodstream or by ascent from the lower urinary tract. In ascending infections the bacteria must gain entry to, survive, and multipy in the successive compartments of the urinary tract. Most infections are auto-infections by normal faecal flora (commonest *Escherichia coli, Staphylococcus albus, Proteus* or *Klebsiella* species; *Enterobacter* and *Klebsiella* are commonest in neonates; *Staphylococcus* commonest in adolescent girls). Firm adhesion (via **adhesin** which recognizes a carbohydrate receptor on the epithelial cell) of pathogenic *E. coli* species to the epithelium is of particular importance in their pathogenicity.

Pathogenesis   Entry of bacteria may be associated with instrumentation, but there is usually no initiating event. In females infection is facilitated by the short urethra. Males have protection from antibacterial action of prostatic secretions. Survival and multiplication of organisms in the bladder is favoured by increased residual urine, pregnancy (associated with decreased detrusor muscle tone) and diabetes mellitus. Entry of bacteria into the ureter is facilitated by vesico-ureteric reflux and entry into the renal parenchyma from the calyces may be associated with the presence of concave (compound) papillae at the poles of the kidney. Multiplication of organisms in the medulla is facilitated by the relatively poor blood supply and the high ammonia concentrations (interferes with the activation of the classical pathway of complement activation by interfering with activation of C4).

Clinical features Commonest complaint is sudden onset lumbar pain and tenderness, fever, rigor and malaise.

Laboratory findings Organisms are cultured from the urine. If greater than 10^5/ml then there is almost certainly a urinary tract infection but when the bacterial count is less than this only one-third will have such an infection and in two-thirds this will be a contaminant.

Macroscopy The kidney is slightly enlarged and reddened. There may be small abscesses on the sub-capsular surface. Cut surface shows streaks of pus in the medullary rays. In blood-borne infections there are multiple parenchymal abscesses.

Microscopy Interstitial oedema and florid intratubular and interstitial inflammatory cell infiltrate associated with necrosis of some tubular epithelium and in some cases the tips of the papillae.

....

CHRONIC TUBULOINTERSTITIAL DISEASE
Chronic pyelonephritis

Definition A chronic disorder characterized by coarse asymmetric scarring affecting the renal pelvis, tubules and interstitium.

Epidemiology Common, accounts for 15% of adults and 25% of children requiring dialysis or renal transplantation.

Aetiology It is not clear whether infection is necessary for the development of chronic pyelonephritis. Urinary outflow obstruction is associated with the condition in some instances but vesico-ureteric reflux is probably the most important factor.

Macroscopy If there has been obstruction with high intra-calyceal pressure and infection there is dilation of the renal pelvis and many or all of the calyces may be deformed and dilated. Frequently both kidneys are involved but this is often asymmetrical. Coarse flat scars alternate with normal parenchyma and the scars are related to a dilated calyx with a deformed pyramid. In vesico-ureteric reflux the scars are usually polar in distribution.

Microscopy Interstitial tissue is increased and scarred with a patchy infiltrate of lymphocytes and plasma cells. The tubules are either collapsed or atrophic with thickened basement membrane (commonest appearance) or greatly distended and lined by flattened epithelium (thyroidiza-tion). The glomeruli in some areas appear normal while in other areas there is periglomerular concentric fibrosis. A complication of chronic pyelonephritis is the development of focal segment glomerulosclerosis once extensive damage has occurred. The medulla and pyramids show scarring with atrophic collecting tubules. In cases with obstruction there may be squamous metaplasia of the transitional epithelium. Blood vessel changes are frequent but inconsistent; in some instances arcuate and interlobular arteries show intimal thickening.

Xanthogranulomatous pyelonephritis

Aetiology A variant of chronic pyelonephritis. Most common in cases associated with obstruction which in most instances is associated with renal stones.

Macroscopy Usually unilateral. Kidney has yellow areas on cut surface.

Microscopy Many lipid-laden macrophages are present in the interstitial tissue and may extend into perirenal fat.

RENAL PAPILLARY NECROSIS
Chronic analgesic abuse

Epidemiology Peak incidence in 5th decade, M:F 1:4.

Aetiology Strongest association with mixtures containing phenacetin. Other drugs that can cause papillary necrosis include aspirin and acetaminophen (particularly in daily users). Large cumulative doses are required to induce papillary disease (minimal requirement 1–3 kg over a period of three years).

Pathogenesis Not clear but thought to be related to the presence of reactive intermediate products from the co-oxidation of acetaminophen (metabolite of phenacetin) with arachadonic acid by cyclo-oxygenase and hydroperoxidase which cause damage to tubular epithelial cells.

Laboratory findings Defects related to urinary concentration, acidification and sodium conservation leading to metabolic acidodis and volume depletion.

Macroscopy Bilateral and equal contraction of kidneys (weight 45–65 g). Scars are present on the sub-capsular surface related to necrotic papillae. The papillae range from normal to focal necrosis of the tip, shrinkage associated with brown discolouration or if severe complete detachment of necrotic papillae.

Microscopy The earliest lesion is in the loops of Henle, at the tips of the papillae where necrotic epithelial cells are seen. Necrosis of the loops becomes more pronounced and extensive. Necrosis of renal papillae is not associated with any accompanying inflammatory reaction between viable kidney and necrotic papillae. In the late stages a clear demarcation zone between viable and non-viable tissue develops and dystrophic calcification may appear. With sloughing the calyx edge becomes ragged and tissue proximally is scarred and shows an interstitial chronic inflammatory response.

Renal papillary necrosis associated with acute urinary infections and diabetes mellitus

Macroscopy Markedly inflamed pelvices may be filled with purulent debris. Abscesses may be present in both medulla and cortex with some or all of the papillae necrotic.

Microscopy   There is a brisk, acute inflammatory infiltrate in the demarcation zone.

Acute renal papillary necrosis in infancy

Epidemiology   Rare.

Aetiology   Associated with shock due to severe dehydration following gastroenteritis.

Sickle cell disease-associated renal papillary necrosis

Epidemiology   Not uncommon complication of sickle cell disease.

Pathogenesis   The renal medulla is thought to favour red-cell sickling, resulting in increased blood viscosity, increased risk of microthrombus in the vasa recta and ischaemic damage to the papillae.

ACUTE RENAL FAILURE

Definition   Loosely defined as a syndrome characterized by significant decline in renal function over hours or days. There is a functional component and recovery is possible.

Pre-renal aetiology

- pump failure (e.g. cardiogenic shock following myocardial infarction)
- decreased circulatory volume (blood loss, plasma loss or loss of salt and water)
- microvascular dilatation and damage (e.g. septicaemic shock).

Anuria/oliguria is characteristic. Urine shows low sodium (< 20 mmol/l) high osmolality (urine:plasma osmolality > 1.5:1) and high urea and creatinine concentrations (urine:plasma urea concentration > 10:1).

Renal aetiology

Acute tubular necrosis.

1. Ischaemia (similar causes to those of pre-renal disease as well as associated with crush trauma to soft tissues).
2. Toxic damage to renal tubules (e.g. with heavy metal poisoning, organic solvent poisoning, antibiotic-mediated damage, snake venoms and tubular deposition of Bence-Jones proteins.

Most commonly occurs against a background of established disease or following surgery or obstetric disorders.

Pathogenesis Mechanisms additional to ischaemia have been suggested, including prolonged vasoconstriction of intrarenal afferent arterioles, leakage of tubular fluid across tubular basement membrane, tubular obstruction by casts and secondary changes in glomerular flow.

Laboratory findings Not associated with anuria, but may be associated with polyuria. Urine sodium is high and urine osmolality approaches that of plasma due to impaired concentration. Granular and cellular casts are numerous and epithelial cells may be seen.

Macroscopy Kidneys are enlarged and swollen. The cut surface bulges slightly and there is cortical pallor.

Microscopy Most changes are seen in the distal convoluted tubule. Necrotic epithelial cells tend to separate from the basement membrane which appears bare. Rarely (about 5%) there are breaks in the tubular basement membrane (tubulorrhexis). Casts can be seen in affected distal tubules. The presence of regeneration suggests tubular epithelial necrosis. Secondary effects are seen in the glomeruli (swelling of the epithelial cells of Bowman's capsule and hyperplastic juxta-glomerular apparatus) and the interstitium (oedema and mixed inflammatory infiltrate). In cases caused by drugs and poisons the necrosis of epithelial cells is more obvious and widespread.

• damage to blood vessels (persisting vaso-constriction, renal artery occlusion, microvascular diseases such as thrombotic/thrombocytopenic purpura, malignant hypertension and bilateral cortical necrosis associated with separation of the placenta

- damage to glomeruli (especially crescentic glomerulonephritis)
- interstitial damage (acute interstitial nephritis of various types)
- tubular lumen damage (crystal deposition e.g. oxalates, sulphonamides).

Reversal of the under-perfused state does not rapidly improve function (as it does in pre-renal renal failure).

Post-renal aetiology

Acute outflow obstruction.

SYSTEMIC HYPERTENSION

Definition The WHO suggests that hypertension is present when systolic pressure exceeds 160 mmHG or diastolic pressure exceeds 95 mmHg and borderline hypertension is present with pressures of 140–160 mmHg systolic or 90–95 mmHg diastolic.

Epidemiology Using the higher level, about 18% of the adult population would be regarded as hypertensive, rising to 25% if the borderline levels are used as the diagnostic cut-off.

Classification
- essential (95%) – initially there may be increased cardiac output but the elevation in blood pressure is sustained by increased tone in the resistance vessels of the arterial tree (small arteries and arterioles)
- secondary (5%) – associated with chronic renal parenchymal or vascular disease, an aldosterone secreting adrenal tumour, a phaeochromocytoma, acromegaly, thyrotoxicosis, hyperparathyroidism, renin-secreting tumour, pre-eclampsia/eclampsia or excessive alcohol intake.

Essential hypertension

Aetiology There is an association between hypertension and high dietary sodium intake, but a genetic effect is involved in variations in susceptibility to high-salt diets.

Increased tone may also be the result of abnormalities of sodium and potassium transport across cell membranes of vascular smooth muscle or an increase in vasoconstrictor signals (e.g. mediated by sympathetic nervous system). Vasoconstriction could also be the result of release of compounds synthesized within the wall (e.g. endothelins) or a decrease in the synthesis and release of nitric oxide.

Non-renal pathological effects (Table 36.5)

Renal effects (nephrosclerosis)

Macroscopy May be normal or reduced in size. Sub-capsular surface is finely granular because of small scars related to ischaemia due to small vessel disease. Cut surface shows reduced parenchymal mass and apparently increased hilar adipose tissue.

Microscopy There is arteriolar hyalinization together with ischaemic changes in the glomeruli consisting of collapse and shrinkage of the capillary tuft, obliteration of glomerular capillary lumen and laying down of collagen fibres on the inner aspect of Bowman's capsule. Ultimately there is complete glomerular sclerosis. The tubules related to these glomeruli become atrophic and eventually disappear. Tubules related to intact nephrons hypertrophy.

Natural history and prognosis Classified into **benign** and **malignant** types on the basis of natural history. Benign

Table 36.5 Non-renal pathological effects of systemic hypertension

Heart	• concentric left ventricular hypertrophy
	• decreased diastolic compliance of left ventricle
	• greater thickness of left ventricle wall leading to decreased perfusion of sub-endocardial region of the myocardium
Arteries	• increased atherogenesis and increased risk of coronary heart disease
	• decreased arterial compliance
	• increased shearing stresses leading to risk of aortic dissection
	• microaneurysm formation in small penetrating vessel within the brain (Charcot–Bouchard aneurysms).
Arterioles	• hyaline arteriosclerosis
	• fibrinoid necrosis in patients with malignant hypertension

hypertension is associated with a long clinical course while the malignant form is characterized by rapidly rising blood pressure (accounts for 5% of patients with hypertension, more common in the young, in males and in blacks).

Malignant hypertension

Clinical features   Patients with malignant hypertension have very high diastolic pressure (> 130 mmHg). Patients with malignant hypertension present with headache, nausea and vomiting, visual disturbances and rarely hypertensive encephalopathy (fits and disturbance of consciousness).

Macroscopy   Kidney size depends on the duration of hypertension. If malignant hypertension has supervened on long-standing benign disease, the changes are similar to those of the benign variant. If accelerated hypertension has been present from the start the kidneys will be of normal size, unscarred and show focal petechial haemorrhages.

Microscopy   The archetypal change is **fibrinoid necrosis**. On light microscopy this is seen as a smudgy, intensely eosinophilic change in the vessel wall. This has been shown to be due to fibrin and other plasma proteins and is associated with necrosis of arteriolar smooth muscle cells. If this change affects the afferent arteriole there may be extension into the glomerular capillaries which might additionally become thrombosed. In small arteries (e.g. interlobular arteries) in the kidney proliferative endarteritis (thickening of the intima due to concentric layers of smooth muscle with intervening collagen) occurs.

Natural history and prognosis   Renal failure is the commonest cause of death (90%).

Unilateral renal artery stenosis

Aetiology   May be due to an atherosclerotic plaque (accounts for 70%) or there may be fibromuscular dysplasia of the renal artery (fibromuscular thickening of the vessel wall at any layer but most commonly the media).

Pathogenesis   There is decreased renal blood flow and decreased glomerular filtration rate. There is increased secretion of renin and therefore increased plasma levels of angiotensin II which causes increased peripheral resistance and increased output of aldosterone resulting in increased resorption of sodium in the distal tubules and increased plasma volume.

GLOMERULAR DISEASE ASSOCIATED WITH SYSTEMIC DISEASE

SYSTEMIC LUPUS ERYTHEMATOSUS (SLE)

Definition Autoimmune disease leading to the formation of circulating immune complexes which may be deposited at a number of sites triggering an inflammatory and tissue damaging response.

Aetiology Prevalence in USA is about 0.02%, M:F 1:9 rising to 1:15 in childbearing age. Commoner in blacks.

Pathogenesis The chief sites of complex deposition are in the small vessels (causing vasculitis), glomeruli (causing glomerulonephritis, present in 40% at diagnosis and up to 75% during the course of the disease), synovium (causing arthritis, particularly of the small joints of the fingers, the wrist and the knee), skin (characteristic eruption over 'butterfly' area of the face, pain and tenderness, splinter haemorrhages in nails and patchy baldness; present in 20–50%), brain (eventually occurring in 20%), lung and pleura (with pleuritic pain in 40–60% and effusions interstitial fibrosis, interstitial pneumonitis and pulmonary vasculitis in 20–30%) and heart (causing pericarditis and Libman–Sacks endocarditis).

Laboratory findings Urine shows proteinuria (50%) and microscopic haematuria. A wide range of auto-antibodies can be found (Table 36.6).

Microscopy
In 1982, the World Health Organization published a classification specifying six classes of glomerular change associated with SLE, some of which can be seen in combination in single biopsies (Table 36.7).

Table 36.6 Antibodies seen in SLE

Antigen	Function
Nuclear antigens	
Double-stranded DNA	Present in > 60%. Highly specific for SLE
Single-stranded DNA	Not specific but useful measure of disease activity
Histones	Present in both spontaneous and drug-induced SLE
Smith (Sm) antigen	An extractable nuclear antigen. Present in 30% black and Chinese SLA patients but 7% whites
Ribonucleoprotein (RNP)	Present in 25% SLE patients, associated with Raynaud's phenomenon
Ro (another ribonucleoprotein)	Positive in 24% SLE patients. Presence in pregnant SLE patients; is associated with congenital heart block in offspring
Phospholipid	
Cardiolipin	Positive in 30–40%. Antibody known as lupus anticoagulant. Not specific for SLE and not actually an anticoagulant. Thrombosis is the major problem and there is a high risk of recurrent abortion. Gives false positive VDRL test for syphilis
Immunoglobulins	
Altered IgG	Antibodies known as rheumatoid factors. Common in SLE
Blood cells	
Lymphocytes and neutrophils	Cytotoxic antibodies found in almost 50% of SLE patients

Table 36.7 WHO classification of SLE

Class	Disorder	Frequency in patients with SLE	Pathological features
I	Minor abnormalities	16	Normal on light microscopy, complexes seen with EM or immunohistology
II	Mesangial changes	16	Increased number of mesangial cells and mesangial matrix affecting most glomeruli. Usually correlates with mild clinical disease and periods of remission
III	Focal segmental glomerulonephritis	20	Segmental distribution of mesangial cell proliferation associated with capillary thrombosis or scarring. Often seen in association with class II lesions
IV	Diffuse proliferative glomerulonephritis	40	• Mesangial proliferative glomerulonephritis – mesangial cell proliferation associated with scarring. Some segments of the glomerular capillary wall are thickened (due to immune complexes) and eosinophilic ('wire looping'). In necrotic areas nuclear debris can be seen (haematoxyphil bodies) • Diffuse endocapillary proliferative glomerulonephritis – resembles post-streptococcal glomerulonephritis but there may be wire-loops, focal necrosis and intracapillary thrombi to suggest SLE • Diffuse mesangiocapillary glomerulonephritis • Diffuse crescentic glomerulonephritis
V	Diffuse membranous glomerulonephritis	10	May occur in pure form (indistinguishable from primary type) or in combination with lesions of other classes
VI	Sclerosing glomerulonephritis	–	As renal disease progresses glomeruli become scarred and many may be replaced by fibrous tissue

Natural history and prognosis

Renal failure is the cause of death in about 20%. The 5-year survival depends on the class of lesion present, being 100% for class II, 73% for class III, 60% for class IV and 90% for class V.

....

SYSTEMIC SCLEROSIS

Definition   Disease characterized by excessive collagen deposits affecting many organs and a marked thickening of the intima of small and medium sized arteries which eventually leads to obliteration of the lumen.

Epidemiology   More common in females than males. Peak incidence 20–50 years.

Clinical features   Presents with localized skin disease (acrosclerosis/scleroderma) which may be part of the CREST syndrome (**C**alcinosis, **R**aynaud's phenomenon, o**E**sophageal dysfunction, **S**clerodactyly and **T**elangiectasia) or as diffuse or progressive systemic sclerosis which shows extensive skin involvement with early visceral involvement including kidneys, heart, lungs, gut and musculoskeletal system.

Aetiology   There is a genetic factor involved in progressive type with association of HLA-DR5 and DRw8.

Clinical features   Presents with Raynaud's phenomenon in majority followed by thickening of the skin. There may be weakness and difficulty swallowing, cough and dyspnoea (if lung involvement), myocardial fibrosis causing dysrhythmias and conduction defects. Renal involvement is the manifestation most likely to be fatal. About 50% of patients have high blood pressure (25% with malignant hypertension) with associated renal and cardiac failure and fits (hypertensive encephalopathy). Chronic renal failure develops in about 25% patients with renal involvement.

Macroscopy of kidneys   There may be many small infarcts.

Microscopy of kidneys   Interlobular arteries show marked intimal thickening with the cells of the neo-intima arranged in concentric layers. There is reduplication of the internal elastic lamina. In patients with malignant hypertension the afferent arterioles may show fibrinoid necrosis and the glomeruli show ischaemic changes. In patients with rapidly progressive course there are frequently thrombi in the small arteries and arterioles.

Laboratory findings Anti-nuclear antibodies are found with two being only found in systemic sclerosis.

- anti-DNA topoisomerase 1 (scl-70) – present in 40% patients with progressive systemic sclerosis
- antibody reacting with centromeres – present in 50–70% of patients with CREST syndrome. There may also be hypergammaglobulinaemia (50%), rheumatoid factors (25%) and increased plasma concentration of complement fragments C3d and C4d (50%).

OTHER RENAL VASCULAR DISORDERS

RENAL INFARCTION

Aetiology Mostly due to emboli in renal artery or branches. Thrombo-emboli arise from the left atrium (e.g. in atrial fibrillation), the left ventricle (e.g. following myocardial infarction) or from damaged valves. Occasional emboli are derived from atheromatous plaques.

Clinical features Unless large most are asymptomatic. If large there is sudden onset of loin pain followed by haematuria and proteinuria. If both renal arteries are occluded there is acute renal failure.

Macroscopy Most measure 1–3 cm along longest axis and are wedge-shaped with the base on the sub-capsular surface. In the first few hours the infarct is red, firm and swollen, but becomes yellowish-grey later with a narrow red zone at the interface between infarcted and viable tissue. By 7–10 days the infarct is depressed below the surrounding surface and over months develops into a V-shaped scar. If the embolus causing the infarct is infected then the centre of the infarct breaks down and an abscess forms.

Microscopy The sequence of changes is:
- red cells become sludged and lose haemoglobin
- tubular epithelial cell nuclei condense
- neutrophils accumulate

- tubular epithelial and mesangial cell nuclei lyse but basement membranes remain intact
- fibrous tissue replaces infarcted area.

Renal cortical necrosis

Aetiology Widespread spasm of vessels due to haemorrhage (most often associated with abortion, placental abruption or placenta praevia, 50% bilateral cases of cortical necrosis) septicaemia with endotoxin shock (30–40%) or severe dehydrating illness.

Clinical features Usually bilateral and therefore causes acute renal failure with profound oliguria.

Macroscopy Somewhat enlarged kidneys with pallor and yellow colouration of the whole cortex with the exception of a rim just below the capsule and the juxta-medullary areas.

Microscopy Coagulative necrosis and thrombi in small vessels. In some cases islands of nephrons may survive.

Renal vein thrombosis

Epidemiology About 50% of cases occur in infants and neonates.

Aetiology May be associated with severe dehydrating illness in young children. In older children and adults it may develop as a consequence of the nephrotic syndrome.

Clinical features Affected children present with acute loin swelling, haematuria, non- or poorly functioning kidney.

Macroscopy Correlates to size and number of veins occluded. If main renal vein is blocked the kidney is swollen and congested.

Microscopy Haemorrhagic necrosis.

Natural history and prognosis Mortality rate of 60%. Survivors may develop hypertension, nephrotic syndrome or tubular dysfunction.

Haemolytic uraemic syndrome

Epidemiology More common in infancy than adulthood. Commonest cause of acute renal failure in children. May be sporadic, endemic or epidemic and in 3% it is familial.

Childhood form

Aetiology May be associated with infection by *E. coli* species which produce the exotoxin verotoxin.

Clinical features In the acute form it presents usually after gastrointestinal or respiratory tract infection with severe oliguric renal failure, bleeding (usually gastrointestinal), haematuria, a haemolytic anaemia, thrombocytopenia and hypertension.

Microscopy There is patchy ischaemic necrosis which in fatal cases can amount to cortical necrosis. Small vessels show fibrin and red cells within the walls of interlobular arteries, arterioles and glomerular capillaries, associated with thrombosis. There is mucoid intimal thickening and sub-endothelial and mesangial accumulation of electron-lucent material in the glomeruli.

Adult form

Aetiology Less often associated with infections, more commonly seen in pregnancy complicated by haemorrhage, in the post-partum period following normal pregnancy and delivery and with the use of contraceptive compounds.

Natural history and prognosis Worse for adults than for children.

....

THROMBOTIC THROMBOCYTOPENIC PURPURA

Epidemiology Uncommon. M:F 2:3. Peak incidence in 4th decade. Other sites involved: Apart from the kidney, the brain, abdominal viscera and heart may be involved.

Aetiology Unknown, but there may be an abnormal chemical in the plasma or a chemical species missing from the plasma which would explain the response to exchange plasmaphoresis. Candidates include abnormal circulating von Willebrand factor, relative deficiency of prostaglandin 1–2 (prostacyclin), or a relative deficiency of platelet activating factor.

Clinical features Classically there is microangiopathic haemolyic anaemia, thrombocytopenia, neurological symptoms (predominant in 92% of cases, including headache, confusion, stupor, coma, hemiparesis, cranial nerve palsies and fits), fever and renal dysfunction although not all are present in every case.

Microscopy Platelet-rich thrombi in arterioles and capillaries. Sub-endothelial deposits are seen in arterioles and capillaries and micro-aneurysms may be seen.

RENAL STONES

Epidemiology Third most common renal disease in industrialized countries. In developing countries they are comparatively rare. Approximately 12% males and 5% females will have an attack of stone-related ureteric colic by age 70.

Biochemistry Composed of mucoprotein (3–5%) and aggregated crystal material derived from precipitated urine solutes. The commonest is calcium oxalate/mixed calcium oxalate/phosphate (75%) followed by magnesium ammonium phosphate (approximately 15%), urate (6–7%), cystine (3–4%) and rarely other types.

Calcium oxalate and mixed calcium oxalate/phosphate stones

Epidemiology M:F 4:1.

Biochemistry Urine is supersaturated with calcium oxalate and so increases in calcium or oxalate in the urine may cause stone formation. Factors include hypercalciuria (present in 70% with these stones), hyperoxaluria (5%) or a decrease in volume resulting in increased solute concentration.

Aetiology In 25% no predisposing factor is found. Hypercalciuria may be associated with hypercalcaemia as in primary hyperparathyroidism, neoplasia-associated hypercalcaemia, sarcoidosis, excessive calcium intake and the milk-alkali syndrome or prolonged immobilization or without hypercalcaemia as in idiopathic hypercalciuria, medullary sponge kidney, renal tubular acidosis (type 1), cadmium poisoning and possibly diets high in protein.

Hyperoxaluria is seen as a primary, inherited disorder or associated with intestinal disease causing failure of resorption of bile acids or in excessive oxalate intake from foods (rhubarb, spinach, strawberries, beetroot, tea, cocoa, peanuts and orange, lemon or grapefruit juice.

Clinical features Ureteric colic when stone passes down ureter.

Macroscopy Yellowish-brown colour. Oxalate predominant stones are nodular with spikes on surface (mulberry stone) but with more phosphate the surface is smooth.

Complications Related to outflow obstruction such as pyelonephritis (acute or chronic) and hydronephrosis.

Magnesium ammonium phosphate (struvite) stones

Epidemiology Accounts for 15% renal stones. M:F 1:2.

Biochemistry Matrix of normal mucoproteins and a carbohydrate-rich glycocalyx secreted by urease-producing bacteria.

Pathogenesis Urease from bacteria (notably *Proteus* species) splits urea to make urine alkaline leading to supersaturation of urine by the stone constituents.

Macroscopy Whitish-grey colour and often have irregular shape filling the calyceal system (stag-horn calculus).

Natural history and prognosis Infection and outflow obstruction may lead to abscess formation and pyonephrolithiasis (pus, stones in kidney). If not removed there is a substantial chance of loss of most or all function in that kidney and 60% patients dying in 15 years. Failure to remove bilateral stones results in death in 50% by 5 years.

Uric acid stones

Epidemiology Account for 5% renal calculi in UK. About 10% patients with gout develop ureteric colic. Geographical variations occur and may be explained by climactic features. M:F 9:1.

Aetiology A minority have true gout (25%). Increased purine breakdown such as seen following treatment of myeloproliferative disorders may raise uric acid levels and high levels are seen in inherited metabolic disorders such as deficiency of enzyme hypoxanthine-guanine phosphoribosyl transferase, increased acivity of 5-phosphoribosyl pyrophosphate and von Gierke-type glycogen storage disease (glucose-6-phosphatase deficiency).

Pathogenesis   Related to increased urinary uric acid, low urine pH and low urinary volumes.

Macroscopy   Hard yellowish-brown stones with smooth outer surface. May be large (> 2 cm). Frequently multiple.

Cystine stones

Epidemiology   Account for 3% of all stones. Occur in patients with primary cystinuria (autosomal recessive disorder with failure to resorb cystine, lysine, ornithine and arginine from filtrate in proximal tubule).

Macroscopy   Stones are yellowish-white and waxy. Usually multiple, small and round. May form stag-horn calculi.

TUMOURS OF THE KIDNEY

....

BENIGN NEOPLASMS
Cortical adenoma

Epidemiology   Commonest benign tumour of kidney.

Macroscopy   Usually small (< 2 cm diameter). Discrete yellow-grey nodules.

Microscopy   Uniform cuboidal epithelial cells, many containing abundant glycogen. A number of architectural patterns may be seen including papillary, solid alveolar, tubular or glandular. Distinction from well-differentiated adenocarcinoma may not be easy but by convention those less than 3 cm are classified as adenoma and those greater than 3 cm as carcinoma.

Natural history and prognosis   They do not behave in an aggressive fashion.

ANGIOMYOLIPOMA

Definition

May be best considered as a hamartoma.

Epidemiology Present in adult life. About 40% are associated with tuberous sclerosis (autosomal dominant inherited disorder with lesions in cerebral cortex causing epilepsy and mental retardation, adenoma sebaceum in skin and other visceral lesions including rhabdomyoma of the heart and pancreatic cysts).

Clinical features May be painful if there is intralesional haemorrhage.

MALIGNANT NEOPLASMS

Renal cell carcinomas (adenocarcinoma, hypernephroma)

Epidemiology Account for 1–3% of all visceral malignancies and 90% of all primary malignant renal tumours in adult life. Disease of middle/later life with peak in 6th and 7th decades. M:F 3:1.

Aetiology Increased risk in smokers and patients with von Hippel–Lindau syndrome (incidence of 28% in patients with this condition). There is an increased incidence in acquired cystic disease associated with dialysis for renal failure who have a 50-fold increase in risk for developing renal adenocarcinoma and in whom 10–20% have microscopic adenomas at 3 years and another 3% have carcinoma at 5 years. There is a geographic variation with an incidence of 12.2/100 000 per annum in Iceland, 3.5/100 000 per annum in the United Kingdom and less than 3/100 000 per annum in Africa, South America, Spain and Asia.

Genetics Associated with translocations t(3,8) and t(3,11) with the breakpoint at the proximal end of the short arm of chromosome 3 (3p). The loss of one allele from 3p occurs in 96% of sporadic renal cell carcinomas.

Clinical features The classic presentation is with flank pain, a mass in the loin and haematuria. Radiological evidence of metastases is present in 25% at diagnosis. There may be associated systemic symptoms including fever, hypercalcaemia (related to parathyroid hormone-related peptide production), erythrocytosis (4%, associated with increased erythropoietin), amyloidosis (3%, due to SAA production in liver), hypertension (increased renin), galact- orrhoea (ectopic prolactin) and gynaecomastia.

Macroscopy Occur in any part but commonly arise at poles with slight predilection for upper pole. Roughly spherical, 3–15 cm diameter with heterogenous cut surface of yellow areas intemixed with areas of haemorrhage and necrosis. There may be bulging and eventual ulceration into the calyceal system. There is a marked tendency to invasion of the renal vein and occasionally a solid cord of tumour can be seen extending along the renal vein and up the vena cava.

Microscopy Different architectural patterns can be seen with cells arranged in tubular, solid alveolar or papillary patterns. A combination of these can be seen in individual tumours. The commonest cell type is polygonal with a clear cytoplasm (glycogen and lipid). About 14% are composed of spindle shaped cells and in 12% the cells have granular cytoplasm. Atypia and mitotic activity is variable (Table 36.8).

Table 36.8 Microscopic variants of renal cell carcinoma

Papillary renal cell carcinoma	Sarcomatoid renal cell carcinoma
Macroscopy Often more necrosis than typical renal carcinoma	*Microscopy* Largely composed of malignant spindle cells with many mitoses
Microscopy The pattern is clearly papillary with vascularized central stalks covered by tubular epithelium. The stalks contain lipid-laden macrophages	*Epidemiology* About 2% of renal carcinomas
Genetics Not associated with abnormalities of the short arm of chromosome 3. Trisomy of chromosome 7 and 17 and loss of the Y chromosome is seen	*Natural history and prognosis* Very poor
Natural history and prognosis Better than ordinary renal carcinoma	

Natural history and prognosis Staging gives more prognostic information than any other single criterion with the most important factor being invasion of perinephric fat. Stage I (confined to kidey) has 65% 5-year survival and 56% 10-year survival dropping to 47% and 20% for stage II (through capsule but not renal [Gerota's] fascia), 51% and 37% for stage III (into regional lymph nodes, renal vein or both without perinephric fat involvement) and 8% and 7% for stage IV (distant metastasis or through renal fascia). The commonest site of spread is lung (30%) and bone (35%) followed by regional lymph node, liver, adrenals and brain. Complications: there may be systemic amyloidosis (about 3% of cases) and mesangial proliferative glomerulonephritis.

Renal oncocytoma

Definition Tumour composed mainly of cells with large amounts of eosinophilic, finely granular cytoplasm.

Epidemiology M:F 3:1.

Macroscopy Well-circumscribed tan coloured tumours which often have a central scarred area and dilated vessels at the periphery.

Microscopy Sheets and islands of large cells with central nuclei and granular cytoplasm.

Natural history and prognosis Generally behave in a benign fashion.

Nephroblastoma (Wilms' tumour)

Epidemiology Commonest renal tumour of childhood constituting 6% of all malignancies in children 0–14 years. Peak incidence 1–4 years. Occasionally seen in adults.

Associations Some children have aniridia (absence of the iris, 1%) and genitourinary abnormalities (5%). Wilms' tumour is also seen in association with hemi-hypertrophy, pseudo-hermaphroditism and Drash syndrome, Beckwith–Wiedemann syndrome and nephroblastomatosis. Familial cases are seen.

Genetics Deletion of material on the short arm of chromosome 11 (11p13) may be seen which is believed to be associated with the loss of tumour suppressor gene activity.

Clinical features Presentation is usually with abdominal mass, fever and abdominal pain.

Macroscopy Large greyish-white masses growing in expansile fashion. Usually unilateral but bilateral in 5–10%.

Microscopy The classic triphasic nephroblastoma has three components: blastema, stroma (may show striated muscle, cartilage bone or adipose tissue differentiation) and epithelium (primitive tubules in a spindle cell background). Occasionally poorly formed glomeruli are seen. Marked atypia and extension through the kidney capsule indicates a poorer than usual prognosis.

Natural history and prognosis In many cases pulmonary metastases are present at diagnosis. Until recently prognosis was poor (5-year survival 10–40%) but with a combination of surgery, radiotherapy and chemotherapy results have improved. Prognosis is determined by stage with stage I tumours (confined to kidney, completely excised) having a 4-year survival of 96.5%, stage II (extending through capsule but without renal vein or periaortic node involvement, completely resected) 92.2%, stage III (residual tumour confined to abdomen) 86.9%, stage IV (blood-borne metastases) 73% and stage V (bilateral renal tumours) a 3-year survival of 76%.

Congenital mesoblastic nephroma

Definition Variant of nephroblastoma.

Epidemiology Accounts for 3% childhood renal tumours tending to occur in first few months of life.

Clinical features Large mass, may be present at birth.

Microscopy Spindle cells arranged in sheets between collagen fibres. Most are fibroblasts but smooth muscle differentiation may be seen.

Natural history and prognosis Good prognosis if removed with rim of normal tissue.

Rhabdoid tumour of kidney

Definition Variant of nephroblastoma.

Epidemiology Acounts for 2% childhood renal tumours. Occurs in early life (within first year). Males more than females.

Microscopy Cells have abundant cytoplasm and hyaline inclusions.

Natural history and prognosis Poor prognosis. More than 75% die within two years. May be associated with cerebellar medulloblastoma.

Clear cell sarcoma of kidney

Definition Variant of nephroblastoma.

Epidemiology Accounts for 4% childhood renal tumours.

Microscopy Islands of polygonal cells with small round nuclei and vacuolated cytoplasm with indistinct cell borders.

Natural history and prognosis Characteristically spreads via bloodstream and lymphatics and unlike classic nephroblastoma, bone metastases are common (bone metastasizing renal tumour of childhood).

Urothelial tumours of the pelvis and ureter

Epidemiology Transitional carcinoma accounts for 5–10% renal tumours.

Aetiology Similar to factors for bladder variety but also associated with analgesic-related nephropathy and Balkan nephropathy.

Microscopy More or less identical to those seen in the bladder.

THE PATHOLOGY OF RENAL TRANSPLANTATION

Biopsies from the donor kidney may show signs of:

- immunological rejection of the graft
- changes that have occured in the donor kidney prior to transplantation (usually related to ischaemia and manifested by tubular necrosis)
- changes due to immunosuppressive drugs (e.g. cyclosporin A)
- changes associated with pre-existing disease in the donor kidney

- changes associated with the development in the donor kidney of a pre-existing disease in the recipient (the commonest being linear dense deposit disease, IgA nephropathy, mesangio-capillar [type I], focal segmental glomerulonephritis and amyloidosis)
- changes associated with new disease in the donor kidney after transplantation.

The lower urinary tract

THE URINARY BLADDER

ANATOMY

Site Extraperitoneal. In the child the bladder is an abdomino-pelvic organ palpable through the lower anterior abdominal wall. In the adult the pelvis is enlarged and it becomes a pelvic organ. When empty it has a pyramidal shape with an apex, base, superior and two infero-lateral surfaces. The apex is behind the margin of the symphysis pubis and is joined to the umbilicus by a fibrous cord in the extraperitoneal fat (the urachus). The neck of the bladder rests on the upper surface of the prostate where the muscle fibres of the two organs merge. The trigone of the bladder is an area of the base where there are no mucosal folds when the bladder is empty due to adherence of the mucosa to underlying muscle. This area is delineated superiorly by a muscular ridge joining the orifices of the ureters.

HISTOLOGY

The urothelium

This consists of three layers, a superficial layer of 'umbrella cells' which are large and flat, an intermediate zone up to four cells thick of cells with their long axis perpendicular to the basement membrane which flatten when the bladder distends and a basal layer of cuboidal cells that also become flattened during bladder distention.

Urothelial variants

1. Brunn's nests: invaginations of urothelium into lamina propria. Loss of continuity with surface leads to appearance of epithelial islands.
2. Cystitis cystica: results from breakdown of the centre of Brunn's nests to form cysts.
3. Cystitis glandularis: columnar/cuboidal or goblet-cell changes in cystitis cystica resembling large intestinal crypts.

The lamina propria

Well-vascularized connective tissue with some smooth muscle which may be continuous to constitute a muscularis mucosae.

Muscularis propria

The bladder neck has three distinct muscle layers (inner longitudinal central circular and outer longitudinal). Elsewhere the layers mix with no discernible orientation. The muscle fibres make up the detrusor muscle which together with relaxation of the sphincters is essential for micturition.

....

DEVELOPMENTAL ABNORMALITIES

Exstrophy of the bladder

Definition Failure of normal migration of mesoderm into the cloacal membrane to reach the midline leading to failure of development of the anterior wall of the bladder and that part of the anterior abdominal wall below the umbilicus.

Epidemiology 1/20,000–1/40,00 live births. M:F 2:1.

Associations In males the penis shows abnormalities (small and epispadias). In females the clitoris maybe abnormal. In other sexes abnormal development of symphysis pubis leads to a waddling gait.

Macroscopy In the most severe form the bladder lacks its anterior wall and presents as a reddened mass on anterior abdominal wall.

Microscopy Inflammation is always present due to recurrent trauma and infection. Squamous or glandular metaplasia of urothelium is common.

Clinical features Infection may extend to upper urinary tract. In surviving individuals carcinoma (more frequently adeno- than transitional carcinoma) may develop.

Persistence of part or all of urachal lumen

Clinical features Urine leaks from umbilicus if complete. Partial patency leads to urachal sinus (umbilical end), bladder diverticulum (bladder end) or urachal cyst (central part).

Outflow obstruction

Causes May be physical (prostatic enlargement, urethral stricture or congenital urethral rings) or related to the nervous system (spina bifida, multiple sclerosis, tabes dorsalis or spinal cord damage).

Macroscopy In the short term, the bladder becomes dilated. Later muscle hypertrophy and increased interstitial fibrous tissue supervenes, resulting in trabeculation of lining and possible diverticulum formation. Sustained high intravesical pressure results in decompensation and return of bladder dilatation with possible extention into the ureters (hydroureter) with reflux of urine and risk of infection.

INFLAMMATION OF THE BLADDER (CYSTITIS)

Causes

Bacterial infection

Epidemiology 20–30% of women will have bacterial cystitis at some time.

Pathogenesis Mostly due to retrograde spread of organisms along urethra.

Bacteriology Most frequently coliforms such as *Escherichia coli*, *Proteus* and *Klebsiella* species.

Viral infections

Virology Organisms include adenovirus type II (particularly bone-marrow recipients and children), herpes simplex, herpes zoster, papova and cytomegalovirus.

Metazoal parasites

Parasitology Mostly schistosomal and most commonly *Schistosoma haematobium*. *S. haematobium* is found in the Nile and other African rivers. An asexual cycle in the fresh water snail (*Bulinus contortus*) culminates in the release of motile larvae (cerariar) into the water which can penetrate the human epidermis. Maturation occurs in the portal circulation from where schistosomes migrate to the systemic circulation.

Pathogenesis The adult worm does not injure the host tissues but the eggs elicit a florid granulomatous reaction.

Macroscopy Bladder mucosa appears granular.

Microscopy Numerous granulomas with prominent eosinophils. The presence of ova makes the diagnosis which for *S. haematobium* are oval, have a terminal spine and stain with Ziehl–Nielson stain.

Complication Well-differentiated squamous cell carcinoma is common in areas such as Egypt where schistosomiasis is common.

Non-infectious causes

Causes Chemical irritants, drugs (e.g. cylcophosphamide), irradiation and trauma.

Macroscopy Mucosa appears red and velvety in acute cystitis but in chronic cystitis may be thickened.

Microscopy Acute cystitis shows oedema, dilation of blood vesels and a predominantly neutrophilic inflammatory cell infiltrate. In chronic cystitis there is thickened urothelium, possibly squamous metaplasia, scarring of the lamina propria and a mixed chronic inflammatory cell infiltrate.

Specific variants of cystitis

1. **Follicular cystitis**: Lymphoid aggregates in lamina propria some of which contain germinal centres.

2. **Haemorrhagic cystitis**: Usually associated with cyclophosphamide therapy.
3. **Eosinophilic cystitis**: Rare. Occurs in children and young adults in association with allergy and high peripheral eosinophil count. Occurs in elderly males associated with prostatic cancer.
4. **Malakoplakia**: Peak incidence in sixth decade, M:F 1:4. Macroscopically yellow/brown plaques. Microscopically there is an infiltrate of large macrophages some containing concentric bodies (Michaelis–Gutmann bodies) containing iron, calcium and PAS positive material. Ultrastructurally there are intracellular bacteria. Disease is thought to be abnormal macrophage response to bacteria – usually Gram-negative coliforms.
5. **Interstitial cystitis**: Chronic inflammatory disorder of unknown cause usually seen in middle-aged and elderly women. Presents with frequency, suprapubic discomfort, pain (pelvic, suprapubic or perineal) and dyspareunia. Two forms are recognized:

   - ulcerated (**Hunner's ulcer**, 10% cases) with bleeding from multiply ulcerated urothelium in a distended bladder and
   - non-ulcerated, with scarring and a mixed chronic inflammatory infiltrate in which mast cells are prominent.

....

BLADDER TUMOURS

Epidemiology About 95% of bladder tumours are transitional carcinoma. Bladder cancer accounts for 4–7% of malignant tumours in males and 2–3% in females in the UK. Rare in first five decades.

Prognosis May be associated with long survival. Only about 50% die of their disease.

Transitional carcinoma

Aetiology Chemical carcinogenesis related to occupation (particularly related to β-naphthylamines in the dye, rubber, cable and chemical industries), cigarette smoking, cyclophosphamide and analgesics. Chronic inflammation such as seen in schistosomiasis or patients with bladder diverticulae.

Genetics Several non-random abnormalities have been identified including abnormalities of chromosomes 1, 5 (isochromosome of short arm in 40%), 7 (trisomy in a few cases), 9 (in 50% superficial papillary tumours), 11 (deletions of short arm in 40%) and 17 (deletions related to p53 tumour suppressor gene on short arm).

Microscopy May be superficial (70%) or deeply invasive (30%). Three patterns – papillary, solid non-papillary or flat in-situ which may occur in combination. Pathological examination provides details of grade (3 grades of carcinoma if true papillomas are excluded) and stage (complex and determined by depth of invasion and invasion of perivesical tissues). Grade 1 papillary tumours show an increased number of urothelial layers with loss of orientation and hyperchromasia. Grade 2 lesions show higher proliferation and more loss of polarity. Grade 3 lesions show more abnormalities which in some cases lead to difficulty in the recognition of transitional nature. Carcinoma in situ may be seen adjacent to invasive tumour or in the absence of overt invasive tumour and shows increased thickness of the urothelium, marked cellular pleomorphism and increased mitoses.

Behaviour Carcinoma in situ is followed by invasive disease in 55–80% within 5 years. Superficial tumours recur after treatment in 80% but only 20–30% develop deeply invasive tumours and these are high grade from the start with early lamina propria invasion and have areas of carcinoma in situ. Deeply invasive tumours are aggressive and if untreated will result in death. Even if treated 50% die of metastatic disease.

URETHRA

ANATOMY

In the male the urethra runs for 20 cm from the neck of the bladder to the external meatus on the glans penis and is divided into three parts:

- prostatic (within the prostate)
- membranous (within the urogenital diaphragm)
- penile (enclosed within the corpus spongiosum).

In the female the urethra is about 4 cm long, opening about 2.5 cm below the clitoris. It traverses the sphincter urethrae and lies immediately anterior to the vagina.

....

HISTOLOGY

In the male the prostatic urethra is lined by transitional epithelium and the remainder by stratified columnar epithelium with the exception of the area near the urethral orifice, which is lined by stratified squamous epithelium. In the female the urethra is also lined successively by transitional, stratified columnar and stratified squamous epithelium.

....

CONGENITAL DISORDERS
Posterior urethral valves

Epidemiology   Commonest cause of urinary obstruction in infancy and childhood. Almost exclusive to males.

Pathogenesis   Abnormally large folds at the end of the inferior urethral crest balloon forwards during micturition causing obstruction.

Clinical features   Depends on severity of obstruction. About 50% present in first year of life many in the neonatal period. Clinical features include failure to thrive, vomiting, easily palpable kidneys and bladder due to dilation of bladder, ureters and pelvicalyceal system, urinary retention, urinary tract infections and chronic renal failure. In severely affected children there may be retroperitoneal leak of urine.

   Natural history and prognosis: early diagnosis and treatment has improved mortality from 10–40% (50–78% in neonates) to 0–3%.

INFLAMMATORY DISORDERS

Gonococcal urethritis

Epidemiology Accounts for one-third of cases of urethritis.

Aetiology *Neisseria gonorrhoeae.*

Pathogenesis Adherence of bacteria is crucial. Following adherence bacteria enter the bacterial cells, multiply and are released into the sub-epithelial tissues which elicits an acute inflammatory reaction. This inflammation spreads to peri-urethral glands, may involve the corpora spongiosa and cavernosa, the seminal vesicles, prostate, Cowper's gland, penile lymphatics and prepuce.

Clinical features Yellow urethral discharge.

Natural history and prognosis Before antibiotics the damaged surface epithelium was replaced by stratified squamous epithelium; the inflammatory response became chronic and resulted in scarring leading to urethral stricture formation.

Non-gonococcal urethritis

Epidemiology Usually young men.

Clinical features Mild dysuria and clear mucoid urethral discharge.

Aetiology *Chlamydia trachomatis* (30–50%) *Ureaplasma urealyticum* (a mycoplasma, 30%) and rarely *trichomonas vaginalis*, yeasts and herpes simplex. The cause is unknown in the remaining 20%.

Microscopy In chlamydial urethritis there is a sub-epithelial lymphoid infiltrate which persists even after the organisms have been eliminated. The overlying epithelium is undamaged.

Reiter's syndrome

Definition Triad of symptoms including urethritis, conjunctivitis and arthritis (particularly weight-bearing joints such as sacro-iliac joint).

Epidemiology Strong association with HLA-B27 which carries a 37-fold increased risk above normal. Marked male predominance, mostly 18–40 years.

Clinical features Often presents following infection of the gut or genital tract. A majority of patients have prostatitis with 20% additionally having haemorrhagic cystitis.

Microscopy Earliest manifestation is urethritis accompanied by many neutrophils in the urine.

Natural history and prognosis There is complete recovery in 25%, occasional recrudescence in 50% and recurrent chronic manifestations in 25%.

Urethral caruncle

Definition Polypoid lesion occurring at urethral meatus.

Epidemiology Exclusively females, usually in post-menopausal period.

Clinical features May be asymptomatic or cause dysuria or mild bleeding.

Microscopy Three basic patterns with overlap:
- papillomatous – irregular clefted surface covered by thickened transitional or squamous epithelium.
- angiomatous – numerous cavernous vascular spaces in sub-epithelial tissue.
- granulomatous – thin surface epithelium and florid inflammatory cell infiltrate in sub-epithelial tissue with granulation tissue-type capillaries.

TUMOURS OF THE URETHRA

Urethral carcinoma

Epidemiology Rare. Mostly elderly.

Site Commonest in anterior portion between meatal squamous epithelium and transitional epithelium of urethra.

Microscopy Most are squamous but transitional and adenocarcinomas have been described.

The male reproductive system

ANATOMY

Size   The adult testis weighs 15–19 g. The right is usually 10% heavier than the left.

Organization   The testis is covered by a fibrous capsule (tunica albuginea). Fibrous septa divide the testis into about 250 lobules each containing 2–4 seminiferous tubules. The seminiferous tubules of the testis are coiled loops (total length of the 1000 tubules in each testis is about 980 m). Groups of seminiferous tubules merge to form six efferent ductules which drain via a series of straight tubules into the epididymis. The epididymis lies on the posterior and lateral surfaces as a coiled structure divided into three regions – head, body and tail – and is responsible for sperm transport, part of the process of sperm maturation, sperm concentration and storage.

HISTOLOGY

Each seminiferous tubule is surrounded by a limiting membrane. The cellular lining consists of germ cells in different stages of development and **Sertoli cells.**

The Sertoli cells do not divide. They are columnar cells with cytoplasmic extensions surrounding germ cells and nuclei with prominent nucleoli. The cytoplasm contains cellular debris and crystalloid bodies made up of bundles of filaments.

The germ cells form the largest cellular component of the seminiferous tubules. Maturation takes about 10 weeks from undifferentiated spermatogonia to primary spermatocytes, secondary spermatocytes (following the first meiotic division) to spermatids (following another meiotic division) which mature by shedding cytoplasm of (phagocytosed by Sertoli cells) to become spermatozoa. In the normal adult testis about 50% of the germ cells should be at the spermatid stage and there should be no more than an average of 12 Sertoli cells in a tubule cross-section.

The **Leydig cells** (which secrete testosterone) occupy the interstium between the tubules in groups or singly. They have abundant intensely eosinophilic cytoplasm and frequently contain lipid and lipofuscin pigment. Some will contain crystalloid bodies (Reinke's crystalloids).

DEVELOPMENT

The testes develop from a urogenital ridge on the posterior wall of the abdomen and descend into the scrotum at about the 28th week of gestation, bringing with them an invagination of peritoneum (tunical vaginalis). The germ cells originate in the yolk sac and migrate to the gonadal ridge in early fetal life. The Leydig cells are present in large numbers in the fetal testes in weeks 1–20, after which their numbers decline sharply although some Leydig precursors are seen in the infant. At about 7 years the precursors start to differentiate into mature Leydig cells.

THE PRE-PUBERTAL TESTIS

The testis in infancy and childhood is characterized by small seminiferous tubules (50 µm at birth, increasing to 65 µm at 12 years), a predominance of Sertoli cells in the tubules and a small number of germ cells. At birth spermatogonia and their precursors, gonocytes, are seen but by 5 years the gonocytes have disappeared and primary spermatocytes are emerging. About 10% of boys have undescended testes at birth but most will descend in the first year.

The ageing testis

Decline in testicular function with age is mirrored by decreased spermatogenesis, peritubular fibrosis, hyalinization of basement membranes and thickening of arterial walls.

....

ABNORMALITIES OF DEVELOPMENT

Cryptorchidism

Definition   Arrest of testes along path of normal descent.

Epidemiology   Occurs in about 1% of male children.

Site   Arrest is most common in the inguinal canal followed by superficially in the inguinal region and then within the abdomen.

Macroscopy   In the adult undescended testes are smaller than normal and have a brown colour on cross section.

Microscopy   The seminiferous tubules are smaller than normal with increased interstitial fibrous tissue. There are decreased germ cells and relatively greater number of Sertoli cells with some in nodules (congeries). The tubular basement membrane is thickened. Leydig cells appear more prominent due to tubular shrinkage.

Natural history and prognosis   If uncorrected there is decreased fertility (if bilateral) and an increased risk for the development of germ cell tumours of the order of 30–50 times. Even following surgical correction the risk of germ cell tumour is increased, particularly if corrected after 6 years.

Ectopic testes

Definition   Testes at a site away from the path of normal descent.

Site   The commonest site is the perineum but also seen in thigh, pelvis and root of penis.

PATHOLOGY OF MALE INFERTILITY

Inadequate FSH/LH (hypogonadotrophic hypogonadism)

Epidemiology Accounts for about 1% of cases of male infertility.

Physiology Germ cell development requires adequate quantities of FSH; Leydig cell secretion of testosterone requires adequate concentrations of LH. Normal quantities of these hormones in turn require normal secretion of gonadotrophin-releasing substances by the hypothalamus, a normal hypothalamic–pituitary axis and normal pituitary function.

Aetiology In children craniopharyngioma is the commonest; in adults, disease of the hypothalamus and pituitary tumours. Decreased gonadotrophin secretion can be seen in chronic renal failure, severe inflammatory bowel disease and in the presence of functioning adrenal cortical tumours. The Prader–Willi syndrome consists of hypogonadism with short stature, hypotonic muscles and small hands and feet.

Clinical features In pre-pubertal cases there is other evidence of hypogonadism such as under-sized phallus, small prostate, high-pitched voice and absent or scanty pubic and axillary hair.

Microscopy If absence of hormones occurs before puberty the testicular morphology is identical to the pre-pubertal testis. In adult patients there are atrophic changes.

Inadequate testosterone

Aetiology The majority have Klinefelter's syndrome – eunuchoidism, gynaecomastia (50%), small firm testes, complete absence of sperm from ejaculate, elevated FSH and mental dullness.

Epidemiology Klinefelter's syndrome occurs in 1/1000–1/1400 live births.

Genetics There is an extra X chromosome in a phenotypic male, classically 47XXY.

Physiology Absence of testosterone, which is necessary for germ cell growth and maturation.

Microscopy The tubules are small, germ cells are rare, the tubule basement membrane is hyalinized and Leydig cells are prominent but deficient in Reinke's crystalloids.

Hormone receptor failure

Physiology Binding of androgens to their appropriate receptors is required for normal biological effects. Testosterone enters cells by passive diffusion and is converted to dihydro-testosterone which binds to a high affinity receptor. This complex enters the nucleus where it exerts its androgenic effect. Dihydo-testosterone mediates normal embryological development of male external genitalia and is responsible for virilization at puberty. Testosterone induces embryological development of Wolffian duct derivatives (seminal vesicles and ductus deferens) and takes part in stimulation and regulation of spermatogenesis. Failure of the androgens to bind to their receptors leads to failure of these functions.

Androgen resistance syndromes

Testicular feminization (male pseudo-hermaphroditism)

Genetics Mutation in the gene coding for androgen receptors. Normal 46XY karyotype.

Clinical features In its complete form the patients appear to be phenotypically normal females. Incomplete forms occur in which the external genitalia may be ambiguous.

Laboratory findings Testosterone levels are normal.

Macroscopy Testes are always present though they usually either inguinal or intra-abdominal.

Reifenstein's syndrome

Genetics Patients have 46XY karyotype.

Physiology Normal binding of androgens to the receptor indicating post-receptor failure.

Clinical features Phenotypic males with gynaecomastia, deficient virilization, cryptorchidism, complete absence or severely reduced numbers of sperm in the ejaculate and a severe degree of penile abnormality in the form of hypospadias.

Lack of testicular tissue

Aetiology Atrophy or destruction of testicular tissue may be due to:

- inflammatory disease – orchitis associated with mumps, mycobacterial infections, bacterial or granulomatous orchitis
- radiation
- chemotherapy
- severe trauma
- increased serum oestrogen levels – seen in liver cirrhosis and in patients with prostatic carcinoma treated with oestrogenic effects
- intrinsic failure in spermatogenesis – associated with germ cell aplasia, maturation arrest, generalized fibrosis or obstruction within efferent ductules.

Post-testicular causes

Aetiology Obstruction which may be congenital, post-inflammatory or post-surgical or due to faults in either the last stages of sperm maturation in the epididymis or in sperm storage.

....

INFLAMMATORY DISEASES OF THE TESTIS (ORCHITIS)

Infective orchitis

Aetiology Many bacteria, viruses, fungi and parasites.

Pathogenesis In a few instances orchitis can be an extension of epididymitis both in non-sexually (e.g. *E. coli*, *Pseudomonas*, *Brucella*) and sexually (e.g. gonorrhoea and chlamydia) transmitted conditions.

Macroscopy Testes and epididymis are enlarged, tense and painful.

Microscopy Acute non-specific inflammatory reaction initially confined to the interstitium spreading to involve tubules. Tissue breakdown with pus formation may occur. Oedema leading to swelling leads to increased intra-testicular pressure leading to ischaemic damage. There may be scarring.

Tuberculosis

Site The epididymis is the primary target of intrascrotal tuberculosis.

Pathogenesis Usually reflection of haematogenous spread.

Microscopy In the epididymis the features are the same as seen in other organs. Caseation necrosis is usually severe. The testis is relatively resistant to tuberculous involvement.

Syphilis

Two types of lesion may be seen, both of which result in scarring of the testicular parenchyma leading to sterility.

- a gumma characterized by an area of coagulative necrosis associated with a macrophage and plasma cell reaction. The necrotic areas show ghost outlines of the tissue architecture
- as a diffuse plasma cell infiltrate associated with obliterative endarteritis in which there is marked intimal thickening in small blood vessels.

Mumps

Organism A paramyxovirus.

Clinical features Associated with inflammation of one or both parotids. Orchitis is seen in about 20% cases in males over the age of 13 years. Orchitis develops when parotid swelling is subsiding. There is severe pain and testicular swelling.

Macroscopy Up to 85% of cases are unilateral.

Microscopy Initially a mild neutrophil infiltrate which spreads to involve the seminiferous tubules. The interstitial infiltrate becomes predominantly lymphocytic and the tubules show neutrophils and macrophages admixed with necrotic germ cells.

Natural history and prognosis Inflammation resolves with some residual scarring. Testicular atrophy occurs in about 50%.

Non-infective orchitis

Granulomatous orchitis

Epidemiology Predominantly in middle-aged men.

Aetiology Unclear. May be associated with trauma.

Clinical features Painless testicular enlargement.

Macroscopy Nodular testis which is firm and rubbery. The tunica vaginalis is thickened. The testis is lobulated and greyish-white in colour.

Microscopy Many epithelioid cell granulomas centred on seminiferous tubules. No necrosis but germ cell degeneration is prominent.

....

TUMOURS OF THE TESTIS

Germ cell tumours

Epidemiology More than 90% of testicular neoplasms accounting for 1% of all malignancies in males excluding leukaemia and lymphoma. Commonest malignant disorder in men 15–34 years. Incidence is 8 × higher in Denmark than in Japan. In the USA whites are affected about 4 × as often as blacks.

Clinical features Most present with increasing painless testicular enlargement. Occasionally the tumour may present with symptoms related to metastases (such as in lung or mediastinum). Manifestations of endocrine disturbance may be present – most frequently gynaecomastia. Most tumours are unilateral, although 1–2.5% are bilateral rising to 15% in men with undescended testes.

Classification   Divided into three groups:
- seminomas (40% germ cell tumours)
- non-seminomatous germ cell tumours
- combination of both.

Natural history and prognosis   Spread first to the iliac and periaortic nodes, then to the supra-diaphragmatic nodes. In most cases nodal deposits are ipsilateral to the tumour but may be bilateral in 15% of cases. Blood-borne metastases are mostly found in the lungs, liver, brain and bones. With the introduction of cisplatin-based chemotherapy the majority of tumours with the exception of trophoblastic tumours can be cured. Prognosis is related to tumour type (good for seminomas, differentiated teratomas and pure yolk sac tumours in infants but poor for undifferentiated teratomas and choriocarcinomas) and stage.

Intratubular germ cell neoplasia (ITGCN)

Microscopy   Normal germ cells are replaced by large vacuolated cells with irregular nuclei and prominent nucleoli. Immunocytochemical features are common to those of the gonocyte e.g. placental alkaline phosphatase synthesis. Tubules involved by ITGCN do not show spermatogenesis

Natural history and prognosis   With the exception of spermatocytic seminoma ITGCN is thought to precede all types of germ cell tumour. Patients in whom ITGCN is seen on biopsy have a 50% chance of developing a germ cell tumour within 5 years.

Classic seminoma

Epidemiology   Accounts for 90% seminomas. Broad age range with peak at 30–50 years.

Laboratory findings   In about 40% plasma placental alkaline phosphatase is raised. Occasionally serum levels of the β sub-unit of human chorionic gonadotrophin may be raised.

Macroscopy   Well-defined masses with greyish-white cut surface. Occasional areas of necrosis may be present.

Microscopy   Sheets of primitive germ cells divided into lobules by fine connective tissue bands. In about 80% the connective tissue shows infiltration by lymphocytes and plasma cells and occasionally granulomas some of which may contain giant cells of Langhan's type. The tumour cells are large and have abundant clear cytoplasm and well defined plasma membranes. The nuclei contain one or two nucleoliand-clumped chromatin. Occasionally multiply-nucleated tumour cells resembling syncytiotrophoblasts are seen and these secrete the β sub-unit of human chorionic gonadotrophin.

Spermatocytic seminoma

Epidemiology   Differs from the classic type in that it occurs at an older age with median age being 55 years.

Macroscopy   Tends to be large and gelatinous.

Microscopy   Always occurs in pure form. Marked variation in size and appearance of the cells which are arranged in sheets. The lymphocyte-rich stroma of classic seminomas is missing. The tumour cell nuclei characteristically have a thread-like chromatin pattern and the cytoplasm is like that of a plasma cell. Cells with 2–4 nuclei are common. Mitoses are frequent. The cells do not produce placental alkaline phosphatase. No ITGCN is seen in the surrounding testis.

Natural history and prognosis   Less aggressive than classic type and metastases are rare.

Anaplastic seminoma

Microscopy   Basically these are classic-type seminomas but with **three or more mitoses per high-power field**. There is nuclear and cellular pleomorphism and more necrosis.

Natural history and prognosis   It is not clear if these are more aggressive than the classic type but appear to present at a more advanced stage.

Teratoma

Definition   This is different between the UK and USA. In the UK the term relates to germ-cell tumours with the potential to differentiate into tissues of ectodermal, meso-dermal or endodermal types while in the USA the term is confined to those tumours in which such differentiation has actually occurred.

Site May be gonadal or extragonadal.

Malignant teratoma differentiated (MTD; WHO classification: teratoma)

Epidemiology Accounts for 3% of testicular teratomas but is the commonest type in childhood.

Microscopy Differentiation into cell types of more than one pattern (ectoderm, mesoderm or endoderm). A single tumour may contain skin, sweat gland, sebaceous gland, bronchus, gut, brain retina, muscle and cartilage. Frequently small areas of frankly malignant tumour can be found in adults if the tumour is well sampled.

Natural history and prognosis In children the potential for spread is low but in adults this may not be the case. Metastases show the same tendency to differentiation as the primary lesions.

Malignant teratoma undifferentiated (MTU; WHO classification: embryonal carcinoma)

Epidemiology Pure undifferentiated teratomas account for 10% of testicular neoplasms. Peak age is 20–30 years.

Macroscopy Cut surface has a variegated appearance with areas of haemorrhage and necrosis which may be extensive.

Microscopy There are sheets of undifferentiated cells with marked variation in size and shape. Mitoses are frequent.

Malignant teratoma intermediate (MTI; WHO classification: embryonal carcinoma with teratoma)

Epidemiology Commonest type of testicular teratoma.

Microscopy Features of both MTD and MTU with a wide range of appearances dependent on the proportion of each.

Natural history and prognosis In general the more undifferentiated the component the more aggressive the tumour.

Malignant teratoma trophoblastic (MTT; WHO classification: choriocarcinoma)

Definition   In the WHO classification the presence of syncytiotrophoblast accompanied by cytotrophoblast is the defining criteria for choriocarcinoma. In the UK for a tumour to be classified as MTT there must be a papillary pattern with syncytiotrophoblast forming a surface layer over cytotrophoblast.

Epidemiology   Pure MTT is very rare.

Macroscopy   The tumours are usually haemorrhagic and show foci of necrosis.

Natural history and prognosis   Choriocarcinoma and MTT are aggressive tumours with a marked tendency to metastasize.

Yolk sac tumour

Definition   Extra-embryonic growth pattern resembling human yolk sac.

Epidemiology   The pure form is seen in infancy and early childhood (< 2 years). It can be seen as part of a mixed germ-cell tumour in adults (up to 65–75% of adult teratomas).

Laboratory findings   There may be raised levels of α-fetoprotein.

Macroscopy   Pure yolk sac tumours are soft and white or yellowish tumours, often with small cystic spaces on the cut surface.

Microscopy   Resembles adenocarcinoma with tubular or papillary structures lined by cuboidal or columnar structures. Schiller–Duval bodies are a helpful diagnostic feature and are formed of one or more tumour cell layers around a central blood vessel.

Natural history and prognosis   Some suggestion that focal yolk sac tumour is an indicator of lower incidence of relapse after treatment in adult teratomas.

Leydig cell tumour

Epidemiology   Accounts for 1–3% of testicular tumours. Occurs at any age.

Clinical features Testicular swelling, gynaecomastia (30%) and sexual pseudo-precocity (secondary sex characteristics in the absence of spermatocyte maturation) in pre-pubertal patients.

Macroscopy Usually unilateral. Well circumscribed with brown colour.

Microscopy Tumour cells resemble normal Leydig cells arranged in sheets or trabeculae. Reinke crystalloids are seen in about one-third of cells.

Natural history and prognosis Malignant behaviour is seen in about 10% with metastases seen up to 9 years after removal of tumour. Malignancy is associated with older age group and is not seen in the pre-pubertal tumours.

Sex cord-stromal tumours

Definition Tumours composed of Sertoli cells and gonadal stroma.

Epidemiology Rare. Can occur at any age but more are seen in children (40%). Frequently associated with other endocrine disturbances and may be associated with Peutz–Jeghers syndrome.

Clinical features Gynaecomastia is seen in the pre-pubertal group and those over 50 years.

Microscopy Tumours may resemble granulosa cell tumours of the ovary (patients usually less than 6 months old) or be Sertoli-cell tumours of various types.

Natural history and prognosis Malignant behaviour is seen in up to 40% of sex-cord stromal tumours in patients older than 10 years at presentation.

Mixed germ cell–sex cord-stromal tumours
Gonadoblastoma

Epidemiology Usually under 20 years.

Clinical features Associated with hypospadias; most have pseudo-hermaphroditism or mixed gonadal dysgenesis. Patients often have a uterus.

Microscopy Combination of germ-cell tumour resembling seminoma and immature sex-cord components

535

showing either granulosa cell or Sertoli-cell differentiation which are arranged in discrete packets separated by fibrous stroma.

Malignant lymphoma

Epidemiology Accounts for 5% testicular tumours. Commonest in men older than 55 years.

Clinical features Most present with testicular enlargement, bilateral in 40%.

Microscopy The majority are non-Hodgkin's lymphoma of B cell type. There is infiltration of the testis by malignant lymphoid cells which surround and infiltrate seminiferous tubules.

Adenomatoid tumour

Epidemiology Most in males aged 30–40 years.

Origin Thought to be of mesothelial derivation.

Clinical Present with a small firm lump which may be painful just above the superior pole of the testis.

Macroscopy Greyish-white nodule 1–2 cm diameter. The cut surface may show small cystic spaces.

Microscopy Cells arranged in solid cord or as a lining of channels.

Natural history and prognosis Benign tumour but may extend into adjacent testis.

··

SPERM GRANULOMA

Epidemiology Most occur in men following vasectomy.

Pathogenesis Disruption of basement membrane leads to leak of spermatozoa into interstitial tissue causing acute inflammatory reaction followed by granulomatous response with giant cells. This is followed by scarring.

Clinical features Pain and some swelling.

Site Most commonly affects epididymis and spermatic cord but can rarely affect testis.

Macroscopy Firm yellowish nodule up to 3 cm diameter.

Microscopy   Macrophages are admixed with spermatozoa, some of which have been engulfed by the macrophages.

Vascular disturbances of the testis: torsion of the spermatic cord

Definition   Twisting of the spermatic cord resulting in testicular ischaemia.

Epidemiology   Occurs mostly in first year of life and in immediate pre-pubertal period.

Aetiology   Abnormal mobility of testis is predisposing factor and may be due to absence of scrotal ligaments, absence of gubernaculum, incomplete testicular descent into scrotum or an abnormally high attachment of the tunica vaginalis around the spermatic cord ('bell-clapper' deformity). Often associated with a history of trauma.

Pathogenesis   Initially twisting results in cutting off the venous drainage causing congestion followed by irreversible ischaemic necrosis of germ cells after about 10 hours.

Varicocele

Definition   Dilated and tortuous veins of the pampiniform plexus.

Epidemiology   Present in 15–20% male population.

Site   Usually unilateral, left > right.

Clinical features   May cause infertility.

Clinical features   Rapid onset of severe pain and testicular swelling associated with nausea, vomiting and abdominal pain.

THE PENIS AND SCROTUM

....

ANATOMY

Site   The root of the penis is in the superficial perineal pouch. The body hangs free and is composed of three cylinders of erectile tissue – two dorsally placed corpora cavernosa and a single corpus spongiosum on their ventral surfaces. At the distal extremity the corpus spongiosum expands to form the glans penis. The urethra runs in the corpus spongiosum. The penis is covered by skin with a hood-like covering of the glans (the prepuce). The scrotum is a pouch of skin containing the testes and lower spermatic cords.

<hr>

CONGENITAL DISORDERS
Abnormalities of penile size

Definition   The commonest is an abnormally short penis (micropenis) – more than 2.5 standard deviations shorter that the mean.

Aetiology   Causes of micropenis are the same as for hypogonadism, such as pituitary or hypothalamic failure, failure of testosterone secretion in fetal development and end-organ androgen resistance.

Abnormalities of penile and urethral development
Hypospadias

Definition   Urethral opening on penile shaft or perineum.

Epidemiology   Occurs in roughly 1/300 live male births.

Clinical features   Commonly associated with unde-scended testis and inguinal hernia. When urethral meatus is situated on ventral aspect there may be abnormal penile curvature (chordee).

Aetiology   Often associated with defective androgen pro-duction in fetal life. More severe forms are associated with intersex disorders including male pseudohermaphroditism, true hermaphroditism, mixed gonadal dysgenesis and Klinefelter's syndrome.

Pathogenesis   Failure of closure of the urethral folds over the urogenital sinus.

Epispadias

Definition   Urethral opening on to dorsal surface of the penis.

Pathogenesis   Failure of precursors of the genital tubercle to meet dorsally in the midline.

Clinical features   Dorsally directed chordee may develop due to abnormally short corpora. Occasionally associated with exstrophy of the urinary bladder.

Abnormalities of penile number

Diphallus

Definition   Double penis.

Epidemiology   Very rare.

Macroscopy   Three types: bifid glans penis, partial separation of whole or part of the shaft, or complete separation with two penises both of which may be malformed.

Abnormalities of lymphatic drainage

Aetiology   May be part of a syndrome including lymphoedema of lower limbs or may effect penis and scrotum alone.

Clinical features   May obstruct urinary outflow.

Peyronie's disease

Definition   A progressive scarring process involving the corpora cavernosa.

Epidemiology   Middle-aged men.

Aetiology   Unknown. Some are associated with Dupuytren's contracture and so may be the result of minimal trauma in men predisposed to fibrosis.

Clinical features   Curvature of the erect penis and pain on erection which may render intercourse impossible. A mass may be felt on the dorsal aspect of the penile shaft.

Microscopy   Scarring of the zone between the corpora cavernosa and the tunica albuginea associated with a chronic inflammatory cell infiltrate and in some cases metaplastic bone.

INFLAMMATORY DISORDERS

The penis can be the site of many inflammatory dermatoses seen affecting skin elsewhere including lichen planus, psoriasis and pityriasis rosea.

Non-infective inflammatory disorders specific to the penis

Balanoposthitis

Definition   Non-infective inflammation of the glans (balanitis) and the prepuce (posthitis).

Aetiology   Occurs in non-circumcised males in whom smegma accumulates between the prepuce and the glans.

Balanitis xerotica obliterans

Definition   Chronic disorder – homologue of chronic vulval dystrophy (**lichen sclerosus et atrophicus**).

Site   Surface of glans and mucosal aspect of prepuce.

Macroscopy   White plaques.

Microscopy   There is hyperkeratosis, thinning of the epidermis and atrophy of the rete pegs, homogenization of the dermal collagen, dilated capillaries and a chronic inflammatory cell infiltrate under the zone of altered dermis.

Natural history and prognosis   There is controversy about the risk of subsequent carcinoma but there is no evidence to suggest that this is the case. Retraction of the tissues may lead to the adherence of the prepuce to the glans (phimosis).

Balanitis of Zoon

Aetiology   Unknown.

Macroscopy   Shiny or velvety patches on the glans and prepuce.

Microscopy   The epidermis is slightly thinned with loss of rete ridges and granular layer. The epidermal cells become diamond shaped and lie with their long axis parallel to the surface and separated from each other by oedema. The dermis contains dilated capillaries and a dense plasma cell infiltrate.

Behçet's syndrome

Definition Syndrome comprising recurring mouth ulcers, recurring ulcers on penis and scrotum (vulva and vagina in females), an acute self-limiting arthritis and cutaneous vasculitis.

Epidemiology Young males. More common in Middle East than western Europe.

Aetiology Unknown.

Pathogenesis Vasculitis leading to ischaemic necrosis of epidermis.

Clinical features Painful ulcers that heal spontaneously and reappear.

Macroscopy Penile ulcers 2–10 mm.

Microscopy A marked perivascular chronic inflammatory infiltrate (lymphocytes and macrophages) in the early stages. Affected vessels show endothelial cell swelling and fibrinoid necrosis.

Infective inflammatory disorders

Syphilis

Definition The natural history of syphilis falls into three phases – primary, secondary and tertiary. The penis is usually involved in the primary phase and may be involved in secondary syphilis.

Organism *Treponema pallidum* (spirochaete).

Clinical features A small nodular lesion (chancre) appears usually 3 weeks after infection. Ulceration occurs a few days later and a thin serous fluid rich in spirochaetes exudes from the surface. The chancre is usually painless. Healing occurs after 3–6 weeks with scarring. In secondary syphilis the glans may be covered by flat papules (mucous patches) which contain large numbers of organisms and, like the fluid from chancres, are highly infective.

Microscopy Chancres show thinning of the epidermis with central erosion. Dermal capillaries show endothelial cell swelling and there is a dense perivascular infiltrate of lymphocytes and plasma cells. The mucous patches of secondary syphilis show epidermal thickening with a florid dermal infiltrate very rich in plasma cells. Dermal vessels show endothelial swelling. Organisms can be demonstrated in both lesions using silver stains (e.g. Warthin–Starry stain).

Chancroid

Organism *Haemophilus ducreyi* (Gram-negative bacillus).

Clinical features A small pustule appears about 5 days after infection which breaks down to form a painful ulcer. In some this heals with scarring but in others there is destructive inflammation, with tender inguinal lymph-node enlargement. The skin over these nodes might break down.

Microscopy The ulcer surface shows necrotic tissue, fibrin and neutrophils and may contain organisms. Deep to this is a zone of palisaded new capillaries and deep to this layer is a striking chronic inflammatory infiltrate rich in lymphocytes and plasma cells.

Granuloma inguinale

Organism *Calymmatobacterium granulomatis* (Gram-negative bacillus of the *Klebsiella* family).

Clinical features Initially a raised ulcer on the glans or prepuce. These may be painless, can bleed and tend to heal with considerable scarring.

Microscopy Thickening of the epidermis at the ulcer margins, a macrophage and plasma cell infiltrate in the dermis. Organisms (Donovan bodies) can be demonstrated in the cytoplasm of some macrophages using silver stains.

Lymphogranuloma venereum

Organism *Chlamydia trachomatis* serotypes L1–L3 (serotype different from those causing urethritis).

Clinical features Both males and females may be asymptomatic carriers (approximately 11% of sexually active heterosexual males). In symptomatic infections the initial lesion is a red papule usually on the coronal sulcus which heals without scarring. The next stage is enlargement of inguinal lymph nodes which soften, become attached to the overlying skin and form sinuses.

Microscopy The ulcer floor shows necrotic debris and neutrophils deep to which there is a chronic inflammatory cell infiltrate with macrophages invading small blood vessels and forming granulomas leading to vascular occlusion and local ischaemia. A similar process occurs in the lymph nodes with large stellate abscesses containing necrotic debris and a variable amount of neutrophils.

Viral infections

Herpes simplex

Organism   Herpes simplex types 1 or 2.

Clinical features   Initially painful blisters which rupture with increased pain. Primary infection usually lasts 2–3 weeks. Recurrence occurs in the absence of new infections and is more common in HSV-2 infection (90%) than in HSV-1 (50%).

Microscopy   Intraepithelial vesicles due to separation of swollen epithelial cells. The cells have characteristic eosinophilic nuclear inclusions with a surrounding clear halo. Multi-nucleate forms may be present. There is acute and chronic inflammatory cells in the underlying dermis.

Tumours and tumour-like lesions

Condyloma acuminata

Organism   Human papilloma virus, usually types 6 and 11.

Clinical features   Development of warty lesions 1–2 months after infection.

Site   Most common on the glans, mostly the penile meatus or fossa navicularis but can involve the shaft.

Macroscopy   Reddish cauliflower-like lesions which may be single or multiple. Multiple lesions may coalesce to cover large areas of the penis.

Microscopy   There is marked papillary thickening of the epithelium without atypia. Clearing of the cytoplasm and shrinkage or wrinkling of the nucleus (koilocytosis).

Fournier's gangrene

Definition   Necrotizing fasciitis of the scrotal skin and occasionally the penis.

Epidemiology Seen in any age group.

Organism Most cases associated with pseudomonas and β-haemolytic streptococci.

Clinical features Pain in genital area with fever. The scrotal skin becomes blackened and sloughs.

Microscopy Extensive necrosis associated with bacterial invaion of small vessels which causes thrombosis.

....

TUMOURS OF THE PENIS

Intraepithelial neoplasia

Erythroplasia of Queyrat and Bowen's disease

Definition Both are similar conditions showing intra-epithelial neoplasia conventionally separated by their site of origin.

Site Erythroplasia of Queryat involves the glans and prepuce. Bowen's disease involves the true skin of the penile shaft and scrotum.

Macroscopy Modified by the site – erythroplasia of Queyrat appears as red velvety patches while Bowen's disease presents as a well-demarcated scaly plaque.

Microscopy There are epithelial cells with large hyper-chromatic nuclei, individual cell keratinization and increased and atypical mitoses involving the full thickness of the epithelium.

Natural history and prognosis About 5% progress to inva-sive squamous carcinoma.

Bowenoid papulosis

Epidemiology Tends to be in younger males than erythro-plasia of Queyrat or Bowen's disease.

Aetiology Most associated with human papilloma virus type 16.

Site Both glans and shaft but commoner on shaft.

Macroscopy Fleshy, usually pigmented nodules.

Microscopy Resembles erythroplasia of Queyrat and Bowen's disease but degree of epithelial disturbance is less severe.

Natural history and prognosis May resolve spontaneously and in any event are unlikely to progress to invasive carcinomas.

Squamous carcinoma

Epidemiology Relatively rare in Western countries, more frequent in some parts of Asia, Africa and Latin America (10–18% of all cancers). Age range 40–70 years.

Aetiology Risk is inversely related to circumcision particularly if carried out in early life. The presence of phimosis (inability to retract prepuce) is an additional risk factor. Also associated with human papilloma infection with type 16 found in 50% and type 18 in just under 10% of cases.

Macroscopy Either a papillary mass (more common on glans) or ulcerating tumour (more common on prepuce).

Microscopy Papillary tumours tend to be well-differentiated keratinizing carcinomas while the ulcerated lesions are poorly differentiated and highly invasive.

Natural history and prognosis Spread is predominantly lymphatic with metastases present in 15% of cases.

Verrucous carcinoma

Epidemiology About 5% of penile carcinomas.

Macroscopy Large cauliflower-like growth with unpleasant smell.

Microscopy Well-differentiated throughout. Individual cells are large and the tumour shows very large rete pegs with a bulbous pattern. True invasion occurs at a late stage.

THE PROSTATE

ANATOMY

Site Pyramidal-shaped organ lying between the neck of the bladder and the urogenital diaphragm surrounding the prostatic urethra. The prostatic urethra is divided into two roughly equal parts by an angulation at which the verumontanum arises. The ejaculatory ducts and the ducts from the glandular elements of the prostate enter the distal portion of the prostatic urethra.

Size About 3 cm long and in the young adult weighs about 20 g.

Organization Divided into three zones:
- central zone (25% gland volume)
- peripheral zone (70% gland volume)
- transitional zone (5% gland volume).

HISTOLOGY

The prostate is made up of glandular components in a fibromuscular stroma. In the central zone the glands are complex, large and polygonal with intraluminal ridges and in the transitional and peripheral zones the glands are simple, small and rounded. The glands are lined by an inner layer of cuboidal/columnar cells with an outer layer of less distinct flattened cells. The stroma in the central and transitional zones is dense but in the peripheral zone is loose and open. The major component of the stroma is smooth muscle.

DISORDERS OF THE PROSTATE

Inflammatory disorders

Acute prostatitis

Aetiology May be bacterial or abacterial. Bacterial causes include *E. coli* (80%), *Serratia* and *Klebsiella* (10–15%), *Enterococci* (5–10%) and *Pseudomonas*. Gonococcal prostatitis was common before the antibiotic era and is now rare.

Clinical features Fever, rigors, lower back pain and dysuria. On rectal examination the prostate is enlarged, tender, a little firmer than normal and warm.

Laboratory findings As prostatic massage may lead to bacteraemia urine culture is normally used.

Microscopy An acute inflammatory infiltrate is present in and around ducts. Absesses may occur.

Chronic prostatitis

Aetiology   May be bacterial, abacterial or granulomatous. Most cases of chronic bacterial prostatitis are caused by *E. coli* while some abacterial cases are thought to be caused by *Chlamydia* and *Ureaplasma*. Granulomatous prostatitis may be associated with tuberculosis (rare), brucellosis, disseminated fungal infections, helminth infestation (e.g. schistosomiasias), post-trauma (e.g. surgery, irradiation), anti-bladder cancer, BCG therapy or can be idiopathic (nearly 70% of cases). Occasional cases are associated with malakoplakia and allergic syndromes (including asthma and Churg–Strauss syndrome).

Laboratory findings   Bacterial infections can be diagnosed by culture of urine following prostatic massage.

Nodular prostatic hyperplasia

Epidemiology   Very common. Seldom presents before 50 years but by this age morphological evidence of hyperplasia is present in 50% of males rising to 75% or more by the eighth decade.

Aetiology   No definite predisposing factors but is not seen in the absence of intact testes.

Site   Frequent in the transitional and periurethral zones and rare in the peripheral zone.

Clinical features   Symptoms can be divided into those relating to bladder outflow obstruction such as poor urinary stream, terminal dribbling, hesitancy and sense of incomplete bladder emptying, and those symptoms related to bladder irritation such as nocturia, frequency, urgency and incontinence.

Macroscopy   The gland may weigh in the range 100–800 g and be smooth or nodular. If nodular the cut surface may show a 'honeycomb' appearance with milky fluid expressable from the cystic spaces and some spaces can contain small calculi or yellow casts (corpora amylacea).

Microscopy   Nodules contain both fibromuscular and glandular elements with the relative proportions being variable. Within individual nodules the number of acini are increased, are dilated and show infoldings, but show the normal two cellular components of the lining. Secondary changes include inflammatory changes related to ducts and infarction (about 25% cases) showing coagulative necrosis and surrounding squamous metaplasia at the infarct periphery in some cases.

Natural history and prognosis Presence of bladder outflow obstruction can lead to urinary retention which in some patients will present as acute retention, particularly in elderly patients following some unrelated surgical procedure. The presence of residual urine in the bladder following voiding increases the risk of infection. Some patients may develop 'high pressure chronic retention' with dilation of the upper urinary tract and renal failure and this may be associated with hypertrophy of the muscle of the bladder wall.

TUMOURS OF THE PROSTATE

Carcinoma

Epidemiology Second commonest cause of death from cancer in males in USA (18% of all male cancer deaths). In USA 50% higher in blacks than in whites but while the incidence of prostatic cancer is very high in North American blacks it is rare in Nigeria and Senegal. Geographically the highest incidences are found in North America and the Caribbean and lowest in China and Japan. Most patients present after 50 years with a progressive increased incidence with increasing age.

Aetiology Unknown but prostatic carcinoma is rare in eunuchs and patients with Klinefelter's syndrome (phenotypic males with two X chromosomes) and is low in patients with liver cirrhosis. Regression of prostatic cancer can be seen following orchidectomy and following oestrogen therapy.

Laboratory findings About 60% patients with localized tumour and 80% with bone metastases have raised serum prostatic acid phosphatase. Serum levels of prostate specific antigen may also be raised in 40–60% patients with localized tumours. However raised prostate specific antigen is *not* specific for carcinoma and can be seen in 30–40% males with nodular hyperplasia. Both these products can be identified in tumour cells by immunocytochemistry on tissue sections.

Site   Most arise in the peripheral zones.

Clinical features   Four categories may be identified on the basis of natural history and presentation.
- latent carcinomas: found incidentally at autopsy in 25–37% males
- incidental carcinomas: unsuspected finding in 6–20% of samples removed for bladder outflow obstruction
- occult carcinomas: presentation with symptoms relating to metastatic disease with no prostatic related problems
- clinical carcinomas: presentation with prostatism and found to have a hard nodular prostate on rectal examination.

Macroscopy   There may not be prostatic enlargement. On cut surface tumour can be difficult to see, is grey or yellow, poorly demarcated and usually firmer than surrounding tisuue.

Microscopy   Virtually all are adenocarcinomas but with considerable variation in appearance. Four patterns of infiltration are recognized.
- a cribriform pattern
- a diffuse infiltrative pattern
- a carcinoma consisting of medium-sized glands lined by malignant cells
- a carcinoma composed of small glands with much cellular atypia.

Microscopic grading of prostatic adenocarcinoma gives prognostic information. The most widely used scheme is the Gleason grade which divides tumours into groups on the basis of glandular differentiation and pattern of infiltration, with grade 1 the most differentiated and grade 5 the poorest. The Gleason score is given as two figures (giving a possible total score of 2–10) by assigning a grade to the predominant pattern and to the pattern with the second greatest area.

Natural history and prognosis   Prognosis is related to the average of the two Gleason grades rather than the worst area. Prostatic carcinoma spreads either directly through the capsule to the seminal vesicles, prostatic urethra, bladder peri-prostatic tissue or rectum or via lymphatics (about 40% at time of diagnosis) or via the bloodstream to distant sites (most commonly to bone where thay are classically osteosclerotic).

The female reproductive system

THE FEMALE GENITAL TRACT

NORMAL DEVELOPMENT

At about 6th week of gestation two ducts develop on the anterolateral aspects of the gonadal ridges lying lateral to the mesonephric duct – the **müllerian ducts**. These grow down to the urogenital sinus and towards the midline separated from each other by a septum, breakdown of which leads to formation of uterine canal. The unfused cephalad portions remain unfused and form the **fallopian tubes**. The **vagina** develops from a downgrowth of a solid cylindrical mass of cells (vaginal plate) which becomes cavitated by ingrowth of cells from the urogenital sinus.

Ovarian development begins with the appearance of primitive germ cells within the yolk sac at the 4th week of gestation. At the 6th week these migrate to the gonadal ridges. At this stage the gonad is neither ovary nor testis. Testicular development will proceed under the influence of a testis-determining factor encoded on the Y chromosome; otherwise ovarian development will proceed. The mesoderm of the gonadal ridge proliferates to form ovarian stroma and surface epithelium.

Failure of structural development

Failure of the müllerian ducts to come together results in:

- **uterus didelphys** (two uterine bodies, two cervices and two vaginas)
- **uterus bicornis bicollis** (two uterine bodies, two cervices and one vagina)
- **uterus bicornis unicollis** (two uterine bodies, one cervix and one vagina)
- **arcuate uterus** (uterus with a deep notch in the fundus).

551

Failure of the septum to break down results in a uterine cavity divided by a septum.

Epidemiology Found in 0.25–0.5 of females.

Clinical features Result in difficulties in childbirth including recurrent abortions, early onset of labour, abnormal fetal presentation and uterine rupture during labour. Dysfunctional uterine bleeding, dysmenorrhoea and infertility may occur.

....

ABNORMALITIES OF SEXUAL DEVELOPMENT

Anomalies associated with abnormal sex chromosomes

Turner's syndrome

Genetics Absence of all or part of one X chromosome. Most are 45XO and the majority of the remainder lack part of the short arm. A small number show mosaicism 45XO/46XX.

Epidemiology Occurs in about 1/3500 live births.

Development Ovarian development in early embryonic life is normal. There is rapid fall in oocyte numbers which is almost complete by two years with the ovary reduced to a fibrous streak.

Clinical features Characteristically there is short stature, broad chest, increase cubital carrying angle (cubitus valgus) and webbing of the neck. There maybe lymphoedema of dorsum of hands and feet, bicuspid aortic valve, coarctation of the aorta and increased berry aneurysms in the circle of Willis. At puberty there is failure to develop secondary sex characteristics.

True hermaphroditism

Definition Presence of both ovarian and testicular tissue.

Genetics Mostly a disorder of gonadal rather than chromosomal sex (60% 46XX, remainder showing various mosaicisms).

Appearance An ovary may be present on one side and testis on the other or a mixed gonad may be seen. In most cases the uterus is present but external genitalia are ambiguous.

Clinical features Increased risk of gonadal germ cell tumours. Virilization is likely at puberty.

Mixed gonadal dysgenesis

Appearance Despite a Y chromosome individuals usually have female phenotype but with masculinization of external genitalia (chiefly clitoral hypertrophy). Testis is present on one side with streak gonad on the other.

Clinical features Virilization at puberty. High risk of gonadal germ cell tumours.

Anomalies associated with normal sex chromosomes

Normal gonads

Appearance Pseudo-hermaphroditism – gonads and genotype of one gender with external genitalia appropriate for the opposite gender.

Genetics Either 46XY or 46XX.

Pathogenesis Female pseudo-hermaphroditism is due to exposure of a 46XX fetus to virilizing influences in embryonic life. The commonest cause is congenital adrenal hyperplasia due to lack of one or other enzyme in the cortisol synthesis pathway – most frequently 21-hydroxylase which results in accumulation of 17-hydroxyprogesterone which is converted to testosterone via androstenedione. Other causes of virilizing effects are maternal ingestion of androgens and progestogens or the presence of a virilizing ovarian tumour during pregnancy.

Abnormal gonads

The commonest disorder in this group is pure gonadal dysgenesis.

Appearance Gonads are fibrous streaks. Female phenotype with infantile external genitalia. Stature is normal.

Hypogonadotrophic hypogonadism

Failure of ovarian stimulation by gonadotrophic hormones e.g. Kallman's syndrome (isolated deficiency of gonadotrophic-releasing hormone) which is either an X-linked or autosomal inherited defect. It is associated with hypogonadism, hyposmia, colour blindness (some cases) and there may be renal agenesis and movement disorders.

THE ENDOMETRIUM

ANATOMY

Site   Lines endometrial cavity.

HISTOLOGY

Tubular glands in a well-vascularized stroma both of which undergo changes associated with ageing and with the cyclic hormonal fluctuations involved in the preparation of the endometrium for blastocyst implantation if fertilization occurs.

PHYSIOLOGY

The normal menstrual cycle lasts 21–34 days and menstruation itself lasts about 5 days. Day 1 of the cycle is the onset of menstruation (see Table 39.1).

If fertilization occurs gestational hyperplasia follows with continued presence of pre-decidual cells, reappearance of glandular secretions and stromal oedema. In some instances there is hypersecretion by the glands, epithelial cell vacuolation and the presence of large darkly staining pleomorphic epithelial cell nuclei (Arias–Stella phenomenon).

In the peri-menopausal period anovulatory cycles occur and may result in simple hyperplasia. The endometrium becomes inactive (mitoses should not be seen after three post-menopausal years) and atrophic. There may be cystic dilation of glands which can be focal or diffuse.

Table 39.1 The menstrual cycle

Menstrual phase	Day 1–5. Sharp drop in oestrogen and progesterone as corpus luteum degenerates. Necrosis of the endometrium associated with haemorrhage.
Proliferative phase	Day 6–21. Secretion of large amounts of oestrogen from follicle under influence of FSH. Endometrial glands increase in length and become tortuous. Mitoses in glandular epithelium and stroma with pseudo-stratification in late stages.
Early secretory phase	Lasts 4–5 days post ovulation. Following release of ovum the follicle becomes a corpus luteum secreting oestrogen and progesterone under the influence of LH. Appearance of sub-nuclear glycogen containing vacuoles in glandular epithelial cells.
Mid-secretory phase	Lasts from 5th–9th post-ovulatory day. Vacuoles become supranuclear. Glands become tortuous and dilated with some secretions. Stroma shows oedema.
Late secretory phase	Begins at about 10th post-ovulatory day. Marked tortuosity of glands with epithelial lining in folds. Glandular secretion lessens. Stromal cells become round with increased eosinophilic cytoplasm (pre-decidual cells). Neutrophils appear in stroma on about 12th post-ovulatory day with granular lymphocytes. Breakdown of endometrium begins.

....

DISORDERS OF FUNCTION

Low oestrogen concentrations

Aetiology Absence of normal ovarian follicle (e.g. streak gonads), absence of hormonal drive (e.g. lack of FSH) or increased resistance to FSH.

Microscopy Endometrium is thin with small inactive glands and compact stroma similar to basal non-functioning or post-menopausal endometrium.

Increased oestrogen concentrations

Epidemiology Anovulatory cycles occur around menarche and menopause.

Aetiology Anovulatory cycles (lack of corpus luteum formation), prolonged proliferative phase, exogenous oestrogens, presence of oestrogen secreting tumour (e.g. granulosa cell tumour or thecoma) or polycystic ovary syndrome.

Low progesterone concentrations

Aetiology Failure of development or function of corpus luteum associated with inadequate follicle development, inadequate LH concentrations or elevated prolactin levels.

Microscopy Delay in morphological evolution of glands and stroma and loss of coupling of gland and stromal maturation (glands appear more mature) and irregular maturation across endometrium (irregular ripening).

Clinical features Small amounts of bleeding before menstruation, prolonged menstruation and infertility or risk of early abortion.

High progesterone concentrations

Aetiology Usually exogenous progesterones.

Microscopy Induction of secretory type changes followed by atrophy of glands and stromal pseudo-decidual change.

....

INFLAMMATION (ENDOMETRITIS)

Acute endometritis

Epidemiology Rare, because of cervical mucus barrier and regular endometrial shedding.

Aetiology Blockage of uterine drainage (e.g. polyp, tumour or cervical scarring), interference with mucus barrier and post-abortional retention of products of conception.

Chronic non-granulomatous endometritis

Aetiology Most frequently associated with intrauterine contraceptive devices (IUCDs) or retained products of conception.

Microscopy The presence of plasma cells is the hallmark. Foamy macrophages may be present in xanthomatous endometritis which is associated with cervical obstruction.

Chronic granulomatous endometritis

Aetiology Almost always tuberculosis.

Microscopy Granulomas (usually non-caseating) are present in late secretory phase. In post-menopausal women caseation may be a feature as there is no endometrial shedding.

Endometrial metaplasia

Aetiology May be associated with chronic endometritis, oestrogen treatments and hyperplasia.

Pathogenesis Müllerian derived tissues (except ovarian) have considerable metaplastic ability.

Microscopy Glands may show squamous (commonest) tubal or mucinous epithelial metaplasia.

Prognosis No clinical significance.

Endometrial hyperplasia

Simple hyperplasia

Epidemiology Most around menarche and in peri-menopausal period.

Aetiology Associated with high oestrogenic stimulus seen in repeated anovulatory cycles, unopposed oestrogen therapy, oestrogen-secreting tumours and polycystic ovary syndrome.

Clinical features Irregular, prolonged bleeding.

Microscopy Simple hyperplasia affects stroma and glands. Glands show varying size but a mostly smooth outline with only a few outpouchings. The glandular epithelium may show multi-layering but no atypia. Mitoses are present in epithelium and stroma.

Natural history Does not develop into atypical hyperplasia and carries no increased risk of carcinoma. Regresses with progesterone therapy or if ovulation commences.

Complex hyperplasia

Aetiology　Similar to simple hyperplasia. Can be seen in women with normal cycles.

Microscopy　Usually focal. Glands appear crowded, are larger but with variable size and have outpouchings into both stroma and gland lumen. No epithelial atypia.

Atypical hyperplasia

Aetiology　Hyperoestrogenism similar to other types of hyperplasia.

Microscopy　Only the glands are affected. May be focal. Marked gland crowding with little intervening stroma. Variable gland size with irregular outline and complex outpouchings. Epithelial cells show atypia, loss of nuclear polarity and mitoses.

Natural history and prognosis　Increased risk for developing carcinoma which develops in 14–35% cases.

....

ENDOMETRIOSIS

Definition　Presence of endometrial glands and stroma outside the uterus.

Epidemiology　Common, affects 10% women in reproductive life. Mean age at diagnosis 25–29 years but also found in adolescence (e.g. 45–60% women under 20 presenting with pelvic pain or dyspareunia).

Pathogenesis　Several theories including metaplasia of pelvic peritoneum, translocation of endometrial tissue to ectopic site and retrograde menstruation, implantation of endometrial tissue after surgery and blood-borne spread of endometrial tissue.

Clinical features　May be asymptomatic or associated with infertility (14–30% cases), pelvic pain or episodic features relating to presence of tissue at ectopic sites including lung and even brain.

Macroscopy　On serosa appear as bluish nodules up to 2 cm diameter which are often cystic containing altered blood (chocolate cysts).

Microscopy Endometrial glands and stroma which undergo normal cyclical changes or may be inactive. Bleeding frequently results in destruction of the glands and accumulation of haemosiderin-laden macrophages.

Natural history and prognosis May develop hyperplasia, atypia or malignancy. In the ovary thought to account for 10–15% ovarian carcinomas, mostly endometrioid (not all endometrioid ovarian carcinomas are associated with endometriosis).

Adenomyosis

Definition Presence of endometrial tissue in myometrium.

Pathogenesis Believed to be downgrowth of endometrial tissue. Not associated with endometriosis.

Macroscopy May be focal or diffuse in the myometrium. Associated with thickening of myometrium and a coarse, trabeculated cut surface.

Microscopy Glands and stroma deep in myometrium. May show cyclical change and can show hyperplasia and occasionally atypia.

Endometrial polyps

Definition Non-neoplastic sessile or polypoid over-growths of endometrium in uterine cavity.

Macroscopy May be single or multiple and of variable size. Superficial parts may show haemorrhage or necrosis.

Microscopy There is inactive basal and functional endometrium, cystic dilation of glands and hyperplastic endometrium.

Natural history Entirely benign. May be associated with haemorrhage or torsion (resulting in infarction).

....

TUMOURS OF THE ENDOMETRIUM
Endometrial carcinoma

Epidemiology One of the commonest invasive gynae-cological malignancies. About 80% patients are post-menopausal. Peak incidence 55–65 years.

Aetiology Associated with nulliparity, obesity, diabetes mellitus, a history of anovulatory cycles, prolonged exogenous oestrogen use or oestrogen-secreting tumours (e.g. granulosa cell tumour or thecoma) and polycystic ovary syndrome.

Macroscopy May be a polypoid mass on broad base (usually fundal) or diffusely infiltrating.

Microscopy About 80% resemble endometrial glands (endometrioid). There is irregularity of gland shape with epithelial tufts and a cribriform pattern. Atypia is present of variable severity with multi-layering of epithelium and mitoses (some atypical). Stroma is scanty and glands appear back-to-back. Histological grading depends on growth pattern and degree of atypia with grade I (about 50%) showing up to 5% solid growth pattern, grade II (35%) 5–50% solid pattern and grade III (15%) with more than 50% solid pattern. The grade is modified by the degree of atypia. Extensive squamous metaplasia is present in 10–20% endometrioid tumours (tumours termed adenoacanthoma) and some cases may have a papillary pattern.

Natural history and prognosis Direct spread occurs into myometrium and through the uterine wall to involve pouch of Douglas and parametrial tissues. Distant spread via lymphatics is to para-aortic and pelvic nodes. Haematogenous spread is a late event to involve lungs, liver, adrenals and bone. Prognosis depends on tumour type, steroid receptor state, vascular invasion and tumour cell ploidy. Overall 5-year survival is 65%.

Non-endometrioid endometrial carcinoma

Serous papillary carcinoma

Microscopy Similar to ovarian papillary serous carcinoma. Complex papillary growth pattern, marked cellular atypia, numerous mitoses, presence of psammoma bodies and patchy necrosis.

Natural history and prognosis Aggressive with prominent deep invasion of myometrium.

Clear cell carcinoma

Microscopy Large cells with clear (glycogen filled) cytoplasm. Papillary arrangement is common covered by cells with 'hobnail' appearance.

Adenosquamous carcinoma

Epidemiology Older women.

Microscopy Both malignant glandular and squamous areas are present.

Natural history and prognosis More aggressive with fewer than 40% surviving 5 years.

....

ENDOMETRIAL STROMAL TUMOURS

Stromal sarcoma

Macroscopy Low grade stromal sarcomas grow via myometrial blood vessels and lymphatics giving a worm-like appearance while high grade sarcomas tend to be soft fleshy masses within the uterine cavity.

Microscopy Spindle-cell mass resembling endometrial stromal cells. High-grade stromal sarcomas show more pleomorphism and frequent mitoses.

Natural history and prognosis Low-grade stromal sarcomas run a long indolent course which may last 20 years with low metastasis rate. High-grade sarcomas show rapid spread both locally and to distant sites and has a 5-year survival of only 15–25%.

Mixed müllerian tumours

Definition Endometrial tumour showing both epithelial and mysenchymal differentiation.

Epidemiology Rare tumours. Tend to occur in elderly.

Macroscopy Bulky masses protruding into uterine cavity often extending to cervical canal.

Microscopy Variable spectrum of malignancy of each component. Tumours can have benign appearing epithelium and stroma (adenofibroma) or benign epithelium and malignant stroma (adenosarcoma) or both the epithelial and stromal components can be malignant (carcinosarcoma). In the latter the stroma may contain only components normal to the uterus (homologous) or elements not normally present such as bone or cartilage (heterologous).

Natural history and prognosis Carcinosarcomas are very aggressive and have usually spread beyond uterus at diagnosis. Prognosis not affected by presence of heterologous elements.

CERVIX

ANATOMY

Location Distal part of uterus. Outer surface is intravaginal (ectocervix). Upper margin in continuity with lower segment of uterus. The endocervical canal leads from the external os distally to the internal os proximally (not a distinct orifice but change from cervical to endometrial tissue).

HISTOLOGY

The ectocervix is covered by non-keratinizing stratified squamous epithelium. The endocervical canal is lined by mucin-secreting columnar epithelium which penetrates the underlying connective tissue to form 'glands'. The two regions meet at the squamo-columnar junction.

PHYSIOLOGY

In 65% female infants endocervical-type epithelium is present on the ectocervix. Soon after birth the squamo-columnar junction retreats into the cervical canal. At menarche hormone-induced swelling of the cervix results in the squamo-columnar junction rolling out on to the ectocervix. As the exposed glandular epithelium appears reddened it is called a 'cervical erosion'. During reproductive life the everted glandular epithelium undergoes squamous metaplasia on the surface and this area is referred to as the transformation zone. In later reproductive life the tranformation zone backs towards the canal and by the menopause is concealed within the canal.

INFLAMMATORY DISORDERS

Infective cervicitis

Aetiology May be viral (particularly herpes), bacterial (e.g. *Neisseria gonorrhoeae*), chlamydial, spirochaetal, protozoal (e.g. *Trichomonas vaginalis*) or due to helminths such as schistosomiasis.

Non-infective cervicitis

Aetiology Post-surgical or obstetric trauma, diathermy or use of intrauterine contraceptive devices.

Cervical polyp

Aetiology Not neoplastic, may be related to inflammation.

Macroscopy Usually small but may measure several centimetres in length.

Microscopy Endocervical glands embedded in inflamed oedematous stroma occasionally accompanied by squamous metaplasia.

Microglandular hyperplasia

Site Endocervical epithelium.

Aetiology Associated with oral contraceptives and pregnancy.

Microscopy Complex proliferation of small glands lined by flat epithelium.

Decidual reaction of cervical stroma

Definition Stromal reaction during pregnancy similar to that at uterine implantation site.

Macroscopy May be multiple. Small yellow or red nodules on cervical mucosa.

Microscopy Stromal cells show enlargement with eosinophilic cytoplasm.

....

TUMOURS OF THE CERVIX

Cervical intraepithelial neoplasia (CIN)

Definition Spectrum of morphological changes ranging from mild to severe dysplasia and carcinoma in situ.

Location Almost always in transformation zone.

Microscopy Combination of abnormal cellular organization (loss of polarity and normal stratification) and cellular changes (hyperchromatic nuclei, nuclear pleomorphism, increased nuclear/cytoplasmic ratio, supra-basal or abnormal mitoses). CIN is graded by extent of changes – CIN I involves the lower third, CIN II extends between lower third to two-thirds and CIN III extends to the upper third. With CIN I and II there is often morphological evidence of human papilloma virus infection (koilocytosis, multi-nucleation and individual cell keratinization).

Natural history and prognosis Failure to treat CIN III will lead to invasive disease in one-third after 20 years.

Screening Mass screening has produced a striking decrease (60% or more) in invasive cervical carcinoma in some countries. Screening at 3-yearly intervals reduces the cumulative risk of developing cervical carcinoma at age 35–64 by about 90%. Annual screening has a very small additional effect.

Microinvasive squamous carcinoma

Definition Tumour which has breached the basement membrane but only extends to a depth of 5 mm or less.

Natural history and prognosis Similar to intraepithelial disease.

Squamous cell carcinoma

Epidemiology Second most common malignancy behind breast. Accounts for 70% cervical carcinomas. Peak incidence around 40 years.

Site Usually in the transformation zone and therefore on the ectocervix in young adults but in the cervical canal in older women.

Aetiology Several factors have been implicated.
- sexual history: early age of first intercourse (2.5-fold increase if below 18 years compared with after 21 years) and increased number of partners (2.8-fold increase for five or more compared with one) or if the partner is promiscuous
- cigarette smoking
- oral contraceptive: although previously suggested this is not thought to be an important independent factor.

Pathogenesis Human papilloma virus (HPV) has been implicated in cervical carcinogenesis. While types 6, 11, 31, 35, 42 and 50 are associated with condylomata acuminata, low grade non-progressive cervical intra-epithelial neoplasia (CIN) and very rarely invasive carcinoma, types 16 and 18 are associated with low-grade progressive CIN, high-grade CIN and invasive carcinoma. Types 16 and 18 have oncogenic properties (transform cells in culture) relating to two viral proteins E6 and E7. The E7 protein binds to the gene product of the retino-blastoma gene (important in cell cycle regulation) and E6 binds to p53. As HPV type 16 can be present in a normal cervix other factors must help promote neoplastic transformation.

Macroscopy Ectocervical tumours are either exophytic with bulky and friable polypoid appearance or ulcerated lesions. Canal lesions tend to expand the cervix forming a firm cylindrical mass.

Microscopy Three patterns are recognized.
- well differentiated (20%): cellular islands with obvious squamous differentiation and keratinization
- moderately differentiated (60%): cells appear squamous. More atypia present. No well-formed keratin whorls

• poorly differentiated (large or small cell non-keratinizing 20%): sheets of uniform either large or small cells with hyperchromatic nuclei. No keratin. Presence of mucin needs to be excluded.

Natural history and prognosis   Local spread occurs through tissue planes either upwards to uterine body, downwards to vagina, laterally into the soft tissues, anteriorly into the bladder or posteriorly into the rectum. Lymph-node spread is first to the ilial, hypogastric and obturator nodes and later to sacral, aortic and inguinal groups. Blood-borne spread is usually a late manifestation and involves lungs, liver and bone. Prognosis depends on fraction of cervix involved (< 20% carries 5-year survival of 70% dropping to 54% with > 60% involvement) stage (5-year survival for stage I = 85–90%, stage II = 70–75%, stage III = 30–35% and stage IV = 10%), and presence of lymphatic permeation. Tumour grade is of lower significance. Overall 5-year survival is 55%.

Adenocarcinoma of cervix

Epidemiology   About 30% of cervical carcinomas have some evidence of adenocarcinomatous areas.

Microscopy   Identification of epithelial mucins is the hallmark.

Natural history and prognosis   More aggressive and worse prognosis compared to pure squamous carcinoma.

MYOMETRIUM

Almost all disorders of the myometrium are neoplastic.

....

TUMOURS OF THE MYOMETRIUM

Benign neoplasms

Leiomyoma

Epidemiology   Commonest uterine tumour found in 20% women over 35 years.

Aetiology   Suggests that oestrogen binding is important which might explain their occurrence in reproductive life, enlargement in pregnancy and regression in menopause.

Site May be entirely within myometrium (intramural), immediately beneath the endometrium (sub-mucosal) or beneath the uterine peritoneal covering (sub-serosal). Some polypoid sub-mucosal leiomyomas can become attached to other structures from which they derive a new blood supply (parasitic leiomyoma). Hyaline change (63%), mucoid/myxoid degeneration (19%), calcification (8%), cystic change (4%) fatty change (3%) and red degeneration (3%) may be seen.

Macroscopy Frequently multiple. Vary in size from < 1 cm to > 20 cm. Expansile growth pattern with well-defined edges and pseudocapsule of compressed myometrium. Cut surface is whorled.

Microscopy Tumours are composed of interlacing bundles of smooth muscle cells separated by well-vascularized fibrous tissue. In some cases the cells are more rounded and polygonal with clear cytoplasm. Occasional tumours show bizarre cells with nuclei which are hyperchromatic, vary in size and may be multiple but without mitoses (atypical or pleomorphic leiomyoma).

Natural history Malignant transformation is very rare.

Intravenous leiomyomatosis
In this variant of leiomyoma the neoplastic cells extend into veins in the uterine wall and adjacent connective tissue and may extend to the inferior vena cava. Distant metastases are very rare.

Benign metastasizing leiomyoma
In this very rare variant of leiomyoma the histology is benign but metastatic deposits with identical benign histology are found in the lung. The possible explanations include synchronous development of pulmonary and myometrial tumours or dissemination of tumour cells in those cases that follow curettage.

Disseminated peritoneal leiomyomatosis
This is a rare benign variant in which typical myometrial leiomyomas are associated with small nodules of smooth muscle in omentum and peritoneum. This is possibly due to in situ change in peritoneal connective tissue and is strongly associated with pregnancy.

Adenomatoid tumour

Epidemiology   Found in 1% uteri.

Site   Usually sub-serosally in cornual region.

Macroscopy   Usually small (mean diameter 2 cm) and ill-defined.

Microscopy   Complex spaces lined by flattened or low cuboidal cells. Between the spaces is connective tissue which may contain abundant smooth muscle.

Natural history   Entirely benign.

Malignant neoplasms

Leiomyosarcoma

Epidemiology   Accounts for 1% malignant uterine tumours. Tend to occur in older women, mean age 54 years.

Aetiology   Most are thought to be de novo tumours rather than malignant transformation of leiomyoma.

Macroscopy   Usually single (two-thirds of cases). Some resemble ordinary benign leiomyomas but most are soft and fleshy with haemorrhage, necrosis and macroscopic invasion.

Microscopy   Hypercellular tumours which may or may not resemble smooth muscle. There can be difficulty in distinguishing well-differentiated sarcomas from benign tumours but mitotic activity is related to behaviour although the exact criteria for classification remains controversial. It has been suggested that tumours with < 5 mitoses/10 high power fields (even if there is pleomorphism) are benign, 5–9 mitoses/10 high power fields are of uncertain malignant potential, while those with > 10 mitoses/10 high power fields are malignant even with minimal atypia. Others suggest that 15 mitoses or less/10 high power fields with bland cytology denotes leiomyoma, those with > 15 mitoses/10 high power fields and bland cytology or 2–4 mitoses/10 high power fields and significant pleomorphism are termed smooth muscle tumours of uncertain malignant potential and those with > 4 mitoses/10 high power fields and cellular pleomorphism are best regarded as leiomyosarcoma.

Natural history and prognosis Invade pelvic organs and show haematogenous dissemination particularly to the lung. Overall 20–30% 5-year survival but worse if in premenopausal period.

THE OVARIES

ANATOMY

Size Each ovary is almond-shaped measuring 4 × 2 cm.

Site Attached to the back of the broad ligament in a depression in the lateral wall of the pelvis (the ovarian fossa).

HISTOLOGY

The ovary is divided into a cortex and medulla. The medulla is composed of connective tissue with vessels. The cortex is composed of cellular stroma containing ovarian follicles. The ovary is covered by simple cuboidal (germinal) epithelium.

DISORDERS OF THE OVARY

Primary ovarian failure

Definition Depletion of oocytes and follicles prior to the time of normal atresia at the time of the menopause.

Aetiology Radiation and some forms of chemotherapy. Viral infections (e.g. mumps), some metabolic diseases (e.g. galactosaemia) and accumulation of toxins (e.g. nicotine metabolites) and in some autoimmune disease.

Pathogenesis The ovary contains a finite number of germ cells and only a few hundred oocytes are involved in ovulation. Most atresia occurs in fetal life and this is greatly increased in some circumstances (e.g. Turner's syndrome).

Clinical features Related to infertility and oestrogen deficiency.

THE POLYCYSTIC OVARY SYNDROME

Epidemiology   Presentation in 2nd–3rd decade.

Clinical features   Presentation with hyperandrogenization (e.g. hirsutism), menstrual disturbance, infertility and obesity.

Laboratory findings   Hypersecretion of LH, normal FSH, prolactin and thyroxine and in some raised testosterone.

Pathogenesis   Unknown.

Macroscopy   Ovaries are large (3 × normal) and contain many 6–8 mm diameter peripheral cysts.

Microscopy   The cysts are cystic follicles with luteinization of theca interna cells. The ovary is covered by a thick fibrous capsule.

Treatment   Some patients respond favourably to wedge resection of ovary or clomiphene treatment.

TUMOURS OF THE OVARY

Ovarian cancer is the cause of up to 4000 deaths in the UK per year being the fifth highest cause of cancer deaths in women. Around 65% arise from the epithelium, 20% are germ cell tumours and the remainder are from the sex cord/stroma.

TUMOURS OF THE SURFACE EPITHELIUM
General

Epidemiology   Epithelial tumours are associated with nulliparity, early menarche and late menopause while multiparity, first child before 25 years and oral contraceptive use appear to be protective. About 1% of ovarian cancer patients have one or more close relatives with ovarian cancer.

Classification   Biological behaviour predicted by the division of tumours into three general morphological categories:

- benign: In epithelial tumours the cysts are lined by single layer of well-differentiated cells. If papillary projections are present these have a fibrovascular core and are covered by similar cells.
- borderline (proliferating): These are highly proliferative with epithelium of two or more layers with papillary tufts. There is moderate dysplasia but no stromal invasion.
- malignant: Anaplastic epithelial component which invades stroma of tumour and neighbouring structures.

Clinical features Presentation is often associated with symptoms related to spread beyond the pelvis including non-metastatic manifestations e.g. hypercalcaemia, cerebellar degeneration, recurrent thrombosis and the appearance of seborrhoeic keratoses (basal cell papillomas).

Laboratory findings Serum tumour markers may be detectable.

- CA125 – increased pre-operatively in 80–85% patients with epithelial ovarian malignancy. Not specific and seen in pregnancy, endometriosis, pelvic infections, liver failure and other tumours such as endometrial, breast and colon cancer.
- inhibin – Elevated serum concentrations in up to 82% of patients with invasive or borderline mucinous tumours and only 17% with equivalent serous tumours. However 27% patients with non-neoplastic ovarian disease also have raised levels.

Natural history and prognosis Depends on stage and grade/degree of differentiation. Cell type is less important but stage for stage clear-cell and mucinous tumours have worse prognosis. Other adverse prognostic factors include older age, the presence of residual tumour after primary surgery and over-expression of epidermal growth factor and of HER-2/neu proto-oncogene.

There is an overall survival of 90% at 5 years and 70% at 15 years for borderline tumours compared with 15% 5-year survival for malignant tumours.

Serous tumours

Definition Show differentiation towards epithelial pattern of fallopian tube.

Epidemiology Commonest ovarian neoplasm accounting for about 40% of ovarian cancers.

Site Bilateral in one-third to half of cases.

Macroscopy Dependent on the relative proportion of cyst formation, papilla formation and stroma.

Microscopy
- benign (serous cystadenoma) – usually cystic and unilocular containing clear fluid. Papillary projections are common either into the cyst lumen or on the external surface. The cells are usually cilliated. About 30% tumours contain calcified spherical bodies (psammoma bodies). A fibrous stroma is always present which in some cases is prominent leading to plump papillae and large fibrous areas. This variant is usually termed cystadenofibroma
- borderline (about 15%). Often multi-locular with complex closely packed papillae covered by 2–3 layers of epithelium showing variable atypia. There is *no* invasion
- malignant (serous cystadenocarcinoma). Often partly cystic and partly solid. The defining criteria is the presence of invasion. There is also a complex glandular and papillary pattern, multi-layering of the epithelim and a marked degree of cellular atypia

Mucinous tumours

Definition Show differentiation towards endocervical (commonest) or intestinal pattern.

Epidemiology Less common than serous tumours. Constitute 10–20% of ovarian neoplasms.

Macroscopy Tend to be larger than serous tumours often as big as 15–30 cm. Benign tumours are usually cystic being multi-locular and filled by clear mucoid material.

Microscopic Tall columnar cells with basally situated nuclei and supra-nuclear collections of mucin. In intestinal types Paneth, neuroendocrine and goblet cells can be seen. In malignant tumours there is stromal invasion and the tumours often have solid areas with focal haemorrhage and necrosis.

Complications Spillage of cyst contents following rupture may lead to pseudomyxoma peritonei in which large amounts of mucoid material accumulate in the abdominal cavity.

Endometrioid tumours

Definition Tumours with endometrial differentiation and resembling endometrial carcinoma.

Epidemiology Constitute 10–25% primary ovarian tumours.

Pathogenesis In 10–20% of cases endometriosis is present in the same ovary. In others the tumour is thought to arise from the covering epithelium.

Macroscopy Moderate size with partly solid, partly cystic areas. Cystic fluid is often brown or bloodstained. Papillae are inconspicuous.

Microscopy Benign and borderline tumours are rare. The tumour is composed of glandular structures similar to those seen in typical endometrioid endometrial adenocarcinoma. Focal squamous metaplasia is seen in about 50% which in most cases is benign.

Associations Co-existence of endometrial carcinoma with endometrioid ovarian carcinoma is quite common and are thought to be independent primaries.

Natural history and prognosis Twice as good as mucinous and serous tumours.

Clear cell (mesonephroid) carcinoma

Pathogenesis Endometriosis is common (6 × as common as compared with other ovarian carcinomas) and transition between these lesions and the carcinoma can be seen in some cases.

Microscopy Fewer than 10% are bilateral. Grossly spongy and often cystic appearance.

Microscopy Solid, tubulo-cystic or papillary arrangements of epithelial cells with abundant clear cytoplasm (mostly glycogen but some fat). In some areas there is a 'hobnail' appearance due to projection of nuclei into the tubule lumen.

Brenner tumour

Epidemiology Rare, accounting for 1–2% ovarian neoplasms. Most patients are over 40 years at presentation.

Macroscopy Most are less than 2 cm in diameter and are firm and fibrous with a grey whorled cut surface.

Microscopy Most are benign. There are sharply demarcated nests of epithelial cells in a fibrous stroma. The cells are round/oval with clear cytoplasm and nuclei which have a characteristic longitudinal groove. The nests resemble urothelium. In about one-third, mucin-filled spaces are seen in the nests and 20% of Brenner tumours are associated with mucinous cystadenomas.

Clinical features Some patients will present with postmenopausal bleeding as Brenner tumours can cause endometrial hyperplasia.

··

GERM-CELL TUMOURS

Dysgerminoma

Definition Undifferentiated germ-cell tumour. Homologue of testicular seminoma.

Epidemiology Accounts for about 1% of all ovarian neoplasms and about 5% of ovarian malignancies. Occurs in young women with more than 80% occurring below 30 years.

Site Bilateral in 15% and of the remainder the right is more commonly affected than the left.

Aetiology About 5% arise in a previously abnormal gonad.

Macroscopy Large tumour, mean diameter about 15 cm. fleshy grey-white cut surface with occasional haemorrhagic or necrotic foci.

Microscopy Closely resemble seminoma. Tumours cells are large round/ovoid with well-defined plasma membranes and central nuclei. The cells are arranged in islands separated from each other by fibrous-tissue stroma rich in lymphocytes. Sarcoid-like granulomata and occasional human chrionic gonadotrophin-containing multi-nucleated giant cells are seen. In about 5% cases there is microscopic involvement of the contralateral ovary which is macroscopically normal.

Natural history and prognosis Overall 5-year survival is 70–90% and is unaltered by the presence of giant cells. The tumours are radiosensitive.

Yolk sac tumour (endodermal sinus tumour)

Definition Germ-cell tumour showing extra-embryonic differentiation.

Epidemiology Tumour of the young, mean age 19 years with almost 25% pre-pubertal.

Laboratory findings Raised serum α-fetoprotein (normal product of the yolk sac) which provides a tool for follow-up monitoring.

Macroscopy Large encapsulated tumours which are either smooth or nodular. Cut surface is yellowish-grey and haemorrhage and necrosis can be prominent.

Microscopy Variable and complex microscopic appearances. A loose network of microcysts lined by flattened cells are frequently seen, as are Schiller–Duval bodies (papillary structures with mesenchymal core containing a blood vessel). Hyaline PAS-positive globules may be seen in tumour cells and extracellular space (globules of α-fetoprotein)

Natural history and prognosis In the past the 3-year survival rate was about 13% but this has improved with chemotherapy so that stage I tumours have a 5-year survival of 80% while advanced disease has a 50% 5-year survival.

Choriocarcinoma

Pathogenesis Can be primary ovarian (rare) or secondary to gestational choriocarcinoma.

Clinical features In pre-pubertal girls may be associated with precocious sexual development.

Macroscopy Variable size. Extensive areas of heamorrhage and necrosis are present.

Microscopy Primary tumours may be seen in a pure form but more often are part of a mixed tumour. The tumours are similar to those of gestational choriocarcinoma.

Natural history and prognosis Response to chemotherapy is poor.

Mature cystic teratoma (dermoid cyst)

Definition Tumour composed of elements recognized to have differentiated along ectodermal, mesodermal and endodermal lines.

Epidemiology Commonest ovarian tumour of childhood accounting for about 50% of all childhood ovarian tumours. Can be at any age but peak at 20–40 years.

Site Usually unilateral.

Clinical features Usually associated with intrapelvic mass. Rarely teratomas may present with haemolytic anaemia.

Macroscopy Usually multi-loculated with the cysts containing hair, keratin and sebum. In some instances the cyst formation is inconspicuous (mature solid teratoma).

Microscopy The most prominent differentiated element in the majority of cases is epidermis and skin adnexae but other tissues frequently seen include adipose tissue, bone, cartilage, neural tissue, bronchi, salivary gland, retina, pancreas, smooth-muscle thyroid and teeth. In occasional cases organogenesis may progess so far that for example a well-formed miniature cerebellum may be seen maroscopically.

Natural history and prognosis Malignant transformation of any one element can occur but the commonest is epidermoid carcinoma (85% of such cases), carcinoid tumour and adenocarcinoma. Occasionally torsion can result in ischaemic necrosis of the cyst wall, rupture and spillage of contents of the cyst. Some solid teratomas may be complicated by peritoneal implants of mature glial tissue (peritoneal gliomatosis). This does not alter the prognosis.

Immature teratoma

Definition The presence of embryonic-type tissue within a teratoma.

Epidemiology Rare. Most frequent in first two decades.

Macroscopy Usually large nodular lesions with a predominantly solid cut surface with some small cysts.

Microscopy A mixture of immature and well-differentiated elements. Neural tissue is often conspicuous.

Natural history and prognosis Depends on the amount and degree of differentiation of embryonal components and best in those lesions in which neural elements predominate. Until recently the prognosis was bleak (5-year survival less than 20%) but with newer chemotherapeutic agents complete remission may be expected in a significant proportion.

Monodermal teratoma

Definition Germ cell tumour that differentiates along only one pathway or in which one element predominates or obliterates others.

Microscopy The commonest type is a cyst lined purely by intestinal mucinous epithelium. In other cases the tumour is composed of thyroid tissue (**struma ovarii**) which can be functionally normal and produce hyperthyroidism. Primary carcinoid tumours of the ovary may be seen either in a teratoma or alone.

Natural history and prognosis Struma ovarii are always benign but may be associated with ascites or pleural effusions.

....

SEX-CORD STROMAL TUMOURS
Adult granulosa cell tumours

Epidemiology Account for about 1.5% of ovarian tumours. Most frequent after the menopause with only 33% occurring in reproductive life and 5% in pre-pubertal girls.

Site Unilateral in more than 90% of cases.

Laboratory findings About 75% produce steroid hormones, mostly oestrogen.

Clinical features Depends on the age. In pre-pubertal cases the oestrogen causes precocious puberty while in post-pubertal females endometrial hyperplasia presenting with abnormal vaginal bleeding occurs.

Macroscopy Variable size from microscopic to over 40 cm with an average of 12 cm. Usually solid or partly solid, partly cystic with a rubbery consistency. Focal haemorrhage and necrosis is frequent.

Microscopy The cells are round or oval with a 'coffee-bean' nucleus that has a longitudinal groove. Architectural patterns are variable, with a micro-follicular pattern with small tumour rosettes containing eosinophilic material and nuclear debris (Call–Exner bodies), a macro-follicular pattern or a follicular pattern resembling ovarian follicles of the newborn.

Natural history and prognosis In 6–10% patients with endometrial hyperplasia endometrial adenocarcinoma may supervene. These are indolent tumours and the 20-year survival rate is 50–60% making assessment of unequivocal malignancy difficult.

Juvenile granulosa cell tumour

Epidemiology Accounts for 85% of pre-pubertal granulosa cell tumours. About 45% occur before 10 years; 32% 11–20 years; 20% 21–30 years and 3% over age 30.

Site Usually unilateral.

Macroscopy Mostly solid.

Microscopy Islands or sheets of tumour cells containing granulosa cell-lined follicles in an oedematous stroma. The cells have nuclei without longitudinal grooves. Luteinization of tumour cells and stroma may occur.

Natural history and prognosis About 5% are malignant with rapid recurrence and metastatic spread the rule in this group.

Thecoma

Definition Tumours arising from ovarian stroma.

Epidemiology About one-third as frequent as granulosa cell tumours. Commonly in post-menopausal women.

Laboratory findings Frequently produce oestrogens, but occasionally androgens.

Macroscopy Solid tumours with a yellow cut surface.

Microscopy Bundles of interlacing spindle cells, some of which are plump and contain lipid.

Natural history and prognosis Thecomas are benign tumours.

Fibroma of the ovary

Epidemiology   Account for 5% of ovarian neoplasms.

Clinical features   No endocrine abnormality. May be associated with ascites or pleural effusion (Meigs' syndrome).

Macroscopy   Large solid tumours which may have a whorled cut surface.

Microscopy   Tumour consists of well-differentiated fibrous tissue.

Natural history and prognosis   Fibromas are benign. Meigs' syndrome resolves with tumour removal.

Androblastoma (arrhenoblastoma)

Definition   Tumours of sex-cord origin with presence of Sertoli and Leydig cells either alone or in combination.

Epidemiology   Tumours consisting of both Sertoli and Leydig cells are very rare accounting for 0.2% of ovarian neoplasms and occur mostly in young women (mean age 25 years).

Laboratory findings   About 10% show no endocrine activity but 20% are androgenic and 70% oestrogenic. The Sertoli–Leydig tumours are usually androgenic.

Macroscopy   Sertoli cell-only tumours are usually not large, mean diameter 9 cm with a yellow or orange cut surface.

Microscopy   Most Sertoli cell tumours consist of well-formed tubules lined by a single layer of columnar on cuboidal cells most of which contain large amount of lipid. Sertoli–Leydig cell tumours have in addition variable numbers of Leydig cells in the intertubular spaces. These tumours are divided into well-, intermediate and poorly differentiated types.

Steroid cell (lipid cell) tumours

Clinical features   Most are virilizing but some patients develop Cushing's syndrome.

Microscopy   Tumour cells show differentiation towards Leydig cells or into cells resembling adrenal cortical cells. In some cases it is only possible to say the cells are steroido-genic.

Natural history and prognosis   Most are benign.

Gonadoblastoma

Definition   Mixed germ-cell–sex cord stromal tumour.

Epidemiology   Very rare. Tends to occur in dysgenic gonads.

Clinical features   For the most part (85%) patients are phenotypically female and genotypically male (have Y chromosome).

Microscopy   Immature germ cells and sex-cord stromal elements (resembling granulosa or Sertoli cells) with the sex cords arranged in nests. Leydig cells are often present. Focal calcification is common.

Natural history and prognosis   Gonadoblastomas are benign but there is a 50% chance of developing a malignant germ cell tumour.

....

OTHER TUMOURS

Lymphoma

The ovary is a common site of involvement of disseminated non-Hodgkin's lymphoma. It is a site of predilection for developing Burkitt's lymphoma.

Metastatic tumours

Present in up to 75% of women dying of malignant disease and accounting for 7% of ovarian neoplasms. The common-est primary sites are breast, the gastrointestinal tract and uterus. A 'Krukenberg tumour' is normally used to describe a metastatic mucin-secreting carcinoma which is usually bilateral, consisting of strands, clumps or sheets of signet-ring cells in an active connective tissue stroma. Prognosis for patients with metastatic disease in the ovary is bleak, with a 2-year survival of not more than 10%.

ANATOMY

Regions Includes the mons pubis, labia majora and minora, the clitoris, the vaginal vestibule and bulb and the greater vestibular (Bartholin's) glands.

Covering Mostly skin, some hair-bearing and some with sebaceous glands.

NON-NEOPLASTIC DISORDERS OF VULVA

The vulva may be affected by dermatological disorders which occur at other sites e.g. allergic dermatitis, psoriasis, intertrigo and lichen planus. A common presentation is vulval itching which may be associated with hyperkeratosis and consequently the development of macroscopic white plaques (leukoplakia).

Lichen sclerosus

Epidemiology Commonest cause of vulval irritation in elderly. Also occurs in young women and children.

Aetiology Unknown. About 10% have thyroid disease, pernicious anaemia or diabetes.

Macroscopy White area with thin and wrinkly skin. If the area has been rubbed the skin will be thickened (lichenified).

Microscopy There is hyperkeratosis, epithelial atrophy with loss of rete ridges, liquefaction degeneration of the basal epidermal layer (not always), hyalinization (homogenization) of papillary and reticular dermis and a band-like chronic inflammatory infiltrate at the deep margin of abnormal dermis.

Squamous hyperplasia

Aetiology May be expression of dermatosis such as lichen simplex, psoriasis or candida infection. Frequently no cause is found. May be seen in conjunction with lichen sclerosus.

Microscopy Hyperkeratosis, epithelial proliferation involving Malpighian layer (acanthosis) without atypia, elongation of rete ridges and dermal chronic inflammatory infiltrate.

Vulval ulceration

Vulva ulceration is seen in a number of conditions.

* herpes virus (herpes genitalis) infection: painful ulceration may be associated with fever and inguinal lymphadenopathy
* primary syphilis
* Crohn's disease: seen in 25–30% of cases
* Behçet's syndrome
* aphthous ulcers: small painful ulcers with yellow base similar to those in the mouth
* Lipschütz ulcers: acute and painful ulceration of labia minora associated with fever and inguinal lymphadenopathy. Unknown cause.

....

NON-NEOPLASTIC CYSTS OF THE VULVA

A proportion of these are cysts which can occur in the skin at any site, such as epidermoid cysts, but some are specific to the vulva.

Cysts from developmental remnants

Origin Mesonephric duct or peritoneal remnants.

Site Those derived from mesonephric origin are in the posterior part of the labia majora. Those from peritoneal remnants (cysts of canal of Nuck) in anterior part.

Cysts of vulval glands

Aetiology Obstruction of mucus secreting glands.

Site Lesser vestibular, Skene's and greater vestibular (Bartholin's) glands. Bartholin's glands are in posterior third of vulva.

Clinical features Bartholin's cysts may become second-arily infected leading to a painful tense swelling.

Treatment Laying open and drainage.

....

TUMOURS OF THE VULVA

Benign tumours

Counterparts of those occuring in the skin elsewhere.

Malignant tumours

Vulvar intraepithelial neoplasia (VIN)

Aetiology Thought to be associated with sexually trans-mitted agent particularly human papilloma virus type 16. About 25% will also have cervical intraepithelial neoplasia.

Clinical features May present with pruritus vulvae but can be asymptomatic incidental finding at routine gynae-cologial examination.

Macroscopy Depends on degree of keratinization. May be multicentric. Recognition helped by application of 5% acetic acid where affected areas show as white patches after 2–3 minutes.

Microscopy Abnormal stratification pattern and matura-tion. May show upwards extension of basal/parabasal cells (basiloid pattern) or premature cellular maturation with abnormal mitoses (Bowenoid pattern). Three grades, similar to those for cervical intraepithelial neoplasia.

Natural history Variable. Risk for development of inva-sive cancer associated with high age, immunocompromised state and basaloid rather than Bowenoid pattern. About 5% progress to invasive carcinoma and about 5% regress spontaneously.

Paget's disease of the vulva

Definition Expression of adenocarcinoma in situ.

Associations Minority (20–30%) are associated with lesions in adnexal structures, Bartholin's glands, urinary tract or anorectal area. Most are purely intraepidermal.

Aetiology Possibly from multi-potent basal cells or intra-epidermal portion of sweat ducts.

Macroscopy Crusting red scaly area.

Microscopy Large, round or oval Paget cells with abundant pale cytoplasm which in most cases stains for mucin. Cells may be single or in nests.

Invasive squamous cell carcinoma

Epidemiology Annual incidence of 3/100 000 in England and Wales (750 new cases per year) accounting for 5% gynaecological cancers. Of vulval carcinoma 90% are squamous.

Aetiology and pathogenesis Some develop in pre-existing VIN. Others are associated with sexually transmitted disease (e.g. syphilis, lymphogranuloma venereum or granuloma inguinale). An association with cigarette smoking has been suggested (associated with carcinogenic metabolites in urine).

Site Most 75% occur on labia majora with the clitoris the second commonest site followed by labia minora, posterior fourchette and perineum.

Clinical features Itching or irritation is present in 71%, a mass or ulcer in 57%, bleeding in 28% and discharge in 23%.

Macroscopy Lesions appear as an intact plaque or mass but often there is an ulcer with raised indurated edges.

Microscopy Most are well-differentiated squamous carcinoma with many keratin pearls.

Natural history and prognosis The most important prognostic factor is extent at time of excision. Lymphatic drainage from the vulva is bilateral to inguinal glands then to femoral and external iliac nodes. Bilateral metastases are present in about 25% of those with nodal involvement. Overall 70% 5-year survival but 90% if no nodal metastasis falling to 25% if there is pelvic nodal involvement.

Verrucous carcinoma

Microscopy Extremely well-differentiated variant of squamous carcinoma. Difficult to distinguish from condyloma.

Natural history Slow growing.

Malignant melanoma

Epidemiology   Second commonest vulval malignancy. About 5% of melanomas in women occur on vulva.

Macroscopy   Similar to those seen elsewhere.

Microscopy   Similar to those seen elsewhere.

Natural history and prognosis   Early dissemination to inguinal lymph nodes. Poor prognosis with 30–40% 5-year survival.

VAGINA

ANATOMY

Site   From vestibule of vulva to uterine cervix. Long axis forms angle > 90° with uterus.

Size   Ventral wall 8 cm and dorsal wall 11 cm long.

HISTOLOGY

Three layers. Vagina is lined by non-keratinizing stratified squamous epithelium and has a muscular coat with surrounding connective tissue adventitia.

PHYSIOLOGY

Epithelium is responsive to oestrogens (causing glycogenation of superficial layers) and atrophies from menopause. Glycogen is substrate for *Lactobacillus vaginalis*, a normal commensal of the vagina and responsible for low pH (4–5) which is a barrier to pathogenic infection.

INFLAMMATORY DISORDERS
Infective

Causes   Mostly sexually transmitted. May be due to bacteria, viruses (notably herpes), fungi (mostly *Candida*) or protozoa (usually *Trichomonas*). *Gardnerella vaginalis* may cause infection in pre-pubertal or peri-menopausal women.

Clinical features   Vaginal discharge with unpleasant smell which may be frothy in *Trichomonas* infection and may be associated with vulval irritation.

Non-infective

Causes   Trauma, irradiation, surgery or chemical compounds and pessary use.

Vaginal adenosis

Definition   Presence of glandular structures from Müllerian epithelium in vaginal wall.

Aetiology   Strong association with maternal diethylstilboestrol treatment before 8th week gestation.

Pathogenesis   Partial failure of replacement of Müllerian elements by urogential sinus-derived squamous epithelium.

Clinical features   May be asymptomatic or associated with mucoid vaginal discharge.

Macroscopy   Roughened patchy red areas on anterior wall.

Microscopy   Glandular structures usually lined by mucus-secreting epithelium in vaginal wall. Some cases show squamous metaplasia.

Natural history   Precursor of vaginal adenocarcinoma.

....

TUMOURS OF THE VAGINA

Vaginal intraepithelial neoplasia (VAIN)

Aetiology   Probably similar to cervical intraepithelial neoplasia.

Macroscopy   Reddish or white patches.

Microscopy   Similar changes in the epithelial cells organization and morphology to those of cervical intraepithelial neoplasia and graded using similar criteria.

Natural history and prognosis Suggestion that 20% of VAIN III progress to invasive carcinoma.

Squamous cell carcinoma

Epidemiology Rare. Approximately 1% of gynaecological malignancies. Squamous carcinoma accounts for 95% vaginal malignancies. Most frequent in elderly women.

Site Most in upper part.

Macroscopy Usually nodular and may be missed at routine examination in early stages.

Microscopy Most are well- or moderately differentiated carcinomas. Occasionally spindle cell carcinoma is seen.

Natural history and prognosis Direct extension accounts for predominant spread which may be lateral, upwards (to bladder) or posterior (to rectovaginal septum and rectum). Spread from lower lesions is to inguinal nodes but higher tumours metastasize to pelvic lymph nodes. Blood-borne spread is late event, usually to bone and lung. Prognosis is dependent on stage with 5-year survival for stage I of 70%, stage II 30–60%, stage III 24–35% and virtually no % year survival for stage IV.

Clear cell adenocarcinoma

Epidemiology Occurs at young age (mean 17 years) and is rare before 12 or after 30 years.

Aetiology Maternal treatment with diethylstilboestrol in early pregnancy in 75% of patients. Approximately 1/1000 girls with in utero exposure to synthetic oestrogens will develop carcinoma.

Site Usually upper part of anterior wall.

Macroscopy Exophytic mass which may fill vagina.

Microscopy Tubules and cysts lined by clear cells with papillary structures and solid areas. Tumour cells are clear due to intracellular glycogen and some fat. Some cells have hobnail appearance with little cytoplasm and large nuclei.

Natural history and prognosis Relatively good for stage I (80% 5-year survival) poor for stage II (17% 5-year survival) and III/IV (no survivors at 5 years).

Embryonal rhabdomyosarcoma (sarcoma botryoides)

Epidemiology Occurs in infants and young children with 65% before two years and 90% before 5 years.

Site Anterior wall.

Macroscopy Conglomerate of soft polypoid masses resembling a bunch of grapes (botryoides = grape-like).

Microscopy Masses are covered by normal epithelium, underlying which is myoid stroma with tumour cells concentrated in a dense sub-epithelial layer. The cells are round or spindle shaped and some have abundant granular eosinophilic cytoplasm and a racquet or strap-like shape.

Natural history and prognosis Local invasion and recurrence is common. Death is due to local extension within pelvis.

THE FALLOPIAN TUBES

ANATOMY

Site Located in the broad ligament (lateral continuation of anterior and posterior peritoneal covering of uterus) on lateral sides or the uterus.

Length Hollow tubes 11–12 cm.

Structure Four anatomical divisions – intramural segment (about 8 mm), thick-walled narrow calibre isthmic segment (2–3 cm), thin-walled expanded ampulla and trumpet-shaped infundibulum opening into peritoneum. The opening is fringed by about 25 fimbriae which capture the ovum at ovulation.

HISTOLOGY

Epithelium is thrown into folds (plicae) and is lined by ciliated (important in ovum transport, most numerous at infundibulum), secretory (prominent at uterine end, secretions include amylase) and intercalated ('peg') cells.

INFLAMMATORY DISEASE OF THE FALLOPIAN TUBES

Acute salpingitis

Causes   *Chlamydia trachomatis* is frequently implicated, as is *Neisseria gonorrhoeae*.

Pathogenesis   Pathogenic organism can reach the tubes either by direct ascent from the vagina to produce mucosal inflammation (endosalpingitis) in the intramural segment or via the lymphatics to principally affect the submucosa (interstitial salpingitis).

Macroscopy   In endosalpingitis the tube is congested and oedematous with swollen hyperaemic mucosa.

Microscopy   May be focal loss of epithelium and adherent plicae. Sub-epithelial tissues are infiltrated by acute inflammatory cells. Lumen contains acute inflammatory exudate and amorphous debris. In later stages inflammation involves deeper parts with fibrinous exudate on external surface.

Complications   Tubo-ovarian abscess may form. Pus may leak from fimbrial end to cause peritoneal inflammation. Obstruction of the fimbrial end may occur resulting in a pyosalpinx.

Natural history   Depends on severity. Mild cases have complete resolution. If this does not occur the process might become chronic. Scarring may cause adherence of fimbriae giving a multi-cystic appearance (**follicular salpingitis**). This condition is associated with diverticulum formation in the isthmic segment (**salpingitis isthmica nodosa**) in some cases. In both these conditions the risk of ectopic pregnancy is increased. In some cases the tube becomes distended with flattened plicae and fills with clear fluid (**hydrosalpinx**).

Chronic granulomatous salpingitis

Causes   Mostly either tuberculosis or schistosomiasis.

Pathogenesis   Tuberculous salpingitis is secondary to tuberculosis elsewhere usually by blood-borne spread (salpingitis is seen in about 20% fatal cases of tuberculosis in women).

Microscopy In early stages the mucosa shows abundant epithelioid granulomata. There may be epithelial hyperplasia. In later stages the tube is distended by caseous material.

Complications Most frequent complication of tuberculous salpingitis is sterility.

BENIGN CYSTS OF THE FALLOPIAN TUBE

Epidemiology Cysts related to the fibrial ends (hydatid cysts of Morgagni) are common.

Aetiology Hydatid of Morgagni is of paramesonephric origin. Occasionally small inclusion cysts derived from the serosal covering (cystic Walthard nests) are seen.

Clinical features Usually asymptomatic but pain if they undergo torsion.

Macroscopy Cysts contain clear fluid. Walthard nests appear as nodules on serosal surface.

Microscopy Fimbrial cysts are usually lined by ciliated epithelium. Walthard nests show transitional cell metaplasia.

TUMOURS OF THE FALLOPIAN TUBE

Benign

Adenomatoid tumour

Definition Benign tumour derived from mesothelium.

Macroscopy Usually small (1–2 cm) firm yellow-white nodule situated on serosal surface.

Microscopy Cells arranged in solid cords or as lining for channels resembling vascular spaces.

Malignant

Adenocarcinoma

Epidemiology Rare. Accounts for less than 0.3% gynaecological malignancies. Commoner in nulliparous women or those with one child compared with multiparous. Age range 40–60 years with peak in early 50s.

Clinical features Presents with cramping iliac fossa pain, abnormal vaginal bleeding and vaginal discharge which may be profuse.

Macroscopy Usually extensive intralumenal growth with distension by grey-white friable tumour.

Microscopy Most are well-differentiated papillary adeno-carcinomas mimicking ovarian serous carcinomas.

Natural history and prognosis May spread via the fimbriae to the peritoneum, into the uterus, or through the tube wall. Lymphatic spread is to the iliac, lumbar and para-aortic nodes. Overall survival is only about 25% at 5 years ranging from >50% for stage I, 16% for stage II to 10% or less for stages III and IV.

DISORDERS ASSOCIATED WITH PREGNANCY

ECTOPIC PREGNANCY

Definition Implantation of ovum at site other than uterine cavity.

Epidemiology Occurs in approximately 1% of recognized pregnancies.

Site Fallopian tube in 95%, other sites include ovary, peritoneal cavity, broad ligament, cervix and myometrium.

Aetiology Defect in normal tubal transport, most commonly post-infective chronic salpingitis but also following reconstructive or sterilization surgery, with congenital abnormalities, associated with tuberculosis or schistosomiasis or with salpingitis isthmica nodosa. In 35–50% the tube appears normal.

Clinical features Most do not survive due to inability of tube to develop adequate decidua, thinness and relative non-distensibility of the wall. Rupture occurs in at least 50%.

Laboratory findings The finding of a raised serum β-human chorionic gonadotrophin level with an empty uterus and no chorionic villi in curettings should suggest the possibility of an ectopic pregnancy.

PRE-ECLAMPSIA AND ECLAMPSIA (TOXAEMIA OF PREGNANCY)

Definition Pre-eclampsia is a syndrome characterized by hypertension, proteinuria and oedema. Eclampsia is a life-threatening syndrome including convulsions, cerebral oedema and/or haemorrhage, pulmonary and laryngeal oedema, disseminated intravascular coagulation, renal cortical necrosis and retinal detachment.

Epidemiology More common in first compared with subsequent pregnancies.

Pathogenesis The hypertension is thought to be due to increased sensitivity to vasoconstrictor effects of angiotensin II resulting from decreased placental prostaglandin secretion associated with placental ischaemia. Placental ischaemia is due to changes in the intramyometerial portion of the spiral arteries.

Clinical features The fetus shows growth retardation and may die in utero or perinatally. Many maternal tissues are affected (Table 39.2).

TROPHOBLASTIC DISEASE

Hydatidiform mole

Complete mole

Definition Abnormal conceptus **without an embryo**, gross hydropic swelling of placental villi and proliferation of trophoblast (both cyto- and syncytiotrophoblast).

Epidemiology About 1 in 1500 pregnancies is USA and UK. Higher incidence in some parts of Africa, Asia and Latin America. Higher risk if woman < 20 years or > 40 years.

Pathogenesis Fertilization of an ovum from which the nucleus has been lost or inactivated. About 90% have haplotype 46XX with both X chromosomes being of paternal origin. This is due to duplication of a haploid sperm (monospermatic or homozygous mole). The remaining cases are 46XY resulting from the simultaneous fertilization

Table 39.2 Changes in maternal tissues associated with pre-eclampsia/eclampsia

	Liver	Kidney	Central nervous system	Placenta
Macroscopy	Pale yellow due to fatty change with focal haemorrhages	Sub-capsular petechial haemorrhages and pale yellow cortex		Smaller than normal. Placental infarction is increased in incidence and extent. Retroplacental haematoma more common
Microscopy	Earliest change is fibrin deposition in sinusoids particularly in periportal region (zone 1) which may be associated with haemorrhages and ischaemic damage (fatty change to infarction)	Glomeruli are swollen and bloodless. EM shows glomerular endothelial cell cytoplasmic swelling, amorphous deposit between endothelial cells and basement membrane and an increase in mesangial cells. Renal cortical necrosis or acute tubular necrosis may occur. Changes regress if pregnancy ends	There may be arteriolar thrombosis and fibrinoid necrosis, petechial haemorrhages and diffuse microinfarcts	Increased thickness of trophoblast basement membrane, proliferation of cytotrophoblast and smaller villi than normal which are poorly vascularized
Pathogenesis	Likely to be associated with disseminated intravascular coagulation			

of an empty ovum by two haploid sperm (dispermic or heterozygous mole).

Macroscopy   Uterine cavity is filled by mass of grape-like vesicular villi. The mass in greater than a normal placenta of same gestational age. No normal placenta.

Microscopy   Distention of entire villous population to a greater or lesser extent. The swollen villi are rounded and often contain a central cavity (cistern). Fetal vessels in the villi are generally absent. Villi show circumferential trophoblastic hyperplasia with some atypia.

Clinical features   Most present between 8–24 weeks' gestation (peak 14 weeks) with vaginal bleeding which may contain molar tissue. Examination reveals a large-for-dates uterus in 50% of cases. Very high human chorionic gonadotrophin (hCG) levels may lead to bilateral theca lutein cysts causing abdominal pain and hyperthyroidism (due to mild thyroid-stimulating effects).

Natural history and prognosis   About 10% develop persistent trophoblastic disease and 3–5% develop choriocarcinoma (relative risk 1000-fold compared with women following normal pregnancy). Follow-up is monitored by serum or urinary hCG levels.

Incomplete (partial) mole

Pathogenesis   Triploid karyotype usually 69XXY. Triploidy is not always associated with partial mole formation but is common if the extra chromosomes are paternally derived.

Macroscopy   Only a proportion of the villi are effected. Appearances are of essentially normal placenta of normal size with scattered swollen villi.

Microscopy   Vesicular villi are admixed with normal ones. The affected villi are smaller than in complete moles and are frequently irregular in shape with identations. A degree of trophoblastic proliferation is always present but is less marked than in complete mole and is ofter focal rather than circumferential.

Natural history and prognosis   May develop into persistent trophoblastic disease. No increased risk of choriocarcinoma.

Invasive mole

Definition   Penetration of myometrium and its blood vessels by abnormal villi or complete or partial mole.

Clinical features   Vaginal bleeding or brown vaginal discharge after evacuation of mole.

Macroscopy   Degree of invasion varies. Some lesions may be large, deeply penetrating and have haemorrhagic cavities while others are inconspicuous.

Microscopy   Depends on the demonstration of abnormal villi in myometrium or its blood vessels.

Natural history and prognosis   Abnormal molar tissue may be transported in the bloodstream to other sites, notably lungs and vagina.

Choriocarcinoma

Definition   Malignant neoplasm composed entirely of syncytiotrophoblast and cytotrophoblast without placental villi.

Epidemiology   Incidence of 1/50 000 gestations in Western countries.

Aetiology   Associated with molar pregnancy (50%), spontaneous abortion (30%) or normal pregnancy (20%).

Clinical features   Length of time between pregnancy and presentation of tumour varies from a few weeks to 15 years but is within 1 year in the majority. Excessive hCG secretion by the tumour may result in endometrial gland hyperplasia, decidual reaction, bilateral ovarian theca-lutein cysts and hyperplasia of breast lobules.

Macroscopy   Appears as single or multiple soft, dark-red haemorrhagic nodules.

Microscopy   Clusters of cytotrophoblastic cells covered by rim of syncytiotrophoblast with a small degree of atypia. No villi are seen. Haemorrhage and necrosis are often prominent. There is a marked propensity to vascular invasion.

Natural history and prognosis   A highly malignant tumour. Prior to chemotherapy death occurred in months rather than years with a survival of 10–20%. With chemotherapy survival for tumours confined to the uterus approaches 100% falling to about 80% in those with metastatic disease. Metastatic spread is via bloodstream, mostly to lungs, liver, brain, kidneys and gut. Poor prognostic features are age > 39 years, long interval between pregnancy and starting treatment, high serum hCG levels, large size, numerous metastases (> 8), situation of metastases in brain and history of previous chemotherapy.

Placental site trophoblastic tumour

Epidemiology About 100 times less common than mole/ choriocarcinoma.

Aetiology Most occur after full-term pregnancy, 5% follow molar pregnancy.

Pathogenesis Arises from extra-villous trophoblastic cells of the placental bed.

Clinical features Varied. Some present with amenorrhoea; one-third have a positive pregnancy test. Others present with vaginal bleeding.

Macroscopy Myometrial mass which may project into the cavity.

Microscopy Infiltration of the myometrium by cytotrophoblastic tissue with multi-nucleated cells. Haemorrhage and necrosis are not features. A high mitotic count suggests malignancy but a low one is no guarantee of benign behaviour.

Laboratory findings Raised serum placental lactogenic hormone produced by tumour.

Natural history and prognosis Does not respond well to chemotherapy. Around 10–15% are aggressive.

BREAST

....

ANATOMY

Location In the fully formed adult the base of the breast extends from the 2nd to 6th rib and from the lateral margin of the sternum to the mid-axillary line. The majority of the gland lies in the superficial fascia but a small part (axillary tail) extends upwards and laterally, piercing deep fascia to come into close relationship with axillary contents.

Size Variable. In young women breasts protrude forwards on circular bases while in the elderly they become pendulous. Maximum size is achieved during lactation.

Organization Each breast contains 15–20 lobes. Each lobe contains many lobular units comprising approximately 30 acini which are lumenated structures encased in a fibrous sheath and which drain into the intralobular portion of the terminal duct. This in turn drains into the extralobular portion of the terminal duct. Extralobular terminal ducts join to form sub-segmental ducts which in turn join, forming segmental ducts draining into lactiferous ducts which exit at the nipple. The lactiferous ducts show segmental dilations – collecting sinuses.

··

HISTOLOGY

Both acini and terminal ducts are lined by a layer of secretory epithelium and an underlying layer of myoepithelial cells.

··

DEVELOPMENT

Origin From milk streaks. Localized thickenings appear from which nipples emerge, from which cords of cell grow downwards to form the first generation of breast ducts.

Prepubertal/pubertal Ducts elongate and branch. With menarche this is enhanced and the terminal duct lobular unit forms. Adipose tissue within the breast increases.

Adult Changes associated with menstrual cycle. From early proliferative phase ductal and ductular cells proliferate. In secretory phase (following ovulation) the stroma becomes oedematous, peaking a few days before menstruation; terminal duct lobular units proliferate in late secretory phase. At menstruation there is involution of proliferated cells by apoptosis.

Pregnancy During pregnancy the number of acini increase under the influence of oestrogen, progesterone and pro-lactin. Secretory glands become lined by cuboidal epithelium which contain secretory granules. When lactation stops the acini and ducts atrophy.

Menopause Further atrophy takes place, basement membrane thickens and intralobular myxoid stroma condenses.

....

INFLAMMATORY DISORDERS
Mammary ectasia

Definition Abnormal duct dilatation of extralobular ducts.

Epidemiology Disagreement as to peak age. Some believe it is commoner in pre-menopausal parous women, others think more occur after the menopause.

Macroscopy Dilated spaces filled with white material (inspissated colostrum).

Microscopy Dilated ducts surrounded by chronic inflammation and scarring. There is no hyperplasia of the duct lining cells.

Clinical features In severe cases there may be retraction and inversion of the nipple suggesting carcinoma. About one-third of patients complain of nipple discharge. Dystrophic calcification may be seen on mammography. There is no increased risk of developing carcinoma.

Fat necrosis

Definition True fat necrosis affects subcutaneous adipose tissue.

Cause Trauma is thought to be the commonest mechanism but a history of trauma is only found in 50%. A few cases are associated with irradiation or as part of Weber–Christian disease (inflammatory condition of adipose tissue).

Pathogenesis Rupture of fat cell plasma membrane leads to a macrophage response to their fatty contents. Fusion of macrophages to form foreign body giant cells may occur.

The injury elicits a chronic inflammatory response followed by attempted healing with scarring.

Clinical features Most present as a discrete, firm breast lump.

Macroscopy Cut surface is usually orange due to deposition of iron pigment. The lesion is firm and fat droplets can sometimes be expressed.

Microscopy Foamy macrophages, foreign body giant cells, chronic inflammatory cells and fibrous scarring are seen.

Breast abscess

Cause Most common during lactation due to rupture of a mammary duct and subsequent infection.

Macroscopy Pus-filled cavity.

Microscopy Central pus surrounded by zone of inflamed breast tissue which eventually becomes scarred.

Granulomatous inflammation

Causes Rare condition but the commonest cause is tuberculosis (either blood-borne or from direct spread from local lesion). Other infective causes include actinomycosis and fungal infections. Non-infective causes include idiopathic granulomatous mastitis and sarcoidosis.

....

FIBROCYSTIC CHANGES IN THE BREAST

Definition Variable changes in the breast comprising many morphological features that may occur singly or in combination. The changes are so common that some investigators consider the changes as being within the spectrum of normality representing aberrations in the normal cyclical alterations of the breast.

Clinical features Presentation is with the following symptoms alone or in combination; cyclic pain in breast, nodularity to palpation or discrete mass.

Macroscopy May be discrete mass or vague thickening of breast tissue.

Microscopy The following changes affecting the terminal duct lobular unit may be seen alone or in any combination.

- **Fibrosis**: fibrosis of extralobular stroma is common and hyperplasia of the delicate myxoid lobular stroma is also frequent, particularly in involuting post-menopausal breasts.

- **Adenosis**: an increase in the number of acini within individual lobules which in the pure form is not associated with epithelial proliferation.

- **Sclerosing adenosis**: a combination of increased intralobular acini and intralobular fibrosis with preservation of normal lobular pattern.

- **Microglandular adenosis**: a rare form of adenosis in which proliferated acini are not seen in lobules but in extralobular connective tissue or fat. The acini have a single cell layer lacking myoepithelial cells and can thus be mistaken for tubular carcinoma.

- **Radial scar (complex sclerosing lesion)**: consists of a stellate shaped lesion with central fibrous area (some with elastic fibres) and variable degree of epithelial distortion and proliferation. Some reserve the term radial scar for lesions < 10 cm diameter.

- **Cyst formation**: may be due to duct obstruction leading to cysts up to 5 cm diameter containing yellow fluid. Occasionally fluid may contain altered blood and appear bluish macroscopically (Bloodgood's blue-domed cysts).

- **Apocrine metaplasia**: most commonly seen in cysts. Lining cells are tall and columnar with very pink granular cytoplasm and apical snouts (identical to the apocrine sweat glands seen for instance in the axilla).

- **Papilloma formation**.

- **Fibroadenomatoid hyperplasia.**

- **Epithelial hyperplasia**: In the terminal duct-lobular unit this is where there are two or more cells above the acinar/ductal basement membrane. Classified by type (usual or atypical) and site (ductal or lobular). Some epithelial hyperplasias are associated with an increased cancer risk.

- usual hyperplasia: mild (3–4 cell layers; no increased risk of invasive carcinoma) or moderate/florid (more than three cell layers; 1.5–2-fold increase of invasive carcinoma)
- atypical hyperplasia: seen in 4–5% biopsies of benign proliferative conditions. Affected cells show architectural and cytological atypia which is less severe than carcinoma in situ (4–5-fold increased risk of invasive carcinoma).

....

BENIGN NEOPLASMS AND TUMOUR-LIKE CONDITIONS

Fibroadenoma

Definition Some workers consider fibroadenomas as benign neoplasms while others think they are forms of nodular hyperplasia of epithelial and stromal elements.

Epidemiology Commonest form of breast lump in 20–35-year olds.

Clinical Mobile firm masses with well-defined edges. Around 80% are single. Increase in size with pregnancy; regress with ageing.

Macroscopy Firm rubbery masses with sharply demarcated borders seldom larger than 3 cm maximum dimension. Cut surface is grey with whorled appearance and slit-like spaces.

Microscopy Increased epithelial elements with two-layered structure which may be compressed (intracanalicular type) or may retain their lumenal structure (pericanalicular) in a proliferation of loose myxoid stroma. In some cases the edges are blurred and blend into breast tissue with fibrocystic change – fibroadenomatoid hyperplasia.

Natural history Malignant change occurs in only 0.1% cases, usually involving the epithelial elements. If this is confined within the fibroadenoma capsule then prognosis is excellent.

Juvenile fibroadenoma

Epidemiology   Occurs in adolescents especially African or West Indian.

Macroscopy   Large, often 10 cm or more.

Microscopy   Hypercellularity of epithelial or stromal elements. No atypia.

Adenoma

The term adenoma is applied to a small number of lesions some of which are hyperplastic.

Tubular adenoma

Epidemiology   Mainly young adults.

Macroscopy   Well-circumscribed. Tan-coloured cut surface.

Microscopy   Closely packed well-formed tubules with epithelial and myoepithelial layers.

Lactating adenoma

Definition   Hyperplastic lesion occurring in pregnancy and puerperium.

Macroscopy   Well-demarcated mass.

Microscopy   Tightly packed slightly dilated tubules lined by actively secreting epithelium.

Nipple adenoma

Epidemiology   Mostly 30–50-year olds.

Site   Sub-areolar ducts.

Clinical features   Presents with bloody nipple discharge.

Macroscopy   Occasionally overlying nipple is ulcerated.

Microscopy   Complex glandular pattern with florid papillomatosis in affected ducts and scarring.

Intraduct papilloma

Epidemiology   Most in middle age (mean 48 years).

Site   Large or small ducts.

Clinical features If large ducts are affected usually presents with bloodly nipple discharge (commonest cause of this presentation).

Macroscopy Usually solitary (90%), seldom exceed 3 cm, are soft and friable. Duct of origin is dilated.

Microscopy Complex branched appearance with fibrovascular cores covered by well-differentiated epithelium. Some myoepithelial cells also present.

....

CARCINOMA OF THE BREAST

Epidemiology Until recently the commonest malignant disease in women, accounting for 20% of cancer-related female deaths. Approximately 1 in 11 women will develop breast cancer.

....

NON-INVASIVE CARCINOMA (CARCINOMA IN SITU)

Definition Carcinoma confined within the ducts or acini. May be ductal or lobular.

Ductal carcinoma in situ (DCIS)

Epidemiology Incidence is increasing with the advent of mammographic identification of small clinically inpalpable lesions. Variants of DCIS occur which are historically divided into morphological types but for prognostic value are best considered to be high-grade DCIS (comedo and non-comedo solid) and low grade (the remainder).

Natural history Hard to determine as treatment has involved mastectomy. Some patients will develop invasive tumour after biopsy has been performed (7/25 with non-comedo DCIS in one series). In mastectomy specimens performed for DCIS diagnosed 6 months earlier 6–18% will have invasive carcinoma.

Comedo carcinoma

Macroscopy   Can reach quite large size, 50% > 2 cm diameter. About one-third multi-focal. Cut surface shows closely packed thin-walled ducts interspersed with normal tissue. Necrotic tissue can be expressed by squeezing tissue.

Microscopy   Ducts packed with pleomorphic tumour cells with large darkly staining nuclei with prominent nucleoli and frequent mitoses. Central necrosis with focal calcification is defining feature.

Solid non-comedo carcinoma in-situ

Microscopy   Necrosis is absent and cell population is more uniform. Cribriform carcinoma in situ.

Microscopy   Well-demarcated, punched-out round spaces giving sieve-like appearance. Trabecular bars (rigid rows crossing the spaces with cells perpendicular to axis of the row) and Roman bridges (curved bars) may be present.

Micropapillary carcinoma

Microscopy   Long epithelial structures projecting into lumen but without fibrovascular cores which tend not to branch.

Papillary carcinoma in situ

Macroscopy   Papillary lesion which may be localized in duct segment of spread intraductally to involve part or whole of a breast segment.

Microscopy   May be difficult to distinguish from benign papilloma. Features suggesting malignancy include cellular uniformity, absence of myoepithelial cells, large dark nuclei, numerous mitoses, absence of obvious fibrovascular cores and the lack of associated fibrocystic changes.

Lobular carcinoma in situ (LCIS)

Clinical features   Unusual to present as breast lump. Diagnosis most often made on microscopy.

Microscopy Multi-centric in 70%, bilateral in 30–40%. Area of affected acini increased, filled and distended by tumour cells which are uniform, small- to medium-sized with round normochromatic nuclei. The cytoplasm clear and may lead to signet-ring cell appearance. Cells are characteristically non-cohesive. May be pagetoid spread along terminal ducts.

Natural history Invasive malignancy (ductal or lobular) develops in 25–30% cases with increased risk operating for both breasts and irrespective of size of LCIS lesion.

....

INVASIVE CARCINOMA

Risk factors in relation to breast carcinoma

- **Female gender**: breast carcinoma occurs only infrequently in males (< 1% all breast carcinomas).
- **Genetic factors**: first-degree female relative of breast cancer patients have increased risk of developing breast carcinoma. This is thought to be related to BRCA1 gene (discovered in 1990) which is responsible for about 5% of all breast cancers and up to 25% of those occurring in under 35-year-olds. The mutated gene appears to be inherited in an autosomal dominant fashion.
- **Retinoblastoma gene (Rb)**: in as many as 25% of breast carcinomas there is homozygous deletion of the Rb gene.
- **Age at menarche and menopause**: early menarche and late menopause are each associated with increased risk for breast carcinoma development thought to be related to prolonged exposure to oestrogens.
- **Childbirth**: nulliparous woment have a greater risk of developing breast carcinoma than parous women providing that the first pregnancy occurs in the middle of the fourth decade. In women with earlier first pregnancy the protective influence is lost.
- **Geographic factors**: the UK has a high mortality from breast carcinoma (28/100 000 women per year) compared with a very low mortality in Japan (5.8/100 000 women per year). Women in Western

Europe and North America are most commonly affected while those in Asia, Africa and South America are relatively spared. Evidence from migration studies suggests that these are environmentally determined. These factors may include industrialization, diet (high fat and obesity associated with carcinoma development).

Invasive ductal carcinoma

Eighty-five per cent of invasive carcinomas.

Invasive ductal carcinoma NOS (Not Otherwise Specified) (> 85%)

Macroscopy Frequently hard mass (scirrhous) which is retracted below cut surface of whole breast. Lesion often has ill-defined infiltrating edge with streaks of white material through it; cuts like an unripe pear.

Microscopy Cells may be in diffuse sheets, solid islands, form glandular spaces or infiltrate in cords or as single cells. Tumours vary in terms of cellular pleomorphism (more than lobular carcinoma) and number of mitoses. Fibrous tissue varies from case to case, elastic tissue is present in 90% and calcification in 60%. Chronic inflammatory cell infiltrate at tumour-stromal interface is variable. Immunocytochemical markers expressed by the tumours include cytokeratin, epithelial membrane antigen, milk-fat globule protein and lactalbumin (70%). Intralymphatic spread is common.

Natural history The 10-year survival rate is 63%.

Tubular carcinoma (2%)

Macroscopic Usually small (about 1 cm diameter) with gritty cut surface and ill-defined borders.

Microscopy Well-differentiated glands lined by single layer lacking basement membrane and with a haphazard arrangement including invasion of adipose tissue. Intraduct carcinoma is a frequent finding.

Prognosis Better than NOS category. Metastatic deposits/recurrence in about 4% after 7 years.

Natural history   As for ductal carcinoma (p. 603).

Mucinous 'colloid' carcinoma (2–3%)

Epidemiology   Usually post-menopausal women.

Macroscopy   Soft mass with well-defined edges.

Microscopy   Cellular islands seen surrounded by lakes of mucin. Some cells (up to 25%) show some neuroendocrine differentiation.

Natural history   Better prognosis than NOS category, probably related to low incidence of nodal metastases.

Medullary carcinoma (1%)

Macroscopy   Soft fleshy mass with grey cut surface and well-defined edge. May have foci of haemorrhage and necrosis.

Microscopy   Confluent growth of tumour with little inter-cellular stroma, no gland formation. The tumour cells are pleomorphic with large nuclei and prominent nucleoli. Mitoses are common. Extensive necrosis with atypical tumour giant cells and dystrophic calcification are frequent findings. A prominent infiltration of lymphocytes and plasma cells at the periphery is characteristic.

Natural history   Good prognosis. The 10-year survival rate is 84%.

Paget's disease of the nipple

Clinical   Red eczematous lesion involving nipple.

Microscopy   The epidermis of the nipple is infiltrated by carcinoma cells which are large with atypical nuclei frequently in the basal layer and extending into the Malpighian layer. Must be distinguished from malignant melanoma and intraepithelial squamous carcinoma (Bowen's disease).

Associations   Virtually always associated with underlying intraduct carcinoma which may or may not have invasive component.

Inflammatory carcinoma

Clinical Mass associated with signs of inflammation including redness and heat. May be 'peau d'orange' – localized lymphoedema of skin.

Microscopy Extensive permeation of dermal lymphatic channels by tumour cells. No significant acute inflammatory infiltrate.

Natural history Associated with poor prognosis.

Invasive lobular carcinoma

Ten per cent of invasive carcinomas.

Microscopy Tendency to be multi-centric and/or bilateral similar to LCIS. Cells are smaller than ductal carcinoma cells, more uniform and with less atypia. Absence of cellular cohesiveness is characteristic. Cells may have an intracytoplasmic lumen, accumulation of intracellular mucin or a signet-ring appearance. Cells frequently infiltrate in an 'Indian file' pattern and may infiltrate around pre-existing duct structures in a targetoid fashion.

···

GRADING BREAST CARCINOMA

In the UK most commonly by modification of Bloom and Richardson's scheme using three morphological criteria. The higher the grade the worse the prognosis.

1. Degree of tubule formation – varying from extensive (score 1) to minimal (score 3).
2. Nuclear atypia – minimal (score 1) to marked (score 3).
3. Mitoses – score 1–3 with highest score assigned to highest mitotic activity. Grade 1 = score 3–5, grade 2 = score 6–7, grade 3 = score 8–9.

···

STAGING BREAST CARCINOMA

Many systems exist based on tumour size, lymph node involvement, local infiltration and presence of distant metasases. The system most used in UK is a basically clinical scheme recommended by UICC (International Union Against Cancer) using a T (tumour size and local fixation) N (node status) M (distant metastases) nomenclature.

....

PROGNOSIS OF BREAST CARCINOMA

Natural history If tumour is localized at diagnosis without infiltration of local structures then the survival rate is about 73% (60% disease free). With involved regional nodes or invasion of local structures the 5-year survival is about 49% (43% disease free).

Prognostic factors

- Presence of invasion: single most important factor. Non-invasive tumours are curable if all lesion(s) are resected. Due to multicentricity this may require mastectomy.
- Tumour size: the smaller the tumour the higher the survival. Survival falls steadily with increasing size independent of node status.
- Tumour type: tubular, medullary, pure mucinous and papillary are associated with more favourable prognosis.
- Lymph node status: one of the most important factors in predicting cancer-free and non-cancer-free survival. Five-year cancer-free survival of 85% for node-negative patients fell to 60% when 1–3 nodes are involved and survival falls progressively with increasing number of nodes involved (4 nodes = 40%, 4–6 nodes = 30.5%, 7–12 nodes = 28%, > 13 nodes = 16.4%).
- Degree of differentiation.
- Character of tumour margin: 'pushing' margin has better prognosis than infiltrating.
- Expression of hormone (oestrogen and progesterone) receptors: an indication of likely response to anti-oestrogens in some cases.
- Expression of epidermal growth factor receptors (EGFR): poorer prognosis if tumour cells express large amounts of EGFR.

- Expression of product of proto-oncogene erb-B2: amplification of c-erb-B2 (also known as HER-2 or neu) is associated with poorer prognosis.
- Tumour cell ploidy: tumours showing cellular aneuploidy are more aggressive than those that are diploid.

PATTERNS OF SPREAD IN BREAST CARCINOMA

- **Direct**: to involve neighbouring structures such as skin, pectoral fascia and pectoral muscles.
- **Via lymphatics**: most frequently to involve axillary lymph nodes but also the internal mammary nodes, particularly in patients with tumours in upper inner quadrant. Supraclavicular and intra-abdominal nodes may also be involved.
- **Via bloodstream**: particularly to lungs, liver, bones and adrenals.

OTHER BREAST TUMOURS

Stromal tumours

Phyllodes tumour

Previously known as cystosarcoma phyllodes.

Epidemiology Mean age of presentation is 45 years.

Macroscopy Can be very large (up to 45 cm diameter) and are usually well-demarcated from surrounding breast tissue. Cut surface has cleft-like spaces suggesting leaves projecting into cystic space.

Microscopy A lesion involving both epithelium and connective tissue in which the connective tissue stroma is more cellular than fibroadenoma. At the 'benign' end of the morphological spectrum there is little atypia and few mitoses while at the 'malignant' end there is marked atypia and many mitoses. There is stromal overgrowth so that some microscopical fields consist only of the stromal component. There may be metaplastic bone or cartilage.

Natural history Variable. Some are cured by excision but 3–12% metastasize. Prognosis in some instances can be predicted by characteristics of the stromal component of the tumour.

Angiosarcoma

Epidemiology Rare tumour, mostly found in young females.

Microscopy Anastomosing vascular channels lined by plump atypical endothelial cells. Some areas show a papillary appearance.

Natural history Very poor prognosis with average time from diagnosis to death of 1.6–2.6 years.

Stromal sarcoma

Tumour consisting of malignant stromal cells without epithelial component. Most are 'fibrosarcoma' but may have areas of metaplastic bone.

Malignant lymphoma

Usually non-Hodgkin's lymphoma which may be part of generalized disease or may be primary within the breast. The majority of the latter are thought to arise from mucosa-associated lymphoid tissue.

....

THE MALE BREAST

Histology

The male breast differs from the female by the absence of acini. There are scanty ducts which resemble those of pre-pubertal females.

Gynaecomastia

Epidemiology Two-peak incidence in adolescence and the elderly.

Pathogenesis Thought to be related to either increase in oestrogens or relative decline in androgens.

Associations   May occur in association with endocrine disorders (pituitary disorders and hyperthyroidism), hormone secreting neoplasms (Leydig cell tumours, of the testes, germ cell tumours secreting human chorionic gonadotrophin and some ectopic hormone-secreting small-cell tumours of the lung), liver cirrhosis, drugs (chlorpromazine, reserpine, digitalis, spironolactone and epanutin) and after oestrogen treatment for prostatic carcinoma.

Microscopy   Ducts commonly show some epithelial hyperplasia with no atypia. The stroma is abundant and in early cases or adolescents appears oedematous becoming fibrotic later.

Clinical features   Patients present with either unilateral (75%) or bilateral enlargement of the breast.

Carcinoma

Epidemiology   Rare. Accounts for 1% of all breast carcinomas in USA but up to 10% of all breast carcinomas in Egypt possibly due to gynaecomastia related to schistosomiasis related liver cirrhosis.

Associations   Increased risk associated with gynaecomastia and Klinefelter's syndrome.

Macroscopy   Usually firm mass.

Microscopy   Same spectrum of histological types as in the female but lobular carcinoma is very rare. Paget's disease and skin involvement occurs earlier than in females.

Prognosis   Similar prognosis stage for stage and grade for grade as in female.

The endocrine system

THE PITUITARY

ANATOMY

Site In the sella. Covered by the dura mater lining the sella and extending over the top of the sella as a firm sheet through which the stalk penetrates. The hypothalamus is divided longitudinally into a midline zone adjacent to the 3rd ventricle, two medial zones and two lateral zones. The neurohypophysis (posterior lobe) is an extension of the ventral portion of the hypothalamus and is attached to the dorsal and caudal surface of anterior pituitary. It is divided by the diaphragm into an upper portion (median eminence or infundibulum) and lower portion (pars nervosa).

Size Bean-shaped organ; average weight 0.6 g. Size increases during pregnancy and decreases with old age.

Vascular supply The hypothalamus receives blood from the circle of Willis. The posterior pituitary is supplied by the inferior hypophyseal artery. The superficial areas of the anterior pituitary are supplied by arteries penetrating the capsule while the main bulk (70–90% of the remainder) receives its blood supply via a system of portal vessels derived from the capillary network of the median eminence. Further blood comes from another portal system from the distal part of the stalk.

Appearance Anterior portion (80%) is reddish-brown while the posterior portion (20%) is grey.

HISTOLOGY AND FUNCTION
The anterior pituitary

Composed of three cell types distinguished by histochemical staining into acidophil (red with H&E, orange with PAS-

Orange G), basophil (bluish with H&E, pink with PAS-Orange G) and chromophobe (no staining). Immuno-cytochemical staining can identify five cell types responsible for secreting six hormones. Somatotropes (50% cell population, acidophil) secrete growth hormone and are found on the lateral wings of the gland. Lactotropes (15–20% acidophil or chromophobe) secrete prolactin with random distribution. Corticotropes (15–20%, basophil) secrete ACTH mainly in the central wedge. Thyrotropes (5%, basophil) secrete TSH mainly in the antero-medial portion. Gonadotropes (10%, basophil) secrete FSH and LH and are found mainly in the central wedge with a few in the lateral wings.

In the hypothalamus the cells secreting gonadotropin-releasing hormone are in the pre-optic region while those secreting growth hormone-releasing hormone are nerve cells in the median eminence of the pituitary stalk.

The neurohypophysis (posterior pituitary)

Consists of unmyelinated nerve fibres and specialized glial cells (pituicytes) of two types – type A have storage granules (300 nm diameter) containing oxytocin and vasopressin and type B cells have smaller granules (50–100 nm) containing amines. Vasopressin (anti-diuretic hormone) reduces urine output and conserves water by increasing resorbtion of solute-free water from renal distal and collecting tubules. Oxytocin is important in breastfeeding, inducing milk ejection by causing myoepithelial contraction.

DISORDERS OF FUNCTION OF ANTERIOR PITUITARY

HYPOPITUITARISM

Hypopituitarism as a result of lack of functioning tissue

Failure of development of anterior pituitary

Occurs in two situations: either defective formation of its anlage – Rathke's pouch– or in embryos with anencephaly.

Destruction of pituitary tissue

Causes Compression of tissue due to a neoplasm (pituitary adenoma, craniopharyngioma or metastatic tumour), infarction (Sheehan's syndrome is ischaemic necrosis of pituitary following severe fall in blood pressure usually in the late stages of pregnancy, at delivery or in parturition), other mechanical/compressive lesions (surgery, cysts of sella or hypothalamus fractures to base of skull), irradiation, autoimmune destruction or in inflammatory or infiltrative conditions (bacterial and viral infections, tuberculosis, sarcoidosis, haemochromatosis or Langerhans cell histiocytosis [histiocytosis X]).

Clinical features Reflect reduced or absent hormone secretion. In general needs 75% of gland loss to be manifest. Usually selective loss of hormones but can rarely involve all hormones (pan-hypopituitarism). May be expressed as hypothyroidism, hypoadrenalism, short stature, incomplete or delayed puberty, amenorrhoea (primary or secondary), fasting hypoglycaemia (due to loss of ACTH and/or growth hormone) or polyuria (lack of anti-diuretic hormone from the posterior pituitary).

HYPERPITUITARISM

Causes May be due to increased drive from releasing hormones but most often due to a secreting tumour of the anterior pituitary.

Pathogenesis Hyperfunction from a tumour may be due to direct secretion (usually single but may be more than one hormone) or due to interference with dopamine-mediated inhibition of prolactin secretion (causing hyperprolactinaemia).

Over-production of growth hormone (acromegaly and gigantism)

Causes Usually pituitary adenoma, but occasionally there is ectopic production from extrapituitary tumours (e.g. pancreatic islet tumour).

Acromegaly

Excess growth hormone causes increased protein secretion mediated via somatomedins (insulin-like growth factors). There is over-growth of bone and connective tissue with increased size of hands and feet together with skin thickening (98%), oligo/amenorrhoea in females (72%), excessive sweating (64%), headaches (55%), paraesthesias (40%), impotence (36%), hypertension (25–35%) and abnormal glucose tolerence (10–25%). There may be cardiac disease (30%) in addition to hypertension including concentric left ventricular hyperplasia and asymmetric septal hyperplasia. Myocardial ischaemia, cardiac failure and arrythmias are common. Rheumatological changes (50–75%) mainly of degenerative nature may occur.

Gigantism

Mostly due to somatotrope adenoma in childhood or adolescence but may be the result of excess growth hormone-releasing hormone. Affected individuals become very tall.

....

DISORDERS OF FUNCTION OF NEUROHYPOPHYSIS (POSTERIOR PITUITARY)

Deficiency of vasopressin secretion (diabetes insipidus)

Aetiology

Deficiency of vasopressin secretion (hypothalamic diabetes insipidus), decreased sensitivity of renal tubular cells to normal vasopressin levels (nephrogenic diabetes insipidus) or ingestion of excessive quantities of water leading to vaso-pressin supression (primary polydipsia). The commonest is due to damage to or loss of hypothalamic or neurohypophy-seal function which may be familial (either X-linked or auto-somal dominant or as association of diabetes insipidus, diabetes mellitus, optic atrophy, nerve deafness and atonia of bladder and ureters [DIDMOAD]) or acquired due to trauma, compression by tumours, infections (bacterial, viral, tubercu-losis) or infiltrations (sarcoid, Langerhans cell histiocytosis [histiocytosis X]), ischaemic necrosis or autoimmune disease.

Clinical features   Polyuria and blood hyperosmolarity.

Causes Ectopic secretion from tumours outside the pituitary, most commonly small cell bronchogenic carcinoma but also thymoma, mesothelioma, Hodgkin's disease, pancreatic, duodenal, uterine and prostatic carcinomas. Also seen in some primary CNS diseases, following administration of some drugs and in some non-neoplastic pulmonary diseases and during mechanical ventilation.

PITUITARY TUMOURS

Craniopharyngioma

Definition Tumour of the parasellar region thought to arise from squamous cell rests representing remains of Rathke's pouch.

Epidemiology Commonly in children in whom it accounts for 5–10% of all brain tumours. Also occurs in adults with 25% found in those > 40 years.

Clinical features Presents with visual disturbances, endocrine dysfunction (growth retardation, pituitary adrenal dysfunction [40%], loss of libido/impotence/menstrual irregularities, diabetes insipidus or hypothyroidism) or evidence of increased intracranial pressure.

Location Most are suprasellar but some are intrasellar.

Macroscopy Usually 3–4 cm diameter. May be solid or cystic. Focal calcification in 75% which may be seen on skull X-ray.

Microscopy Similar to ameloblastoma of jaw. Interlinked islands of epithelial cells with palisaded outer and stellate inner-cell regions.

Adenomas

Definition Arise from one or more cell types.

Epidemiology Constitute 10–15% all intracranial tumours and found incidentally in 6–24% unselected autopsies.

Classification By size into micro- (< 10 mm) and macroadenomas (> 10 mm), by hormone production (if present) and by growth pattern (expansile or invasive).

Natural history and prognosis Expansile pattern is associated with slow growth. Invasive growth is faster eroding the sella wall to involve other structures including the cavernous sinus, posterior pituitary, hypothalamus, optic chiasma and cranial nerves.

Null-cell adenoma

Epidemiology Commoner in older age. Seventeen per cent of pituitary adenomas.

Clinical features Relate to pressure effects on surrounding tissue notably optic chiasma and cranial nerves.

Macroscopy Mostly macroadenomas (> 10 mm diameter).

Microscopy Usually chromophobe cells. EM shows some secretory granules.

Oncocytic adenoma

Definition Variant of null-cell adenoma. Cells contain numerous mitochondria giving granular eosinophilic appearance.

Laboratory findings May be slight increase in prolactin due to interference with dopamine (inhibitor of prolactin secretion) passage from hypothalamus.

Macroscopy Often very large.

Microscopy Cells are large with granular eosinophilic cytoplasm.

Silent adenoma

Definition Adenomas in which the cells show immunoreactivity for one or other hormone (usually ACTH) but there is no hyperfunction.

Prolactin-producing adenoma

Epidemiology Commonest – 26% pituitary adenomas. Any age but most are young women.

Microscopy Chromophobe cells. Amyloid in stroma is a common finding.

Natural history and prognosis Hyperprolactinaemia of microadenomas can be treated by use of a dopamine agonist (e.g. bromocriptine). In macroadenomas this treatment may cause tumour shrinkage.

Growth-hormone secreting adenoma

Epidemiology Usually sporadic but can be part of MEN type 1.

Clinical features Gigantism if epiphysial union has not occurred or acromegaly if it has occurred.

Microscopy Acidophil or chromophobe cells.

ACTH-secreting adenoma

Associations Cause approximately 70% of cases of Cushing's syndrome and are associated with Nelson's syndrome (ACTH secreting adenoma following bilateral adrenalectomy for Cushing's syndrome).

Microscopy Most are microadenomas and mainly basophil type. Occasionally they may be chromophobe.

Natural history and prognosis Adenomas associated with Nelson's syndrome tend to be fast growing. Patients present with hyperpigmentation and signs of a space-occupying lesion.

Gonadotrope-secreting adenoma

Epidemiology Most common in middle-aged males.

Clinical presentation Most with evidence of a space occupying lesion. Hypogonadism with decreased libido and impotence are relatively frequent.

Laboratory findings Secrete FSH and LH either alone or in combination. FSH secretion is commonest with increased plasma levels of the whole hormone and its α and β subunits. Hypersecretion of LH is less common and is associated with raised plasma testosterone.

Thyrotrope adenoma

Epidemiology Rare. Most common in individuals with primary hypothyroidism.

Microscopy Most are chromophobe cells.

Carcinoma

Epidemiology Very rare.

Microscopy May show nuclear pleomorphism, atypical mitoses and focal necrosis but these features can be absent and show no morphological evidence of malignancy.

Natural history and prognosis Distant metastases occur.

ANATOMY

Weight   Combined weight 4–5 g.

Site   Paired organs.

HISTOLOGY

Divided into two functionally distinct regions.

Cortex

Constitutes peripheral 80% of gland. Divided into three zones:

1. **Zona glomerulosa** (5–10%). Secretes aldosterone. Discontinuous layer of small cells with large nuclei and little cytoplasmic lipid.
2. **Zona fasciculata** (80%). Secretes cortisol and androgens. Cells arranged in columns two cells thick perpendicular to the capsule.
3. **Zona reticularis** (5–10%). Secretes cortisol and androgens. Anastamosing columns one cell thick of smaller cells with less cytoplasmic lipid.

Age-related changes include the appearance of cortical nodules (more frequent in hypertensive and diabetic individuals).

Medulla

About 2 mm thick central portion accounting for about 10% adrenal weight. Single cell type – phaeochromocyte (chromaffin cell).

EMBRYOLOGY

During fetal life the cortex is divided into a large central zone (fetal cortex) which disappears after birth and an outer thin definitive cortex which becomes the adult cortex. This development is dependent on a functional pituitary.

The adrenal medulla arises from the phaeochromoblasts which are part of the primitive cells of the sympathetic nervous system (sympathogonia).

....

FUNCTION
Function of cortex

Secretes upwards of 50 hormones in three main functional groups, produced in the different zones of the cortex and derived from cholesterol as a common precursor.

1. **Mineralocorticoids** (zona glomerulosa). Mainly aldosterone (50% mineralocorticoid activity), 11-deoxycorticosterone and 18-oxocortisol. Target organs are the kidney (particularly the collecting tubules) gut, salivary glands, sweat glands, vascular endothelium and brain. The actions result in maintenance of intravascular volume by retention of sodium and elimination of potassium and hydrogen ions.
2. **Glucocorticoids** (zona fasciculata). Exert actions through effects on metabolism (inhibits action of insulin leading to increased blood sugar by increasing glycogenesis in liver and gluconeogenesis and decreasing glucose uptake in tissues; increases lipids by lipolysis; increases protein breakdown), on the immune system (decreases circulating lymphocytes [T > B]; decreases antibody formation; causes atrophy of thymus and lymphoid tissue; decreases vascular events in acute inflammation, chemotaxis and phagocytosis), on connective tissues (decreases collagen formation and wound healing), on calcium and bone metabolism (decreases serum calcium and increases osteoporosis), on the circulatory system (increases cardiac output and increases sensitivity to catecholamines leading to hypertension in excess), on the kidney (increases blood flow, free water clearance and excretion of potassium and hydrogen ions, decreases vasopressin action), on the CNS (decreasing cerebral oedema and libido and causing mood lability/psychosis), and on the endocrine system

(decreases response to TSH and GRH and decreasing secretion of gonadotrophins). Glucocorticoids show mineralocorticoid activity but about 400 times less than aldosterone.

3. **Adrenal androgens** (zona reticularis). Action exerted following conversion to active androgens (testosterone) and oestrogens (oestrone and oestradiol). In males the adrenal accounts for 2% androgens, in females the proportion is 50%.

Function of medulla   The principal function is production and storage of catecholamines (adrenaline and noradrenaline). Release of these is a result of release of acetylcholine by pre-ganglionic neurones.

REGULATION

Cortisol secretion is regulated by secretion of adreno-corticotrophic hormone (ACTH) from the anterior pituitary. ACTH is stimulated by hypothalamic derived corticotropin-releasing hormone (CRH). Release of both ACTH and CRH is modulated by negative feedback effect of blood cortisol.

DISORDERS OF FUNCTION: HYPOFUNCTION OF ADRENAL CORTEX

Lack of functioning adrenocortical tissue

Addison's disease

Epidemiology   Autoimmune Addison's disease associated with HLA-B8 and DR3.

Causes   Autoimmune disease accounts for 70% of adrenal hypofunction caused by loss of adrenal tissue in the West. In developing countries tuberculosis is the commonest cause and other infective causes include *Histoplasma capsulatum*.

Immunology   In 65% cases antibodies directed against adrenal cortex are found. Other organ specific antibodies are frequently found and Addison's disease may form part of polyglandular autoimmune deficiency syndromes in up to 40% of cases.

Clinical features Symptoms include weakness, fatigue, nausea, abdominal pain, diarrhoea and salt craving. Signs include weight loss, skin hyperpigmentation (due to increased MSH derived from cleavage of ACTH and β-lipotropin secreted in excess due to feedback stimulation of low cortisol).

Laboratory findings Low plasma sodium (95%) associated with high serum potassium (65%). Hypoglycaemia may occur. Low plasma cortisol and low urinary cortisol metabolites (17-ketosteroids). High ACTH levels and lack of response to ACTH infusion.

Microscopy Autoimmune type shows similar appearances to other autoimmune diseases. Tuberculosis shows destruction of the cortex by caseating granulomas.

Waterhouse–Fridrichsen syndrome and acute adrenal failure

Definition Waterhouse–Fridrichsen syndrome is acute adrenal failure in a child with meningococcal meningitis but it may occur in association with *Enterobacteriaceae* and *Pseudomonas* infections.

Clinical features Peripheral circulatory collapse (hypotension and peripheral vasoconstriction), cutaneous petechial haemorrhage, massive adrenal haemorrhage and features of disseminated intravascular coagulation.

Microscopy Haemorragic necrosis of the cortex.

Congenital adrenal hypoplasia

Causes Lack of normal drive in fetal life.

Associations Anencephaly, pituitary hypoplasia and hypothalamic malformations.

Lack of drive to adrenal cortex

Causes Lack of CRH or ACTH which may be caused by any lesion in the pituitary or hypothalamus including space-occupying lesions, inflammation or trauma to the pituitary stalk. The commonest cause is the result of prolonged treatment with glucocorticoids (rare unless the daily dose of hydrocortisone exceeds 15mg/m^2.

Lack of enzymes

Congenital adrenal hyperplasia

Definition   Set of genetically determined disorders caused by enzymatic defects in cortisol synthetic pathways.

Epidemiology   Congenital adrenal hyperplasia due to 21 α-hydroxylase deficiency (90% CAH) is an autosomal recessive genetic disorder present in 1:5000 in white populations with a gene carrier rate of 1:35.

Pathogenesis   Low plasma cortisol results in high CRH and ACTH causing adrenal cortical hyperplasia.

Clinical features   Vary with enzyme defect. Virilization is common. In the commonest form (21 α-hydroxylase deficiency) it presents in the female at birth and in the male during childhood. If the defect is early in the synthesis chain there is lack of androgen causing failure of normal male masculinization. If aldosterone synthesis or secretion is affected there will be hyponatraemia and hyperkalaemia.

Adrenoleukodystrophy

Definition   Syndrome characterized by chronic adrenal insufficiency due to cortical atrophy and diffuse demyelination of cerebral white matter.

Epidemiology   May be X-linked or autosomal recessive disorder.

Pathogenesis   Lack of the enzyme very long chain acyl-COA ligase activity resulting in accumulation of very long chain fatty acids in cells and blood.

Clinical features   X-linked disorders may present either between 5–10 years (commonest, 50% cases) with rapid deterioration of cerebral function leading to death usually within three years or in early adult life with gonadal failure, severe spastic paraparesis, sensory disturbances in lower limbs and disturbances of sphincter function (adreno-myeloneuropathy, 25% cases). The autosomal recessive disorder may present at birth.

Microscopy Progessive destruction of myelin in the brain with sparse macrophage infiltrate. Striations are apparent in the cells of the inner part of the zona fasciculata and the zona reticularis due to accumulation of very long chain fatty acids.

....

HYPERFUNCTION OF THE ADRENAL CORTEX

Glucocorticoid over-secretion (Cushing's syndrome)

History First recognized in 1910 by Harvey Cushing (while a medical student at Johns Hopkins) in a 23-year-old patient with an adrenal tumour.

Causes May be due to exogenous steroid ingestion or to endogenous hypersecretion which may be ACTH independent (cortisol-producing adrenal tumours, bilateral adrenal hyperplasia) or ACTH dependent (75% endogenous cases) usually pituitary adenoma of basophil cells (technically Cushing's disease) but also associated with ectopic ACTH production by other tumours (e.g. small cell carcinoma of lung, thymoma, pancreatic islet cell tumours, bronchial carcinoid, thyroid medullary carcinoma and some gonadal tumours).

Clinical features Centripetal obesity, high blood pressure, proximal muscle weakness, abdominal striae, hirsutism, thinning of scalp hair, backache, purpura and insomnia.

Laboratory findings Increased cortisol secretion is determined by increased 24 h urinary free cortisol (normal < 250 µg) with a disturbance of diurnal pattern (normally mean evening level is less than half mean morning level). The dexamethasone suppression test is positive in 90% pituitary driven hypersecretion cases but negative in ACTH independent hyperfunction. ACTH driven Cushing's will show an increased ACTH level following CRH administration.

Primary aldosterone over-secretion (Conn's syndrome)

Causes Aldosterone-producing adrenal cortical adenoma/carcinoma, associated with bilateral adrenal cortical (zona glomerulosa) hyperplasia or due to dexamethasone-suppressible hyperaldosteronism (autosomal dominant inherited disorder).

Clinical features Hypertension (causes 2% all cases of hypertension), headache, fatigability and muscle weakness.

Laboratory findings High plasma and urinary aldosterone, hypokalaemia and low plasma renin levels. There is usually a high plasma aldosterone/renin ratio following administration of 25–50 mg captopril.

Secondary aldosterone over-secretion

Cause High renin levels due to renal ischaemia, renin-producing tumours or oedema of variety of causes.

Laboratory findings High plasma and urinary aldosterone associated with high plasma renin.

Androgen over-secretion (adrenogenital syndrome)

Cause Commonest is congenital hyperplasia of the adrenal due to 21-hydroxylase or 11-β-hydroxylase deficiency. Some associated with tumours secreting sex steroids.

Clinical features Depends on age of onset and sex. In adult life the males show no obvious signs while females show hirsuitism, oligomenorrhoea and increased muscular development. In childhood males show precocious puberty while females show hirsuitism and clitoral enlargement.

Bilateral nodular adrenal hyperplasia

Cause Abnormal sensitivity of cortical cells to ACTH or as part of the Carney complex (primary nodular dysplasia of the adrenal cortex, myxomas, peripheral nerve tumours, pigmented skin lesions and various endocrine disorders) – an autosomal dominant inherited disorder associated with adrenal cortical stimulating serum immunoglobulins, or the McClune–Albright syndrome (hyperfunctioning nodules in adrenal, thyroid, pituitary and gonads) due to mutation affecting the stimulatory G protein activating adenylate cyclase. Occasionally it may be due to a factor which is not ACTH such as gastric inhibitory peptide (GIP).

···

TUMOURS OF THE ADRENAL CORTEX

Adenoma

Epidemiology   Aldosterone secreting tumours have peak incidence 20–40 years. Androgen-producing adenomas are rare.

Macroscopy   Glucocorticoid-secreting tumours are usually rounded, well-defined and encapsulated. Most are less than 5 cm diameter with yellow colour (some are black). Aldosterone-secreting tumours rarely exceed 2.5 cm, are usually single and unilateral and are bright yellow.

Microscopy   Glucocorticoid and androgen-producing adenomas show a mixture of clear and compact cells arranged in nests or clusters. Surrounding tissue shows suppression atrophy in adenomas secreting glucocorticoids but not in those producing androgens. Aldosterone-secreting adenomas resemble the zona fasciculata.

Carcinoma

Epidemiology   Rare; incidence of 2 per million in USA. Peak incidence 30–50 years.

Laboratory findings   May be functioning or non-functioning. Non-functioning more common in males, functioning more common in females.

Macroscopy   Those producing Cushing's syndrome are usually large and weigh more than 1 kg. The cut surface is yellow with focal haemorrhage or necrosis.

Microscopy   Cells contain less lipid than normal and are arranged in cords and solid alveoli. Pleomorphism is present and nucleoli are prominent. Determination of malignancy may not be easy.

Prognosis   Poor. Most die within three years of presentation. Metasases may occur with lungs and liver most frequent recipient.

TUMOURS OF THE ADRENAL MEDULLA

Phaeochromocytoma

Epidemiology Peak incidence 30–50 years, M:F 1:1. Slightly more common in whites than blacks. About 10–20% are familial, of which 50% are bilateral. Familial cases can be:

- inherited as an isolated autosomal dominant condition
- part of MEN IIa
- part of MEN IIb
- associated with neurofibromatosis
- associated with von Hippel–Lindau syndrome (with retinal and cerebellar haemangioblastomas)
- part of tuberous sclerosis (with sebaceous adenomas, mental deficiency and astrocytomas)
- part of Sturge–Weber syndrome (with haemangiomas).

Site About 10% are extra-adrenal.

Clinical features Hypertenstion (accounting for 0.2% all cases of hypertension) which may be sustained with or without paroxysmal elevations or can be purely paroxysmal. Paroxysms are associated with headache, sweating, anxiety, nausea, palpitations, pallor and abdominal pain. The presence of paroxysms, headache, sweating and palpitations in combination indicate a phaeochromocytoma with 94% specificity and 91% sensitivity.

Laboratory diagnosis Elevated 24 h urinary adrenaline/noradrenaline, vanillylmandelic acid (VMA) and/or metanephrine/normetanephrine in the absence of other causes which increase these urinary products such as amphetamines, methyl-DOPA, nalidixic acid and clonidine-withdrawal. Plasma catecholamines can be examined after collection in carefully controlled circumstances that will not lead to artificial elevation. Around 55% of phaeochromocytomas secrete both adrenaline and noradrenaline, 30% noradrenaline only and 15% adrenaline only.

Macroscopy Vary in size 1 g to 4 kg with average weight 200 g. Cut surface is grey-brown but turns deep brown if exposed to dichromate-containing fixative (due to stored catecholamines).

Microscopy Large cells with abundant rather basophilic cytoplasm which are arranged in nests or trabeculae with sinusoidal blood supply. Benign and malignant tumours are indistinguishable microscopically.

Natural history and prognosis Malignant phaeochromocytomas will manifest themselves by the appearance of metastatic deposits. Approximately 10% are malignant.

THE ENDOCRINE PANCREAS

DIABETES MELLITUS

Definition Set of disorders characterized by an absolute or relative deficiency of insulin or by insulin resistance which is primarily expressed as hyperglycaemia and glycosuria.

Classification At the simplest level diabetes can be divided into primary and secondary (i.e. part of another disease).

Primary diabetes mellitus

Insulin dependent diabetes mellitus (IDDM, juvenile onset or type 1 diabetes)

Epidemiology Accounts for 10% of all cases. Occurs mainly in young people with peak age 12 years.

Genetics In Caucasians 95% of IDDM patients have MHC haplotype HLA-DR3 or DR4 allele or both. HLA-DR2 appears to be protective against IDDM.

Non-genetic factors Support for environmental influences in the aetiology of IDDM is supported by the finding of considerable geographical variation in incidence (the further away from the Equator a population resides the greater the risk of IDDM, and country of origin is also important – risk for a Finnish child is 35 times that of a Japanese child). Changes in IDDM incidence has been too rapid to be accounted for by genetic variation. Migrants from a low-risk area acquire a higher risk when they move to a high-risk area. Also certain environmental agents are known to cause IDDM (e.g. congenital rubella is associated with a 20% chance of developing the disease).

Pathogenesis Characterized by autoimmune destruction of the β-cells in the islets of Langerhans associated with antibodies against these cells and against insulin.

Clinical features Patients typically complain of polyuria, polydipsia, tiredness, loss of appetite and loss of weight. There may be recurrent infections.

Biochemical features Shown in Table 40.1.

Non-insulin dependent diabetes mellitus (NIDDM, maturity onset or type 2 diabetes)

Epidemiology Commoner. Occurs in older people.

Table 40.1 Biochemical features of IDDM

• Effect on fat metabolism	There is increased plasma free fatty acids (FFA), triglycerides and cholesterol. The rise in FFA reflects increased flow of fatty acids from adipose tissue to the liver due to lipolysis resulting from loss of the normal inhibitory effect of insulin on a lipase in the adipose tissue.
• Effect on amino acid/protein metabolism	Severe insulin deficiency is accompanied by negative nitrogen balance and protein wasting (insulin normally stimulates protein synthesis and inhibits protein catabolism and release of amino acids from muscle).
• Diabetic ketoacidosis	In this condition there is a **metabolic acidosis** due to accumulation of ketones (notably β-hydroxybutyric acid and aceto-acetic acid) as a result of accelerated lipolysis, increased β-oxidation of free fatty acids in mitochondria (due to activation of acyl-carnitine transferase system) and decreased utilization of these organic acids in muscle tissue. **Hyperosmolarity** occurs due to hyperglycaemia (resulting from decreased utilization of glucose and increased hepatic glucose production) and water loss. **Dehydration** results from the osmotic diuresis accompanying hyperglycaemia and vomiting which is usually associated with severe metabolic acidosis.

Aetiology Associated with increasing age (in UK rare before age 35 years) and obesity (particularly abdominal obesity) and physical inactivity.

Pathogenesis No evidence for autoimmune disease although amyloid (derived from amylin) deposition in the islets of Langerhans is a frequent finding. Diminished insulin secretion (NB: although there is an absolute increase in insulin in obese diabetic patients there is a greater increase in insulin levels in non-diabetic obese individuals). It has been suggested that there is adequate basal insulin secretion to maintain normal glucose concentrations but that the response to feeding is inadequate, resulting in hypergylcaemia after meals with slow return to normogly-caemia. Basal insulin secretion then decreases. Blood glucose concentrations rise and stimulate insulin secretion and a new steady state is reached where both glucose and insulin levels are increased but the higher insulin levels are insufficient to restore glucose levels to normal. Many patients with NIDDM show insulin insensitivity possibly associated with obesity. Insulin resistance may result from failures in two possible phases. First the binding of insulin to its two unit glycoprotein receptors (i.e. deficiencies in number or function) or second in the post-binding stage in which there is secondary messenger generation.

Other forms of primary diabetes

- **Maturity onset diabetes in the young** (MODY)
  Definition Non-insulin dependent diabetes in the young.
  Genetics Autosomal dominant inheritance.
- **Impaired glucose intolerance**
  Associated with a 20–60% chance of developing diabetes over a 10-year period.
- **Gestational diabetes mellitus.**

Natural history and prognosis of diabetes

With current treatments following the discovery of insulin ketoacidosis with dehydration, coma and death are declining in frequency. Major long-term dangers of diabetes arise due to a marked incremental effect on atherogenesis (the relative risk of coronary heart disease is 1.9, of stroke is 2.5 and of large vessel peripheral vascular disease leading to intermittent claudication and eventually diabetic gangrene is 4.0) and to structural and functional changes in microvasculature particularly affecting the retina, kidney, peripheral and autonomic nervous systems.

Metabolic aspects of diabetic complications

Non-enzymic glycosylation of proteins

This is due to hyperglycaemia. In aqueous solution glucose is a mixture of ring forms and a straight chain aldehyde form. The aldehyde form binds spontaneously and non-enzymatically to the epsilon amino acid groups of lysine residues on the amino terminal of proteins forming **Schiff bases** which can undergo slow but irreversible rearrangement into a ketamine configuration (Amadori rearrangement). Glycosylation of haemoglobin is a very common event especially if diabetic control is not efficient (HbA1c). The measurement of this glycosylated haemoglobin is an effective means of determining the degree of glycaemic control over the preceding 2–3 months.

Glycosylation of serum proteins such as immunoglobulins and albumin can form cross-linkages with glycosylated tissue proteins (possibly contributing to thickening of capillary basement membrane). Glycosylation of fibrin decreases the susceptibility to cleavage by plasmin (possibly increasing the risk of thrombosis) and glycosylation of low-density lipoprotein (LDL) inhibits its binding to the LDL receptor impairing LDL catabolism and leading to an increase in the plasma concentrations of this atherogenic lipoprotein. In addition glycosylated LDL binds to connective tissue matrices within the wall of both large and small blood vessels, contributing to the thickening of the basement membrane.

Sorbitol pathway, myo-inositol and sodium-potassium ATPase

In the sorbitol pathway fructose is produced from circulating glucose by the 'polyol' pathway which consists of 2 steps:

1. Glucose + NADPH → sorbitol + NADP⁺ catalysed by aldose reductase.

2. Sorbitol + NAD$^+$ → fructose + NADH catalysed by sorbitol dehydrogenase.

High levels of intracytoplasmic sorbitol are believed to contribute to some diabetic complications due to increased tissue osmolality (most notably causing cataract).

Diabetics lose excessive amounts of myo-inositol in their urine and lack of this is thought to be associated with reduction in nerve conduction velocity.

Morphological features of diabetic complications

Capillary basement membrane thickening

The basic pathological feature in the chief targets for diabetic complications (kidney, retina and peripheral and autonomic nerves) is the same – hyaline thickening of the walls of arterioles and capillaries. The basement membrane is thickened by structureless eosinophilic material that stains strongly with periodic acid-Schiff stains. This thickening is associated with increased vascular permeability.

The diabetic kidney

Epidemiology　Renal failure is a frequent complication of diabetes causing death in 30–50% of those developing the disease in childhood.

Clinical features　The chief clinical presentations relate to glomerular syndromes (proteinuria, nephrotic syndrome, chronic renal failure), recurrent and chronic pyelonephritis and papillary necrosis.

Diabetic glomerular disease

Epidemiology　Occurs in more than 50% of patients with IDDM and about one-third of patients with NIDDM.

Clinical features　Initial manifestation is proteinuria.

Microscopy　May include one or more of:

- **Diffuse basement membrane thickening**. This is followed by increased mesangial matrix which ultimately obliterates the whole glomerulus. It is associated with hyaline thickening of both afferent and efferent arterioles.

- **Nodular glomerulosclerosis (Kimmelstiel–Wilson lesion)**. Deposition of glycoprotein in a nodular fashion within the mesangium near the periphery of the glomerular lobules. These may be single or multiple. They contain fibrin and low density lipoprotein.

- **Exudative lesions**. Areas, usually involving the tips of the glomerular capillary loops, that show a fuzzy, brightly eosinophilic appearance believed to be due to accumulation of protein, notably fibrin.

- **Capsular 'drop'**. Small hyaline eosinophilic nodule projecting from the capsule into Bowman's space.

Natural history and prognosis   Renal failure may supervene within 4–5 years following development of proteinuria.

Renal papillary necrosis complicating urinary tract infections

Pathogenesis   There may be compromise of the relatively poor blood supply to the medulla due to diabetic small vessel disease. Urinary tract infection combined with relative ischaemia and poor local tissue defences may account for many cases.

Macroscopy   The renal pelvis may be filled with purulent debris. Small abscesses may be present in cortex and medulla. Some or all of the papillae may be necrotic with greyish-yellow colour. In some cases there is detachment of the necrotic papillae leaving a ragged edge to the affected calyx.

Microscopy   Usually complete necrosis of the affected papillae. There is a heavy inflammatory infiltrate at the demarcation zone between necrotic and viable tissue and the tubules in the viable area contain pus.

Diabetic retinopathy

Epidemiology   Causes blindness in about 30–40 000 individual per year in the UK.

Microscopy   The earliest change is loss of capillary pericytes (whose role includes controlling blood flow through retinal vessels and maintaining the stability of these vessels). This is followed by a number of changes including:

- basement membrane thickening
- development of small aneurysms (due to lost pericytes)
- presence of well-defined small yellow-white patches (hard exudates) which are accumulations of lipid
- small haemorrhages ('dot and blot' haemorrhages)
- beaded appearance along vessels
- ischaemic areas in the superficial retina manifested by soft exudates ('cotton-wool' spots)
- Neovascularization elicited by patchy ischaemia of the retina. Extension of the new blood vessel formation into the vitreous may be followed by haemorrhages and scarring in the vitreous.

TUMOURS AND HYPERPLASIAS OF THE ISLETS

- Islet cell tumours and hyperplasias are less common than exocrine tumours. They may be benign or malignant but distinction on histological criteria alone is often difficult or impossible.
- They may be silent (non-secretory) or characterized by enzyme hypersecretion.
- They are commonly referred to as APUDomas following the concept of the APUD (**A**mine **P**recursor **U**ptake and **D**ecarboxylation) system with a supposed common origin from the neural crest.

β-cell tumour (insulinoma)

Epidemiology   Commonest islet cell tumour.

Macroscopy   Variable from tiny to large. May be multiple.

Microscopy   Interlacing cords and ribbons of epithelial cells with a sinusoidal-type pattern of blood vessels. Immunohistochemistry shows the cells to stain with antibodies to insulin.

Ultrastructure   Secretory granules show a rather crystalline core.

Clinical features Hyperinsulinaemia results in hypoglycaemia leading to:

- confusion
- blurred vision
- muscle weakness
- sweating
- palpitations.

Gastrinoma

Epidemiology Second commonest islet cell tumour.

Macroscopy and microscopy Indistinguishable from insulinomas. Diagnosis depends on demonstration of gastrin secretion either by serological studies (before surgery) or by immunohistochemical studies of histological material.

Clinical features Excess gastrin secretion (ectopic hormone secretion as gastrin is not normally secreted by islet cells) results in gastric acid hypersecretion and recurrent peptic ulceration (Zollinger–Ellison syndrome). About 60% behave in a malignant way with spread to regional nodes and liver.

α-cell tumours (glucagonomas)

Epidemiology Rare: most frequent in peri- or postmenopausal women.

Macroscopy and microscopy Indistinguishable from other islet cell tumours. Diagnosis depends on demonstration of glucagon secretion either by serological studies (before surgery) or by immunohistochemical studies of histological material.

Clinical features Patients have anaemia, mild diabetes and a migratory and necrotizing rash mainly over lower body. More than 50% behave malignantly with spread to regional lymph nodes and liver.

VIPomas

Biological features Arise from D_1 cells and secrete vasoactive intestinal peptide. There is over-stimulation of the

Table 40.2 MEN syndromes

MEN I	Tumour or hyperplasia
	Parathyroid
	Pituitary
	Adrenal cortex
	Pancreatic islets
MEN IIa	Phaeochromocytoma
	Medullary carcinoma of thyroid
	Parathyroid hyperplasia or adenoma
MEN IIb	Medullary carcinoma of thyroid
	Phaeochromocytoma
	Mucocutaneous neuromas

adenyl cyclase system in small intestinal epithelial cells resulting in excess transport of water, chloride, sodium and potassium from the cell into the lumen with blocking of the absorption of water, sodium and chloride across villous epithelium.

Clinical features Patients have profuse watery diarrhoea with hypokalaemia and achlorhydria (Verner–Morrison syndrome). The majority behave benignly.

Multiple endocrine neoplasia (MEN) syndromes and the pancreas

Definition Symptom complexes resulting from tumours or hyperplasia in two or more organs (see Table 40.2).

Clinical features A patient with MEN I may present with amenorrhoea and galactorrhoea (due to prolactin producing tumour in pituitary), hypercalcaemia (associated with hyperparathyroidism) and/or Zollinger–Ellison syndrome.

THYROID

ANATOMY

Size Gland consists of two lobes 4 cm in length, 2–2.5 cm in width joined by an isthmus.

Weight 14.5 g in women, 18 g in men.

Position Lower portion of anterior surface of neck.

DEVELOPMENT

Medial portion from foramen caecum beginning descent to adult position at 5th week gestation. Lateral portions from the ultimobranchial body producing the calcitonin-secreting parafollicular C cells.

THYROID HORMONES

Control

Hypothalamic–pituitary–thyroid axis under negative feedback control. Circulating thyroid hormone exerts inhibitory feedback on pituitary. The pituitary receives a tonic stimulation by thyrotropin-releasing hormpone (TRH) from the hypothalamus. In the thyroid hormone production is controlled by TSH, binding to epithelial surface membrane receptors.

Production

Iodide is actively transported from plasma into follicular cells. Approximately 80 μg iodide is needed each day. Iodide is converted to iodine and bound to tyrosyl residues of thyroglobulin. One molecule of di-iodotyrosine fuses either with a mono-iodotyrosine of another di-iodotyrosine molecule to form an iodothyronine. Resorption of this from the follicular lumen is by endocytosis. Thyroglobulin is digested and free hormone is secreted into capillaries adjacent to basement membrane. Plasma levels: 5 ng/dl.

Transport

About 90 μg T4 and 30 μg T3 are secreted daily with 99.7% bound to thyroid binding globulin (TBG, 75% of T4), transthyretin (15% of T4) and albumin (10% T4). TBG levels are increased by pregnancy, oestrogens, oral contraceptives, hepatitis and porphyria and decreased by androgens, liver cirrhosis and the nephrotic syndrome.

Action

Multi-system effects. Probably bind to nuclear receptors leading to changes in gene expression. Important in normal development and growth of infants particularly the central nervous system.

....

ABNORMALITIES OF THYROID DEVELOPMENT

Non-descent   Results in lingual thyroid.

Failure of normal descent   Ectopic thyroid anywhere along normal path of descent.

Abnormally low descent   Retrosternal thyroid.

Failure of fusion of C cell portion.

Lateral aberrant thyroid   Thyroid tissue lateral to the jugular vein. If not in lymph node may be developmental abnormality (within nodes most likely metastatic carcinoma).

....

DISORDERS OF THYROID FUNCTION: HYPOTHYROIDISM

Epidemiology   Affects up to 2% of the population. Disorder of middle age. M:F 1:10.

Clinical features   Lethargy, memory defects, decreased physical ability and libido, constipation and nausea, dry rough skin, hair loss, brittle nails and intolerance of cold.

Congenital hypothyroidism (cretinism) presents in first two months of life with abnormal facial features, decreased growth and general inactivity. If untreated mental retardation develops.

Causes   Loss of thyroid tissue mass (agenesis, destruction by surgery or irradiation [radio-iodine or external], autoimmune destruction or associated with abnormal infiltrates), lack of thyroid drive (TRH or TSH deficiency or block), lack of substrate (iodine deficiency) or lack of enzymes (including enzyme-blocking drugs). Cretinism may be due to abnormal thyroid development, iodine deficiency or enzyme deficiency (e.g. Pendred's syndrome – lack of peroxidase – associated with mild hypothroidism and nerve deafness).

Microscopy In cases without tissue loss as a cause the thyroid shows follicular epithelial hyperplasia due to increased TSH secretion.

Hashimoto's thyroiditis

Epidemiology Commonest cause of hypothyroidism. Disease of middle age with predilection for females. Increased in people with HLA-DR5 haplotype (relative risk 3:2).

Aetiology and pathogenesis Autoimmune disease in which the mechanism of damage is obscure. Theories include escape of sequestered antigens to which immune tolerance has not developed, abnormal presentation of self-antigens, deficiency of suppressor T cells or genetic factors.

Clinical features Presents with goitre (75% of which are euthyroid), hypothyroidism or occasionally hyperthyroidism (possibly combined Hashimoto's and Graves' diseases – Hashitoxicosis).

Laboratory findings Confirmation of diagnosis involves establishing thyroid status and identifying circulating antibodies to thryoglobulin and thyroid epithelial microsomes.

Macroscopy Gland is moderately enlarged, pale and more opaque. Cut surface shows nodularity. In longstanding cases gland may be shrunken and weigh only a few grams.

Microscopy Infiltration by lymphocytes and plasma cells. Lymphoid follicles with germinal centres common. Smaller thyroid follicles with small amounts of dark-staining colloid. Follicular cells become cuboidal with eosinophilic granular cytoplasm due to large numbers of mitochondria (variously called oncocytic, Askanazy or Hurthle cells). In long-standing cases there may be extensive fibrosis with mild or moderate lymphoid infiltrate and virtually complete loss of thyroid follicular tissue.

DISORDERS OF THYROID FUNCTION: HYPERTHYROIDISM

Causes Autoimmune mechanism via thyroid-stimulating antibodies (Graves' disease, 90% cases), functional thyroid tumours, TSH secreting pituitary tumours, iatrogenic (drugs, iodide), sub-acute thyroiditis with transient hyperfunction or mild stimulatory effect of human chorionic gonadotrophin, for example in hydatidiform mole.

Graves's disease (autoimmune thyroid hyperplasia)

Epidemiology Occurs at any age, commonest in women (M:F 1:5) between 20–40 years. Associated with HLA-DR3 (relative risk 3.7) and HLA-B8.

Aetiology and pathogenesis Serum autoantibodies against an epitope of TSH receptor in 90% patients mimicking TSH stimulation. Other antibodies include those that stimulate growth of thyroid epithelium. May be due to genetic factors (often family history, high concordance in twins and increased risk in first-degree relatives), cross-reacting antibodies to infectious agents (e.g. *Yersinia enterocolitica* has TSH binding site) or defects in T-suppressor activity.

Clinical features Usually diffuse enlargement of thyroid which is initially soft but hardens later. Wide-ranging clinical features including nervousness, fatigue, inability to concentrate and irritability, weight loss and tremor. There may be focally increased mucin deposition in the tissues of the legs (pre-tibial myxoedema). Ocular changes are present in 25–50% with lid lag, lid retraction and stare. Increased volume of intraorbital tissue may result in bulging of the eyes (exophthalmos) and is frequently associated with pretibial myxoedema.

Laboratory findings Depends on the demonstration of elevated circulating T3 or T4. A TSH stimulation test may be needed if conventional measurements are not diagnostic. TSH receptors can be assayed by bioassay of the effect of patient's plasma on cell cultures or by immunological binding studies.

Macroscopy Diffusely enlarged gland, reddish-brown colour with meatier than normal cut surface.

Microscopy Hyperplastic follicles with papillary infoldings. Tall columnar lining cells with basal nuclei and often clear cytoplasm. Scanty colloid feebly eosinophilic with scalloped edge where usually in contact with epithelium. Foci of lymphoid cells with occasional germinal centres in stroma.

Toxic nodular goitre

Definition Nodular enlargement of the thyroid with excess production of thyroid hormones.

Epidemiology Usually older age groups.

Macroscopy Large gland in which there may be many nodules or, more rarely, a single nodule.

Clinical features No pre-tibial myxoedema or eye changes.

....

NON-TOXIC GOITRE

Definition Thyroid enlargement not due to neoplasia or infiltrative disease and without hyperthyroidism.

Aetiology Environmental factors (iodide deficiency), intrinsic defects in hormone synthesis, growth promoting plasma immunoglobulins, goitrogenic foodstuffs (e.g. cabbage, turnips and kale) or drugs that inhibit iodide uptake/hormone sythesis/hormone release (e.g. thionamides, amiodarone, lithium, fluoride and carbutamide).

Iodide-deficiency goitre

Epidemiology Increased risk in countries far from the sea such as Switzerland, the Andes and the Himalayas. In some areas affects up to 10% of the population.

Clinical features Often presents at times of increased need e.g. puberty, pregnancy and during lactation. Diffuse colloid goitre is most often seen in adolescence and pregnancy.

Macroscopy May produce a diffuse hyperplastic goitre with little increase in thyroid size, a diffuse colloid goitre with glistening pale yellowish colloid in the distended follicles or a nodular goitre with marked enlargement (up to 2 kg) and irregular nodules. There may be haemorrhage, cystic change and calcification.

Microscopy In the diffuse hyperplastic goitre there is epithelial hyperplasia and little colloid. In the diffuse colloid goitre there are distended follicles containing colloid with flattened epithelium. In the nodular goitre there is marked variability of the appearances in terms of follicle size cell morphology and arrangement (some papillae formations) and there may be evidence of haemorrhage with haemosiderin and cholesterol clefts.

....

THYROIDITIS

Acute bacterial thyroiditis

Aetiology Direct spread from adjacent structures or haematological spread from distant foci. Commonly haemolytic streptococci, *Escherichia coli* and pneumococcus.

Clinical features Severe local pain, tenderness and enlargement accompanied by fever, rigors and malaise. Histological material not usually available.

Sub-acute thyroiditis (De Quervain's or granulomatous thyroiditis)

Aetiology Thought to be viral in origin. Both mumps and human syncytial viruses have been isolated in patients.

Clinical features Painful swollen thyroid gland. May be transient hyperthyroidism early in disease followed by euthyroid phase and then hypothyroidism. Self-limiting in most cases with spontaneous recovery of thyroid function in 6 weeks to 6 months.

Microscopy Granulomas with giant cells are the characteristic finding.

Riedel's thyroiditis

Epidemiology   Very rare.

Aetiology   Unknown.

Macroscopy   Woody hard consistency to thyroid, often fixed to surrounding tissues.

Microscopy   Thyroid replaced by fibrous tissue with focal lymphocytic infiltration. Surviving thyroid tissue often atrophic.

'Silent' thyroiditis

Epidemiology   Often post-partum.

Clinical features   Abrupt onset of hyperthyroidism. Gland is non-tender. Spontaneous resolution after period of weeks or months.

Macroscopy   Minimal enlargement of the gland.

Microscopy   Lymphocytic and plasma cell infiltrate with occasional follicle centres similar to Hashimoto's thyroiditis but lacking all other features of the latter disease.

....

BENIGN TUMOURS
Follicular adenoma

Definition   While several morphological patterns exist almost all benign tumours of the thyroid can be considered to be follicular adenomas. For a nodule to be considered a neoplasm it must be truly solitary and there should be complete encapsulation, follicular architecture that is different from the surrounding gland and compression atrophy of normal gland.

Epidemiology   More common in young adults, M:F 1:5.

Clinical features   Mostly a painless lump although pain may occur if there in intratumoural haemorrhage.

Macroscopy   Round encapsulated nodule up to 10 cm in diameter which often differs in colour and consistency from surrounding thyroid.

Microscopy Follicles are of differing size. Adenomas categorized as trabecular, microfollicular (minute follicles with very little colloid), normo (macro-)follicular, atypical (cellular pleomorphism present) or Hurthle cell (enlarged eosinophilic and granular cells) dependent on the dominant pattern. Categories have no prognostic significance.

....

MALIGNANT TUMOURS

Epidemiology Rare, up to 1% of all malignancies with 10 000 new cases and 1000 cancer-related deaths in the USA per year.

Associations Features suggesting malignancy in a solitary thyroid nodule include previous irradiation (external or radio-iodine), a family history of endocrine neoplasia (multiple endocrine neoplasia syndromes IIa and IIb), rapid growth, dysphagia, signs of local invasion (e.g. Horner's syndrome, hoarseness), cervical lymphadenopathy, male sex and young age.

Diagnosis Once a nodule has been confirmed as solitary, cytological examination of fine needle aspirate of the nodule will give a 90% specificity and 70% sensitivity for the diagnosis of malignancy in suspicious lesions. If cytology reveals a follicular thyroid lesion then radio-iodine will distinguish betwen hot (positive uptake) and cold nodules. Of the cold nodules 20% will be malignant.

Papillary carcinoma

Epidemiology Up to 70% of thyroid carcinomas. Occult tumours found incidentally in 10% autopsies show no peak age incidence and M:F 1:1. Overt tumours are rarer, affecting 1 in 27 000 people per year; peak incidence 20–50 years with M:F 1:2–3.

Aetiology Associated with irradiation in childhood.

Macroscopy Most are well defined but unencapsulated (only 5% show complete encapsulation). Occult tumours are less than 1 cm, star-shaped and show fibrosis.

Microscopy Papillae with fibrovascular cores are covered by neoplastic cells. Some tumours contain more typical follicles giving a mixed papillary-follicular pattern or follicular variant depending on the proportion of follicular pattern. The tumour cells have a characteristic appearance, being columnar or cuboidal. The nuclei are large and pale with an empty appearance on fixed and processed material (so-called 'Orphan Annie' nuclei after the comic-strip character). Nuclei show grooving and may contain pseudoinclusions. Psammoma bodies (spherical calcified nodules) are seen in the stroma of about 50% of cases. Direct extension into surrounding tissues is seen in about 25% and palpable nodal metastases in up to 50% cases.

Natural history and prognosis Cure rate is high and in those not cured this is most frequently an indolent disease. Overall, 90% 10-year survival and 80% 20-year survival. Factors associated with worse prognosis are older age, multi-centric origin in thyroid, undifferentiated foci, large size, extraglandular spread and presence of blood-borne metastases.

Follicular carcinoma

Epidemiology Rarer than papillary carcinoma. About 15% of thyroid malignancies. Occurs later in life (median age 52 years), M:F 1:2–5.

Clinical features Most present as a 'cold' nodule.

Macroscopy Appears well-encapsulated with thick fibrous capsule. Colloid content is variable.

Microscopy In well-differentiated lesions distinction from benign nodules can be difficult. The defining criterion for malignancy is invasion through capsule or intravascular permiation.

Natural history and prognosis Well-differentiated and minimally invasive tumours have good prognosis but overall only 30% 10-year survival after primary treatment. Poor prognostic factors include older age, marked invasion, aneuploid tumour cells and presence of metastatic disease at presentation (seen in about 15%, bone and lung most frequent sites).

Anaplastic (undifferentiated carcinoma)

Epidemiology   Around 10–15% of thyroid malignancies. Any age but peak in 7th decade.

Aetiology   Thought to arise from pre-existing well-differentiated tumour.

Macroscopy   Marked invasion of thyroid and surrounding structures. Necrosis and haemorrhage frequently obvious.

Microscopy   Variable pattern with spindle cells, 'squamoid' epithelial cells and giant cells. Bizarre mitoses frequently seen.

Natural history and prognosis   Very poor prognosis with mean survival 6–8 months from presentation.

Medullary carcinoma of the thyroid

Definition   Malignant tumour of thyrocalcitonin secreting parafollicular (C) cells. May secrete a number of products including calcitonin.

Epidemiology   Accounts for about 10% thyroid malignancies. May be sporadic (90%) or hereditary (autosomal dominant) as part of multiple endocrine neoplasia (MEN) syndrome type IIa (medullary thyroid carcinoma [90%], phaeochromocytoma of adrenal medulla [50%] and hyperparathyroidism [10–20%, mostly hyperplasia]) or MEN type IIb (medullary thyroid carcinoma, phaeochromocytoma, ganglioneuromas and neuromas of tarsal plate, anterior third of tongue, lips and alimentary tract). Occasional hereditary tumours are unrelated to MEN syndromes.

Macroscopy   Sporadic tumours usually single but hereditary ones are frequently multiple and bilateral.

Microscopy   Tumour cells are either spindle-shaped or rounded and arranged in sheets or nests. Amyloid is characteristically seen in the stroma of both primary and metastatic deposits.

Clinical features   May present with thyroid nodule, cervical or mediastinal lymphadenopathy, distant metastases (principally lung, liver, bone and adrenals) or as a result of hormones secreted by tumour causing diarrhoea (seen in

30% patients with widespread tumour) or – rarely – Cushing's syndrome.

Natural history and prognosis More aggressive than papillary carcinoma. Overall 65% 10-year survival. Cervical/ mediastinal lymph node metastases occur in 50% patients. Worse prognosis associated with sporadic tumours, age > 50 years at diagnosis and presence of metastases at presentation.

41

The haemopoietic system

HAEMOPOIESIS AND DISORDERS OF THE BLOOD

NORMAL HAEMOPOIESIS

Sites of haemopoiesis depend on age (Table 41.1).

With maturation active haemopoietic bone marrow is replaced by fatty adipose tissue leaving the axial skeleton (vertebral bodies, ribs, sternum and pelvis) and the proximal ends of of the humerus and femur as normal sites of haemopoiesis. If drive for haemopoiesis increases active marrow can spread down the medullary cavities of the long bones.

Normal maturation

All the cellular elements of the blood are derived from a pluripotent stem cell giving rise to a series of intermediate progenitors from which the individual cell lineages arise. Two main classes of intermediate progenitor exist – a common lymphoid progenitor and a cell which, when appropriately stimulated, gives rise to colonies of cells which show multiple differentiation (colony-forming units capable of giving rise to cells which differentiate into granulocytes, erythroid cells, monocytes and megakaryocytes, CFU_{GEMM}). This is a complex interplay involving many cytokines (Table 41.2).

Table 41.1 Sites of haemopoiesis

Fetal life 0–6 wks	Yolk sac
Fetal life 6 wks–6/7 months	Liver and spleen
Fetal life 6/7 months-term	Liver, spleen and bone marrow
Neonatal period 0–2 wks	Liver, spleen and bone marrow
Childhood and adult life	Bone marrow

Table 41.2 Regulation of haemopoiesis

Factor	Cellular target
M-CSF From endothelial cells, monocytes and fibroblasts	Monocytes
GM-CSF From T cells, endothelial cells and fibroblasts	Granulocytes, megakaryocytes, erythrocytes, stem cells and leukaemic blasts
G-CSF From endothelial cells, placenta and monocytes	Granulocytes, endothelial cells, macrophages, fibroblasts and leukaemic blasts
IL-3 From T cells	Granulocytes, red cells and their precursors, multi-potent stem cells and leukaemic blasts
IL-4 From T cells	B and T cells
IL-5 From T cells	B cells and CFU_{EO}
IL-6 From fibroblasts, leucocytes and epithelial cells	B and T cells, CFU_{GEMM}, CFU_{GM}, BFU_E, macrophages, nerve cells and liver cells
IL-7 From leucocytes	B cells
IL-8 From leucocytes	T cells and neutrophils
IL-9 From lymphocytes	CFU_{GEMM}, and BFU_E
IL-11 From macrophages	B and T cells, CFU_{GEMM} and macrophages
Erythropoietin from kidney (90%) and liver (10%)	BFU_E and CFU_E
Stem cell factor (c-kit ligand) from bone marrow stromal cells	Pluripotent stem cells

IL-1 and TNF-α stimulate haemopoiesis by stimulating production of GM-CSF, G-CSF, M-CSF and IL-6.

RED CELL FUNCTION

Haemoglobin

This mediates the red cell function of transporting oxygen to tissues and carbon dioxide away from them.

Table 41.3 Structure of haemoglobin

Normal adult	Two α chains and two β chains ($\alpha_2\beta_2$)
Early fetal life Haemopoiesis in yolk sac	Two ζ chains and two ε chains ($\zeta_2\varepsilon_2$) – Hb Gower I
Later fetal life	Two α chains and two ε chains ($\alpha_2\varepsilon_2$) – Hb Gower II Two ζ chains and two γ chains ($\zeta_2\gamma_2$) – Hb Portland
3 months' gestation	Two α chains and two γ chains ($\alpha_2\gamma_2$) – fetal Hb (HbF)

Structure (see Table 41.3)

Four globin chains and a haem group form a molecule of haemoglobin. The globin chains vary with maturation.

From three months' gestation the proportion of HbF decreases to 80% at 35 weeks' gestation with the remainder being mostly adult haemoglobin HbA ($\alpha_2\beta_2$). Thereafter the proportion of HbF continues to drop at a rate of about 3–4% per week.

The affinity of haemoglobin for oxygen is decreased by high concentrations of 2,3-diphosphoglycerate, high concentrations of hydrogen ions, high concentration of carbon dioxide and the presence of certain abnormal haemoglobins. Affinity is increased by the presence of large amounts of fetal haemoglobin and the presence of certain abnormal haemoglobins that are associated with polycythaemia.

....

DISORDERS OF RED CELLS

Anaemia

Definition   Haemoglobin concentration in the blood below normal (i.e. below 13.5 g/dl in adult males; below 11.5 g/dl in adult females).

Aetiology   Usually associated with a fall in red cell numbers and total red cell mass but may be associated with increased plasma volume (e.g. in pregnancy).

Clinical features

Effect is produced by decreasing the oxygen-carrying capacity of the blood. This is modulated by the rapidity of onset, degree of anaemia, age of the individual, changes in the oxygen dissociation curve and the capacity of the heart and lungs to compensate for the anaemia. Symptoms of severe anaemia include dyspnoea (may be present at rest) and patients may complain of fatigue, dizziness, weakness and a feeling of faintness (especially on standing). Physical signs include pallor of skin and mucous membranes, tachycardia, full bounding pulse, cardiac enlargement and pulmonary or apical systolic murmurs.

Classification

May be kinetic or morphological.

Kinetic Normally production = destruction. Numbers will decline if there is increased destruction/loss/pooling or decreased production. Destruction may be due to:

- blood loss – acute or chronic haemorrhage
- haemolysis – either due to disorders outside the red cell (antibodies, infections such as malaria, sequestration and destruction in the spleen, drugs, chemicals, physical agents, disorders such as lymphoma or red cell trauma) or intrinsic red cell disorders (hereditary [membrane defects, abnormal haemoglobins, enzyme deficiencies] or acquired [paroxysmal nocturnal haemoglobinuria, lead poisoning]).

Inadequate production of red cells

Table 41.4 lists causes of inadequate red cell production.

Table 41.4 Morphological classification of anaemia

Nutritional deficiencies	Vitamin B_{12}, iron, folic acid, protein, vitamin C, vitamin B_6, copper.
Insufficient erythroblasts	Atrophy of marrow involving all cell lines • idiopathic, • chemicals and drugs • congenital/pure red cell aplasia • thymoma • congenital (Diamond–Blackfan syndrome) • associated with autoimmune disease
Infiltration of marrow	Leukaemia/lymphoma, plasma cell dyscrasias, carcinoma, sarcoma, myelofibrosis
Renal/hepatic/endocrine disease	

Morphological Based on size and haemoglobin content.

Macrocytic Red cells are larger than normal. Red cell numbers are decreased in relation to haemoglobin content and red cell mass.

Microcytic, hypochromic Red cells are smaller than normal. Haemoglobin and red cell mass are decreased in relation to number of red cells.

Normocytic Red cell size unchanged.

Normochromic Red cell haemoglobin concentration is normal.

....

MACROCYTIC ANAEMIA

A macrocyte is a red cell with increased MCV (> 100 fl), increased MCH and normal MCHC. In a blood film the cells exceed 8.5 μm diameter and lack the central pale zone.

Megaloblastic macroctytic anaemia

Definition Megaloblastosis is the morphological expression of retarded red cell DNA synthesis.

Aetiology The commonest cause is deficiency of either vitamin B_{12} (e.g. pernicious anaemia) or folate (nutritional deficiency or malabsorption states such as coeliac sprue). Other causes include rare inherited disorders of DNA synthesis (orotic aciduria) and drug-induced disorders of DNA synthesis.

Pathogenesis Vitamin B_{12} deficiency develops if there is insuffient intake (usually only in vegans), defective absorption due to lack of intrinsic factor (pernicious anaemia, congenital lack/abnormality of IF, gastrectomy) or due to lack of absorptive surface (ileal resection, chronic sprue, blind loop syndrome causing bacterial overgrowth and competition for the vitamin).

Microscopy The bone marrow erythroblasts (megaloblasts are large) with normal haemoglobin synthesis but failure of nuclear maturation. The nuclei have fine stippled chromatin characteristic of less mature stages of erythropoiesis.

Pernicious anaemia

Definition Chronic disorder due to failure of gastric mucosa to produce intrinsic factor (IF) normally secreted by the parietal cells.

Epidemiology Mainly late adult life with mean age in Caucasians of 60 years. Occasionally seen in children when due to congenital failure to produce intrinsic factor (autosomal recessive). In Northern Europe M:F 1.4:1, but elsewhere M:F 1:1. Associated with blue eyes, early greying of the hair, blood group A. There is an increased risk of gastric cancer development.

Pathogenesis Absence of IF means absorption of vitamin B_{12} does not occur. Vitamin B_{12} is usually absorbed in the terminal ileum with the IF remaining on the mucosa. The absorbed vitamin binds to transcobalamin I and II. Lack of IF is associated with loss of all gastric secretions due to gastric atrophy. This is associated with the appearance of auto-antibodies particularly to gastric parietal cells and intrinsic factor.

Normal vitamin B_{12} Body stores are small (2–3 mg). Daily intake required is about 1 mg/day and normal daily diets contain about 20 mg.

Clinical features Insidious onset with features common to all anaemias. May be associated with skin changes (pallor and jaundice), gastrointestinal changes ('beefy red' tongue, diarrhoea) and neurological disturbances (paraesthesiae, difficulty walking, weakness, diminished vibration and position sense, hyperreflexia and the syndrome of sub-acute combined degeneration of the cord [degeneration in posterior and lateral columns of spinal cord and in peripheral nerves]).

Laboratory findings The blood shows variable anaemia, macrocytosis, decreased platelets and hypersegmentation of the neutrophil nuclei. The bone marrow shows hypercellularity with many erythroid precursors with megaloblastic features. Some cells of the myeloid series are larger than normal. There is reduced gastric acid secretion (achlorhydria) and changes in the plasma concentration of some enzymes (rise in lactate dehydrogenase [LDH]). There is a slight increase in unconjugated bilirubin due to increased destruction of red cells.

Folic acid deficiency

Aetiology Deficient dietary intake is the commonest cause but there may be increased demand (e.g. pregnancy, infancy and disorders causing rapid proliferation of blood cells), disordered metabolism (e.g. associated with alcoholism), failure of absorption (e.g. tropical sprue and coeliac disease) or deficiency may be associated with drugs (anti-convulsants and folate antagonists).

HYPOCHROMIC MICROCYTIC ANAEMIA

Definition Characterized by a decrease in red cell size and a decrease in haemoglobin concentration (reflecting impaired haemoglobin synthesis – see Table 41.5).

Laboratory findings There is a lower than normal MCV, lower MCHC and a decrease in mean red-cell diameter with increased central pallor.

Aetiology Normal haemoglobin synthesis requires adequate quantities of iron, protoporphyrin and globin. Anaemias due to impaired haemoglobin synthesis can be divided using this basis (Table 41.5).

Normal iron metabolism

Iron is carried in plasma bound to transferrin. If the level of saturation of transferrin with iron falls to low levels (below

Table 41.5 Anaemias caused by impaired haemoglobin synthesis

Deficient iron metabolism	Iron deficiency anaemia
	Anaemia of chronic disease
Defect in globin synthesis	Thalassaemias
	Haemoglobin E trait and disease
	Haemoglobin C disease
	Unstable haemoglobin disease
Defect in porphyrin and haem synthesis (sideroblastic anaemias)	Defective synthesis of δ-aminolevulinic Acid (vitamin B_6 deficiency, Drugs/toxins/defective ALA synthetase)
	Coproporphyrinogen oxidase deficiency
	Haem synthetase deficiency
	Lead poisoning
	Unknown

16%) production of haemoglobin decreases and anaemia results. About two thirds of the body iron is contained in haemoglobin. Each day about 6 gm of haemoglobin are synthesized requiring about 20 mg of red cells (much of which is recirculated from effete red cells). Only a proportion of the iron is derived from the diet and control of absorption is exerted within the mucosa of the duodenum and jejunum. Excess dietary iron is retained in the mucosal epithelium as complexes with apoferritin and is returned to the gut lumen when the epithelial cells are shed. Iron loss occurs in sweat, faeces and urine (0.5–1 mg per day in total) and menstruating women lose a further 0.5–1 mg per day.

....

IRON DEFICIENCY ANAEMIA

Aetiology There is either prolonged negative balance in respect of iron or the stores of iron are inadequate to cope with increased demand. Causes of negative iron balance include:

1. **Inadequate iron intake**

   - patients with achlorhydria
   - following gastric surgery (gastrectomy, vagotomy and gastroenterostomy)
   - coeliac disease
   - pica (eating clay).

2. **Excessive iron loss**

   - from gastrointestinal tract (peptic ulcer, haemorrhoids, oesophageal varices, hiatus hernia, gastritis associated with non-steroidal anti-inflammatory drugs, neoplasms, diverticular disease, hookworm infestation and angiodysplasia)
   - renal dialysis (occurs in 50% of patients with chronic renal failure on dialysis)
   - excessive uterine loss.

3. **Increased demand for iron in**

   - infancy
   - pregnancy
   - lactation.

Clinical features

This will be a combination of symptoms related to anaemia (e.g. fatigue and weakness) and to the underlying cause of that anaemia. Some features are associated with iron deficiency:

- impaired growth in children
- poor muscular performance
- defective structure and function of epithelial tissues:

  - nails atrophic and flattened. Eventually become spoon-shaped (koilonychia)
  - tongue: atrophy of lingual papillae and sore red smooth tongue
  - mouth: angular stomatitis (ulcers and fissures at the corners of the mouth)
  - hypopharynx/oesophagus: associated with webs (e.g. Plummer–Vinson syndrome)
  - stomach: non-specific gastritis

- effects on immunity:

  - 35% reduction in the number of circulating T cells (both helper and suppressor)
  - impaired bacterial killing by phagocytes – related to decrease in oxidative burst.

Laboratory findings

Symptoms usually occur when haemoglobin falls to 7–8 g/dl. Red cells show decreased MCH and MCV and in longstanding cases MCHC is reduced. Anisocytosis (variation in cell size) is seen. Decreased haemoglobinization results in increased central pallor of red cells. In most cases circulating platelets are increased. The bone marrow shows hyperplasia of red cell precursors with small normoblasts which have scanty and ragged cytoplasm. Stainable iron is much decreased or absent in the marrow. Serum iron concentrations are reduced (mean value 28 µg/dl – about 50% normal). The total iron binding capacity (TIBC) usually rises. Serum ferritin is considerably decreased to about 12 µg/dl (normal for adult male is about 175 µg/dl).

ANAEMIA OF CHRONIC DISEASE

Associated with chronic infections (e.g. tuberculosis, lung abscess, infective endocarditis), non-infective inflammatory disorders (e.g. rheumatoid arthritis, rheumatic fever, SLE, severe trauma), malignancies (e.g. carcinoma, Hodgkin's disease, non-Hodgkin's lymphoma) and other disorders (e.g. alcoholic liver disease, congestive heart failure and thrombophlebitis).

Pathogenesis

Not yet clear. There are three functional components:

- shortened red cell survival
- failure to transfer iron from macrophage stores to serum
- impairment of marrow response.

Clinical features   Usually mild and appear 1–2 months after the onset of the chronic disease.

Laboratory findings   The anaemia is normally normochromic and normocytic though microcytosis and hypochromia may occur. Serum iron and TIBC are increased and saturation of transferrin is below normal. There is no lack of iron in macrophages. There is moderate shortening of red cell survival which is not associated with hyperplasia of red cell precursors in the bone marrow nor with increased reticulocyte count.

Sideroblastic anaemia

Laboratory findings   There is hypochromic microcytic anaemia which is refractory to treatment. Amorphous iron deposits are seen in the mitochondria of erythroblasts (sometimes arranged in a ring-like fashion around the nucleus – ring sideroblasts). Total body iron is increased, transferrin is almost completely saturated and ferritin concentrations are high. There is ineffective erythropoiesis and impaired haem synthesis (see Table 41.6).

Table 41.6 Classification of sideroblastic anaemia

	Hereditary	Acquired
Genetics	Various inheritance patterns including X-linked, autosomal dominant and autosomal recessive	
Aetiology	In some cases of the X-linked form there is a defect in δ-aminolevulicinic acid synthetase	There is an idiopathic form with expansion of a single clone of abnormal erythroblasts, forms associated with myelodysplasia, myeloproliferative disorders and haematological malignancies and reversible sideroblastic anaemia associated with alcoholism and certain drugs, e.g. isoniazid and chloramphenicol

Anaemia associated with lead poisoning

Aetiology Long-standing presence of lead-containing bullets in tissues, inhalation of lead as an atmospheric pollutant or in children licking toys covered by lead-containing paints.

Pathogenesis Interference with haem synthesis at several points together with effects on globin sythesis and interference with breakdown of RNA.

Laboratory findings There is basophilic stippling in red cells (due to accumulation of denatured RNA). Anaemia is of a mild–moderate degree. Red cells are microcytic and hypochromic. The reticulocyte is usually raised. Mean red cell survival is shortened. Markers of haem synthesis are affected (e.g. there is decline in red cell concentrations of aminolevulinic acid dehydrogenase).

HAEMOLYTIC ANAEMIAS

Accelerated red cell destruction with marked shortening of red cell survival and no impairment of the bone marrow to respond to the extra demands.

Pathogenesis Occurs either because of an intrinsic abnormality in the red cell (usually inherited) or due to some factor outside the red cell causing membrane damage (usually acquired).

Clinical features Anaemia with crises occuring when the equilibrium between increased destruction and demand is disturbed (e.g. with human parvovirus B19 infection). Release of excess amounts of haemoglobin from red cells leads to increased plasma concentrations of unconjugated bilirubin (and thus increased risk of developing pigment gallstones). Expansion of the bone marrow may lead to skeletal changes. If the cause of the haemolysis is increased rigidity of the red cells there may be occlusion of small vessels and effects on the tissues downstream of any occlusion.

HEREDITARY HAEMOLYTIC ANAEMIAS

General considerations

Aetiology of hereditary haemolytic anaemias
(Table 41.7)

Clinical features

Anaemia of variable severity. In some severe anaemia may be present at birth. In general the balance between destruction and replacement means that anaemia is mild to moderate. Jaundice again is variable in degree. In neonates there may be severe hyperbilirubinaemia but in others jaundice may be episodic and mild. The bilirubin is unconjugated. Gallstone formation is a not uncommon complication of increased haemoglobin breakdown. Aplastic crisis may occur. This usually develops non-specifically with changes in the blood picture developing 4–7 days after infection with a fall in haemoglobin and no attendant rise in reticulocyte count. Recovery is heralded by raised reticulocytes. The crisis usually lasts 10–14 days (parvovirus colonizes the red cell lines and inhibits red cell formation). Leg ulcers may develop in a small proportion of patients mostly with sickle cell disease or hereditary spherocytosis (prevalence 5%). The ulcers are often bilateral and located on the malleoli. Bony

Table 41.7 Aetiology of hereditary haemolytic anaemias

Defects in red cell membranes	• Hereditary spherocytosis • Hereditary elliptocytosis • Stomatocytosis • Abetalipoproteinaemia • Rh$_{null}$ disease
Deficiencies in glycolytic enzymes	• Pyruvate kinase deficiency
Abnormalities of red cell nucleotide metabolism	
Deficiencies in enzymes of the pentose phosphate pathway	• Glucose-6-phosphate dehydrogenase deficiency • Defect in glutathione synthetase or glutathione reductase
Defects in globin structure or regulation of globin synthesis	• Sickle cell disease • Other homozygous abnormalities of haemoglobin (CC, DD, EE disease) • Various forms of thalassaemia • Unstable haemoglobin disease • Doubly heterozygous diseases (such as a combination of sickle cell and thalassaemia traits or haemoglobin SC disease)

abnormalities are due to expansion of the red marrow and may cause the development of a tower-shaped skull and thickening of the frontal bone (X-ray appearance of hairs standing on end). There may be prominence of the cheek-bones leading to exposure of the upper teeth. There can be thinning of the bony cortex leading to misshapen small bones of the hands and feet.

Laboratory findings

1. Signs of excessive red cell destruction

- shortened red cell survival time – demonstrated by serial measurement of degree of anaemia, reticulocyte response
- increased bilirubin
- decrease in plasma haptoglobin concentrations – haemoglobin released by red cell breakdown binds to haptoglobin and the resulting complex is removed by the liver.

2. Evidence of intravascular haemolysis

Haemoglobin in the plasma occurs either when there is red cell destruction within the circulation or when extravascular destruction is so great or rapid that the ability of the macrophages to engulf the red cell contents is exceeded. This results in:

- haemoglobinaemia
- haemoglobinuria (when the plasma haemoglobin levels exceed the binding capacity of haptoglobin) with urine appearing pale pink to deep red
- iron in the urine
- methaemalbuminaemia giving serum a coffee colour.

3. Signs of compensatory erythropoeisis

- blood shows increased reticulocytes, macrocytosis, presence of nucleated red cells, increased numbers of neutrophils and platelets
- bone marrow shows erythroid hyperplasia
- iron transport rates are 2–8 times higher than normal and erythrocyte turnover rate is increased
- Red cells show decrease in average age which can be measured by red cell creatinine (higher in young red cells).

4. There may be specific abnormalities that point towards particular causes of haemolysis

- spherical red cells – seen in hereditary spherocytosis and also in some acquired forms
- acanthocytes (cells with spicules from cell membrane) – indicate abnormality in lipid composition of red cell membrane as seen in abetalipoproteinaemia and sometimes in liver cirrhosis
- stomatocytes (red cells with central slit or stoma) – due to abnormality of red cell cation metabolism. Seen in hereditary stomatocytosis
- target cells (cells with central zone of pigment) – seen in thalassaemia, homozygous abnormal haemoglobin states, lecithin-cholesterol-acly tranferase deficiency, some non-haemolytic states such as cholestatic jaundice and following splenectomy
- sickle cells

- schistocytes (fragmented red cells) – suggest that haemolysis is due to physical trauma.

5. Changes in osmotic fragility

   Increased osmotic fragility occurs typically in hereditary spherocytosis and there is increased resistance to osmotic stress in thalassaemia and sickle cell anaemia.

6. Antiglobulin (Coombs') test

   Most widely used to diagnose immune-mediated haemolytic anaemia in the form of the direct Coombs' test (positive indicates that the cells are covered by IgG and or complement).

7. Heinz body formation

   Irregularly shaped inclusions due to precipitation of haemoglobin. Seen in certain enzyme deficiencies (notably glucose-6-phosphatase deficiency), thalassaemia, unstable haemoglobin disease and certain types of chemical injury to red cells.

....

HEREDITARY SPHEROCYTOSIS

Epidemiology Commonest familial haemolytic anaemia in persons of northern European extraction.

Genetics Most commonly autosomal dominant inheritance.

Pathogenesis Structural and functional abnormalities of the red cell plasma membrane due to abnormality of the red cell cytoskeleton as a result of absent or defective spectrin. In the autosomal dominant form spectrin is reduced to between 60–80% of normal (the lower the spectrin the greater the severity of the disease).

Clinical features There is anaemia which is not usually severe, intermittent jaundice, splenomegaly, a marked amelioration following splenectomy and occasional aplastic crises. Pigment gallstones are very common and occur in young children.

Laboratory findings Anaemia is accompanied by an increased reticulocyte count (5–20%) and an increase in MCHC. There are microspherocytes and increased fragility of red cells to osmotic stress. There is increased autohaemolysis when blood is incubated at 37°C under sterile conditions for 48 hours (corrected by addition of glucose). An intermittent increase in unconjugated bilirubin is seen. The Coombs' test is negative. The bone marrow shows erythroid hyperplasia.

HEREDITARY ELLIPTOCYTOSIS

Epidemiology Worldwide distribution with incidence 1/1000–1/5000.

Genetics Usually autosomal dominant inheritance.

Pathogenesis Red cell cytoskeletal abnormalities.

Clinical features Disease may be mild but severe haemolytic anaemia can be seen particularly in homozygous patients.

Laboratory findings There is the presence of at least 25% elliptical red cells in the peripheral blood.

DEFECTS IN GLYCOLYTIC ENZYMES
Pyruvate-kinase deficiency

Genetics Autosomal recessive inheritance.

Pathogenesis There is lack of ATP. As energy requirements exceed available ATP the membrane pumps concerned with regulation of the cation gradient start to fail. Potassium loss exceeds sodium gain causing a net loss of water from the cell and membrane distortion promoting destruction by the reticulo-endothelial system.

Clinical features Spectrum of severity ranges from severe neonatal anaemia with splenomegaly and jaundice to a fully compensated anaemia. Most cases are diagnosed in infancy.

Laboratory findings There is a moderate to severe degree of anaemia. Morphological examination shows the presence of poikilocytosis, polychromasia, anisocytosis and the presence of nucleated red cells. Osmotic fragility is normal. Serum unconjugated bilirubin is increased. There is increased autohaemolysis which is not corrected by glucose. Diagnosis depends on the demonstration of the enzyme deficiency.

....

DEFICIENCY IN ENZYMES INVOLVED IN THE PENTOSE PHOSPHATE PATHWAY

Glucose-6-phosphate dehydrogenase (G6PD) deficiency

Epidemiology Worldwide distribution, but variations in frequency occur with the most affected populations in West Africa, countries bordering the Mediterranean, the Middle East and south-east Asia.

Genetics Some cases are X-linked recessive.

Pathogenesis There is decreased intracellular reduced glutathione which is an important defence against oxidative stress. G6PD deficient red cells are therefore more liable to membrane damage by reactive oxygen species (free radicals).

Clinical features G6PD deficiency may be clinically silent, associated with episodic acute acquired haemolytic anaemia, a congenital non-spherocytic haemolytic anaemia or associated with consumption of the broad bean *Vicia fava* (favism).

Acute acquired haemolysis

Aetiology Drugs such as sulphonamides, anti-malarials, sulphones and nitrofurans.

Clinical features A common presentation is with jaundice, pallor and dark urine which may or may not be associated with back or abdominal pain.

Laboratory findings Compatible with intravascular haemolysis. There is a sharp fall in haemoglobin. Morphological abnormalities of the red cells in which there are small portions of the cytoplasm missing (bite cells; these represent cells from which Heinz bodies have been removed). Heinz bodies may be present in some cells.

Congenital non-spherocytic haemolytic anaemia

Clinical features Anaemia and jaundice are usually seen in neonates and the jaundice may be so severe as to require an exchange transfusion.

Favism

Epidemiology Most commonly in young children.

Clinical features Severe intravascular haemolysis within 5–24 h of having eaten the fava beans.

....

DEFECTS IN GLOBIN STRUCTURE OR REGULATION OF GLOBIN SYNTHESIS

Haemoglobinopathies

Haemoglobin S and sickle-cell disease

Definition So-called because cells which contain appreciable amounts of sickle-cell haemoglobin (HbS) undergo a characteristic sickle-shaped deformation in oxygen concentrations below a critical level.

Epidemiology Commonest abnormal haemoglobin especially in tropical Africa where the mutated gene is present in 40–50% of the population. Eight per cent of North American blacks show the presence of the mutation. A high prevalence of the HbS gene is found where malaria is endemic as HbS confers resistance against parasitization by *Plasmodium falciparum*.

Clinical features Heterozygotes do not normally show clinically significant phenotypic abnormalities (sickle cell trait). Homozygotes in whom there is no normal haemoglobin A show a clinical phenotype (sickle cell disease) of differing grades of severity.

Pathogenesis A substitution of thymine for adenine in the 6th codon of the β chain gene results in the substitution of valine for glutamic acid. This causes deoxygenated HbS to polymerize and this causes sickling. Sickled red cells are more adherent to endothelium and macrophages contributing to the haemolytic anaemia. The flow patterns of sickled red cells are different with the result that there is obstruction of small vessels and ischaemic tissue damage.

Haematological abnormalities There is mild anaemia which is usually present by 12 weeks of age. At all ages the effects of the anaemia are offset by the fact that HbS yields its oxygen more readily than normal adult haemoglobin. There is splenomegaly usually by the age of 6 months. Splenic sequestration crisis (rapid enlargement of the spleen with decrease in blood volume which can lead to hypo-volaemic shock) may occur usually between the ages of 6 months and 2 years. These crises may recur up to the age of 5-6 years but by that time the spleen is too fibrotic to expand. Splenic infarction and atrophy then occurs as a result of the occlusion of small vessels. There may be mega-loblastic crisis associated with folate deficiency, aplastic crisis or a haemolytic crisis.

Ischaemic manifestations These may be precipitated by infection, fever, acidosis, hypoxaemia and cold. Acute bone ischaemia may affect the small bones of the hands and feet (hand–foot syndrome) which tends to occur early in the disease. Bone and joint crises may also affect the larger bones associated with severe gnawing pain. There may be manifestations occurring in the central nervous system (stroke), lungs (associated with fever, chest pain, rapid breathing, neutrophil leucocytosis, lung infiltrates on X-ray and sudden decrease in haemoglobin) and abdominal system. More chronic affects of ischaemia include destruc-tive changes in the bones and joints, chronic ulcers of the lower leg, impaired growth or maturation, retinopathy, increased pigment gallstones, haematuria and inability to concentrate the glomerular filtrate and priapism. There is an increased susceptibility to infections.

Laboratory findings There is a decreased haemoglobin concentration with the presence of sickle cells and target cells. Sickling occurs following the addition of sodium metabisulphite or sodium dithionite to blood samples. There is an increased white cell and platelet count and a low ESR (sickled cells fail to form rouleaux).

Haemoglobin electrophoresis Absence of HbA band. Around 80–85% is HbS with the remainder fetal haemoglobin (HbF). In sickle cell trait about 40% is HbS with the remainder HbA.

Haemoglobin C disorders

Genetics   Lysine replaces glutamic acid at the 6th position from the amino terminal end. HbC can be found as a trait with only one allele of the β chain affected.

Pathogenesis   Deoxygenated HbC from intracellular crystals leads to increased intravascular viscosity rendering red cells less deformable and causes them to fragment easily, become sequestrated in the spleen and to form small spherocytes. Some individuals show the presence of HbC and HbS.

Clinical features   Anaemia is mild to moderate with a slightly elevated reticulocyte count but the symptoms of the anaemia are less than expected due to shift of the oxygen dissociation curve to the right.

Laboratory findings   Target cells are characteristic and may make up 90% of the red cells. Red cell survival is shortened and turnover is increased.

THE THALASSAEMIAS

THE α-THALASSAEMIAS

Pathogenesis   Most frequently the result of deletions of the genes encoding the α-globin chain. The presence or absence of anaemia and its severity correlate with the number of genes deleted.

4 α-globin genes deleted

Epidemiology   Most frequent in south-east Asia.

Haemoglobin   There is no synthesis of α chain. The haemoglobin is entirely Hb Barts (tetramers of γ chains) which have a high oxygen affinity.

Clinical features   Death in utero or hydrops fetalis.

Pathology   Placenta is enlarged and oedematous. Infant's liver is enlarged due to extramedullary haemopoesis.

3 α-globin chains deleted

Epidemiology Seen throughout south-east Asia, Middle East and the Mediteranean islands such as Cyprus. Very rare in Africans.

Haemoglobin HbH disease (tetramers of β-globin chains).

Pathology Infants are normal at birth but by the age of 1 year they have developed anaemia and splenomegaly; jaundice and liver enlargement occur at a later stage. Red marrow hyperplasia causes skeletal changes which are seen in about 30% of children with HbH disease.

Laboratory findings Moderate degree of microcytic hypochromic anaemia, raised reticulocytes, some target cells and distorted red cells.

Haemoglobin electrophoresis HbH accounts for 5–40% of haemoglobin. At birth 20–40% of haemoglobin is Hb Barts which is replaced in the first few months of life by HbH.

2 α-globin chains deleted (α-thalassaemia minor)

Clinical features Anaemia, if present, is mild. Haemoglobin concentrations are normal or slightly decreased and also some decrease in MCV and MCH.

Laboratory findings At birth there is an increase in Hb Barts but this is dificult to demonstrate after the first few months.

1 α-globin chain deleted (silent carrier state)

Clinical features No abnormality.

Laboratory findings No abnormality.

....

THE β-THALASSAEMIAS

Pathogenesis Point mutations in the genes encoding the β-globin chain. More than 100 genetic abnormalities have been recorded.

Pathophysiology Sub-normal amounts of HbA (adult haemoglobin) result in the cell being small and hypochromatic. The imbalance between α- and β-globin chains leads to formation of α-chain aggregates within red cells which precipitate as insoluble inclusions. There is therefore destruction of red cell precursors in the marrow (ineffect-ive erythropoiesis, up to 85% normoblasts destroyed). Haemolysis of red cells occurs mostly in the spleen.

Classification By clinical phenotype.

- β-thalassaemia major – most severe form. Severe anaemia requiring repeated blood transfusions leading to iron overload.
- β-thalassaemia intermedia – less degree of anaemia. Repeated blood transfusion is not required.
- β-thalassaemia minor (thalassaemia trait) – asymptomatic. Morphological red cell abnormalities but no anaemia.

Thalassaemia major

Clinical features Affected infants appear normal at birth. Pallor develops with abnormal girth (enlargement of liver and spleen), haemoglobin level falls (to 3–5 g/dl), skeletal abnormalities and growth retardation and other endocrine abnormalities (diabetes mellitus, hypothyroidism and hypoparathyroidism). The most common causes of death are cardiac failure and cardiac dysrhythmias due to iron deposition. Liver enlargement usually occurs early and later there is cirrhosis due to iron overload.

Laboratory findings Severe microcytic hypochromic anaemia. Striking variation in red cell size (anisocytosis), target cells are frequent. There may be basophilic stippling and normoblasts. Reticulocyte count is raised. Osmotic fragility of the red cells is decreased. Leucocyte count is usually raised. Increased unconjugated bilirubin.

Haemoglobin electrophoresis Very little or no HbA, most is HbF.

Molecular analysis Increase in α:β chain ratio (β chain synthesis absent or much reduced).

Natural history and prognosis Bleak. Many children die before 5 years.

Thalassaemia intermedia

Clinical features Growth retardation and pubertal delay not seen. Many individuals are pale with intermittent jaundice and splenomegaly. There are facial and other bony lesions.

Laboratory findings Anaemia less severe than thalassaemia major (6–9 g/dl). Morphological changes in red cells are identical to those of thalassaemia major.

Natural history and prognosis Most survive to adulthood. May be normal life expectancy. Where premature death occurs it is commonly the result of haemosiderin deposition in the myocardium.

Thalassaemia minor

Epidemiology Common.

Clinical features Usually symptomless.

Laboratory findings Anaemia may be mild or absent. Red cell abnormalities are seen in those more severely affected. MCV and MCH are low.

Haemoglobin electrophoresis A number of different patterns of which increase in HbA_2 is the commonest.

....

NON-INHERITED ABNORMALITIES OF RED CELLS LEADING TO HAEMOLYSIS
Paroxysmal nocturnal haemoglobinuria

Definition Rare acquired condition in which there is production of red cells that are abnormally sensitive to lysis by complement occurs.

Pathophysiology Red cells have shortened survival. In a single patient the red cells vary in their susceptibility to complement-mediated destruction and respond in three ways:

- no increased susceptibility (PNH I)
- 3–5 times increased susceptibility (PNH II)
- 15–25 times increased susceptibility (PNH III).

The severity depends on the relative proportions.

Clinical features Classically associated with intravascular haemolysis occurring mainly at night. There is more commonly chronic intravascular haemolysis, pancytopaenia, iron deficiency and recurrent episodes of thrombosis. Haemoglobinuria occurs in only about 25% of patients and need not be nocturnal.

Laboratory findings   Severe anaemia is present in most patients, leucopaenia is often present. Plasma may be golden-brown due to unconjugated bilirubin, haemoglobin and methaemalbumin. Urine shows urobilinogen haemoglobin and heamosiderin. Marrow shows normoblastic hyperplasia. The Ham test (lysis of red cells when acidified human serum is added) is positive.

Natural history and prognosis   Mean survival is about 10 years.

....

HAEMOLYSIS DUE TO ABNORMALITIES OUTSIDE THE RED CELLS

Immune haemolytic anaemias

Alloimmune haemolytic anaemia

Definition   Lytic antibodies are elicited by antigens foreign to affected individual.

Aetiology   Haemolytic transfusion reactions (IgM antibodies) and haemolytic disease of the newborn (IgG antibodies which react with paternal fetal antigens).

Pathogenesis
1. **IgM antibodies and red cell destruction**

   * antibodies elicited by blood group antigens A, B and H and also cold agglutinins
   * agglutinate red cells (complete antibodies)
   * destruction mediated via complement. Starts by binding C1q resulting in red cells coated by C3b being phagocytosed and intravascular lysis through direct membrane attack complex of complement.

2. **IgG antibodies and red cell destruction**

   * in the context of alloimmune haemolysis these are against Rh system
   * no agglutination (incomplete antibodies)

- direct antiglobulin test negative. Indirect agglutinin test positive
- red cells destroyed by adhesion to and phagocytosis by macrophages.

Clinical features
- **Haemolytic transfusion reactions** – patients experience fever, back or chest pain and shortness of breath. Haemoglobinuria and haemoglobinaemia are present. Complications include shock, acute renal failure and disseminated intravascular coagulation.
- **Haemolytic disease of the newborn** – most commonly there is anaemia, jaundice, enlargement of the liver and spleen and bilirubin encephalopathy (kernicterus, due to unconjugated bilirubin). In severe intrauterine haemolysis there is ascites and hypoalbuminaemia. There may be intrauterine portal hypertension leading to high pressures in the umbilical vein, placental oedema and hypertrophy of trophoblast (hydrops fetalis).

Autoimmune haemolytic anaemia (AIHA)

Definition   Antibodies produced against patient's own red cells.

Classification   Based on activity at ambient temperature.

1. Warm antibodies

Definition   Bind most avidly at 37°C.

Epidemiology   Not common. Annual incidence 1/80 000. Females more than males.

Aetiology   May be primary (idiopathic) or associated with autoimmune disease (mostly systemic lupus erythematosus), malignant disease of the lymphoreticular system (accounts for 60% of cases and includes chronic lymphocytic leukaemia and lymphoma), non-haemolytic neoplasms, viral infections (e.g. hepatitis, cytomegalovirus, Epstein–Barr virus, rubella, etc.) and immune deficiency syndromes.

Pathogenesis   Antibodies coating the red cells are most commonly IgG leading to destruction in the spleen with little intravascular haemolysis.

Clinical features   Symptoms include weakness, dizziness and fever. Signs include splenomegaly (80%), hepatomegaly (45%), lymph node enlargement (34%) and jaundice (21%).

Laboratory findings   Degree and duration of anaemia is variable. Blood films show differing degrees of spherocytosis. Reticulocyte count is usually raised. Direct antiglobulin test is positive but is an insensitive test. Serum bilirubin is moderately raised.

2. Cold antibodies

Definition   Bind at body temperature but increased affinity as the temperature approaches 0°C.

Aetiology   Monoclonal cold-reactive antibodies are associated with the chronic idiopathic cold agglutinin syndrome or with lymphoreticular neoplasms (lymphoma, lymphocytic leukaemia, myeloma) and Kaposi's sarcoma. Polyclonal cold-reactive antibodies are associated with infections (most commonly *Mycoplasma pneumoniae* but also mumps, cytomegalovirus, Epstein–Barr virus, trypanosomiasis, malaria, listeria and syphilis), autoimmune diseases, angioimmunoblastic lymphadenopathy.

Pathogenesis   Antibody is usually IgM. Most of the destruction is due to C3b-mediated phagocytosis by cells of the reticuloendothelial system.

Clinical features   Vascular disturbances resulting from agglutination at lower temperatures in small blood vessels in skin and subcutaneous tissues. Intravascular haemolysis or sequestration of C3b-coated cells in the liver. There may be paroxysmal cold haemoglobinuria (passage of haemoglobin in the urine) after the individual has been exposed to cold.

3. Mixed warm and cold antibodies

Drug-induced immune haemolytic anaemia

Three different mechanisms.

- Drug binds to red cell membrane and acts as hapten. Associated with penicillin, tetracyclines and cephalosporins.
- Drug binds to circulating macromolecules. Antibody formation is elicited and a large soluble immune

complex is formed which becomes deposited on red cell membranes. This causes acute intravascular haemolysis. Associated with para-aminosalicylic acid, quinidine, chlorpromazine, thiazides and fluorouracil.
• Drug causes development of autoantibodies directed against red-cell antigens. Associated with α-methyldopa.

Non-immune haemolytic anaemias

Red cell fragmentation syndromes

Direct damage to the red cells may be associated with microangiopathy or as a result of interactions between red cells and foreign surfaces such as vascular grafts.

Haemolytic anaemia due to direct injury of red cells

Associated with infections such as malaria, trypanosomiasis, *Bartonella bacilliformis* infection, clostridial infections (notably gas gangrene due to *Cl. perfringens*) and spirochaete infections (such as those caused by *Borrelia recurrentis* causing relapsing fever and *Leptospira icterohaemorrhagica* causing Weil's disease). Oxidative damage can be caused by chemical agents including sulphonamides sulphones, nitrofurans, salicylates, nitrites, chlorates and resorcin. Chemicals causing non-oxidative damage include arsine, copper, lead, glycerol, propythiouracil, mephenesin and water.

Laboratory findings Oxidant damage to red cells results in characteristic morphological changes:
• Heinz bodies
• bite cells
• presence of 'hemighosts' – red cells in which the haemoglobin appears to have shifted into only one half of the cell leaving the other half clear.

APLASTIC ANAEMIAS

Definition Conditions with pancytopaenia, decreased production of cellular elements of blood in the marrow and absence of primary disease which infiltrates, replaces or suppresses the marrow.

Fanconi's anaemia (familial aplastic anaemia)

Genetics   Autosomal recessive inheritance.

Epidemiology   Manifests at 5–10 years.

Clinical features   Pancytopenia, bone marrow hypoplasia, skeletal abnormalities, increased risk of acute myeloid leukaemia and other neoplasms, variety of other abnormalities (e.g. mental retardation, squint, defective genital development, dwarfism and splenic atrophy) and brown-patch skin pigmentation.

Laboratory findings   There is anaemia (normocytic or slightly macrocytic), reduced absolute reticulocyte count and decreased white cell count. The marrow may be normo- or hypercellular in early stages but becomes hypocellular. Cultured lymphocytes show chromosome fragility.

Acquired aplastic anaemia

Related to drugs or chemical agents.

May be classified as either predictable or idiosyncratic.

1. Predictable (always induces aplasia if dose is large enough).

   - benzene poisoning
   - radiation
   - antitumour chemotherapeutic agents

     — sulphur and nitrogen mustards
     — anti-metabolities (6-mercaptopurine)
     — anti-mitotic agents (vinca alkaloids, colchicine)
     — anthracycline compounds (adriamycin, daunoru-
     · bicin).

2. Idiosyncratic

   - antimicrobials (chloramphenicol, organic arsenicals, quinacrine)
   - anti-convulsants (mesantoin, tridione)
   - analgesics (phenylbutazone)
   - others (e.g. gold).

Clinical features   Manifestations of anaemia and bleeding together with increased infections.

Macroscopy   The marrow appears yellowish-white.

Microscopy   Severe hypoplasia so marrow consists mainly of adipose tissue, fibrous tissue and lymphocytes.

Natural history and prognosis   Poor prognostic signs include bleeding at an early stage, presence of more than 70% non-myeloid cells in initial bone marrow biopsy, male gender and low reticulocyte count.

....

'PURE' RED CELL APLASIA

Congenital erythroid hypoplasia (Diamond–Blackfan syndrome)

Definition   Moderate to severe chronic anaemia beginning in infancy.

Laboratory findings   No erythroblasts in bone marrow. Absolute deficiency of reticulocytes. White blood cells and platelets are normal. Fetal haemaglobin level higher than expected.

Natural history and prognosis   Progessive but 20% go into remission.

Acute transient red cell aplasia

Aetiology   Occurs in a number of circumstances:
- associated with parvovirus B19 infection
- in children with no obvious underlying cause
- in adults associated with hepatitis or other viral infections
- in association with drugs (e.g. aspirin, heparin, glutethimide, tolbutamide and others).

Chronic acquired red cell aplasia

Aetiology   Two types. Either associated with thymoma (accounts for more than 50%, a sixth of these also with myasthenia gravis) or not associated with any thymic abnormality.

Epidemiology   Adults only.

Natural history and prognosis   In those associated with thymoma, remission following thymoma resection occurs in only 25%.

BLOOD VESSELS: NORMAL RESPONSE

In injured areas local blood vessels constrict. The endothelial lining cells synthesize and secrete pro-coagulant factors, anti-coagulant factors, factors that promote platelet adhesion and factors that inhibit platelet adhesion.

BLEEDING DISORDERS DUE TO ABNORMAL BLOOD VESSELS

Hereditary blood vessel disorders

Hereditary haemorrhagic telangiectasia (Osler–Weber–Rendu syndrome)

Genetics Autosomal dominant inheritance.

Pathogenesis Blood vessels become tortuous and dilated. The walls of the affected segments are abnormally thin being lined only by a layer of endothelium.

Clinical features Telangiectasia, most easily seen in the skin and mucous membranes, are present varying in size from pinpoint to 3 mm diameter and appearing as bright red spots. Although lesions may develop in childhood, bleeding is not usually seen until adulthood when it may be severe – especially if the gastrointestinal tract is involved. In some individuals there may be arteriovenous communications in the lungs – these patients have recurrent haemoptysis, recurrent pulmonary infections, secondary polycythaemia, finger clubbing and cyanosis.

Hereditary conditions affecting supporting connective tissue

Abnormal bleeding may complicate several inherited connective tissue disorders including:

- various forms of Ehlers–Danlos syndrome. Type IV is most likely to be associated with severe bleeding
- osteogenesis imperfecta
- pseudoxanthoma elasticum.

These include:

- autoimmune purpura such as Henoch–Schönlein purpura
- bacterial infections such as meningococcal septicaemia, leptospirosis and scarlet fever
- viral and rickettsial infections such as smallpox, Rocky Mountain spotted fever, typhus
- protozoal infection such as malaria
- acquired abnormalities of connective tissue such as scurvy, Cushing's syndrome, senile purpura
- fat embolism.

....

PLATELETS AND HAEMOSTASIS

Normal platelet function

Size and number Normal count is $150–450 \times 10^9$/l. Platelets circulate as flat discs 1–2 microns in diameter. Newly released platelets migrate to the spleen where they remain for 1–2 days. Up to one-third of the platelets may be in the spleen at any one time.

Platelets contribute to haemostasis via a number of steps:

1 Adhesion

The platelet adheres to damaged endothelium or exposed sub-endothelial connective tissue. Collagen binds to glyco-protein receptor (GP Ia) and von Willebrand factor (vWF) synthesized by endothelial cells binds to GP Ib.

2 Release

Adherent platelets undergo shape changes releasing several pre-formed and newly formed molecules. The platelet contains two types of storage granules:

- α granules (containing platelet derived growth factor, thrombospondin, platelet factor 4, β-thromboglobin, fibrinogen, fibronectin, von Willebrand factor, etc.)
- dense bodies (contain ATP, ADP, GDP, GTP, serotonin and calcium).

The release is usually triggered by exposure to collagen or thrombin. Collagen and thrombin also mediate the release of arachidonate from platelet membrane in the first step to the synthesis of prostaglandins including the anti-aggregatory prostacyclin and the pro-aggregatory thromboxane A_2.

3 Aggregation

This is the adhesion of platelets to other platelets to form a mass of activated cells via fibrinogen bridges. The stimuli for aggregation are ADP and thromboxane A_2.

4 Provision of co-factors for clotting

Platelets interact with factors in the clotting cascade (including Factors V, VIII, IX, and X).

ABNORMAL BLEEDING DUE TO PLATELET DISORDERS

Clinical features There are purpura, spontaneous haemorrhages and prolonged bleeding after trauma.

Laboratory findings Prolonged bleeding time.

Thrombocytopenia

Definition A significant decline in circulating platelet numbers.

Aetiology May be due to deficient production, increased destruction/consumption or abnormal distribution of platelets.

Pathogenesis Decreased production is often associated with failure to produce red and white cells and may be idiopathic or due to a well-recognized cause such as cytotoxic drugs, radiotherapy, infiltration of the marrow (e.g. in leukaemia or other malignant disease) or with HIV infection. Isolated thrombocytopenia may be due to drugs and as a complication of some viral infections. Increased destruction or utilization may or may not be immune mediated.

Immune-mediated thrombocytopenia

Aetiology May be idiopathic or may be triggered by drugs or associated with disorders such as systemic lupus erythematosus, various haemolytic anaemias, some lymphoreticular diseases, rheumatoid arthritis and hyperthyroidism.

Non-immunological platelet destruction or utilization

Thrombotic thrombocytopenic purpura (TTP)

Epidemiology Peak incidence 30–40 years. More common in females than males.

Aetiology Unknown. About 85% occur in previously healthy individuals. The remainder are associated with other conditions such as systemic lupus erythematosus, immune-mediated vasculitis, graft rejection and various infections.

Clinical features Widespread thrombosis involving the microcirculation causing ischaemic damage in various tissues (including brain and kidney), thrombocytopenia, fever and haemolytic anaemia (due to red cell damage as a result of their interaction with thrombi).

Microscopy Thrombi occur in terminal arterioles and consist of platelets and fibrin. There are sub-endothelial hyaline deposits associated with endothelial cell proliferation.

Natural history and prognosis Before the introduction of plasmapheresis about 80% died within three months. Now about 80% survive the initial attack and may have long-term remission.

Disseminated intravascular coagulation

Widespread intravascular deposition of fibrin associated with consumption of platelets and clotting factors.

Aetiology Table 41.8 lists the causes.

Clinical features Abnormal bleeding, a degree of shock greater than expected for degree of blood loss and signs of underperfusion of vascular beds notably the kidney, brain, lung and liver.

Table 41.8 Causes of DIC

Obstetric complications	• Amniotic fluid embolism • Abruptio placentae • Septic abortion • Severe eclampsia
Infections	• Viral (e.g. viral haemorrhagic fevers) • Bacterial e.g. meningococcal septicaemia) • Rickettsial (e.g. Rocky Mountain spotted fever) • Fungal (e.g. aspergillosis) • Protozoal (e.g. malaria)
Neoplasms	• Carcinoma (prostate, pancreas, lung, ovary etc.) • Disseminated carcinoid • Neuroblastoma • Others
Blood disorders	• Intravascular haemolysis • Acute leukaemias • Sickle cell disease • Fresh water immersion
Vascular malformations associated with increased platelet activity	• Giant haemangiomas (Kasabach–Merrit syndrome) • Aneurysms • Coarctation of the aorta • Large prosthetic grafts
Vasculitides	• Polyarteritis nodosa • Systemic lupus erythematosus
Hypoxia and underperfusion	• Myocardial infarction • Acute respiratory distress syndrome • Various forms of shock
Massive tissue injury	• Fat embolus • Acute pancreatitis • Hypothermia • Graft versus host disease • Bites of certain venomous snakes

Laboratory findings There is a low platelet count, low plasma fibrinogen, prolonged thrombin time, prothrombin time and activated partial thromboplastin time. Fibrin and fibrinogen degradation products are present in plasma and urine. Fibrin monomer products are present in blood and there is evidence of microangiopathic haemolysis and red cell abnormalities.

Natural history and prognosis Mortality rates are about 54–68%.

ABNORMAL BLEEDING ASSOCIATED WITH QUALITATIVE DISORDERS OF PLATELETS

Thrombasthenia (Glanzmann's disease)

Pathogenesis Deficient or abnormal GP IIb/IIIa surface glycoproteins results in platelet activation not being followed by their rearrangement so there is no heterodimer for fibrinogen to bind. Normal platelet aggregation cannot occur.

Storage pool disease

Definition Deficiency of either α granules or dense bodies.

d-storage disease

Definition Lack of dense bodies.

Pathogenesis Initial stages of aggregation are not amplified due to lack of ADP so stable plugs cannot be formed.

Associations May be associated with albinism, and accumulation of ceroid pigment in macrophages in the Hermansky–Pudlak syndrome (autosomal recessive inheritance).

Laboratory findings There is deficiency of ADP-mediated platelet aggregation and deficient clot retraction.

Grey platelet syndrome

Definition Lack of α-granules.

Laboratory findings Platelets are enlarged and there may be mild thrombocytopenia. Bleeding time is prolonged.

Bernard–Soulier syndrome

Pathogenesis Lack of glycoprotein GP Ib so the interaction between this and von Willebrand factor does not occur and the adhesion phase of platelet plug formation does not occur.

Clinical features There is moderate to severe bleeding such as epistaxis, easy bruising and menorrhagia.

Laboratory findings Giant platelets, mild thrombocytopenia.

Von Willebrand's disease

Genetics Autosomal dominant inheritance.

Laboratory findings Prolonged bleeding time, low plasma von Willebrand factor, low plasma Factor VIII and defective ristocetin-induced platelet aggregation.

Acquired disorders of platelet function

Aspirin

Pathogenesis Interferes with cyclo-oxygenase resulting in deficiency of cyclo-oxygenase catalysed metabolic products of arachidonic acid in particular thromboxane A_2. Production of prostaglandin PGI_2 is affected to a lesser degree. This leads to inhibition of aggregation of platelets by collagen and the normal secondary wave of aggregation. This affect is irreversible and lasts for the complete lifespan of the platelet (7–10 days).

Systemic disorders

Abnormal bleeding may complicate paraproteinaemia and uraemia.

COAGULATION

NORMAL COAGULATION

Clotting factors

Coagulation of the blood is a cascade process in which the participant factors act as both substrates and, following their cleavage, as active enzymes. The cascade is directed towards the formation of thrombin which cleaves fibrinogen to form fibrin. This is polymerized and cross-linked to form the basic structure of a clot.

Vitamin K and clotting factors

Six factors require the presence of vitamin K in order to be activated:

- Factor II
- Factor VII
- Factor IX
- Factor X
- Protein C
- Protein S.

Clotting pathways

The intrinsic pathway

Trigger Contact-mediated activation of **Factor XII (Hageman factor)**. In the vascular system Factor XII activation is brought about by exposure of collagen and basement membrane.

Pathway Activated Factor XII cleaves Factor XI which is promoted by activation of the kinin system by Factor XIIa (pre-kallikrein to kallikrein). The next step is cleavage of Factor IX; activated Factor IX in conjunction with Factor VII and calcium then cleave Factor X.

The extrinsic pathway

Trigger Release of **tissue factor** that binds to and activates Factor VII.

Pathway Activated Factor VII activates Factor X directly thus leading to cleavage of prothrombin. Activated Factor VII also activates Factor IX promoting more activation of Factor X.

The common pathway

Trigger Assembly of activated **Factor X** on the platelet phospholipid (platelet Factor III). Calcium and Factor V are cofactors.

Pathway This complex constitutes a prothombinase which cleaves prothrombin to form thrombin which cleaves fibrinogen.

Tests of coagulation

Bleeding time Prolongation usually indicates **defective platelet function** (either functional or numerical).

Prothrombin time Measured by adding tissue factor and calcium to citrated plasma and noting the time to clot formation. **Normal 10–14 s**. Prolongation indicates deficiency or inhibition of one or more of **Factors VII, V, X, II or fibrinogen (extrinsic or common pathways)**.

Activated partial thromboplastin time Measured by adding calcium, phospholipid and a surface activator (kaolin or celite) to citrated plasma and noting the time to clot formation. **Normal 30–40 s**. Prolongation indicates deficiency or inhibition of one or more of **Factors XII, IX, VIII, X, V, II and fibrinogen (intrinsic and common pathways)**. Most sensitive indicator of deficiencies in Factor VIII and IX.

Thrombin time Measured by adding dilute bovine thrombin to citrated plasma and noting time to clot formation. **Normal 14–16 s.** Prolongation indicates either lack of fibrinogen or presence of an inhibitor to thrombin.

Control of coagulation

Local processes

- dilution of clotting factors once activated
- rapid binding of thrombin by fibrin which has already been polymerized at the site.

Inhibitors of coagulation

- Anti-thrombin III (AT III) – Binds to serine in thrombin and the resulting complex is cleared from the blood by the liver cells. AT III also inactivates Factors X, IX and kallikrein.
- Heparin cofactor II – This is activated by heparin and shows some homology with AT III but is a weaker inhibitor of activated Factor X.
- Protein C–S system – Protein C inhibits coagulation at the interface between blood and endothelial cell. To be activated protein C requires thrombin, thrombomodulin (transmembrane protein on endothelial cells), calcium ions and protein S. The resultant complex inactivates activated Factors V and VIII. Activated protein C also

promotes fibrinolysis by splitting tissue plasminogen activator from its inhibitor plasminogen inhibitor-1 (PAI-1).

Fibrinolysis

Plasmin is formed by conversion of inert blood plasminogen. This is achieved through the actions of **tissue plasminogen activator (TPA)** which is synthesized in the endothelial cells and secreted by macrophages and some malignant cells. Release of TPA is stimulated by trauma, exercise, emotional stress, stasis, ischaemia, thrombin, bacterial toxin and many other factors. Another plasminogen activator is **urokinase**, found in endothelium, kidney cells and certain tumour cells.

Endothelium and platelets (Table 41.9)

INHERITED DISORDERS OF COAGULATION

Haemophilia A

Genetics X-linked recessive inheritance. About one-third have no family history.

Defect Deficiency or abnormality of Factor VIII.

Clinical features Severity depends on the degree of reduction below normal in concentrations of Factor VIII:

> 50%	No abnormal bleeding
20–50%	Prolonged bleeding after severe injury or surgery
5–20%	Prolonged bleeding after minor injury or surgery

Table 41.9 Endothelium and platelets

Nitric oxide	Inhibits platelet activity
Prostaglandin I_2 (PGI$_2$, prostacyclin)	Inhibits platelet aggregation
Tissue factor	Triggers clotting
von Willebrand factor	Mediates platelet adhesion
Antithrombin III	Inhibits clotting
Tissue plasminogen activator	Cleaves plasminogen and thus triggers fibrinolysis
Plasminogen activator inhibitor I	Binds to TPA and inhibits its action
Thrombomodulin	Binds thrombin and leads to activation of protein C which inactivates Factors Va and VIIIa

2–5%   Prolonged bleeding after trivial injury or surgery
          Occasional spontaneous bleeding

< 2%   Spontaneous bleeding into joints and muscle.
          Severe bleeding after injury or surgery. Increased
          risk of spontaneous intracerebral bleeding.

Principal sites of bleeding are joints (into joint space, neighbouring bone or periarticular soft tissues), muscles, mouth/gums/tongue, urinary tract and brain.

Laboratory findings In severe cases there is prolonged activated partial thromboplastin time, prolonged whole blood clotting time and reduced plasma concentrations of Factor VIIIc. The bleeding time is normal and there are normal levels of von Willebrand factor and Factor IX.

Haemophilia B (Christmas disease, Factor IX deficiency)

Genetics X-linked recessive inheritance.

Defect Deficiency of Factor IX.

Clinical features Similar to haemophilia A.

Factor XI deficiency

Epidemiology Common in Ashkenazi Jews.

Genetics Autosomal recessive inheritance.

Clinical features Spectrum of abnormalities ranging from no symptoms to trauma-related haemorrhage requiring multiple transfusions. Spontaneous bleeding is rare.

....

ACQUIRED DISORDERS OF COAGULATION
Deficiency of vitamin K-dependent factors

Epidemiology May occur in adults or in children (**haemorrhagic disease of the newborn**).

Aetiology Haemorrhagic disease of the newborn is due either to immaturity of the liver cells (producing lower levels of Factors II, VII, IX and X) or due to delayed colonization of the gut by vitamin K-producing bacteria. In the adult deficiency may be caused by malabsorption of any cause or to biliary obstruction and lack of bile salts in the gut.

Pathological inhibitors of coagulation

Antibodies to Factor VIII

Epidemiology   Found in 5–21% patients with haemophilia A probably as a result of administration of Factor VIII.

Aetiology   In other individuals it is found in the elderly, rarely in the post-partum state and in patients with chronic inflammatory disease mediated by immune mechanisms (e.g. rheumatoid arthritis, systemic lupus erythematosus and ulcerative colitis).

Clinical features   Bleeding may be severe.

Other acquired defects in coagulation

Associated with:

- Liver disease — deficient/aberrant factor formation
  - impaired clearance of activated factors or plasminogen activator
  - accelerated destruction of clotting factors.

- Acclerated destruction of clotting factors (diffuse intravascular coagulation, DIC)
- Miscellaneous — after massive transfusion
  - after bypass surgery
  - overdose of oral anticoagulants (including agonists of vitamin K such as coumarins)
  - drugs such as antibiotics (alter gut flora and therefore decrease vitamin K) and cholestyramine.

THE HYPERCOAGULABLE STATE

Definition   Normal haemostatic equilibrium tilted to favour thrombosis.

Aetiology May be due to abnormalities of the blood vessel wall, blood constituents or blood flow (Virchow's triad). Aetiological factors include:

- upregulation of platelet/vessel wall interactions
- increase in pro-coagulants (e.g. fibrinogen or Factor VII)
- decrease in natural anti-coagulant factors (e.g. antithrombin III or the protein C–S–thrombomodulin system)
- increased blood viscosity
- presence of anti-cardiolipin antibodies (lupus anticoagulant)
- stasis
- use of oral contraceptives (3–5-fold increased risk)
- nephrotic syndrome (average incidence 35%)
- release of pro-coagulant factors by tumours (e.g. adenocarcinomas)
- thrombocytosis
- increased platelet adhesiveness or aggregatability.

INHERITED DISORDERS WHICH INCREASE RISK OF THROMBOSIS

Abnormalities of anti-thrombin III

Genetics Autosomal dominant inheritance. Most are heterozygous.

Clinical features Recurrent mainly venous thrombosis (commonly leg veins). In females, may present initially in pregnancy or with oral contraceptives. Episodes more frequent with increasing age.

Protein C deficiency

Genetics Autosomal dominant inheritance.

Pathogenesis Two mechanisms: either decrease in amount or a function defect.

Clinical features Lifelong increased risk of thrombosis. In heterozygotes usually deep leg veins with superficial thrombophlebitis also seen. In the rare homozygotes children present with devastating thromboembolic diatheses starting in infancy. Clinical picture may be complicated by purpura fulminans (skin haemorrhages associated with fibrin plugs in small skin vessels).

Protein S deficiency

Genetics   Autosomal dominant inheritance.

Clinical features   Similar to protein C deficiency.

Protein C resistance

Genetics   Autosomal dominant inheritance.

Pathogenesis   Abnormal resistance to normal biological effect of activated protein C.

Clinical features   Recurrent venous thrombosis.

Inherited disorders affecting fibrinolysis

Epidemiology   Rare.

Pathogenesis   Includes:
- dysfibrinogenaemia
- dysplasminogenaemia
- defective release of plasminogen activator from vessel wall.

Elevated plasma fibrinogen and factor VII$_c$ concentrations

Aetiology   Fibrinogen levels increase with increasing age, obesity, use of oral contraceptives, onset of menopause, diabetes and cigarette smoking. With the exception of smoking the same factors increase plasma Factor VII$_c$ with the addition of high dietary fat.

THE LEUKAEMIAS

GENERAL CONSIDERATIONS

Classification   Leukaemias are divided into acute and chronic forms on the basis of proportion of blast cells (acute leukaemias are blastic in nature).

Table 41.10 Factors predisposing to the development of leukaemia

Inherited factors

Down syndrome	20 X risk. Tends to be acute myeloblastic leukaemia before 3 years age and lymphoblastic after this age
Disorders with DNA fragility	Fanconi's anaemia Bloom's syndrome Ataxia telangiectasia
Other inherited disorders	Wiscott–Aldrich syndrome Osteogenesis imperfecta

Acquired factors

Environmental toxins (benzene in particular)	
Radiation (ionizing and non-ionizing)	
Chemotherapeutic agents, particularly nitrosoureas and the alkylating agents such as chlorambucil and melphalan	
Viruses	In humans only the HTLV-1 virus is implicated (adult T cell leukaemia/lymphoma)
Pre-existing haematological disease	Myeloproliferative disorders, myelodysplasia, paroxysmal nocturnal haemoglobinuria, aplastic anaemia and multiple myeloma

Aetiology and pathogenesis Many factors predispose to the development of leukaemia (Table 41.10).

GENETIC EVENTS IN LEUKAEMOGENESIS

Chronic myeloid leukaemia and the Philadelphia chromosome

Virtually all cases of chronic myeloid leukaemia carry a t(9;22) translocation resulting in the presence of a Philadelphia (Ph) chromosome (der(22)). The translocation involve the *c-abl* protoncogene on chromosome 9 and the *bcr* gene on chromosome 22. The resultant hybrid *bcr–abl* gene codes a protein in which the tyrosine kinase activity of *c-abl* is upregulated by the *bcr* sequence converting it into a transforming protein for haemopoietic cells. The abnormality is found in all haemopoietic cell lines suggesting that this is a stem cell tumour. The Ph chromosome is also seen in 20–25% of adults and 5% children with acute lymphoblastic leukaemia.

The retinoic acid receptor

In the promyelocytic variety of acute myeloblastic leukaemia the t(15;17) disrupts the retinoic acid receptor gene. Patients with this condition who are treated with all-*trans*-retinoic acid can go into complete remission and cultured cells from this disease exposed to all-*trans*-retinoic acid differentiate into neutrophils.

Gene mutations in leukaemias

Mutations of the *ras* genes can be seen in 20–30% of cases of acute myeloblastic leukaemia, 15–20% of cases of acute lymphoblastic leukaemia, 20–40% of cases of myelodysplastic syndromes and 20% of cases of myeloma. The gene most often affected is the N-*ras*.

··

ACUTE LEUKAEMIAS

Clinical features

The clinical presentation arises as a consequence of a number of abnormalities

- **Lack of normal haemopoietic cells** This may lead to increased susceptibility to infection as a result of neutropenia, decreased production of immunoglobulins and defects in cell-mediated immunity), haemorrhage (due to thrombocytopenia, DIC in some cases, lack of clotting factor if there is liver disease and increased fibrinolytic activity [promyelocytic leukaemia]) or anaemia.
- **Metabolic disturbances** This may be due to an acute tumour lysis syndrome, high plasma uric acid (due to

increased purine metabolism) or high plasma levels of calcium.

- **Organ infiltration by leukaemia** Nervous system involvement may lead to increased intracranial pressure (meningeal involvement; seen in 26–80% patients with acute lymphoblastic leukaemia) visual disturbances and spinal cord compression. Respiratory tract involvement may cause nasal blockage or interstitial pulmonary infiltrates. There may be hepatomegaly, splenomegaly, renal dysfunction, gum hypertrophy, skin or bone infiltration.

··

ACUTE LYMPHOBLASTIC LEUKAEMIA (ALL)

Epidemiology Commonest malignant disease of childhood with 75% of new cases in the USA being under 15 years. The remainder occur at any age with median 30–40 years.

Classification

Morphological classification (French–American–British [FAB])

Three sub-types recognized on the basis of nuclear size and shape, cell size, number and prominence of nucleoli and amount of and characteristics of the cytoplasm assessed on Romanowsky stained preparations with or without additional cytochemistry.

- **L1** Small cells with regular (sometimes cleaved nucleus, fine or clumped chromatin, indistinct nucleoli, scanty cytoplasm which is slightly basophilic and may contain vacuoles.
- **L2** Large cells with irregular nuclei, fine chromatin with large and prominent nucleoli (may be multiple), moderate amount of cytoplasm which is slightly basophilic and may contain vacuoles.
- **L3** Large cells with regular round to oval nuclei, fine chromatin and large prominent nucleoli (may be multiple), a moderate amount of cytoplasm which is deeply basophilic and vacuolated.

Table 41.11 Immunological markers for ALL

Marker	Common ALL	Null-type AL	Pre-B-ALL	T-ALL	B-ALL
CD10 (CALLA)	+	−	+/−	−	+
CD19	+	+	+	−	+
cytoplasmic CD22	+	+	+	−	+
cytoplasmic μ heavy chains	−	−	+	−	Ig on membrane
CD7	−	−	− & cytoplasmic CD3	+	−
nuclear TdT	+	+	+	+	−

Immunological markers in the classification of ALL

- **Precursor B-ALL** Includes three sub-types – common-ALL, null type-ALL and pre-B-ALL
- **T-ALL**
- **B-ALL**.

About 75% of these fall into the L3 FAB group and therefore have a less favourable prognosis (Table 41.11).

Prognosis The FAB classification provides prognostic information with groups L1 and L2 having the most favourable prognosis.

....

ACUTE MYELOID LEUKAEMIA (AML)

Epidemiology Accounts for about 10–15% of cases of childhood leukaemia but is the commonest form of acute leukaemia in adults and the most likely to complicate other haematological disorders.

Classification

The FAB system recognizes 7 types of AML (Table 41.12)

Table 41.12 The FAB system

M0 AML undifferentiated	No granules or Auer rods
M1 AML minimal differentiation	Scanty granules MPO+, SB+, may be Auer rods and CAE+
M2 AML with maturation myelocytes	Myeloblasts with granules, promyelocytes, few myelocytes
M3 promyelocytic L	Promyelocytes with prominant granules, Auer rods, MPO+, CAE+
M4 acute myelomonocytic L	>20% myeloblasts and promyelocytes, >20% promonoblasts and monoblasts, Auer rods +/–, MPO+, CAE+
M5 acute monoblastic L	Large monoblasts, Auer rods +, MPO+, CAE
M6 acute erythroleukaemia	> 50% megaloblastic erythroid precursors, > 30% myeloblasts
M7 acute megaloblastic L	Megakaryoblasts. No Auer rods or MPO

(MPO = myeloperoxidase; SB = Sudan black; CAE = chloracetate esterase)

THE CHRONIC LEUKAEMIAS

Chronic myeloid leukaemia (CML)

Epidemiology Accounts for a little less than 20% of all leukaemias. Mostly a disease of adult life. Fewer than 5% of patients with CML are children. M:F 3:2.

Genetics Associated with the Philadelphia chromosome in more than 95% of cases (found in all haemopoietic cell lines).

Clinical features Splenomegaly is present in about 95%. Hepatomegaly is present in just under half. There is sternal tenderness (78%), fatigue (81%), weight loss (61%) and in rare cases there may be priapism in males.

Laboratory findings In the blood there is a marked leucocytosis with all stages of neutrophil series present. There is an increase in the absolute number of circulating basophils. Most patients show some degree of anaemia (normochromic normocytic usually). The platelet count is high in about 50%.

Microscopy The bone marrow is grossly hypercellular mainly due to neutrophils and their precursors with an increase in the immature:mature ratio. The cytoplasm of the immature cells appears to mature more rapidly than the nucleus. Megakaryocytes show hypolobation.

Juvenile CML

Epidemiology Most common in children 1–2 years.

Genetic Usually lack the Philadelphia chromosome.

Clinical features Marked splenomegaly and hepatomegaly, lymph node enlargement and a desquamating skin rash.

Laboratory findings Thrombocytopenia, a white count that is lower than classic CML and an increase in the proportion of fetal haemoglobin.

Prognosis Response to treatment is usually poor.

Natural history and prognosis of CML

In chronic phase there is usually good response to therapy (20% survive 10 years). Median survival is 3–4 years. Death may be due to infection, haemorrhage or blast transformation.

Blast transformation (Blast crisis)

Definition Transformation of CML to an acute leukaemic picture.

Laboratory findings A degree of anaemia out of proportion with the white cell count, thrombocytopenia, increased circulating immature cells.

Microscopy The blast crisis is most often myeloblastic but in 30% it is lymphoblastic. In the marrow there are increased blasts (many accept that there have to be >30% for the designation of blast transformation). Fibrosis occurs.

....

CHRONIC LYMPHOCYTIC LEUKAEMIA (CLL)

Definition Proliferation and accumulation of relatively mature lymphocytes in blood, bone marrow, spleen, liver, lymph nodes and other tissues. Mostly a disease of B cells.

Epidemiology Commonest form of leukaemia in the Western world accounting for 30% of all cases. Rare in Asia. Disease of later life mostly over 50 years. M:F 2:1.

Genetics Several chromosomal abnormalities have been described, the commonest being trisomy 12 although it is thought that this might be a secondary phenomenon.

Clinical features In about 25% the diagnosis is made in asymptomatic individuals by the finding of lymphocytosis in the blood. Occasionally patients present with fatigue, lymph node enlargement or evidence of infection. The spleen may be enlarged and there may be tonsillar enlargement. Features of autoimmunity are fairly common – 15–35% have autoimmune haemolytic anaemia while a few have antoimmune neutropenia or thrombocytopenia.

Laboratory findings The International Workshop on CLL has proposed the following criteria for B-CLL:
- lymphocytosis – absolute and sustained blood lymphocyte count of $10 \times 10^9/1$ with most of the cells having the appearance of mature lymphocytes and showing B cell markers
- bone marrow in which lymphocytes account for at least 30% of the nucleated cells.

Variants of CLL

Prolymphocytic leukaemia

Definition Proliferation of lymphocytes larger and of less mature appearance than those of classic CLL.

Clinical features An aggressive disorder with high lymphocyte counts.

Microscopy The cells have condensed nuclear chromatin and rather prominent nucleoli.

Hairy cell leukaemia

Epidemiology Peak age 40–60 years; M:F 4:1. Accounts for about 10% of cases of CLL.

Clinical features Patients present with weakness and fatigue. There is splenomegaly, no lymph node enlargement and differing degrees of pancytopenia.

Microscopy The cells have 'hairy' cytoplasmic projections. The cytoplasm is blue-grey and there are no granules. The cells contain tartrate resistant acid phosphatase (95%).

Natural history and prognosis Treatment by splenectomy reverses some of the pancytopenia (due to pooling in the spleen). Treatment with α-interferon produces a response in 80–90% but remission in only 5–10%.

··

THE MYELODYSPLASTIC SYNDROMES (MDS)

Epidemiology Mostly elderly, median age at diagnosis 65 years.

Characteristics Refractory anaemia and other cytopenias, hypercellular bone marrow with abnormal development in one or more cell line. Some evolve into acute leukaemia.

Classification Depends on the proportion of blasts in blood and bone marrow, presence of ring sideroblasts in marrow, the number of monocytes in the blood and the presence of Auer rods (see Table 41.13).

Genetics Chromosomal abnormalities are found in 50%, the commonest abnormalities being partial or total loss of chromosomes 5,7, and Y and trisomy 8. Loss of part of chromosome 5 occurs in cases of RA (70%), RARS (30%), RAEB and RAEB-t (30%) but <5% of cases of CMML. When there is loss of 5q as the only defect the appearances are characteristic (5q-syndrome).

Clinical features There is usually weakness and fatigue (associated with anaemia), easy bruising (due to thrombocytopenia) and increased susceptibility to infection (due to neutropenia).

Laboratory findings There is anaemia in 90% (associated with thrombocytopenia in 25%) and neutropenia in 5–10%. The neutrophils show abnormal morphology including the Pelger abnormality (bilobed nucleus rather than multilobed) and decreased response to chemotactic factors, phagocytosis and adhesion to appropriate ligands.

5q syndrome

Epidemiology Usually elderly females.

Table 41.13 Classification of the myelodysplastic syndromes

	Blasts in marrow (%)	Blasts in blood (%)	Ring sideroblasts in marrow (%)	Monocytes in blood × 10⁹/l
Refractory anaemia (RA)	<5	<1	<15	–
Refractory anaemia with ring sideroblasts (RARS)	<5	<1	≥15	–
Refractory anaemia with excess blasts (RAEB)	5–20	<5	–	–
Refractory anaemia with excess blasts in transformation (REAB-t)	>20–30 and/or Auer rods	<5	–	–
Chronic myelomonocytic leukaemia (CMML)	≥20	≤5	–	>1

Clinical features There is often a long and usually uneventful natural history but with splenomegaly.

Microscopy In the marrow the megakaryocyte nuclei show fewer lobes than normal.

MYELOPROLIFERATIVE DISORDERS

Definition Set of closely related conditions characterized by proliferation of one or more haemopoetic cell lines. In many cases the proliferations are clonal and neoplastic.

Natural history One entity can become transformed into another and there is a tendency to develop myeloid leukaemia.

POLYCYTHAEMIA RUBRA VERA

Characteristics Increase in red cell numbers as well as other white cells.

Epidemiology Principally in later life, mean age at diagnosis is 60 years. Rare in Afro-Caribbeans. Amongst Caucasians, Jews are more at risk (2-fold).

Clinical features Presentation is associated with increased red cell mass and hyperviscosity and symptoms include headache, dizziness, tinnitus, itching of skin after hot bath, visual disturbances, dyspepsia (increased risk of duodenal ulcer), dyspnoea and red skin. The spleen is enlarged in 65–90% and hepatomegaly occurs in over 40%.

Laboratory findings
- increased red cell count – normal morphology
- increased white cell count – myeloid cells commonly show shift to the left
- increased platelet count
- increased total blood volume and total red cell volume
- increased blood viscosity – 5–10-fold
- hyperuricaemia in 50–75%

Natural history and prognosis Increased risk of arterial and venous thrombosis. Treatment is directed to maintaining normal red cell mass and platelet counts. Survival may be 10–15 years.

Secondary polycythaemia

Definition   Affects only red cells.

Aetiology   Increased erythropoietin which may be appropriate (e.g. those living at high altittudes, congenital heart disease with right–left shunt, hypoxia and smokers) or inappropriate (e.g. associated with massive uterine leiomyomas, some liver cell carcinomas, some renal carcinomas and cerebellar haemangioblastoma).

....

IDIOPATHIC MYELOFIBROSIS

Definition   Clonal neoplastic disorder involving haemopoieitic stem cells associated with marrow fibrosis.

Characteristics   There is stem cell proliferation with spillover into the circulating blood and colonization of tissues leading to extramedullary haemopoiesis.

Epidemiology   Mostly elderly.

Clinical features   Most present with symptoms related either to anaemia or hypersplenism. There is usually hyperuricaemia (due to high cell turnover) and there may be gout or renal calculi. The spleen may be massively enlarged extending to the pelvic brim. Hepatomegaly is present in about 50%. Sternal tenderness is unusual.

Laboratory findings   There is anaemia in most cases. The blood film shows a leucoerythroblastic picture (nucleated red cells and immature neutrophils). The red cells may have a **tear-drop** appearance. Platelets are larger than normal. White cell and platelet counts are raised in 50% but in 25% the white cell count is decreased. Attempts to aspirate the bone marrow frequently fail and in those in whom it is possible the findings are often non-specific. Biochemical changes in the blood include increased lactate dehydrogenase and β-hydroxybutyrate dehydrogenase (reflecting increased cell turnover) and increased alkaline phosphatase (reflecting increased bone formation).

Microscopy There is osteosclerosis with thick and abnormally shaped bony trabeculae. In some areas the marrow space may be obliterated. The spleen shows extramedullary haemopoiesis which may also be present in the liver and almost any other tissue.

Natural history and prognosis Death may be due to infection, evolution into acute leukaemia, haemorrhage, cardiac failure or occasionally portal hypertension (caused by intrasinusoidal haemopoiesis or thrombosis).

ESSENTIAL THROMBOCYTHAEMIA

Definition Abnormal clonal proliferation of megakaryocytes resulting in increased platelet count.

Pathogenesis The pathogenesis of the bleeding tendency is poorly understood but may be related to functional abnormalities in the platelets.

Clinical features There is abnormal bleeding and an increased risk of thromboembolic events. Thrombi are particularly found in the splenic vein, intracranial vessels and small vessels of the fingers and toes. The spleen is significantly enlarged in 80% but atrophy may be a late development. Hepatomegaly may be present.

Laboratory findings There is a greatly increased platelet count and the platelets are of abnormal size and shape. The neutrophil count may be increased and 'shifted left' (more immature forms).

Microscopy Marked proliferation of megakaryocytes.

Natural history and prognosis Treatment is with myelosuppressive therapy (e.g. busulphan, hydroxyurea or α-interferon. The commonest cause of death is thromboembolism but transformation to acute myeloid leukaemia may occur.

The lymphoreticular system

42

THE THYMUS

ANATOMY

Site Flattened bilobed structure lying in the anterior mediastinum between the sternum and the pericardium.

Size Varies with age: 20–30 g at birth with peak of 40–50 g at puberty.

HISTOLOGY

The thymus is partly epithelial and partly lymphoid divided into cortex and medulla. The epithelial component is of four types.

1. Sub-capsular: 1–2 cells thick abutting capsular membrane. Extends along septa to blend with perivascular epithelium
2. Cortical: large cells with prominent nucleoli and cytoplasmic extentions around lymphoid precursors
3. Medullary: spindle-shaped cells with densely staining nuclei and inconspicuous nucleoli
4. Hassall's corpuscles: whorls of epithelial cells which develop keratinized centres as they enlarge.

DEVELOPMENT

The epithelial component is derived from 3rd (and occasionally 4th) pharyngeal pouch and cervical pouch endoderm. Colonization by lymphoid cells begins at about 9 weeks' gestation. By 13 weeks' gestation export of T cells has begun.

The volume of the thymus is not affected by ageing but as life progresses much of the lymphoid tissue is lost and replaced by adipose tissue – half the thymic tissue is lost by 10 years and only 10% remains after 30 years. Inappropriate involution (accidental involution) may occur following acute stress due to apoptosis of cortical thymocytes or in association with a chronic wasting disease or severe malnutrition.

··

PRIMARY IMMUNODEFICIENCY

Di George's syndrome

Definition Thymic hypoplasia associated with cardiac defects, cleft palate, abnormal facies and absence of parathyroids (causing hypocalcaemia).

Immunology Selective T-cell deficiency with defective cell-mediated immunity.

Aetiology Defect in development of 3rd and 4th pharyngeal pouches.

Genetics Not inherited. Deletion of material on chromosome 22.

Macroscopy Absence of thymus is rare. Most have small thymus.

Microscopy Normal thymic histology.

Clinical features May succumb to viral infections.

Nezelof's syndrome

Immunology Selective T-cell deficiency.

Genetics Either autosomal or X-linked inherited disorder.

Macroscopy Only thymus affected.

Clinical features May succumb to viral infections.

Severe combined immunodeficiency diseases (SCID)

Definition Set of disorders characterized by defects in both cellular and humoral immunity. Usually associated with lymphopenia.

Genetics Inherited as either autosomal or X-linked recessive disorder.

Pathogenesis Usually abnormal B and T cell development from bone marrow stem cells.

Autosomal recessive SCID

1. Adenosine deaminase (ADA) deficiency

Epidemiology Accounts for 50% autosomal recessive and 20% of all cases.

Pathogenesis Accumulation of metabolites toxic to lymphocytes and blocks DNA synthesis.

Treatment Either with transfusions of enzyme containing red cells or the enzyme itself. In the future may be a candidate for gene therapy.

2. Purine nucleoside phosphorylase (PNP) deficiency

Pathogenesis Accumulation of toxic metabolites. T cells more affected than B cells.

3. Bare lymphocyte syndrome

Pathogenesis Failure to express HLA class II antigens on surface of lymphocytes, macrophages and dendritic cells leading to failure of antigen presentation to T helper cells.

Many cases of SCID do not fit into these categories. Some of these may be due to T and T cell receptor abnormalities. Further cases may be due to bone-marrow stem-cell production defects (reticular dysgenesis) resulting in deficiency of B- and T-cell precursors.

Macroscopy Thymus is usually normally sited but small (0.5–4 g).

Microscopy Loss of cortico-medullary differentiation, absent Hassall's corpuscles and lymphoid cell depletion.

....

SECONDARY IMMUNODEFICIENCY

Aetiology Allogeneic bone marrow transplantation (due to pre-transplant treatment and/or graft-versus-host disease) and AIDS are the most common causes.

Definition Myasthenia gravis is an autoimmune disorder characterized by progressive muscular weakness.

Immunology Autoantibodies react with acetylcholine receptor. In addition 50% have antibodies to the A band of striated muscle (90% of cases with thymic epithelial tumour).

Pathogenesis Around 75–85% of patients have thymic abnormalities.

Microscopy There may be one of three patterns:

1. Lymphoid follicular hyperplasia (thymitis): associated with 50–60% cases of mysthenia. Commonest between 10–40 years. M:F 1:3. Associated with HLA types A1, B8 and DR3. Lymphoid follicles with germinal centres are present. Antigen is found on myoid cells in the thymus.
2. Thymic epithelial tumours.
3. Normal or mildly atrophic thymus.

....

TUMOURS OF THE THYMUS

Thymic epithelial tumours

Thymoma

Epidemiology Commonest epithelial tumour of thymus and commonest neoplasm of anterior mediastinum (45% tumours at this site). Most common in middle to later life with mean age at diagnosis 50 years. M:F 1:1.

Clinical features May be asymptomatic, associated with myasthenia gravis or non-mysthenic para-neoplastic syndromes or can present with symptoms related to anterior mediastinal mass.

Classification Difficult and controversial. Rosai and Levine (1976; see Table 42.1) classified the tumours by invasiveness and metastatic potential into category I (minimal cytological atypia, local invasion only and rare lymphovascular invasion) and category II (cytologically malignant). More recently Muller–Hermelink have related thymomas to their counterpart in the normal thymus resulting in a greater correlation with clinical features and behaviour.

Table 42.1 Rosai and Levine's classification

Type	Frequency (%)	M:F 3	Association with myasthenia (%)	Rosai and Levine classification	Stage I (%)	Stage II (%)	Stage III (%)	Stage IV (%)
Medullary thymoma	5.0	1:1.7	33	non-invasive (benign)	66	34	0	0
Mixed thymoma	20.0	1:2.1	39	non-invasive (benign)	66	34	0	0
Predominantly cortical thymoma	7.7	1:3.5	33	invasive (category I)	44	44	1	0
Cortical thymoma	41.9	1:1.1	66	invasive (category I)	21	32	38	9
Well-differentiated carcinoma	16.8	1:2.1	77	invasive (category I)	0	17	57	26
Other carcinoma	7.7	3:1	0	invasive (category II)	0	8	59	33

Macroscopy Most are well-circumscribed firm lesions. In encapsulated thymomas the capsule is fibrous and the tumours may be lobulated. In invasive thymomas the edges tend to be poorly defined. Size is variable from 150 g to several kg. Cystic degeneration may be present.

Thymic lymphoma

Non-Hodgkin's lymphoma (NHL) Mediastinal involvement is seen in 18–24% of NHL, mostly T-cell lymphoblastic lymphoma. Primary B cell thymic lymphoma.

Synonyms Mediastinal large cell lymphoma with sclerosis.

Epidemiology Commonest in young adult females.

Microscopy Large lymphoid cells often with clear cytoplasm and associated with marked fibrous tissue response.

Clinical features Can present with superior vena caval obstruction. Lymph node involvement is rare. Spread is frequently to other extranodal sites.

Hodgkin's disease The mediastinum is a common site for Hodgkin's disease, often of nodular sclerosis sub-type.

Germ-cell tumours

Pathogenesis Failure of migration of primordial germinal crests from urogenital ridges. Types:

- Seminoma: affects males in third decade.
- Benign teratoma: accounts for 80% mediastinal germ cell tumours. Usually second or third decade.
- Malignant teratoma: almost exclusively young males.

THE LYMPHORETICULAR SYSTEM

NORMAL ANATOMY AND FUNCTION

The immune response results from cellular interactions within peripheral lymphoid tissue which includes:

- lymph nodes – respond to antigens within the tissues transported via the lymphatics

- the spleen – responds to antigens in the blood
- mucosa-associated lymphoid tissue (MALT) – responds to antigens which cross epithelial surfaces.

....

THE LYMPH NODE

Site Situated along lymphatics. Occasionally clustered into groups such as in the groin, axilla, periaortic region, cervical and supraclavicular areas.

Lymph flow **Afferent lymphatics** penetrate the fibrous capsule at several points and drain into the **marginal sinus**. These in turn drain into the **cortical sinuses** which penetrate the node and break up into fine arborizing channels. These then form the **medullary sinuses** which drain into the efferent lymphatic leaving the node at the hilum. The sinuses are lined by phagocytic endothelial cells and macrophages.

Blood flow Blood enters the node at the hilum via a single artery. This branches eventually forming a fine network of capillaries which drain into the **high endothelial venules**. These vessels are the site of **lymphocyte migration**. These venules fuse to eventually form a single vein which leaves the node at the hilum.

Cellular compartments of the lymph node

B lymphocytes

Most of the nodal B-cell population is located in the cortex in the form of lymphoid follicles. In the unstimulated node these are small and consist of small lymphocytes (the primary follicle) resembling the mantle zone population of stimulated follicles (secondary follicles). Secondary follicle centres are divided into zones. At the centre there is the region termed the follicle centre which appears paler than the surrounding regions and contains two main cell populations centroblasts (large actively dividing cells with round nuclei and two or more obvious nucleoli) and centrocytes (smaller with irregular nuclei, coarse chromatin and indistinct nucleoli). These two populations show characteristic clustering with centroblasts mostly found in an area further from the node capsule (the dark zone) and centrocytes nearer the capsule (light zone). Other cells found in the follicle centre include the follicle dendritic cell and macrophages (principally involved in removal of apoptotic lymphocyte debris leading to the term 'tingible body macrophage' being applied to them). The follicle centre is surrounded by the mantle zone which is thicker at the capsular aspect and contains small lymphocytes.

T lymphocytes

T cells are found between the lymphoid follicles in the paracortex.

Antigen-presenting cells

There are two populations within this group. The population found in the follicle centres (folliclular dendritic cells) have enlongated cytoplasmic processes forming a meshwork. They trap immune complexes which are powerful immunogens and provoke B-cell proliferation and activation. The second population of antigen-presenting cells is found in the paracortex (interdigitating reticulum cells) and their function is the stimulation of T cells.

....

NON-NEOPLASTIC DISORDERS OF LYMPH NODES

There are a limited number of morphological appearances that can be seen as a result of stimulation of lymphoid tissue within lymph nodes. Different disease entities stimulate the different cell populations to different extents which results in one or other pattern predominating. This results in particular patterns being characteristically associated with particular diseases.

Acute lymphadenitis

Aetiology Most frequently pyogenic micro-organisms e.g. β haemolytic streptococci (causing pharyngitis) or staphylococci (causing skin lesions).

Clinical features Nodes become enlarged and tender.

Microscopy Since the cause is usually obvious biopsy is seldom performed. The nodes show oedema, hyperaemia and emigration of neutrophils. Suppuration is rare.

Follicular hyperplasia

Aetiology Seen in nodes draining a local inflammatory reaction but is also seen in rheumatoid arthritis, systemic lupus erythematosus and the early phase of HIV infection.

Pathogenesis Immune response mediated predominantly by B lymphocytes.

Microscopy The overall architecture of the node is preserved. The lymphoid follicles are increased in size and number. The follicles vary both in size and shape. The enlarged germinal centres show increased cell turnover with large numbers of tingible body macrophages. There may be large numbers of plasma cells as a result of differentiation of the proliferated cells and these are predominantly found in the medulla.

Paracortical hyperplasia

Aetiology Most frequently associated with viral infections such as Epstein–Barr virus infection (infectious mononucleosis) and in drug reactions (e.g. hydantoin, non-steroidal anti-inflammatory drugs, antiobiotics notably penicillin, and some anti-malarials).

Pathogenesis Immune response mediated predominantly by T lymphocytes.

Microscopy May be diffuse or nodular. The increased population consists of small lymphocytes and T immunoblasts. High endothelial venules become prominent.

Sinus histiocytosis

Aetiology Frequently seen in nodes draining a source of antigens including nodes in the region of malignant tumours.

Microscopy Increased numbers of large macrophages within the sinuses with increased phagocytic activity.

Pulp histiocytosis

Aetiology Insoluble materials e.g. carbon and other dusts.

Microscopy Large numbers of macrophages are seen within the node pulp. The promoting agent may be visible (e.g. carbon dust).

Dermatopathic lymphadenopathy

Aetiology Occurs in superficial nodes of patients with certain skin diseases including psoriasis, chronic exfoliative dermatitis, mycosis fungoides and other skin conditions associated with itching.

Pathogenesis Debris from the breakdown of epidermal cells is taken up by macrophages that migrate to lymph nodes leading to expansion of the paracortical area.

Microscopy Paracortical expansion includes macrophages that contain lipid and melanin pigment. There is expansion of the interdigitating reticulum cell population (clear cells). There may be accompanying follicular hyperplasia and plasmacytosis.

....

SPECIFIC REACTIVE LYMPHADENOPATHIES
Mycobacterium tuberculosis

Site Most frequently pulmonary hilar nodes associated with a lung parenchymal lesion (primary complex). May be seen in cervical nodes associated with ingested organisms that pass to the nodes from the pharynx (scrofula).

Macroscopy The nodes are enlarged and matted together. Sectioning reveals cheesy material (caseation).

Microscopy Numerous granulomas are composed of epithelioid cells. The centres undergo caseation necrosis resulting in featureless areas of eosinophilic material. Giant cells of Langhan's type are almost always present. Granulomas are surrounded by lymphocytes. Organisms may or may not be identifiable using special stains.

Mycobacterium avium intracellulare

Bacteriology These bacteria inhabit the soil and may be inhaled or swallowed.

Clinical features May cause caseating cervical lymph nodes (scrofula), disseminated disease involving macrophages throughout the body (particularly associated with decreased host cell-mediated immunity) or a pulmonary lesion similar to that seen in post-primary tuberculosis.

Yersinial lymphadenitis

Bacteriology   *Yersinia pseudotuberculosis* and *Yersinia entero-colitica*. These are Gram-negative coccoid or oval organisms usually carried by wood pigeons and rats.

Site   Usually mesenteric (frequently ileocaecal) nodes associated with gut infections.

Clinical features   Patients (usually children) present with symptoms mimicking acute appendicitis.

Microscopy   There is oedema and an increase in immuno-blasts and plasma cells in the cortex and paracortex. Follicular hyperplasia is present and if the cause is *Y. pseudotuberculosis* there may be small granulomas and abscesses.

Cat-scratch disease

Bacteriology   *Bartonella henselae*. An extracellular coc-cobacillus.

Clinical features   The organism is transferred to humans through the skin following a scratch or bite from a cat.

Microscopy   The features are only characteristic in the later stages. There are abscesses with a star-like outline and central necrosis. The necrotic areas contain neutrophils and neutrophil debris and this area is surrounded by palisaded histiocytes. Similar abscesses are seen in patients with **lymphogranuloma venereum**. There may be expansion of monocytoid B cells.

Infectious mononucleosis

Epidemiology   Worldwide distribution. Presents as a clini-cal disease most frequently in adolescents.

Virology   Epstein–Barr virus is the aetiological agent.

Clinical features   Many cases may be sub-clinical or asso-ciated with non-specific viral-type symptoms. In addition to nodal involvement there may be splenomegaly and hepatitis.

Laboratory findings   The blood film shows large atypical lymphocytes which are T cells that have undergone blast transformation. Paul–Bunnell test (recognizes heterophile antibodies) is positive.

Microscopy Most cases are diagnosed without recourse to biopsy. The node shows a very marked proliferative expansion of the paracortex which may blur the normal architecture and may be confused with a neoplastic proliferation. The cells are predominantly immunoblasts (some of which will be within the sinuses) and immature plasma cells. There may be infiltration of the node capsule and surrounding adipose tissue. Follicular hyperplasia may be present.

HIV-related lymphadenopathy

Virology HIV is a C-type retrovirus.

Clinical features Lymph node disease can be present in the early stages of the disease in the absence of other pathology such as opportunistic infections. Patients present with persistent widespread lymphadenopathy (**persistent generalized lymphadenopathy**) which may be accompanied by fatigue.

Microscopy There may be striking lymphoid follicular hyperplasia. Monocytoid B cells may be prominent. In may cases there is folliculolysis with the germinal centres infiltrated and broken up by small lymphocytes. With time there is atrophy of the follicles and the node adopts an 'empty' appearance.

Toxoplasma lymphadenitis

Parasitology Infection by the protozoon *Toxoplasma gondii*. In the UK the reservoir is the domestic cat.

Clinical features Many cases are asymptomatic. The commonest presentation is with painless lymphadenopathy commonly affecting the posterior triangle of the neck. Infection in pregnancy can induce serious eye and brain defects in the fetus. Individuals with decreased immunity (e.g. AIDS patients) can develop severe and sometimes fatal complications including encephalitis, pneumonitis and choroidoretinitis.

Microscopy The features are not specific but are characterized by the presence of follicular hyperplasia, small epithelioid granulomas both within lymphoid follicles and at the periphery of the node and the presence of monocytoid B cells.

Sinus histiocytosis with massive lymphadenopathy (Rosai–Dorfman disease)

Site   In addition to lymph nodes, other sites may be involved in up to 25% of cases including the orbit, upper respiratory tract central nervous system, salivary gland, skin and bones.

Epidemiology   Usually occurs in first two decades of life. More common in black Afro-Caribbeans than whites.

Aetiology   Unknown.

Clinical features   Characteristically there is massive painless bilateral lymph node enlargement in the neck. There might be fever, leucocytosis, raised erythrocyte sedimentation rate and polyclonal hypergammaglobinopathy.

Microscopy   The affected nodes are enlarged and the capsule is thickened. There is enormous distention of the sinuses by macrophages with large vesicular nuclei and abundant cytoplasm. Within the cytoplasm intact lymphocytes can be seen (emperipolesis).

Natural history and prognosis   There is spontaneous resolution in most cases.

Sarcoidosis

Site   The disease may occur in virtually any tissue within the body.

Epidemiology   More common in Scandinavians in Europe and in the USA the disease is 10–15 times more frequent in blacks than in whites.

Aetiology   Unknown.

Clinical features   Depend on the sites involved.

Macroscopy   The node may have a grey cut surface.

Microscopy   There are small well-defined and non-caseating granulomas with epithelioid cells and occasional Langhans' giant cells. Necrosis is not a prominent feature and if present in the centre of the granulomas is of the fibrinoid type. The giant cells may contain Schaumann bodies (rounded laminated bodies containing iron and calcium), asteroid bodies (star-shaped bodies of collagen) or crystals of calcium oxalate – none of which are specific for sarcoid.

Histiocytic necrotizing lymphadenitis without granulocytic infiltration (Kikuchi's disease)

Epidemiology   Most frequently seen in young females in Japan but is also seen in Europe and North America.

Aetiology   Unknown.

Clinical features   Patients present with painless enlargement of lymph nodes in the neck associated with mild fever.

Microscopy   The nodes show well-demarcated foci of necrosis in the paracortical zone containing much apoptotic debris. This is surrounded by transformed T cells and macrophages. Neutrophils are absent.

Natural history and prognosis   Usually spontaneous recovery. Very rarely there may be relapse.

Mucocutaneous lymph node syndrome (Kawasaki's disease)

Epidemiology   Disease of infancy and early childhood.

Microscopy   The affected nodes are enlarged and contain areas of necrosis. There are thrombi in the small intranodal vessels.

Angiofolicular lymph node hyperplasia (Castleman's disease, giant lymph node hyperplasia)

Site   May involve a single site (frequently the mediastinum but also in the lung, neck, axilla retroperitoneum and limbs) or be multi-focal with widespread involvement.

Clinical features   There may be associated features such as fever, anaemia, joint pain, sweating, skin rashes hypergammaglobinopathy, amyloidosis and endocrine disturbances (more common in the multi-centric form).

Microscopy   There are two morphological forms.

1. **Hyaline vascular type**
   There are large follicle structures in which blood vessels are prominent which are surrounded by hyaline material. The B cells component of the follicles are decreased

and the follicular dendritic cells are prominent. The mantle zone lymphocytes are arranged in concentric layers (onion-skin pattern). There is prominent interfollicular stroma with conspicuous post-capillary venules. The cells in the interfollicular area include plasma cells, eosinophils and immunoblasts. This is the commonest variant seen in the localized type.

2. **Plasma cell type**
   Characterized by a diffuse plasma cell proliferation in the interfollicular area. The prominent vascular changes in the interfollicular area and hyalinization of vessels is not seen. Amorphous eosinophilic material may be seen in follicle centres.

Natural history and prognosis Surgical removal of localized lesions causes remission of symptoms. The prognosis of the multi-centric form is poor with median survival 2–2.5 years. About 20–30% of patients with multi-centric Castleman's disease develop Kaposi's sarcoma or B cell non-Hodgkin's lymphoma.

....

TUMOURS OF THE LYMPH NODES: PRIMARY TUMOURS (LYMPHOMA)

Hodgkin's disease

Epidemiology Accounts for about 50% of all cases of lymphoma. Bimodal age distribution with the early peak in young adults and a second peak in old age (except in less-developed countries when the early peak is attenuated or absent and there is a greater frequency in children).

Aetiology It has been suggested that the first peak may be related to an environmental (possibly infectious) factor. The most canvassed agent is Epstein–Barr virus (EBV) which is suggested by an increased risk associated with infectious mononucleosis, high frequency of anti-EBV antibodies and the presence of EBV genome in some tumour cells.

Clinical features First, there is usually enlargement of a single lymph node group (most commonly cervical nodes).

Macroscopy Individual nodes tend to remain discrete. The cut surfaces may be greyish or a pale tan colour. The consistency depends on the degree of sclerosis (increased sclerosis is associated with firmer nodes).

Microscopy The most reliable feature in so-called 'classical' Hodgkin's disease is the presence of Reed–Sternberg cells in an appropriate background.

The Reed–Sternberg cell

This is believed to be the neoplastic cell of Hodgkin's disease. It has a large bilobed nucleus with a central prominent nucleolus surrounded by a clear zone. The nuclear membrane is well demarcated and there is abundant cytoplasm. Mononuclear variants (Hodgkin cells) can be seen. The origin of the Reed–Sternberg cell is the source of much debate. It is agreed by most that it is of lymphoid origin and at present the most likely candidate is the B cell. The Reed–Sternberg cell characteristically expresses the CD30 antigen (a marker associated with activated B and T cells). A proportion may express the CD15 antigen (X-hapten, more characteristically associated with myeloid cells) and CD25 (IL-2 receptor). In some series up to 60% express B-cell associated antigens although antigens associated with T cells and other lymphoid cell lineages have been described. In different series molecular studies have shown rearrangement of the immunoglobulin genes and the T-cell receptor genes. EBV genome can be seen in up to 35% of cases.

The cellular background

In most cases there is distortion or loss of the normal nodal structure either involving the whole node or just the T or B zones. Several cell types are seen including lymphocytes, plasma cells, eosinophils, macrophages and granulocytes. In general the lymphocytes are small and mature and mostly T cells.

Classification A histological classification based on a modification of the Rye classification.

- Lymphocyte predominance (10%):

  - nodular
  - diffuse
  - mixed

- nodular sclerosis (50–75%)
- mixed cellularity (17%)
- lymphocyte depleted (4%).

Move recently the classification has been updated by WHO and a further category of lymphocyte rich classical Hodgkin's has been added.

Most investigators now accept that lymphocyte predominance HD is a separate entity with the other three groups constituting 'classical' HD.

Lymphocyte predominance Hodgkin's disease

Definition In this type there are no classic Reed–Sternberg cells. The putative neoplastic cells are variously termed L&H or 'popcorn' cells. They have multi-lobated nuclei and small nucleoli with scanty cytoplasm. These cells express lymphocyte-related antigens (CD45-leucocyte common antigen) together with antigens associated with B cells (CD20, CD79a, J chain) but rarely express CD30 in paraffin tissue and never CD15.

Nodular lymphocyte predominance HD

Site Lymph nodes of neck, axilla and inguinal regions. Rare if ever in mediastinum.

Epidemiology This is the commonest form. Occurs at any age but peaks in fourth decade and rare after 40 years. Males affected more than females.

Microscopy Nodules are present but may be poorly - delineated. Nodules contain L&H cells sometimes in con- siderable numbers, with small lymphocytes and macrophages.

Diffuse lymphocyte predominance HD

Microscopy Nodal structure is effaced by diffuse infiltrate of small lymphocytes. Macrophages are distributed randomly or in small granulomas. L&H cells are scattered and in some cases do not express B-cell markers.

Nodular sclerosis Hodgkin's disease

Epidemiology Commonest type of HD in developed countries. Arises typically in young adults less than 40 years. Females more than males.

Site Anterior mediastinum is a common site but arises in other node groups as well.

Microscopy There is a striking fibrous tissue (hyaline collagen rich fibrosis) response in the node-delineating cellular nodules. A variant of Reed–Sternberg cell is often present with a multi-lobed nucleus and small amount of cytoplasm (**lacunar cell**) which appears to sit in a lacuna when the tissue has been fixed in formalin (fixation related shrinkage artefact). Classic Reed–Sternberg cells may be difficult to find and the reactive cell population is variable but granulomas and necrosis may be present. Histologically some investigators have divided this type into two types depending on the reactive population in the nodules (type 1 with lymphocytes or mixed pattern; type 2 with relative depletion of reactive cells) and the presence of necrosis.

Mixed cellularity Hodgkin's disease

Epidemiology Accounts for about 17% cases in the UK. Tends to occur in older individuals in Western countries but in Third World countries occurs in younger individuals.

Microscopy There are a substantial number of Reed–Sternberg and Hodgkin cells with a cellular response that is rich in plasma cells, neutrophils and eosinophils. The connective tissue response is not banded and hyalinized.

Lymphocyte depleted Hodgkin's disease

Epidemiology Rarest form in the UK but more common in less developed countries. Mostly affects those in late adult life.

Site May be extranodal (including liver and bone marrow).

Microscopy Two histological patterns; reticular with sheets of pleomorphic Reed–Sternberg and Hodgkin cells and a lymphocyte poor reactive infiltrate but with many macrophages and a diffuse fibrosing type characterized by pleomorphic and classic Reed–Sternberg cells set in an amorphous collagen-poor background depleted of reactive cells.

Staging of Hodgkin's disease

Staging is most widely performed using the Ann Arbor system (Table 42.2).

Clinical features The disease is sub-classified by the absence (A) or presence (B) of one or more of the following clinical symptoms – unexplained fever >38°C; night sweats; loss of ≥10% of body weight in 6 months.

Natural history and prognosis Determined by histological sub-type (lymphocyte predominance better than nodular sclerosis better than mixed cellularity better than lymphocyte depleted; nodular sclerosis type 1 better than type 2), stage and presence of disease bulk (nodal mass greater than 10 cm or increased mediastinal width by more than one third). There is a significant down-regulation of cellular immune response in HD resulting in increased risk of infection especially by opportunistic pathogens such as fungi, viruses and mycobacteria.

Table 42.2 Ann Arbor staging system

Stage I	Involvement of single nodal region (or extranodal site [IE])
Stage II	Involvement of two or more nodal regions on the same side of the diaphragm (or an extranodal site plus other nodal groups on the same side of the diaphragm [IIE])
Stage III	Involvement of nodal regions on each side of the diaphragm (or involvement of extranodal site plus nodal regions on each side of the diphragm [IIIE] or involvement of spleen [IIIS] or both spleen and one other extranodal site [IIISE])
Stage IV	Diffuse or disseminated involvement of one or more extranodal site with or without node involvement.

NON-HODGKIN'S LYMPHOMA
General considerations

Classification Many classification schemes exist for tumours which are derived from lymphocytes. It is fairly well established that the non-Hodgkin's lymphomas recapitulate the various stages in the ontogeny of lymphocytes and more recent classifications have tried to include clinico-pathological entities and relate them to their normal lymphoid counterpart. The most commonly used classification systems in the past were the Kiel classification and the Working Formulation for Clinical Usage. More recently new classification systems have been proposed and are being gradually adopted: the Revised European–American Classification of Lymphoid Neoplasms (REAL Classification) and the WHO classification.

Kiel classification
Originally proposed in 1974, modified in 1978 and updated in 1988 this classification relies on the distinction between tumours derived from B and T cells. The tumours are further sub-divided into histologically low- and high-grade lesions on the basis of the number of blasts and transformed cells. Entities within the B-cell arm of the classification are named for the putative normal counterpart in lymphoid ontogeny from which they are thought to arise while the T-cell arm relies more on pattern and cell morphology. While there is interobserver consistency in the diagnosis of low-grade B-cell lymphomas using this classification there is some doubt about the reliability of the use of groups within the T-cell arm and high-grade B-cell lymphoma groups.

The working formulation for clinical usage
Following the failure of pathologists and clinicians to agree on a single lymphoma classification that could be used worldwide a method of translating between various existing classifications was proposed based on the study of the pathology and clinical characteristics of a large number of lymphoma cases. Although not intended as a de facto classification it has now been established in this mould. The classification relies on the assessment of clinical behaviour

(low, intermediate or high grade) and the morphological characteristics of the tumour cells and in particular the size of the cell and presence or absence of nuclear cleaves. This takes no account of cell lineage or the presence of distinct clinicopathological entities and some distinct entities are split between groups.

The revised European–American classification of lymphoid neoplasms (REAL)

Proposed in 1994 by an international group of pathologists with a special interest in lymphoma pathology this classification attempted to list those lymphoma entities which the participants could diagnose confidently in their routine practice (i.e. what lymphoma pathologists *do* do, rather than *should* do). The result was a classification scheme loosely based on the Kiel classification (i.e. recognizing B and T cell groups and attempting to relate tumours to the cell of origin) with the recognition of precursor (lymphoblastic) and peripheral lymphomas. Within these broad categories there were established entities about which there was general agreement that they had a characteristic clinical behaviour, morphology, immunophenotype and in some cases genotype. The criteria that there should be low interobserver variability resulted in the grouping together of many of the high-grade B-cell lymphomas and T-cell lymphomas recognized in the Kiel classification. In addition there were several provisional entities whose existence as separate lymphoma groups was not absolutely established. The classification also included Hodgkin's disease but this differed little from the existing classification schemes.

The WHO classification

Following studies confirming the appropriateness of the REAL classification, the WHO produced its own classification as part of a wider review of all tumour types. the classification includes all haemopoietic and lymphoreticular tumours and for lymphoma is largerly based on the REAL classification.

Laboratory methods

Many techniques are used for the classification of lymphoma. This is possible due to knowledge of the antigen profile of lymphocytes in the different stages of differentiation during B and T cell ontogeny and the availability of antibodies to recognize these antigens in processed tissue specimens. Molecular techniques have also been developed to identify cytogenetic abnormalities and the presence of genetic rearrangements of the immunoglobulin and T-cell receptor genes. These two groups of genes are rearranged during normal B (immunoglobulin genes) and T (T-cell receptor genes) development and give rise to the diversity of the immune system.

Immunophenotyping

A very large number of individual leucocyte antigens exist which can be identified in tissue sections by antibodies. Many of these antibodies have been grouped together with respect to the antigenic determinants that they recognize and give a CD (cluster of differentiation) number. The application of these antibodies allows the identification of cell type (B, T, macrophage, myeloid, red cell, platelet etc.), stage of differentiation, state of activation and presence of associated ligands or membrane-bound enzymes.

Molecular genetics

While immunophenotyping can reveal information about cell lineage, confirmation of clonality is more problematical. In B-cell tumours the demonstration of the secretion of a single immunoglobulin light chain (light chain restriction) by the cell population is taken to imply clonality but this is a crude measure. For T cells there is no equivalent immunophenotypic marker. Using molecular techniques the demonstration of identical rearrangement of immunoglobin/T-cell receptor genes by the cell population is very good evidence of clonality as cells within a reactive population would be expected to be immunologically diverse and therefore have different gene rearrangements. The techniques used include Southern blot and the polymerase chain reaction (PCR) both of which can detect clones making up as little as 2–5% of the lymphoid population.

Chromosomal analysis of non-Hodgkin's lymphomas has identified several abnormalities that appear characteristically associated with particular lymphoma entities.

Translocations in Burkitt's lymphoma

Characteristic cytogenetic changes involving a breakpoint in the site of the *c-myc* oncogene on the long arm of chomosome 8 are associated with this lymphoma. This results in the translocation of the *c-myc* region most commonly into the region of the immunoglobulin heavy chain gene on chromosome 14 (t(8;14)) and less commonly into the region of the light chain genes on chromosome 2 or 22. The result is loss of normal regulation of *c-myc* expression and increased cellular proliferation.

Translocations in follicular lymphoma (follicle centre centroblastic/centrocytic)

A translocation between chromosome 18 and the immunoglobulin heavy chain gene on chromosome 14 occurs in these tumours in up to 90% of cases in USA, 70% in the UK and somewhat less in Japan. The gene involved in this case is the *bcl-2* gene which encodes a protein believed to inhibit apoptosis thus giving the tumour population a survival advantage.

Translocations in mantle cell lymphoma (centrocytic; intermediate lymphocytic)

This is associated with translocations involving the *bcl-1* or PRAD-1 oncogene on chromosome 11 which is again translocated into the region of the immunoglobulin heavy chain gene. The gene product appears to activate a protein kinase (*cdc2*) which regulates progress through the cell cycle.

Aetiology

Several circumstances are thought to predispose to the development of non-Hodgkin's lymphoma.

Epstein–Barr virus (EBV)

In African-endemic Burkitt's lymphoma EBV DNA can be found in the neoplastic B cells in up to 95% of cases (compared with 15% of non-endemic cases). It is thought that EBV infection causes B-cell proliferation which is not ultimately halted by T cells in individuals in whom cell-mediated immunity is suppressed (possibly due to co-infection by malaria). This provides favourable circumstances for *c-myc* abnormalities and thus increases the risk for the development of this tumour.

Human lymphotropic virus (HTLV-1)

This is an oncogenic C-type retrovirus found in parts of south-western Japan, the Caribbean, New Guinea and parts of South and Central America. Transmission is via contaminated body fluids (blood transfusion, needle sharing, sexual intercourse, breastmilk) and rarely transplacental. The effect of infection is to enhance expression of genes encoding IL-2 receptor and IL-2 itself resulting in deregulated T-cell proliferation.

Primary immunodeficiency

Several causes of primary immunodeficiency have been associated with the development of lymphoma:

- Ataxia telangiectasia – autosomal recessive inheritance. Associated with chromosomal instability. Up to 20% develop non-Hodgkin's lymphoma of B and T cell types.
- Wiskott–Aldrich syndrome – X-linked recessive inheritance. Cells lack surface CD43. Almost 75% of malignancies in boys with this syndrome are non-Hodgkin's lymphomas often B-cell type and frequently involving the CNS.
- Common variable immunodeficiency.
- Severe combined immunodeficiency.
- X-linked lymphoproliferative syndrome (XLP).

EBV plays an important role. Around 65–70% of XLP patients develop fulminating infectious mononucleosis and 25–35% develop a B-cell lymphoma usually at an extra-nodal site (e.g. intestine).

Secondary immunodeficiency (Table 42.3)

Histological low-grade B cell non-Hodgkin's malignant lymphoma (ML)

Kiel ML lymphocytic.

WF ML small lymphocytic consistent with CLL.

WHO/Real Small lymphocytic.

Cell of origin Small mature B lymphocyte.

Table 42.3 Secondary immunodeficiency

Organ transplantation	This is followed by a 30–40 fold increase in risk of developing malignant lymphoma. Related to EBV infection
Acquired immunodeficiency syndrome (AIDS)	Prevalence of non-Hodgkin's lymphoma is 3–4% in this group usually either systemic/peripheral or involving the CNS. Most are high grade and many are associated with EBV
Autoimmune diseases (such as Sjögren's disease and Hashimoto's thyroiditis)	Promotes the acquisition of extranodal lymphoid tissue within which lymphoma may develop
Hodgkin's disease	Non-Hodgkin's lymphoma may follow Hodgkin's disease in about 1–5% of cases possibly due to defects in cell-mediated immunity or related to treatment

Microscopy Diffuse infiltrate of small lymphocytes with scattered collections of larger cells (proliferation centres or pseudo-follicles) which contain prolymphocytes and paraimmunoblasts. High grade transformation may occur (Richter's syndrome) when the cells are large, bizarre and may be multi-nucleate.

Immunophenotype Express B-cell associated antigens (CD 19, 20, 79a) as well as CD23. Usually express IgM and IgD. Also express CD5 (normally associated with T cells).

Natural history and prognosis Usually generalized (equivalent to B chronic lymphocytic leukaemia). Slowly progressive and indolent. Hypogammaglobulinaemia may be present.

Kiel ML immunocytoma.

WF ML small lymphocytic plasmacytoid.

Real Lymphoplasmacytoid lymphoma.

WHO Lymphoplasmacytic lymphoma.

Definition Tumour resembling ML lymphocytic but showing plasmacytic or plasmacytoid differentiation.

Epidemiology Most commonly middle aged and elderly.

Microscopy Effacement of the architecture may not be complete and the proliferation may be confined to interfollicular regions. Predominantly small lymphocytes with some tumour cells showing plasmacytic or plasmacytoid differentiation. Plasmacytoid cells may contain characteristic intranuclear inclusions (Dutcher bodies) of immunoglobulin. Mast cells may be numerous.

Immunophenotype There are large amounts of intracellular IgM in the plasmacytic/cytoid cells. IgD is not usually seen.

Natural history and prognosis Often associated with serum IgM paraprotein (Waldenstrom's macroglobulinaemia). The disease is indolent but generally not curable.

Kiel ML centroblastic/centrocytic.

WF Follicular mixed small cleaved and large cell.

Real Follicle centre lymphoma.

WHO Follicular lymphoma.

Epidemiology Commonest non-Hodgkin's lymphoma in developed countries (40% of all cases in USA). Predominantly late adult life but may occur in young adults.

Cell of origin Follicle centre cell.

Microscopy There are closely packed follicles with obliteration of the sinuses. Mantle zones are inconspicuous or absent. The relative proportion of centrocytes and centroblasts is variable but centrocytes tend to predominate. In contast to reactive follicle centres there is no zoning, mitotic activity is scarce, tingible body macrophages are rare and the distinction between follicle centre and mantle is blurred.

Immunophenotype The cells express B-cell associated antigens (CD19, CD20, CD79a) as well as CD10. The cells do not express CD5. In contrast to reactive follicle centres the cells express the *bcl*-2 protein in the majority of cases and proliferation as marked by staining with the cell cycle-related protein *Ki-67* is low.

Natural history and prognosis Usually disseminated at diagnosis. Clinical course is long and usually indolent with good response to therapy. Over time the histology may worsen with transformation to a more aggressive type.

Kiel ML centrocytic.

WF ML diffuse small cleaved cell.

WHO/Real Mantle cell lymphoma.

Cell of origin   A sub-set of cells in the follicle mantle.

Microscopy   In most cases there is a diffuse infiltrate of small lymphocytes with irregular nuclear outline. In other instances it may be nodular or perifollicular. There are no blasts.

Immunophenotype   The cells express IgM and IgD, B-cell associated antigens and CD5 but not CD10. Cells over-express cyclin D1 as a result of t(11; 14).

Natural history and prognosis   The disease may present with isolated lymphadenopathy or primary involvement of spleen or intestine. There may be a leukaemic phase. This tends to be more aggressive than other low grade B-cell lymphomas (WF intermediate grade).

Histological high-grade B-cell non-Hodgkin's lymphoma

Kiel   ML centroblastic.

WF   ML diffuse large non-cleaved cell.

WHO/Real   diffuse large B cell lymphoma.

Epidemiology   Accounts for about 30–40% of non-Hodgkin's lymphoma in adults.

Aetiology   May develop de novo or as a high-grade trans-formation of a low-grade lymphoma.

Site   Commonly presents with regional lymphadenopathy but may have extranodal involvement.

Microscopy   Diffuse infiltrate of cells with large nuclei and two or three nucleoli which are characteristically seen touching the nuclear membrane.

Immunophenotype   Express B cell antigens (CD19, CD20, CD22, CD79a). May show surface immunoglobulin.

Natural history and prognosis   Depends on the degree of dissemination at diagnosis. If localized (stages I and II) the chances of cure are substantial.

Kiel   ML immunoblastic.

WK   ML large cell immunoblastic.

Real   diffuse large B cell lymphoma.

Epidemiology   Tumour of adult life median age in fourth decade. Females more common than males.

Microscopy   Diffuse infiltrate of uniform large cells with abundant cytoplasm and a large nucleus and single cen-trally placed nucleolus.

Immunophenotype Cells express B cell antigens. Surface immunoglobulin is weak.

Kiel ML Burkitt's.

WF ML small non-cleaved cell, Burkitt's.

WHO/Real Burkitt's lymphoma.

Epidemiology Commonly affects children. Occurs in endemic and non-endemic forms. The endemic form occurs in a belt stretching across equatorial Africa. The median age at diagnosis is 7 years. Non-endemic Burkitt's presents in children of slightly older age.

Aetiology Good evidence for the role of EBV in the endemic form. Both forms have the characteristic t(8:14) translocation or one of the variants.

Site Endemic Burkitt's commonly presents with enlargement and deformation of the jaw. May involve the retroperitoneum, gonads or other viscera. In non-endemic cases their target tissues are the lymph node, intestine and bone marrow but rarely the jaw.

Cell of origin B cell at unknown stage of differentiation.

Microscopy Diffuse infiltrate by uniform population of medium-sized cells with round nuclei and 2–3 nucleoli. There is considerable mitotic activity and cell death. Macrophages containing apoptotic debris appear as clear areas in the infiltrate (giving a 'starry sky' appearance).

Immunophenotype Cells express B-cell associated antigens and CD10. Usually IgM positive.

Natural history and prognosis About 40% can be cured with modern chemotherapy.

Kiel ML lymphoblastic.

WF ML lymphoblastic.

WHO/Real Precursor B-lymphoblastic lymphoma/leukaemia.

Epidemiology Most patients are children and will be leukaemic.

Cell of origin Bone marrow derived precursor B cell.

Microscopy Cells are slightly larger than small lymphocytes with round or convoluted nuclei, fine chromatin and scanty cytoplasm. Mitoses are frequent and a starry-sky pattern may be seen.

Immunophenotype Cells express B-cell antigens (CD19, CD79a and sometimes CD20) and may express CD10. They are TdT positive and express HLA-DR.

Histological low-grade T cell non-Hodgkin's lymphoma

Kiel – ML lymphocytic.

WF – ML small lymphocytic.

WHO/Real – T chronic lymphocytic and prolymphocytic leukaemia; large granular lymphocyte leukaemia, T cell and NK cell types.

Epidemiology Rare.

Microscopy Diffuse infiltration by small lymphocytes with irregular nuclei.

Immunophenotype Cells commonly express CD2. T-cell varieties mark for CD3.

Kiel – ML small cerebriform cell.

WF – Mycosis fungoides.

WHO/Real – Mycosis fungoides; Sézary syndrome.

Definition The term cerebriform is derived from the convoluted nature of the nuclear outline. Occurs in two forms.

Mycosis fungoides

Clinical features A cutaneous lymphoma which in general follows a long clinical course divided into three stages:

1. Patch stage. The lesions are flat, scaly and reddish-brown.
2. Plaque stage. The skin lesions are thickened and plaque-like.
3. Tumour stage. Large ulcerated tumour nodules.

Lymph node enlargement is frequent in mycosis fungoides but may be reactive (dermatopathic lymphadenopathy) or due to infiltration by lymphoma.

Microscopy There is an infiltrate of cerebriform cells in the upper dermis admixed with macrophages and eosinophils. The infiltrate breaches the dermoepidermal junction and extends into the epidermis ocasionally in clusters (Pautrier microabscess). There is no spongiosis.

Immunophenotype The cells are usually CD3 and CD4 positive and very rarely CD8 positive.

Sézary syndrome

Clinical features There is red scaly skin, baldness and a leukaemic blood picture in which cerebriform cells are prominent.

Kiel ML lymphoepithelioid (Lennert's lymphoma).

WF ML large cell immunoblastic.

Real Peripheral T cell lymphoma.

Site Usually presents with regional lymphadenopathy but is often accompanied by involvement of the tonsillar region.

Microscopy Mixed infiltrate in which T cells predominate. Some cells resemble Reed–Sternberg cells. There are clusters of macrophages with a granulomatous appearance.

Natural history and prognosis May behave in an aggressive fashion.

Kiel ML angioimmunoblastic.

WF ML large cell immunoblastic.

WHO/Real Angioimmunoblastic T-cell lymphoma.

Definition Also known as angioimmunoblastic lymphadenopathy with dysproteinaemia (AILD).

Epidemiology Fairly common in Japan.

Clinical features Formerly thought to be a reactive condition due to variable clinical outcomes including apparent spontaneous cure, death due to immunodeficiency and sometimes appearance of overt lymphoma.

Microscopy There is a striking proliferation of high endothelial venules with an intervening mixed-cell infiltrate including large immunoblastic cells with a clear cytoplasm. There is also a proliferation of follicular dendritic cells.

Kiel ML T-zone type.

WF ML large cell polymorphous.

WHO/Real peripheral T-cell lymphoma.

Microscopy The B-cell follicles are preserved. There is an infiltrate in the paracortex similar to that seen in angio-immunoblastic lymphoma.

Natural history and prognosis May evolve into a diffuse high-grade T-cell lymphoma.

Histological high grade T-cell non-Hodgkin's lymphoma

Kiel ML lymphoblastic.

WF ML lymphoblastic, convoluted or non-convoluted.

WHO/Real Precursor T-lymphoblastic lymphoma/leukaemia.

Epidemiology Mostly age less than 20 years. Males more than females.

Clinical features Lymphadenopathy is common and a mediastinal mass is seen in 50%.

Microscopy Diffuse infiltration by cells slightly larger than lymphocytes with irregular nuclei.

Immunophenotype TdT is expressed in all cases. In some cases the tumour will mark for CD2, 5 and 7.

Natural history and prognosis Aggressive and if untreated is rapidly fatal. Dissemination to bone marrow and meninges may occur.

Kiel ML pleomorphic T cell (HTLV-1 positive or negative).

WF ML large cell immunoblastic polymorphous.

WHO/Real Peripheral T cell lymphoma.

Microscopy Diffuse infiltrate of large cells with pleomorphic nuclei and prominent nucleoli.

Immunophenotype Cells are CD4 positive and CD7 negative.

Natural history and prognosis Very aggressive disease. May be associated with hypercalcaemia.

Kiel ML large cell anaplastic.

WF ML large immunoblastic.

WHO/Real Anaplastic large cell lymphoma T- and null-cell types.

Epidemiology Often found in young individuals and children.

Microscopy Large cells with pale cytoplasm and atypical pleomorphic nuclei. The tumour cells are frequently seen in lymph node sinuses.

Immunophenotype The defining criteria is that the tumour cells are CD30 positive. They may express T-cell antigens (occasionally B-cell antigens) and are positive for epithelial membrane antigen.

Genotype   There is frequently a t(2;5) translocation.

Natural history and prognosis   Prognosis is better than other high-grade T-cell lymphomas.

....

TUMOURS OF HISTIOCYTES

Langerhans cell histiocytosis (histiocytosis X)

Clinical features   Depends on the location and type of disease (see Table 42.4).

Microscopy   Characteristically there are large cells with deep clefts in the nucleus. Eosinophils are prominent in the background.

Electron microscopy   The cells contain characteristic rod-shaped structures with a terminal ovoid swelling (looking like a tennis racket) – the **Birbeck granule**.

Immunophenotype   The cells express S100 protein and CD1 and they bind peanut agglutinin.

Table 42.4 Clinical features of Langerhans cell histiocytosis

Hand–Schüller–Christian disease	Characteristically has enlarged liver and spleen with lymphadenopathy, osteolytic lesions and polyuria due to diabetes insipidus
Letterer–Siwe disease	Enlargement of liver and spleen with lymphadenopathy, osteolytic lesions, involvement of bone marrow and a skin rash. There is fever
Eosinophilic granuloma	Multiple osteolytic bone lesions in the absence of visceral involvement
Congenital self-healing histiocytosis (Hashimoto–Pritzker syndrome)	Very rare. Skin lesions are similar to the disseminated form and appear at birth or within 2–3 weeks. Spontaneous regression occurs within 3 months

....

PLASMA CELL DYSCRASIAS

Multiple myeloma

Definition   Neoplastic proliferation of mature and immature plasma cells with osteolytic lesions and M protein in serum and urine.

Epidemiology   1–2 per 100,000 in Caucasians in USA but double in Afro-Americans. Chiefly middle aged and elderly.

Clinical features   Characterized by:

- bone pain due to lytic lesions. May be associated with pathological fractures
- infections. Usually due to virulent encapsulated organisms (e.g. *Streptococcus pneumoniae*) in early stages. Later infection with *Staphylococcus aureus* predominates
- involvement of the nervous system. May be associated with direct spread from lesion in vertebral body. Can be associated with amyloid deposition but 2–3% of patients develop polyneuropathy with unknown pathogenesis
- renal complications.

Chronic renal failure is a common endpoint of myeloma. Several factors contribute:

- Bence Jones Protein – immunoglobulin light chains filtered into the urine. Much is endocytosed by tubular epithelial cells but remainder forms casts in tubules.
- hypercalciuria – associated with bone resorption from lytic bone lesions.
- high urinary acid – associated with increased cell turnover – may be associated amyloid deposition.

Laboratory findings   Monotypic peak on serum electrophoresis. 75% of this is intact immunoglobulin (commonest is IgG, followed by IgA). Normal immunoglobulin production is depressed. Urine shows light chains in about 65% of patients. β_2-microglobulin is frequently increased. There is frequently anaemia and an increased erythrocyte sedimentation rate.

Microscropy   Abnormal plasma cells in the bone marrow. May be in nodules of purely interstitial.

Waldenström's macroglobulinaemia

Definition   Monoclonal proliferation of B cells with production of monotypic IgM or macroglobulin.

Epidemiology   Mostly elderly. Peak in 6–7th decade. Males more than females.

Clinical features Onset is often insidious. May present with anaemia, bleeding tendency, hyperviscosity syndrome, neuropathy or intestinal problems.

Laboratory findings Raised erythrocyte sedimentation rate, monotypic IgM on serum electrophoresis.

Microscropy Similar to lymphoplasmocytic non-Hodgkin's lymphoma.

Benign monoclonal gammopathies (monoclonal gammopathies of unknown significance; MGUS)

Definition Abnormal clonal immunoglobulin in serum without clinical or laboratory evidence of malignant plasma cell disorder.

Epidemiology Benign monoclonal gammopathy is not uncommon; seen in 1% of individuals >25 years and 3% of individuals over 70.

Clinical associations Features suggesting a diagnosis of MGUS includes

- an M protein concentration usually less than 20 g/l that does not increase in size
- absence of light chains in urine
- normal polyclonal immunoglobulins in background
- absence of bone lesions
- plasma cells not exceeding 10% in bone marrow.

Natural history and prognosis Less than 5% develop myeloma in the first year but up to 22% may develop myeloma after longer follow up. Median time to diagnosis of myeloma is just under 10 years.

THE SPLEEN

ANATOMY

Location Right hypochondrium.

Size About the size of a clenched adult fist.

Mean weight Male – 125 g; female – 105 g.

Blood supply Arterial blood is derived from the splenic artery entering the spleen at the hilum. This divides into smaller arteries which are found in the fibrous septa derived from the capsule. These leave the trabecul entering the spleen as the central arterioles. The adventitial coat of these gives way to a sheath of lymphoid cells which widens to become a lymphoid follicle and may contain a follicle centre. These arterioles divide into capillaries which either enter the sinuses directly (closed circulation) or into the splenic cords (open circulation) re-entering the sinuses through fenestrations in the sinus epithelium.

Accessory spleens

Frequency About 20–30%.

Location Tail of pancreas or gastrosplenic ligament. Rarely omentum or mesentery.

Size Usually less than 1 cm.

Significance Important in cases of hypersplenism, idiopathic thrombocytopenia and hereditory spherocytosis where failure to remove these may result in failure of surgical treatment.

FUNCTION

1. Filtration of obsolescent and abnormal red blood cells, removal of abnormal red cell inclusions and phagocytosis of bacteria.
2. Immunological responses to antigens and formation and emigration of lymphoid cells from white pulp.
3. Haemopoiesis in embryological life and in severe anaemia or bone marrow infiltration (extra medullary haemopoiesis).
4. Storage reservoir for blood elements.

Phagocytosis within the splenic cords

About 1/120 of the circulating red cells are destroyed each day as they get to the end of their 120-day lifespan. About 50% of this is accomplished by the splenic macrophages. Damaged or abnormal cells (such as in sickle cell disease or hereditary spherocytosis) are also removed. Within the spleen the passage of the red blood cells between the cords and the sinuses depends on a degree of deformity. If this deformity is diminished either as a result of damage, an intrinsic abnormality or obsolescence then the flow is slowed and phagocytosis of that component increased. In the case of cells with inclusions such as Heinz bodies (oxidized and denatured haemoglobulin) or Howell–Jolly bodies (DNA remnants) these are removed leaving the red cell intact in a process known as pitting).

Macrophages also phagocytose bacteria and particulate material produced from cell debris.

···

HISTOLOGY

The spleen can be divided into two functional areas which are integrated functionally and anatomically by the vascular system.

The white pulp

Periarterial lymphoid sheaths known as Malpighian corpuscles measuring 2–3 mm in diameter seen macroscopically as a white dot against the deep red background of the splenic cut surface.

Three functional compartments:

1. T cell area surrounding central artery (periarteriolar lymphoid sheath). About 70% of these cells are helper T cells (CD4 positive), the remainder are suppressor/cytotoxic T cells (CD8 positive) together with some antigen-presenting cells.
2. B-cell areas occupying the expanded area of the lymphoid sheath. May contain germinal centres.
3. A zone surrounding the follicle composed of a meshwork of reticulin fibres with a moderate number of IgM expressing B lymphocytes in which about 50% of the splenic lymphoid traffic occurs.

The red pulp

Consists essentially of sinuses and the splenic cords between them.

....

DISORDERS OF FUNCTION

Hypersplenism

Definition Pathological increase in some splenic functions as a result of splenomegaly.

Features Splenomegaly, deficiency of one or more constituent blood constituents, normal or hypercellular bone marrow and reversal of the abnormalities following splenectomy.

Mechanism Poorly understood. As a result of pooling – up to 50% of the red cell mass can be pooled in the spleen. Up to 90% of the platelet population can be found in a grossly enlarged spleen (normal = 10%). Higher proportion of blood becomes plasma.

Hyposplenism

Definition Usually absence of spleen but occasionally due to inadequate development or splenic atrophy.

Causes Absence of the spleen is most often following surgical removal. May be absent from birth (associated with other congenital cardiac abormalities) or hypoplastic (may be seen in Fanconi's anaemia). Splenic atrophy is seen in association with coeliac sprue and in sickle cell anaemia and essential thrombocythaemia (due to splenic infarctions).

Associated blood changes Loss of phagocytosis of abnormal constituents results in the appearance of nucleated red blood cells, target cells, red cells containing Howell–Jolly bodies and Pappenheimer bodies (iron-containing granules), a high platelet count and the appearance of giant platelets.

Effects of splenectomy

In addition to haematological disorders absence of the spleen gives rise to other effects.

1. Immune effects – fall in plasma IgM and defect in antibodies directed against carbohydrate containing antigens such as capsules of certain bacteria (e.g. *Streptococcus pneumoniae*). Although risk of infection by capsulated bacteria in adults is small, in children there is a significant increase in risk particularly for pneumococcal infections. These may present as septicaemia or meningitis. Other organisms with substantial increased risk include *Haemophilus influenzae* and *Neisseria meningitidis*. Immunization for *Strep. pneumoniae* is available.

2. Platelet number and function.
   Platelet numbers are increased following splenectomy and may show increased adhesiveness leading to risk of thrombosis.

3. White cell changes.
   Transient increase in circulating neutrophil numbers and permanant small increase in monocyte and lymphocyte numbers.

....

SPLENOMEGALY

Almost all diseases involving the spleen result in splenomegaly.

Congestive splenomegaly

Causes Portal hypertension which may be pre-hepatic (e.g. thrombosis or other obstructions of splenic or portal veins), hepatic (e.g. portal fibrosis or cirrhosis) or post-hepatic (e.g. Budd–Chiari syndrome).

Macroscopy Gross enlargement (500–1000 g). Firm dark red cut surface. Thickened capsule. May be small brown nodules (Gamna–Gandy bodies).

Microscopy Thickened capsule and fibrous septae. Dilation of sinuses. Areas of scarring with iron-containing macrophages (Gamna–Gandy bodies) which may become calcified and are due to sinus rupture and intraparenchymal haemorrhage.

Clinical features Hypersplenism and pooling of blood. Increased collagen in sinus basement membranes slows red cell transport and increases red cell destruction.

Splenomegaly associated with storage diseases

Massive splenomegaly may be encountered in some of the over 30 types of lysosomal storage diseases. Genetic defects lead to the absence of a lysosomal enzyme which may result in accumulation of an intermediate metabolite with associated increase in storage cells (tissue macrophages), absence of a normal end product or increased activation of a subsidiary metabolite.

Storage diseases are categorized by the accumulated metabolite type.

Sphingolipids

Accumulation of compounds containing ceramides.

Gaucher's disease   Rare. Autosomal recessive. Seen frequently in Jews from the Baltic regions. Deficiency of B-glucocerebrosidase leading to intracellular accumulation of glucocerebroside. Three types: **Type I (adult Gaucher's disease)** is commonest, may be seen in childhood and does not effect the central nervous system.

Clinical features   Splenomegaly (up to 1 kg is common), bone deformities and bone pain (50% patients with bone involvement) and yellowish-brown skin pigmentation affecting face neck and hands (45–70% patients).

Microscopy   Glucocerebroside laden macrophages (Gaucher cells) are large (20–80 microns). Cells appear faintly pink and striated on H&E-stained sections and pale blue with Romanowsky stains.

Electron microscopy   Clear elongated membrane-bound spaces with lysosomes distended by cerebroside.

Niemann–Pick disease   Deficiency of sphingomyelinase leads to accumulation of sphingomyelin. Three types (A,B and C) all involve the spleen and liver. Types A and C involve the central nervous system.

Microscopy   Presence of foamy macrophages that are blue on Giemsa-stained smears – sky blue histiocytes (also seen in familial condition called sea-blue histiocytosis and as a secondary phenomenon in idiopathic thrombocytopenic

purpura, chronic myeloid leukaemia, thalassaemia, polycythaemia, sickle cell disease and various chronic granulomatous diseases.

INFLAMMATORY DISORDERS

Acute and sub-acute inflammatory disorders

A variety of disorders, particularly those associated with
suppuration, cause enlargement of the spleen.

Macroscopy   Spleen may be 2–3 times normal weight and
is soft with a dull greyish cut surface.

Microscopy   Infiltration of the splenic cords by neutrophils
if the underlying cause is suppurative in nature. In typhoid
there are increased macrophages. In infectious mononucleosis there are atypical lymphocytes.

Chronic inflammatory disorders

Granulomatous inflammatory diseases

Splenic enlargement is seen in miliary tuberculosis, secondary and tertiary syphilis, tularaemia, brucellosis and
rarely in the septicaemic form of yersinial infection.

Fungal infections

A wide variety of fungal infections can involve the spleen
including infection by *Histoplasma capsulatum* with the end
result of multiple small foci of calcification.

Protozoal infections

Malaria and leishmaniasis are the commonest.

1. **Acute falciparum malaria**

Macroscopy   Spleen up to three times normal weight; congested and dark brown.

Microscopy   Abundant haemazoin (haematin-like) pigment.

2. **Chronic malaria**

Macroscopy   Spleen may weigh up to 1–2 kg. Firm but
rather friable with increased risk of rupture. Slate grey colour.

Microscopy   Haemazoin in macrophages in splenic cords.

3. **Tropical splenomegaly**

Seen in young adults living in areas where falciparum malaria is endemic. Associated with high plasma IgM levels.

Clinical features Associated with hypersplenism. Anti-malarial therapy usually causes reduction of splenic size.

Macroscopy Massive enlargement up to 3–4 kg.

Microscopy Little disturbance of normal architecture. No haemazoin-laden macrophages.

4. **Leishmanial splenomegaly** (visceral leishmaniasis, kala-azar)

Cause *Leishmania donovani*, endemic in many parts of the world. Up to 12 million people infected worldwide.

Clinical presentation Insidious with fever, anaemia, hepatosplenomegaly and increased skin pigmentation (kala-azar = black fever in Hindi).

Macroscopy Massive splenomegaly up to 4 kg.

Microscopy Splenic cords full of macrophages loaded with leishmania with numerous plasma cells. Distinction between red and white pulp may be difficult to appreciate.

....

AUTOIMMUNE CHRONIC INFLAMMATORY DISEASE

Rheumatoid arthritis

In some patients with deforming rheumatoid arthritis Felty's syndrome (rheumatoid arthritis, splenomegaly and leukopenia) will occur.

Macroscopy Moderate splenomegaly (mean weight 900 g).

Microscopy Expansion of the splenic cords by macro-phages. Some hyperplasia of white pulp in some cases. Vessels of white pulp may show fibrinoid necrosis and lam-inated peri-arteriolar fibrosis.

In a small proportion of rheumatoid cases (0.6%) the splenomegaly is due to proliferation of large granular lym-phocytes which are monoclonal and show clonal rearrangement of the T-cell receptor gene. This condition can be difficult to distinguish from Felty's syndrome.

Treatment Splenectomy returns white cell count to normal but leucopaenia recurs in some patients.

··

AMYLOIDOSIS

May be focal or diffuse. If extensive there is an increased risk of splenic rupture.

Macroscopy Mild to moderate splenomegaly. Cut surface shows numerous small (2–3 mm) white nodules so-called sago spleen.

Microscopy Amyloid chiefly found in white pulp. Amyloid may be of either reactive (AA) or immune (AL) type but extensive deposition is more common in reactive amyloidosis.

··

NON-NEOPLASTIC HAEMATOLOGICAL DISORDERS

Haemolytic anaemias

Splenomegaly may occur in a number of diseases resulting in haemolysis either due to an intrinsic abnormality (hereditary spherocytosis, sickle cell disease, thalassaemia) or because they are coated by antibody (autoimmune haemolytic anaemia).

Microscopy Splenic cords are congested but sinuses appear empty and are lined by plump cells.

Idiopathic thrombocytopenic purpura (ITP)

Definition Thrombocytopenia due to immune mediated destruction with no identifiable specific cause.

Epidemiology Young adults (two-thirds under 21 years) with female preponderance. More frequent in autumn and winter.

Aetiology Possibly related to respiratory tract infections. IgG antibody in plasma.

Haematology Decreased survival time of platelets.

Microscopy Hyperplastic germinal centres in Malphigian corpuscles in about 50% cases. Cords contain macrophages many of which are enlarged and vacuolated similar to sea-blue histiocytes.

Clinical features Splenectomy returns platelet count to normal.

THE SPLEEN IN MYELOPROLIFERATIVE DISORDERS

Diseases Polycythaemia rubra vera, myelofibrosis, essential thrombocythaemia.

Macroscopy Spenomegaly that is frequently massive in patients with myelofibrosis (up to 7 kg).

Microscopy Extramedullary haematopoiesis involving all three cell lines is conspicuous.

RUPTURE OF THE SPLEEN

Aetiology Most commonly blunt trauma to normal spleen. Occasionally due to minimal trauma to enlarged spleen (e.g. infectious mononucleosis, the commonest cause, measles, pregnancy).

Macroscopy May have large laceration in the splenic capsule.

NEOPLASTIC DISORDERS OF THE SPLEEN
Hodgkin's disease and non-Hodgkin's lymphoma

All types may involve the spleen. Involvement may be microscopic or massive leading to splenomegaly. Usually involves and follows the architecture of the white pulp.

WHO/Real – Splenic marginal zone lymphoma

Other – Splenic lymphoma with villous lymphocytes

Epidemiology Accounts for about 1% of non-Hodgkin's lymphoma. Most patients are over 50. Equal sex incidence

Site Usually confined to spleen and hilar lymph nodes with bone marrow infiltration and circulating lymphocytes.

Clinical features Commonly presents with splenomegaly. Maybe autoimmune thrombocytopenia or anaemia.

Microscopy The splenic white pulp is surrounded or replaced by a population of neoplastic cells consisting of an inner layer of small lymphocytes and an outer layer consisting of larger cells with more abundant cytoplasm and scattered large, nuleolated cells. The red pulp shows small nodules and occasional sheets of similar cells that also infiltrate sinuses. Often associated with abnormal lymphoid cells in peripheral blood to have short surface villi (villous lymphocytes).

Immunophenotype Express pan-B cell antigens (CD20 & CD79a) but are negative for CD5 and CD10. Usually express IgD and IgM.

Cell of origin Originally thought to be the marginal zone B cell. Now origin is uncertain but may be from subset mantle cells.

Natural history and prognosis Indolent clinical course. Often responds to splenectomy alone.

Leukaemia

Most frequent in chronic myeloid leukaemia (CML) where splenomegaly is seen in up to 95% which may be massive.

....

NON-HAEMATOLOGICAL MASSES IN THE SPLEEN

Splenic cysts

Definition Parasitic or non-parasitic.

Aetiology

1) Parasitic: commonest is hydatid (*Echinococcus granulosus*) found in many areas particularly North Africa and Middle East but also in sheep-rearing communities such as Wales and New Zealand.

2) Non-parasitic: Divided into two groups on the basis of presence or absence of an epithelial lining. A minority (20%) have a squamous epithelial lining. The cysts without an epithelial lining may be post-traumatic or secondary to liquefaction of splenic infarcts.

Splenic hamartomas

Epidemiology Rare.

Macroscopy Intrasplenic nodules 2–4 cm diameter compressing normal spleen.

Microscopy Contain tissue arranged like normal white pulp or have a complex array of small blood vessels with lymphocyte infiltrated fibrous tissue.

....

BENIGN NEOPLASMS

Most are vascular in type, usually small and found incidentally.

....

MALIGNANT NEOPLASMS

Angiosarcoma

Epidemiology Commonest non-haemopoietic tumour of spleen.

Microscopy Solid areas of sarcomatous stroma interspersed with cystically dilated vascular channels.

Associations Macrocytic anaemia, disseminated intravascular coagulation (DIC), consumptive coagulopathy and micro-angiopathic anaemia.

Natural history A highly malignant tumour. Most patients die within 1 year of diagnosis.

METASTATIC TUMOURS IN THE SPLEEN

Macroscopic tumour deposits are seen in the spleen in 4–8% patients with malignant disease. Common primary sites are melanoma, lung carcinoma, ovarian carcinoma and malignant trophoblastic tumours.

The skin

THE SKIN AND ITS DISORDERS

HISTOLOGY

Epidermis

Embryology   Derived from ectoderm.

Organization   Consists predominantly of stratified squamous cells in small numbers of melanocytes (responsible for melanin synthesis), Langerhans cells (specialized antigen-presenting cells) and Merkel cells (neuroendocrine cells). The superficial surface is flat but the deep surface is undulating due to papillary folds extending into the upper dermis. The keratinocytes are arranged in four layers (deep to superficial).

- **Basal layer**   Mitotically active. Cuboidal/columnar with large nuclei and prominent nucleoli. Basophilic cytoplasm. Frequently pigmented due to uptake of melanin from melanocytes (usually situated within the basal layer). A basement membrane separates this layer from the dermis.
- **Squamous layer**   Stratum spinosum or prickle-cell layer. Several layers of polyhedral cells. In the lower layers the cells are rounded and basophilic, in the upper layers the cells are flattened and orientated with their long axis parallel to the surface. The term 'prickle cell' is used to describe these cells due to the appearance of short processes joining adjacent cells which are seen by light microscopy (due to retraction of cytoplasmic membranes except where held together by desmosomes).
- **Granular layer**   Normally 1–3 layers of flattened cells in the cytoplasm of which are basophilic keratohyaline granules.

- **Cornified layer**   Stratum corneum. Cells contain no nuclei or organelles leaving only a keratinous skeleton. Normally 3–4 cells thick with a basket-weave appearance. Keratin is usually shed.

Dermis

Organization   Two zones.
- **Upper zone (papillary dermis)**   Series of papillae separated by downward projections of epidermis (rete ridges). Loose meshwork of collagen with some elastin fibres arranged more or less perpendicular to the skin surface. Within this there are loops of blood vessels and nerve fibres (responsible for touch, pain and temperature sensations).
- **Lower zone (reticular dermis)**   Beneath the level of the tips of the rete ridges. Thick collagen bundles arranged parallel to the skin surface with thick elastin fibres which often show fragmentation. Embedded within this region are adnexal structures including eccrine and appocrine sweat glands, sebaceous glands and hair follicles with associated arrectores pilorum muscles.

Subcutaneous tissue

Organization   Predominantly mature adipose tissue arranged in lobules separated from each other by bands of connective tissue (interlobular septa).

....

FUNCTION

- physical barrier to micro-organisms and antigens
- prevention of excessive water loss or absorption
- prevention of injury from UV-light
- synthesis of vitamin D
- regulation of temperature
- mediation of senses of light, touch, pain and temperature
- mediation of immunological reactions through the Langerhans cells.

Table 43.1 provides a glossary of terms used in dermatology; Table 43.2 provides a list of microscopic abnormalities.

....

DISORDERS OF THE SKIN

Psoriasis

Epidemiology One of the commonest disorders of the skin. Affects 0.9–2.8% of Western populations. It is geneti-

Table 43.1 Glossary of terms used in dermatology/dermatopathology

Lesion	Single area of skin pathology. Usually analysed in terms of number, size, shape and colour.
Rash	The totality of the lesion present. Often applied to lesions that are widespread, red and only slightly (if at all) raised.
Macule	A small area of colour change. Not palpable. Usually < 1.5 cm diameter.
Papule	A small palpable lesion < 1.5 cm diameter. A sub-type is a wheal (non-loculated interstitial fluid).
Nodule	A lesion resulting from enlargement of a papule in length and width and height.
Plaque	A lesion resulting from enlargement of a papule in length and width but not height.
Vesicle	A small blister < 1.5 cm diameter.
Pustule	A vesicle filled with pus (neutrophils).
Bulla	A blister ≥ 1.5 cm diameter.
Crust	Dried proteinaceous material resulting from exudation of plasma on to the surface. Rough to palpation and yellow colour (red/violet/black if associated with bleeding).
Scale	Formed as a result of increased thickness of keratin layer (stratum corneum). May be **psoriatic** (easily visible silvery flakes large enough to be picked individually), **pityriasis-type** (too small to be picked individually, cannot be seen unless lesions are scraped when they appear as fine white powder) or **lichen-type** (slight roughness of skin surface, tightly adherent, shiny appearance).
Erosion	Loss of epidermal surface of all or part of the lesion. **Fissures** are cracks between islands of epidermis.
Ulcer	Focal loss of epidermis associated with dermal damage (deeper than erosion).

Table 43.2 Microscopic abnormalities

43

Disorders of the skin

Acantholysis	Loss of cohesion between keratinocytes. Results in the formation of intraepidermal clefts, vesicles and bullae.
Acanthosis	Increase in size and number of cells in the prickle-cell layer. May be due to elongation of rete ridges (as in a psoriasiform reaction) or whole epidermis (as in lichenification).
Ballooning degeneration	Marked swelling and pallor of individual keratinocytes with loss of intercellular bridging
Basal cell Liquefaction	Small droplets or vesicles develop within and between basal cells. May lead to sub-epidermal blister. Melanin from affected cell is released and taken up by dermal macrophages (melanin incontinence).
Bullae	A fluid-filled cavity situated within or below the epidermis. May be the result of spongiosis, reticular degeneration, acantholysis or keratinocyte destruction.
Crusting	Dried plasma protein either on the surface or replacing lost epidermis.
Cytoid, colloid or Civatte bodies	Homogenous rounded eosinophilic bodies resulting from apoptosis of a keratinocyte. Most often in basal layers.
Dyskeratosis	Abnormality of keratinization usually in association with malignant, pre-malignant or acantholytic disorders.
Microabscesses	Small collections of inflammatory cells within the epidermis or at the tips of the papillae: • Munroe microabscesses – collections of neutrophils usually in the stratum corneum (psoriasis) • Pautrier microabscesses – collections of atypical lymphocytes in epidermis (cutaneous T-cell lymphoma [mycosis fungoides]) • Papillary tip abscesses – collections of neutrophils (rarely eosinophils) within the tips of the dermal papillae (dermatitis herpetiformis and other bullous conditions).
Orthokeratosis	Increased thickness of stratum corneum without retention of keratinocyte nuclei.
Parakeratosis	Retention of keratinocyte nuclei in stratum corneum. Usually associated with reduction in thickness or absence of granular layer.
Spongiosis	Widening of intercellular spaces in the epidermis due to oedema.
Saw-toothing	Tips of the dermal papillae are widened and the tips of the rete ridges are pointed rather than rounded.
Vesicles	A collection of fluid that is smaller than a bulla.

caly determined to a considerable extent with a strong link to HLA-CW6 (13 × risk of developing psoriasis).

Pathogenesis   There appears to be an increase in proliferation and decreased turnover time (3–4 days compared with a normal turnover time of 28 days) of keratinocytes. The proliferation may be due to increased drive or increased transduction of normal drive.

Clinical features   Well-defined pink/red plaque-like lesions covered by large silvery-white scales, removal of which sometimes shows small bleeding points. Lesions especially likely on extensor surfaces, the trunk and scalp. Lesions characteristically occur at sites of trauma (Koebner phenomenon). In 5–10% there is a severe arthropathy (not associated with rheumatoid factor). The nail-bed, nail matrix (pitting of nail plates) and mucous membranes can be affected.

Microscopy   The epidermis is thickened due to increased number and size of cells in the stratum spongiosum. The granular layer is absent. The rete ridges are thickened and club-shaped and adjacent ridges may fuse. There is an increased epidermal cell mitotic rate (10 ×). The suprapapillary epidermis is usually atrophic and shows parakeratosis. Neutrophils may be present in the epidermis and collect in small foci (Munro microabscesses). The dermal papillae show a mild to moderate inflammatory infiltrate, including macrophages, around dilated and tortuous blood vessels.

Seborrhoeic dermatitis

Epidemiology   Infants are commonly affected in whom it frequently involves the scalp (cradle cap) and remits spontaneously after 1 year. The disease is then rare before puberty.

Aetiology   Unknown.

Clinical features   Scaly rash in areas where seborrhoeic glands are present (notably scalp, eyebrows, paranasal areas, naso-labial folds, pre-sternal area, central back and the folds behind the ears). The scales may be dry or greasy.

Microscopy   Similar to psoriasis particularly with respect to the parakeratosis in the supra-papillary areas. Munro microabscesses are rare and tiny.

Table 43.3 Blistering (bullous) diseases caused by immune mechanisms

Location	Disease
Intraepidermal	• Pemphigus foliaceus
Stratum corneum/stratum granulosum	• Fogo selvagem
Intraepidermal	• Pemphigus vulgaris
Suprabasal	• Pemphigus vegetans
Sub-epidermal	• Bullous pemphigoid
	• Cicatricial pemphigoid
Sub-epidermal	• Dermatitis herpetiformis
Associated with micoabscesses at tips of papillae	
Sub-epidermal	• Erythema multiforme
Associated with necrosis of keratinocytes	

Blistering diseases caused by immune mechanisms (Table 43.3)

Pemphigus vulgaris

Epidemiology Commonest of the four varieties of pemphigus. There is a worldwide distribution but it is particularly common in Ashkenazi Jews. Increased association with HLA antigens A10, A26, Bw38 and DR4.

Pathogenesis The pemphigus vulgaris antigen is a normal component of the keratinocyte plasma membrane.

Clinical features Presents with generalized blistering which in early stages is most marked in the skin folds. Rupture of the blisters is associated with extensive crusting. Decreased cohesion between epidermal cells of apparently normal skin means separation of epidermis from underlying tissue can be induced with sliding pressure (Nikolsky's sign). The mouth is frequently affected in the early stages which may be associated with considerable pain.

Microscopy The blister occurs just above the basal layer so the floor of the blister shows a line of basal cells which appear like tombstones. Within the blister there are a moderate number of acantholytic keratinocytes. In general inflammation is absent but in early lesions there may be some spongiosis associated with an eosinophil infiltrate.

Immunofluorescence IgG is seen in a linear fashion on the keratinocyte membrane sometimes associated with C3. In patients with active disease there may be serum IgG which will bind to the keratinocyte antigen.

Pemphigus vegetans

Definition   Variant of pemphigus vulgaris and rarest of all varieties of pemphigus.

Clinical features   In the early stages there are flaccid blisters (similar to pemphigus vulgaris). They rupture easily and as they heal warty hyperplastic masses are seen at the sites of erosion.

Microscopy   There is hyperkeratosis and epidermal hyperplasia with downgrowths of the rete ridges and a particular tendency for the epithelium of the hair follicles to be involved.

Pemphigus foliaceus

Aetiology   May occur sporadically (idiopathic variety) or endemically in certain parts of South America (notably Brazil) where the disorder is called *fogo selvagem* (wild fire) and may be caused by a virus (possibly via insect bite). Cases can also be seen associated with drugs (e.g. penicillamine, piroxicam, captopril, rifampicin and phenobarbitone).

Clinical features   The blisters are smaller than in pemphigus vulgaris and rupture more easily with crusting. Itching is prominent and Nikolsky's sign is positive. The face and upper trunk are frequently involved. In fogo selvagem the distribution tends to be generalized.

Microscopy   Sub-corneal acantholysis.

Immunofluorescence   IgG and C3 are found in a linear pattern in relation to the keratinocytes of the upper layers of the epidermis. Autoantibodies bind to a normal component of the keratinocyte desmosome, desmoglein 1.

Pemphigus erythematosus (Senear–Usher syndrome)

Definition   Variant of pemphigus foliaceus.

Clinical features   In addition to the features of pemphigus foliaceus there are features of SLE.

Microscopy Features of both pemphigus foliaceus and SLE are present.

Immunofluorescence Serum contains antibody to the lupus erythematosus antibody in the basement membrane as well as desmoglein 1.

Bullous pemphigoid

Epidemiology Chiefly middle-aged and elderly individuals with some degree of female preponderance.

Clinical features Flexural areas are particularly affected with the inguinal regions being a site of predilection. Blisters may occur on a background of normal or erythematous skin and are large and more tense than seen in pemphigus. They rupture less easily. Nikolsky sign is negative. Lesions usually heal without scarring but milium cysts may occur at the site of the blisters. In the variant cicatricial pemphigoid, in which the mouth, eyes and genital areas are involved, scarring is prominent.

Microscopy Bullae lie between the dermis and epidermis. The roof consists of full thickness epidermis without keratinocyte necrosis or acantholysis. The cavities contain large numbers of eosinophils. Healing occurs by extension of epidermal cells along the exposed dermo-epidermal junction.

Immunofluorescence Linear IgG along the lamina lucida of the basement membrane. IgM and IgA in small amounts are occasionally seen. The autoantibody appears to be a protein component of hemidesmosomes.

Dermatitis herpetiformis

Epidemiology Not seen in blacks or Asiatics. Associated with HLA A1, B8 and DR3.

Associations Most patients have gluten-sensitive enteropathy (may be asymptomatic).

Clinical features Intensely itchy condition with small vesicles on the scalp, scapulae and extensor surfaces of limbs and buttocks. Vesicles contain blood and are often excoriated due to scratching. Characteristically symmetrical.

Microscopy There are small neutrophil-rich abscesses at the tips of the dermal papillae and multi-locular sub-epidermal bullae.

Immunofluorescence Granular deposits of IgA along the dermo-epidermal junction.

Natural history and prognosis Cutaneous lesions respond to gluten-free diet.

Erythema multiforme (Table 43.4)

Clinical features Round fixed erythematous lesions. Self-limiting or recurrent.

Pathogenesis No evidence of immune complex-related damage or autoantibodies. May be associated with cell-mediated damage.

Clinical features Three main forms are recognized with some degree of overlap:

- Iris type Commonest. Symmetrically distributed round, red or purplish, lesions with central slightly raised and more erythematous areas and a less severely affected periphery. Usually self-limiting and lasts only a few weeks. Lesions tend to occur on the hands, feet, forearms and legs.
- Vesico-bullous type Centre of the lesion becomes vesicular or bullous. Lesions tend to rupture leaving painful ulcers. Involvement of genitalia and mouth may occur.
- Stevens–Johnson syndrome Rare but potentially lethal. Skin and mucous membranes are extensively involved by blistering ulceration. Patient may be febrile and unable to eat, due to oral involvement. Conjunctival involvement may lead to corneal scarring and blindness.

Microscopy The upper dermis shows dilatation of small blood vessels and there is oedema of the papillary dermis. There is an inflammatory infiltrate predominantly of lymphocytes and macrophages around vessels but most severe at the dermo-epidermal junction. Some degree of keratinocyte necrosis is always present ranging from single cell to the full thickness of the epidermis.

Immunofluorescence There is granular C3 along the dermo-epidermal junction and in small blood vessels in the papillary dermis. This may be associated with IgM.

Table 43.4 Aetiology and associations of erythema multiforme

Viral infections	• Herpes simplex • Epstein–Barr • Vaccinia
Bacterial infections	• Streptococci • Yersinia • Mycobacterium tuberculosis • Treponema pallidum (syphilis)
Protozoal infections	• Trichomonas
Mycoplasma infections	• Primary atypical pneumonia
Fungal infections	• Histoplasmosis • Coccidiomycosis
Immunizations	• Horse serum • Various other vaccinations
Drugs	• Sulphonamides • Anti-convulsants • Penicillins • Tetracyclines • Methotrexate • Quinine • Dapsone • Cocaine • Isoniazid • Clindamycin • Chlorpropamide • Oestrogens
Contact dermatitis	• Nickel • Primula • Terpenes
Neoplasms	• Leukaemia • Lymphoma • Leiomyoma
Connective tissue diseases	• SLE
Physical agents	• Sunlight • X-radiation
Foods	• Emulsifying agents in margarines
Inhalants	• Methylparathion
Other diseases	• Sarcoidosis • Inflammatory bowel disease

NON-IMMUNE BLISTERING DISORDERS

Darier's disease (follicular keratosis)

Genetics Autosomal dominant inheritance.

Clinical features Dark brown warty nodules on hands, trunk, scalp, groins, axilla and neck. Associated with a degree of immunodeficiency and susceptability to infections.

Microscopy   Supra-basal cleft due to acantholytic separation of keratinocytes. Some cells of stratum spinosum undergo premature keratinization to form **corps ronds** which have centrally placed shrunken basophilic nuclei surrounded by a clear halo. Later forms of corps ronds are found in the stratum corneum as eosinophilic bodies with no nuclear remnants (**grains**). There is hyperkeratosis and parakeratosis of the epidermis above the clefts. Papillary downgrowths of epidermis are seen especially in relation to sweat glands and hair follicles.

Immunofluorescence   No antibody deposition.

Benign familial pemphigus (Hailey–Hailey disease)

Epidemiology   Presentation is usually in adolescence.

Genetics   Autosomal dominant inheritance.

Clinical features   Large flaccid blisters form in areas of friction. These become eroded and crust over.

Microscopy   Acantholysis starts supra-basally with acantholysis affecting the upper layers of the stratum spinosum as well. The clefts are much larger than in Darier's disease. The acantholysis appears incomplete and the effect is likened to a 'dilapidated brick wall'. Hyperkeratosis and concentration on hair follicles seen in Darier's disease are also absent.

Immunofluorescence   No antibody deposition.

Acantholytic dermatosis (Grover's disease)

Epidemiology   Not inherited. Particularly seen in middle-aged men.

Clinical features   An eruption of papules and vesicles. May be precipitated by heat, sunlight exposure and sweating.

Microscopy   Focal acantholysis and dyskeratosis.

Epidermolysis bullosa

Definition   A set of disorders of skin or mucous membranes (all but one inherited) in which blister formation follows an inappropriately small dgree of trauma. Blisters occur at the dermo-epidermal junction but exact location varies with each variant so electron microscopy may be required for classification.

Classification Classified on the basis of inheritance pattern, parts of the skin affected, precise level of clefting and age of onset. There are three principal forms of inherited epidermolysis bullosa (Table 43.5).

Acquired epidermolysis bullosa

Associations Inflammatory bowel disease, various autoimmune diseases and internal malignancies.

Microscopy Clefting below the lamina densa of the basement membrane.

....

ECZEMA (Table 43.6)

Definition A set of different disorders of the skin which share certain clinical and histological features in common.

Histological features

- spongiosis – which may result in vesicle formation if severe
- acanthosis
- hyperkeratosis and focal parakeratosis
- predominantly lymphocytic perivascular infiltrate in the upper dermis
- there are almost invariably superimposed effects of scratching and/or infection.

Aetiology

May be due to exposure to allergens or irritating substances (contact dermatitis) or some endogenous problem (see Table 43.7).

Atopic eczema

Epidemiology Significant genetic component. Common disease affecting moore than 1% of children in UK. Skin lesions appear about aged 3 months.

Table 43.5 Principal forms of epidermolysis bullosa

	Genetics	Clinical features	Microscopy
Epidermolysis bullosa simplex	Autosomal dominant inheritance	Many variants, the commonest being Weber–Cockayne syndrome which usually appears a short time after birth and principally affects the hands and feet. Blisters are large, contain clear fluid and heal without scarring or hyperpigmentations	Clefting at or just above level of basal cells
Junctional epidermolysis bullosa	Autosomal recessive inheritance	In the more severe forms there is involvement of tissues outside the skin (e.g. gastrointestinal tract). Nails may be abnormal or absent. Pitting of the teeth is frequent	Clefting at the level of the lamina lucida
Dystrophic epidermolysis bullosa	2 types: autosomal dominant and autosomal recessive inheritance	Both may cause extensive and widespread blistering. Healing is associated with scarring and the formation of tiny white milium cysts. In general the autosomal recessive variant is associated with more severe symptoms and extracutaneous manifestations. An unusual but characteristic appearance seen in the recessive form is fusion of the skin between the digits. If this is not corrected early then the fingers and toes become encased in a keratinous wrapping (mitten deformity).	Clefting in the upper part of the papillary dermis

Table 43.6 Clinical features of eczema

- **Acute**   Intensely itchy papules, vesicles and blisters filled with watery fluid
- **Sub-acute**   Redness, scaling and crusting
- **Chronic**   Thickened, dry, scaly and sometimes fissured skin in which the normal landmarks are exaggerated (lichenification). In some cases fibrotic nodules are present (prurigo nodularis). There may be increased or decreased pigmentation.

Table 43.7 Aetiology of ecyema

Endogenous eczematous reactions	Eczematous reactions due to exposure to allergens or irritants
Atopic eczema	Dermatitis due to repeated contact with irritants, e.g. urine (nappy rash in infants) or cleansing agents (shampoo). A variant occurs in elderly people who develop excessive drying and fissuring under conditions of cold or following frequent washing (asteatotic eczema).
Discoid eczema	
Pompholyx eczema – confined to hands and feet and characterized by blistering	
Juvenile plantar dermatosis	Allergic contact dermatitis – delayed hypersensitivity due to cell-mediated immunity. Once the individual is sensitized to a skin allergen the allergen must be avoided as the potential to react is permanent.
Lichen simplex	
Lichen striatus	
Eczematous reactions due to venous stasis	

Associations Associated with other features of atopy such as asthma, urticaria or hay fever.

Pathogenesis Atopy is a form of Gell and Coombes' type I hypersensitivity with an inappropriate degree of IgE response to one or more of a number of intrinsically harmless antigens such as pollens, grasses or animal dander. In patients with atopic eczema a combination of elevated IgE levels and decreased numbers of T-suppressor cells is frequently seen. Water within the stratum corneum enhances the barrier functions and so an abnormal degree of drying of the skin is likely to be associated with increased permeability. Patients with atopic eczema have dry skin and increased water loss across the epidermis.

Clinical features   Initial lesions affect principally the face, skin flexures and the posterior gluteal folds. The eruption is usually symmetrical and itchy.

Complications   Children with atopic eczema are prone to develop bacterial infections: herpes simplex (Kaposi's vari-celliform eruption/eczema herpeticum), papilloma virus and molluscum contagiosum are the commonest.

Contact dermatitis

Pathogenesis   Either a cell-mediated type of allergic reaction to an exogenous allergen which is usually of low molecular weight and acts as a hapten or as a result of exposure to an irritant but without involvement of the immune system (e.g. may cause drying of the skin).

CONTACT URTICARIA

Definition   Group of conditions which produce an exaggerated wheal and flare reaction.

Aetiology   A number of agents, all of which are chemicals.

Microscopy   There is dilation of blood vessels in the upper dermis accompanied by increased permeability leading to dermal oedema.

Non-immunological urticaria

Aetiology   Insect bites, stinging nettles, various marine organisms, chemicals used as preserving agents in foods and medicines (e.g. benzoic acid and cinnamic acid).

Pathogenesis   Agent penetrates skin and directly affects dermal mast cells which release preformed histamine and tryptase, activating the alternate pathway of the complement system through cleaving C3. There is associated synthesis and release of prostaglandins, leukotrienes and platelet activating factor.

Clinical features Usually mild and localized to the site of exposure. Lesions occur without previous exposure to the agent.

Immunologically-mediated urticaria

Pathogenesis Due to an IgE mediated type I hypersensitivity.

Clinical features Occurs only after previous sensitization. Lesions may be local or generalized. There may be a systemic anaphylactic response.

....

PAPULOSQUAMOUS DISORDERS

Lichen planus

Epidemiology Common. Peak incidence between 30–60 years, M:F 1:1. All races affected (possible that Nigerians have particular susceptibility).

Pathogenesis An immune reaction is suggested by the prominence of antigen-presenting Langerhans cells and helper T cells. There may be a genetic association with HLA-DR1 and Dqw1.

Clinical features Intensely itchy polygonal, flat-topped purplish (violaceous) papules covered by a network of white lines (Wickham's striae). Trauma leads to the Koebner phenomenon. Particularly affects the wrists, forearms, ankles, lumbosacral region, genitalia in males, the pre-tibial regions and the dorsa of the hands. Mucous membrane involvement is very common (oral mucosa involved in 50%).

Microscopy There is hyperkeratosis but *no* parakeratosis. There is focal and irregular thickening of the granular layer and irregular acanthosis with a saw-tooth appearance. Degeneration of the basal layers may lead to clefting and blister formation. Civatte bodies (eosinophilic colloid bodies) are seen in the basal layer. A band-like infiltrate of inflammatory cells (mostly lymphocytes) hugs the dermo-epidermal junction. Melanin released from damaged melanocytes is seen in dermal macrophages (melanin incontinence) and there is often a linear deposit of fibrin along the dermo-epidermal junction. IgM and C3 may be seen in the Civatte bodies. Although these features are characteristic they are not specific and can be seen in graft-versus-host disease, lupus erythematosus, in drug-induced lichenoid reactions (e.g. with gold and mepacrine) and dermatomyositis.

Natural history and prognosis About 50% clear within 9 months and most clear within 18 months but where there is erosive disease of mucous membranes the course may be more prolonged.

Lupus erythematosus

Definition Autoimmune disease which affects many organs including the skin. It is characterized by autoantibodies against nuclear antigens resulting in the formation of circulating immune complexes which are deposited in a number of sites and result in tissue damage.

Epidemiology At some time the skin is involved in 70–80% of patients with lupus and is the site of presentation in 25%.

Clinical presentation

There are three major types of skin disease:
- Discoid lupus erythematosus – a chronic scarring eruption usually in those with little or no systemic symptoms.
- Acute cutaneous lupus erythematosus – tends to occur in patients with active systemic disease.
- Sub-acute cutaneous lupus erythematosus – prolonged course and associated with milder forms of systemic disease. The eruption is photosensitive and heals without scarring.

Discoid lupus erythematosus (DLE)

Epidemiology Tends to occur in early adult life. M:F 1:2. May be associated with HLA B7, B8, Cw7, Dr2 and DQW1 (if any of these are combined the risk for the individual is increased).

Clinical features Largely confined to face, scalp and ears most commonly occuring in the 'butterfly' area across the bridge of the nose and on the cheeks. The lesions are red occasionally with hyperpigmentation at the edges and central hypopigmentation. There is plugging of follicles and scarring associated with atrophy of the skin and in areas of the scalp this scarring is associated with permanent loss of hair (scarring alopecia).

Microscopy Hyperkeratosis with follicular plugging and atrophy of the pilo-sebaceous apparatus. Focal epidermal atrophy due to damage to basal cells (with focal basal liquefaction and apoptotic bodies) associated with focal lymphoid infiltrates. Lymphocytic infiltrate affecting any level of the dermis but usually the middle third. Thickening of the basement membrane and degenerative changes in the dermal connective tissue.

Immunofluorescence Linear IgG and IgM at the dermo-epidermal junction. In 70% cases properdin may be seen together with C3. C1q is seen in 25% of immunofluorescence positive cases (compared to 90% in SLE).

Sub-acute cutaneous lupus erythematosus

Clinical features The skin lesions are either non-scarring papulosquamous eruption (two-thirds of patients) or ring-shaped lesions involving neck, trunk and outer arms. Follicular plugging is uncommon and the lesions heal without scarring although there may be residual areas of hypopigmentation. In about 50% the skin lesions appear to be sensitive to sunlight. There is non-scarring alopecia in 50%. Mouth ulceration is not uncommon. About half satisfy the criteria of the American Rheumatism Association for a diagnosis of SLE.

Microscopy There is a greater degree of epidermal atrophy than seen in DLE but other features are less severe than DLE.

Immunofluorescence Deposition of immunoglobulin at the dermo-epidermal junction is seen in about 60%.

Pityriasis rosea

Epidemiology Commonly affects children and young adults but can occur at any age.

Aetiology Unknown but may be viral. Similar lesions can be seen as a reaction to drugs (e.g. gold, barbiturates, captopril, β-blockers, isoniazid, non-steroidal anti-inflammatory agents and metronidazole.

Clinical features　An eruption affecting the 'vest and underpants' area is preceded by a single red papular or plaque-like lesion larger than those that subsequently appear (a **herald patch**). This starts as a reddish papule that enlarges to 2–10 cm diameter and most commonly occurs on the trunk. After 3–14 days crops of erythematous lesions erupt involving the trunk and proximal parts of the limbs. The lesions are round to oval with a frilly border (collarette).

Microscopy　Similar to those of eczema. There is mild acanthosis, spongiosis and a dermal infiltrate of lympho-cytes and macrophages.

Pityriasis rubra pilaris

Epidemiology　Uncommon. Found in 1/3500–5000 patients in skin clinics. M:F 1:1. Bimodal age distribution affecting 1st and 5th decades in particular.

Pathogenesis　There is increased proliferative activity in the affected areas.

Clinical features　Red plaques with prominent scaling, hyperkeratosis of palms and soles and follicular plugging are seen.

Microscopy　There are keratin plugs in the follicles with parakeratosis of the perifollicular epidermis with diffuse hyperkeratosis and acanthosis affecting the areas between the follicles. There is a mild perivascular chronic inflamma-tory cell infiltrate in the upper dermis.

ACNE VULGARIS

Epidemiology　Common. Particularly seen in adolescents. M:F 1:1 but males more severely affected.

Pathogenesis　Chronic disorder of the pilo-sebaceous unit associated with increased sebum secretion and blockage of pilo-sebaceous ducts by sebum and keratin.

Clinical features   There is a polymorphic skin eruption in which there are papules, pustules, dermal nodules and cystic lesions.

Non-inflammatory lesions in acne

- Open comedones: Pilo-sebaceous orifices are widely distended by keratin plugs which contain abundant oxidized melanin pigment (hence the term 'blackhead').
- Closed comedones: Follicular plug appears to be trapped in the duct. The distended pilo-sebaceous duct may rupture into the surrounding tissue and set up an inflammatory reaction ('whitehead').

Inflammatory lesions of acne

These may be superficial consisting of reddened papules and pustules or deep with cysts, nodules or pustules.

Nodulocystic acne

Chronic condition with deep and painful papules and nodules. Healing is associated with excessive scarring. This type does not remit in early 20s and goes on into middle life.

ROSACEA

Epidemiology   Tends to appear at any time from 4th decade onwards. M:F 1:1.

Aetiology   Unknown. Exacerbated by vasodilators, of which the commonest is alcohol.

Clinical features   There are four sequential clinical phases.
- frequent episodes of flushing
- persistent erythema
- development of small papules and pustules in affected areas
- hypertrophy of the sebaceous glands and surrounding connective tissue. The lower portion of the nose may be affected (**rhinophyma**) but the changes may occur on the cheek, ears, chin and forehead.

In most cases the disorder does not progress beyond the second phase. In some cases there may be involvement of the eyes (conjunctivitis, blepharitis or keratitis).

Microscopy In all stages there is dilatation of dermal blood vessels. There is dermal fibrosis and a mixed lymphocytic and macrophage infiltrate around blood vessels. With the exception of rhinophyma the sebaceous glands and hair follicles are not involved.

....

INFECTIONS OF THE SKIN

Acute bacterial infections

Impetigo

Epidemiology Usually affects children, especially in hot climates.

Microbiology Caused by either *Streptococcus pyogenes*, *Staphylococcus aureus* or both. Highly infectious.

Clinical features Small thin-walled pus-containing vesicles which rupture with the formation of yellow brown crusts. Heals without scarring. Responds well to antibiotics. A bullous form (bullous impetigo) is the result of a toxin produced by some strains of staphylococcus (causes splitting of the epidermis just below stratum corneum). Occasionally infection with a nephritogenic streptococcus is associated with the development of acute proliferative glomerulonephritis.

Staphylococcal scalded skin syndrome (Lyell–Ritter's disease)

Epidemiology Uncommon. Affects infants and young children.

Microbiology caused by group 2 staphylococcus (phage type 71) which produces a toxin that damages the granular layer without an inflammatory response.

Clinical features There is acute diffuse tenderness of the skin followed by redness and widespread desquamation of the superficial parts of the epidermis leaving red underlying surface.

Furuncles and carbuncles

Definition   Staphylococcal infections affecting hair follicles and causing inflammation that spreads to the surrounding dermis.

Epidemiology   Carbuncles are more common in diabetics than the general population.

Clinical features   Furuncles (boils) affect a single hair follicle with a pustular centre through which the hair passes. A carbuncle occurs most commonly on the back of the neck and affects several adjacent hair follicles with pus discharging from many of these orifices.

Folliculitis

Definition   Inflammatory process involving the opening of the hair follicle associated with blockage and formation of pustules confined to the follicles.

Clinical features   In children folliculitis occurs mainly on the scalp while in adults the limbs and beard area are involved.

Erysipelas and cellulitis

Definition   Distinguised by the level of the skin involved. Erysipelas involves the dermis and the most superficial parts of the subcutaneous tissue. Cellulitis may involve the entire thickness of the subcutaneous tissue.

Microbiology   Both are caused in most cases by β-haemolytic streptococci.

Pathogenesis   The spread of these lesions is associated with the secretion of enzymes (e.g. hyaluronidases) by the streptococci.

Clinical features   There are systemic symptoms including high fever, tachycardia, confusion and low blood pressure. The involved skin is red, tender and oedematous and there is lymphangitis and enlargement of the regional lymph nodes.

Necrotizing fasciitis

Definition   Infection that is associated with necrosis of the connective tissue and the underlying connective tissue fascia. Where the male genitalia is involved the term **Fournier's gangrene** may be applied.

Microbiology May be due to β-haemolytic streptococci alone but frequently there is associated anaerobic bacteria.

Clinical features Most commonly affects the extremities with the second commonest region being the perineum where it may be associated with earlier surgery, perirectal abscess or infection of the periurethral glands. There is severe pain. There is associated fever and evidence of toxaemia. The skin of the affected area is red, hot tender and oedematous. The inflammation spreads rapidly to surrounding areas and the skin may show purple discolouration, bullae, dermal crepitus (due to gas bubbles in necrotic tissues) and superficial gangrene. Treatment involves surgical removal of affected tissues.

CHRONIC BACTERIAL INFECTIONS

Cutaneous tuberculosis (Table 43.8)

Tuberculous chancre

Epidemiology More common in children and in communities with high prevalence of TB.

Aetiology Direct inoculation into the skin of non-immune individual with *Mycobacterium tuberculosis*.

Clinical features May follow ritual circumcision, ear-piercing or other types of minor trauma. The lesion starts as a papule which undergoes ulceration and then heals over several months in the absence of treatment. The local lesion is associated with enlargement of the draining lymph nodes.

Microscopy First there is a neutrophil infiltration followed by necrosis at which time there are numerous bacilli. Over the next 3–6 weeks a typical macrophage granuloma forms with caseation at which time the organisms are not found in the lesion.

Warty tuberculosis

Definition Manifestation of direct infection into the skin of an individual with moderate to high immunity to *Mycobacterium tuberculosis*.

Aetiology Most from accidental infection from an external source (e.g. during butchery or while performing a post-

Table 43.8 Classification of cutaneous tuberculosis

Type	Route of infection	Type of lesion	Individual's immunity
I	Inoculation TB (exogenous infection)	• Tuberculous chancre • Warty tuberculosis • Lupus vulgaris	• No immunity • Previous infection and moderate to high immunity • Moderate to high immunity
II	Endogenous infection in previously infected individuals	• Scrofuloderma • Lupus vulgaris • Miliary TB	Spread from adjacent caseous lymph nodes
III	Blood spread from primary focus	• Tuberculous 'gumma'	
IV	Eruptive TB (tuberculides)	• Lichen scrofulosorum • Papular or papulonecrotic tuberculides • Erythema induratum (Bazin's disease)	All of these represent skin reactions to an internal tuberculous focus

mortem examination). Patients with active tuberculosis may develop the condition following exposure to their own infected sputum.

Clinical features   Warty plaque-like lesion.

Microscopy   Intense mixed inflammatory cell infiltrate within the dermis. Well-formed granulomas are scanty. There is marked hyperplasia of the overlying epidermis (pseudoepitheliomatous hyperplasia).

Lupus vulgaris

Definition   Occurs in individuals (particularly women) with a moderate to high degree of immunity to *Mycobacterium tuberculosis*.

Aetiology   Bacilli gain access to skin via inoculation from outside, spread from adjacent nodes, via the bloodstream, or through lymphatic spread from a lesion in the mucous membrane of the nose or throat.

Clinical features   Reddish-brown well-demarcated plaque on the face. When this is pressed with a glass slide small translucent nodules can be seen ('apple jelly'). There is extensive tissue destruction and scarring. Squamous carcinoma may be a late complication.

Microscopy   In most cases there are well-formed granulomas but the organism is usually not seen (can be cultured in only 6% of cases).

The tuberculides

Definition   A set of disorders seen in the presence of internal infection. Thought to be reactive rather than result of direct infection. Clear on anti-tuberculous therapy.

Papulonecrotic tuberculide

Epidemiology   Young adults are most likely to be affected.

Pathogenesis   May be due to dissemination of mycobacterial antigens.

Clinical features   Crops of papules mostly on the extremities (mostly legs, elbows, hands and feet but also face, buttocks and genitalia) and frequently symmetrical. The papule centres become necrotic and breakdown.

Microscopy Central coagulative necrosis surrounded by chronic inflammatory cells. Affects the dermis but may spread to involve the overlying epidermis and the superficial parts of the subcutaneous tissue. In large lesions palisaded activated macrophages surround necrotic centre. The surrounding blood vessels show changes ranging from lymphocytic infiltration to vasculitis with fibrinoid necrosis and secondary thrombosis. Mycobacteria are never seen or and cannot be cultured.

Nodular tuberculide (erythema induratum, Bazin's disease)

Epidemiology Most common in females.

Pathogenesis Uncertain but may be due to immune complex deposition.

Clinical features Persistent or recurrent nodular lesions most commonly localized on the backs of the lower legs.

Microscopy Similar to nodular vasculitis with inflammatory involvement of small and medium-sized blood vessels in the connective tissue of the subcutaneous adipose tissue. There is extensive necrosis. Tuberculoid granulomas are seen.

Fish tank and swimming pool granuloma

Microbiology *Mycobacterium marinum.*

Clinical features Itchy purplish-red nodules appearing at the site of some trivial skin injury. The lesions may be warty and frequently ulcerate. Additional lesions may appear along the line of lymphatic drainage.

Microscopy Non-specific chronic inflammation in early stages followed by granuloma formation in which a few acid-fast bacilli can be seen.

....

VIRAL INFECTIONS

Herpes simplex

Virology Commonest to find herpes simplex virus (HSV)-1 in infections of the mouth and lips and HSV-2 in lesions around the genitals.

Clinical features There are small painful vesicles on an erythematous base.

- **Primary infection** – usually sudden onset with appearance of a group of macules. These become vesiculated and painful. Rupture is associated with crusting. In HSV-2 infection there may be fever and enlargement of the draining lymph nodes. A variant of primary infection follows acquisition of infection on the fingers and frequently affects healthcare workers (herpetic whitlow). Newborn infants can acquire infection from infected mothers during passage down the birth canal and in known cases of maternal genital herpes a caesarian section may be appropriate.
- **Recurrent infection** – HSV can enter into a lifelong latency stage within the nuclei of neural ganglia. During an episode of reactivation the individual experiences tingling or discomfort of the skin followed by eruption of a crop of painful vesicles. An attack lasts for 5–10 days and heals without scarring although there may be some hyperpigmentation.

Microscopy There is ballooning and reticular degeneration with the production of intraepidermal vesicles containing a meshwork of cellular debris. Intranuclear inclusions which stain red with eosin (Cowdry type A) are commonly present as are large multinucleated cells.

Herpes zoster (shingles)

Pathogenesis Reactivation of latent varicella zoster virus in neural ganglia.

Clinical features Small painful vesicles on an erythematous base usually restricted to one or two dermatomes. Lesions do not cross the midline. The first symptom is discomfort on one side which is followed by the development of vesicles. Widespread dissemination can occur (associated with 15% mortality, mostly from varicella pneumonia). The lesions contain virus and may be source of chicken pox for those not immune. Cranial nerves may be involved (most commonly the trigeminal). If the ophthalmic branch of the trigeminal nerve is involved ocular complications can develop in 30–50%. Post-herpetic neuralgia (pain lasting for more than 1 month) may be seen in 10–15%, which resolves in 2 months in 50%, and within 1 year in 75%, but may persist in a small proportion.

Microscopy In the vesicular stage the features are similar to those of HSV infection but there may be additional acute inflammation in the sensory nerves of the affected dermatome with some evidence of necrosis.

Varicella (chicken pox)

Virology Primary infection with the varicella zoster virus (herpes virus 3). Infection is thought to be via the respiratory tract followed by a viraemic stage and then localization of the virus in the skin. Visceral involvement can occur. The incubation period is 14–21 days.

Clinical features The earliest symptoms are malaise and fever followed by crops of lesions that are papular at first then vesicular. Lesions are distributed for the most part in a centripetal fashion with the trunk and face affected first. Successive crops develop so that lesions of varying ages can be seen at any instant in time.

Microscopy Similar to those in HSV infections.

Natural history and prognosis Complications are rare although encephalitis can occur (about 10%). Neonatal varicella contracted from the mother just before or at the time of delivery has a mortality of 20%.

Viral warts

Epidemiology Very common. Peak incidence 12–16 years.

Virology Mostly due to direct innoculation with human papilloma virus (HPV), a DNA virus with a circular genome and up to 50 different sub-types some of which appear to be oncogenic.

Microscopy There is acanthosis, papillomatosis, hyperkeratosis and koilocytosis. Inclusion bodies may be seen in the stratum corneum.

Common warts (verruca vulgaris)
Virology HPV-1 and 2.

Clinical features Usually the hand and feet. Lesions appear as flesh-coloured papules with a rough surface.

Microscopy There is epidermal hyperplasia with cone-shaped projections and intervening 'valleys'. The granular layer of the valleys shows a hyperplasia while the papillae are covered by a thin layer of parakeratotic epidermis. The rete ridges appear to be orientated towards the centre of the area of underlying dermis.

Plane warts

Virology HPV-3.

Clinical features Commonly occur on the face, hands and fingers. Less papillomatous giving the lesion a smoother appearance. They are either flesh-coloured or light brown and are only slightly raised above the surface of the skin. May occur in areas following minor skin trauma (Koebner phenomenon).

Mosaic warts

Virology HPV-2.

Clinical features Roughened skin usually found on the soles, heels, palmar surfaces of the hands or in relation to the nails.

Plantar warts

Virology HPV-1.

Clinical features Discrete lesions raised just above the surface. Commonly seen on the foot where they penetrate more deeply due to pressure of body weight. The proliferated epidermis is surrounded by a collar of thick translucent keratin.

Epidermodysplasia verruciformis

Epidemiology Variable inheritance pattern mostly autosomal recessive.

Clinical features Individuals show a marked predisposition to widespread and persistent infections with multiple types of HPV giving rise to a complex picture with plane warts, reddish plaques and lesions resembling pityriasis versicolor.

Natural history and prognosis   Malignant transformation of some lesions occurs in 30% of patients most commonly to squamous carcinoma on sun-exposed areas.

....

FUNGAL INFECTIONS
Superficial fungal infections

Superficial layers of skin including hair and nails.

Pityriasis versicolor

Mycology   *Pityrosporum orbiculare*, a unicellular yeast which is a normal skin commensal and only become pathogenic when budding occurs.

Pathogenesis   Budding is favoured by high environmental temperature.

Clinical features   Lesions are usually distributed over the torso as small patches with either hyper- or hypopigmentation and associated fine scales.

Microscopy   Skin scrapings show spherical yeasts and elongated hyphae ('spaghetti and meatballs').

Diseases caused by dermatophytes

Mycology   Fungi with an ability to colonize keratinized tissue (including hair, nails and stratum corneum). Include *Microsporum*, *Trichophyton* and *Epidermophytes*.

1. **Tinea capitis**

Epidemiology   Rare in adults. More common in black than white children in USA.

Organism   *Microsporum canis, Trichophyton tonsurans*.

Area of skin   Scalp hair.

Appearance of lesion   Non-inflammatory lesions are well-dermarcated patches of scaling. The hair appears grey and lustreless black dots are seen at the centre where hair shafts have broken off level with the skin surface. Inflammatory lesions vary from small pustules to large boggy suppurating lesions (kerions).

2. Tinea corporis (ringworm)

Organism *Trichophyton rubrum, Trichophyton mentagrophytes.*

Area of skin Non-hairy smooth skin. Affects the trunk and limbs.

Appearance of lesion Single or multiple circular papulo-squamous lesions with raised red-scaling edge and central clearing with scale formation. In some cases there is a greater inflammatory component with vesicle and pustule formation.

3. Tinea pedis (athlete's foot)

Organism *Trichophyton rubrum, Trychophyton mentagrophytes, Epidermophyton floccosum.*

Area of skin Interdigital spaces on feet. Only in those people who wear shoes.

Appearance of lesion Variable. Commonest is a boggy fissured lesion involving toe webs (especially between 4th and 5th toes). The lesion may extend on to the upper surface of the foot. Inflammatory lesions with vesicles and pustules may develop and these are prone to secondary bacterial infection.

Candida albicans infection (candidiasis)

Aetiology *Candida albicans* is a normal commensal of the oropharynx gut and vagina in 80% of individuals but does not normally colonize the skin. Infections are associated with a predisposing cause that may be systemic leading to defect in cell-mediated immunity (e.g. diabetes mellitus, Cushing's syndrome, corticosteroid administration or malignancy), neutropenia or to alteration of normal flora by antiobiotic administration. Local factors such as damage to the stratum corneum (e.g. associated with obesity, friction in skin folds or the presence of indwelling devices such as catheters) also predispose to infection.

Pathogenesis Virulence is associated with ability to adhere to epithelial surfaces associated with adhesion molecules on *Candida* (including a β_1 integrin, lectins and carbohydrates), with ability of the organism to secrete a proteinase and secretion of adenosine, that interferes with neutrophil function.

Clinical features   In addition to oral candidiasis there are a number of presentations.

Candida intertrigo

Site   Keratinized skin of skin folds such as gluteal, perineal and inguinal folds, the scrotum, axillae and the folds below the female breasts and in the abdominal wall of the obese. A variant is 'nappy' dermatitis in young infants beginning in the perianal region and extending to involve the groin, buttocks and medial aspect of the thigh.

Pathogenesis   Friction and moistness causes maceration of stratum corneum.

Appearance of lesions   Affected areas are reddened and eroded. Scales are often present. Vesicles and pustules may develop, often as satellites to the main lesion.

Candida affecting the nail and nail-beds

Epidemiology   Associated with occupations involving prolonged and frequent immersion of the hands in water.

Appearance of lesion   Nail-folds become swollen, reddened and painful. Serous or purulent exudate may ooze from the folds.

Chronic mucocutaneous candidiasis syndrome

Definition   Candidiasis involving the skin, nails, oral or genital mucosa that is resistant to treatment and is associated with a defect in anti-candidal cell-mediated immunity.

Epidemiology   Predilection for children under 6 years (65% cases) but can also be seen in adults.

Clinical features   Spectrum of presentations.

Chronic oropharyngeal type

Genetics   No specific inheritance pattern.

Site   Oral mucosa with or without oesophageal involvement. Skin and nails spared.

Chronic candidiasis with endocrine abnormalities

Genetics   Autosomal recessive inheritance.

Site   Mucous membranes and skin.

Associations Classic triad is candidiasis, Addison's disease and hypoparathyroidism. Autoantibodies may be present in serum.

Localized mucocutaneous candidiasis

Genetics No specific inheritance pattern.

Epidemiology Usually appears in childhood.

Appearance of lesion Hyperkeratotic, granulomatous and vegetating features.

Associations Recurrent bacterial pneumonias.

Chronic diffuse mucocutaneous candidiasis

Genetics Variable inheritance pattern.

Epidemiology Onset in childhood.

Site Widespread.

Associations No endocrine abnormality.

Adult-onset chronic candidiasis

Epidemiology Onset usually after 3rd decade.

Site Diffuse resistant infections of mucosae, skin and nails.

Associations High incidence of thymic tumours.

....

INFESTATIONS
Scabies

Parasitology Infestation is by *Sarcoptes scabiei*, an 8-legged acarid mite. Infection is by intimate contact with infected individuals or rarely via inanimate objects such as sleeping bags. Mature mites secrete keratinolytic substance which burrows into the stratum corneum. Gravid females lay eggs within the stratum corneum (rate of two per day for two months). The larvae hatch out and leave the burrow, pass through a nymph stage and mature. The cycle then restarts.

Clinical features There is intense itching, worse at night, and a polymorphic erythematous papular eruption. The burrows appear as serpiginous linear tracts a few millimetres long and slightly raised above the skin surface. At one end of the burrow a black spot is often seen.

(Table 43.9)

NON-INFECTIOUS GRANULOMATOUS DISORDERS OF THE SKIN

Granuloma annulare

Epidemiology   Frequently seen in children and young adults. Increased risk in females.

Aetiology   Unknown. May be associated with diabetes mellitus.

Clinical features   Ring-shaped reddish lesions with individual papules at the margins. Most commonly affects the backs of the hands, knees, ankles and elbows but can present as a widespread papular eruption.

Microscopy   Granulomatous process affecting the mid and upper dermis. The centres contain degenerate collagen which appears bluish on H&E staining which is surrounded by macrophages, fibroblasts and lymphocytes in a palisaded arrangement. A small amount of mucin may be present in the central zone. In some instances there is a perforation from where the process extends through the epidermis. In others the process may involve the subcutaneous adipose tissue.

Necrobiosis lipoidica diabeticorum

Epidemiology   Occurs in about 0.3% of all diabetics who account for about 75% of cases of this condition. M:F 1:3.

Clinical features   The diabetes is usually well developed but in 14% of the diabetic cases the skin lesions predate the development of overt diabetes mellitus. The lesions are reddish-brown to yellow plaques with firm waxy consistency. Sites of predilection are the shins and feet.

Microscopy   There is necrosis of dermal collagen with an appearance identical to *Granuloma annulare*. There may be a predominantly granulomatous reaction with activated macrophages and giant cells associated with scarring but without the central necrosis of collagen.

Table 43.9 Types of pediculosis

	Parasitology	Epidemiology	Clinical features
Pediculosis capitis	*Pediculosis humanus*	Principally in school children	Eggs (nits) can be seen on hair shafts. Lice are usually apparent to the naked eye. There is intense itching and often a papular rash occurring particularly behind the ears and in the occipital region which can be the site of secondary bacterial infection
Pediculosis corporis	*Pediculosis humanus.* While similar to the head louse, this louse is about twice as large and moves more slowly	Rare in normal practice. Associated with war, enforced movements of populations, gross overcrowding and poor hygiene	The eggs adhere to clothing. Bites cause an itchy red, * papular rash associated with wheal formation most often clustered on the trunk and thighs
Pubic lice	*Phthirus pubis*	Usually sexually transmitted	While the pubic hair is primarily infected other hair-bearing sites may be involved including axilla, eyebrows and eyelashes. Eggs attached to pubic hair can be seen but require close examination. Bites are associated with an intensely itchy eruption

* Associations: Vector for **typhus** (*Rickettsia prowazeki*), **trench fever** (*Rickettsia quintana*) and **relapsing fever** (*Borrelia recurrentis*).

Aetiology

Sun exposure

In malignant tumours derived from keratinocytes and some derived from melanocytes tumour development is associated with increased exposure to ultraviolet light and decreased skin pigmentation (including albinism).

Microscopy Following sun exposure over a long time period there may be atrophy of the epidermis, aberrant differentiation, atypia and hyperplasia together with degenerative changes in the dermis with fragmentation and basophilia of the collagen fibres. The orderly maturation of the epidermis is disturbed with hyper- and parakeratosis. The areas over the follicles and intraepidermal parts of the sweat glands are usually spared.

Inability to repair DNA (Xeroderma pigmentosa)

Genetics Autosomal recessive inheritance.

Pathogenesis The basic defect is an inability to excise and repair segments of DNA altered by exposure to ultraviolet light due to lack of endonucleases.

Clinical features Individuals are normal at birth but develop large numbers of freckles on skin exposed to sunlight. Freckles are associated with dryness of the skin and abnormal dilatation of blood vessels. There is often photophobia, conjunctival inflammation and ulceration.

Natural history and prognosis The risk of developing either squamous or basal cell carcinoma is increased 1000-fold and there is a greatly increased risk of developing malignant melanoma. Keratinocyte tumours develop during childhood (median age 8 years).

Exposure to chemical carcinogens

History First observed by Percival Pott in 1775 when he noted a high prevalence of cancer of the scrotal skin in chimney sweeps.

Chemicals Polycyclic hydrocarbons have carcinogenic potential which is associated with the generation of active epoxides that bind DNA. Other carcinogenic substances include arsenic (widely taken orally in the early part of the twentieth century) and PUVA (psoralen and long wavelength ultraviolet light [UVA], used as treatment for psoriasis and mycosis fungoides [cutaneous T cell lymphoma]).

Radiation-induced tumours

History There was noted to be an increased frequency of squamous cell carcinoma of the skin of the hand in radiologists in the early years of X-ray examination (when the exposure was determined by the radiologist X-raying his own hand).

Pathogenesis X-rays induce breaks in DNA in cells and incorrect excision and repair leads to mutations which may be oncogenic.

Chronic inflammatory processes associated with a severe degree of scarring (Marjolin's ulcer)

Epidemiology The mean interval between sustaining an injury and developing a cancer at the same site is about 36 years but there is an enormous scatter in the duration of such intervals.

Aetiology The two most common precursor lesions are burns and chronic stasis ulcers associated with venous insufficiency.

Renal transplantation

Epidemiology About 7.5% of renal allograft recipients develop neoplasms of which about 75% affect the skin. Incidence is related to length of time from transplantation and to degree of exposure to sunlight.

....

BENIGN EPIDERMAL TUMOURS AND TUMOUR-LIKE LESIONS

Epidermal cyst

Site Most frequently found on the face and trunk.

Clinical features Presents as a smooth dome-shaped rubbery nodule often with a central punctum from which cheesy cyst contents (largely keratin) may be expressed.

Microscopy Cyst wall is keratinizing squamous epithelium and cyst cavity is filled by keratin lamellae. Rupture of the cyst (associated with squeezing) releases keratinous content into the surrounding dermis and excites a florid chronic inflammatory reaction in which multi-nucleate giant cells are prominent.

Pilar cyst (trichilemmal cyst)

Derivation Outer root sheath of hair follicle.

Site Scalp, face and neck.

Clinical features Similar to epidermal cyst but no punctum.

Microscopy Cyst wall consists of a tough basement membrane and a stratified epithelial lining with a pattern of keratinization characteristic of the hair sheath (abrupt transition from epidermal cell to keratin in the absence of a granular layer).

Steatocystoma multiplex

Genetics Autosomal dominant inheritance.

Clinical features Presents with multiple cystic lesions about the time of puberty occuring on the neck, sternal region, axillae and scrotum.

Microscopy Cysts are lined by keratinizing stratified squamous epithelium but can be distinguished from other epidermal cysts by the presence of sebaceous epithelium in the wall.

Basal cell papilloma (seborrhoeic keratosis)

Epidemiology Mostly middle-aged or elderly adults.

Site Commonly the trunk.

Clinical features May be single or multiple. The lesion has a 'stuck-on' appearance and protrudes above the surface. Pigmentation is frequent but of variable intensity. Sudden appearance of a lesion or an increase in size or number may be a signal of internal malignancy (**the Leser–Trélat sign**).

Microscopy The lesion consists mainly of basal cells with interspersed keratin-filled cystic spaces. Some of the basal cells contain melanin pigment. 'Eddies' of mature squamous cells are not infrequent and are especially seen when the lesion has been 'irritiated'.

....

POTENTIALLY MALIGNANT EPIDERMAL CONDITIONS
Bowen's disease

Definition A form of intraepidermal squamous neoplasia. Lesions occuring in sun-exposed areas are more appropriately labelled **actinic keratoses of bowenoid type**.

Site Predominantly not sun-exposed areas.

Clinical features Indolent scaly red patches.

Microscopy Varying forms of keratinocyte atypia including nuclear hyperchromatism, individual cell keratinization and increased or abnormal mitoses. The change may involve virtually the entire epidermal thickness but a little surface maturation is usually present.

....

MALIGNANT EPIDERMAL TUMOURS
Squamous cell carcinoma

Aetiology Most are related to exposure to sunlight.

Site Most common sites are the backs of the hands, face and lips.

Microscopy Over 80% are well differentiated with easily identifiable 'prickles'. Variants occur e.g. with pseudo-glandular or spindle-shaped arrangement.

Basal cell carcinoma

Epidemiology Most common type of skin cancer. About 500 000 cases per year in the USA.

Aetiology Strong association with sun exposure although may occur in non-exposed areas associated with venous stasis in lower limbs, scars, irradiation and ingestion of small doses of arsenic.

Pathogenesis Arise from the basal layer of the epidermis and pilo-sebaceous unit and differentiate incompletely in the direction of various adnexal structures.

Clinical features Variable including superficial, nodular, ulcerative erythematous, sclerosing and pigmented subtypes.

Microscopy Variable. The tumour cells are small and darkly staining with palisading of the cells at the periphery of the cellular islands.

Associations Multiple basal cell carcinomas may occur as part of the basal cell naevus (Gorlin) syndrome whch also shows palmar pits, dural calcification, keratinous cysts of the jaws, skeletal anomalies and occasional abnormalities of the central nervous system. In this syndrome the tumours tend to be superficial and multi-centric in type and have osteoid metaplasia of the stroma.

Natural history and prognosis Most show no tendency to metastasize. Growth tends to be slow. They invade locally and if left cause extensive tissue destruction.

Adnexal tumours

There are a wide variety of adnexal tumours showing differentiation towards hair follicles, apocrine and eccrine sweat glands and ducts.

Keratoacanthoma

Definition Thought to arise from the infundibular portion of the hair follicle which may be confused clinically and microscopically with squamous cell carcinoma.

Epidemiology M:F 3–4:1.

Clinical features Dome-shaped lesion with central keratin-filled crater. Normally arises from normal skin, waxes over 4–6 weeks and then regresses over 4–6 weeks leaving a depressed scar. However there is considerable variation.

Microscopy The lesion has a half-moon shape with over-hanging edges and a large crater filled with keratin. Most of the proliferating epithelium is well differentiated and the cells have a glassy cytoplasm. The growing aspect is usually pushing rather than infiltrating. Differentiation from squamous carcinoma can be difficult.

Tumours derived from neuroendocrine cells

Merkel cell tumour

Epidemiology Rare. Mostly middle-aged or elderly patients.

Site Usually face or extremities.

Clinical features Commonly presents as a reddish or violet nodule which may ulcerate.

Microscopy Uniform population of small round cells with high nuclear-cytoplasmic ratio. Histochemically the cells are argyrophilic and express neurone specific enolase. Rarely they may contain peptide hormones.

Natural history and prognosis Aggressive behaviour with spread to regional lymph nodes being common. Lung, liver and bones may be involved by metastases.

....

TUMOURS OF MELANOCYTIC ORIGIN

Melanocytic naevi (moles)

Epidemiology Most people have melanocytic naevi and these are often multiple (up to 20–40) and usually appear age 2–6 years.

Site Most commonly face, neck and trunk.

Classification Based for the most part on the level in the skin where the proliferation occurs with some additional rarer types.

Junctional naevi

Clinical features Flat or slightly raised brown patches usually < 5 mm diameter.

Microscopy In the earliest stages there is an increase in the number of melanocytes in the basal layer with no clustering (a lentiginous proliferation). As the lesion progresses the cells form clusters or nests at the tips of the rete pegs on the epidermal side of the basement membrane.

Natural history and prognosis Most are benign but malignant transformation can occur.

Intradermal naevi

Microscopy Small clusters of well-differentiated melanocytes are present within the dermis without any evidence of basal layer proliferation or junctional activity. The cellularity and degree of pigmentation varies from lesion to lesion. With time the deepest parts tend to become less cellular and with spindle-shaped cells reminiscent of nerve sheath.

Compound naevi

Clinical features As age increases the junctional component tends to decrease with the exception of the skin of the soles of the feet and palms of the hand where age does not influence junctional activity.

Microscopy These combine features of both junctional and intradermal naevi.

Blue naevus

Site Commonly head, neck and upper limbs.

Clinical features Small darkly pigmented lesion.

Microscopy Ill-defined intradermal proliferation of elongated melanocytes in which melanin pigment is present in large amounts. There is a band of uninvolved dermis between the lesion and overlying epidermis. Junctional activity is never seen.

Cellular blue naevus

Definition Variant of blue naevus.

Site Most commonly buttock and sacrococcygeal region.

Clinical features Tend to be larger and intensely pigmented.

Microscopy Extremely cellular. No junctional activity, cellular atypia or abnormal mitoses.

Natural history and prognosis Invariably have a benign behaviour but a few show local recurrence and regional lymph node involvement has occurred.

Spitz naevus (previously known as juvenile melanoma)

Epidemiology Characteristically occurs before puberty but can be seen in adults.

Site Most often on face.

Clinical features Commonest appearance is of a pink or red nodule.

Microscopy Most have a compound pattern with prominent intraepidermal component but 5–10% are purely junctional and 20% are intradermal. They are composed either of spindle cells arranged vertically (raining down from surface) or large and polygonal (epithelioid) cells with abundant eosinophilc cytoplasm. Multi-nucleate giant melanocytes are seen and mitoses are found in up to 50% of cases although atypical mitoses are rare.

Natural history and prognosis Almost always benign but a few cases with aggressive behaviour have been reported with local and distant spread.

Dysplastic naevus syndrome

Genetics Autosomal dominant inheritance.

Sites In addition to those for benign naevi these are found on the scalp, buttocks and breast.

Clinical features Lesions are absent at birth. Increased number of abnormal naevi present between 5–8 years with a change in number and appearance at puberty. Dysplastic naevi are typically larger than benign naevi (range 6–15 mm) and usually number 25–75 per person (but may be as many as 100). Atypical naevi increase throughout adult life. The lesions have an irregular border and margin that fades into the normal surrounding skin. The surface is 'pebbly'. The pigmentation is often mixed with tan, brown, dark-brown and pink areas.

Natural history and prognosis Very high risk of developing malignant melanoma. Estimated that 5–10% melanoma arises on a familial basis.

Malignant melanoma

Aetiology Risk factors for melanoma are shown in Table 43.10.

Characteristics

Radial growth phase (RGP)

Definition Presence of a component adjacent to the main mass.

Microscopy Tumours may be present in the epidermis alone (in situ lesion) or in the dermis as well. The tumour cells in the dermis closely resemble those in the epidermis, are usually confined to the papillary dermis, are dispersed in clusters 10–15 cells wide, shows no evidence of growth advantage in one or other of these nests and the nests very uncommonly form clusters that are larger than the epidermal nests.

Biological characteristics Cell lines can only be established with difficulty and the cultured cells are not

Table 43.10 Risk factors for malignant melanoma

• Adulthood	Melanoma is rare before 15 years. Median age is 53 years. Adults have an 88-fold risk for melanoma compared with children.
• Pre-existing melanocytic naevus	1. **Dysplastic naevus with a history of familial melanoma**. Autosomal dominant inherited syndrome. Relative risk 148-fold.
	2. **Dysplastic naevus with no history of melanoma**. Wide range of relative risk (7–70 fold) quoted for this syndrome.
	3. **Presence of large congenital mole**. Relative risk 17–21-fold.
	4. **Presence of lentigo maligna.** Relative risk 10-fold.
	5. **Presence of a large number of benign melanocytic naevi.** Wide range of relative risk quoted for this factor.
• Being white rather than black	Relative risk 12-fold.
• Sun exposure and sun sensitivity	Sun-related burning is a critical factor if it occurs during childhood or adolescence and if it is intermittent.
• Others	Including immunosuppression, previous history of melanoma in the individual concerned, a parent or sibling.

tumourigenic in nude mice. The cells show non-random abnormalities on chromosome 6.

Frequency Present in 67% superficial spreading melanomas, 9% lentigo malignant melanoma and 4% acral lentiginous. Absent in nodular melanomas.

Natural history and prognosis If only a radial growth phase then no metastases might be expected to lymph node or distant site 7 years after diagnosis.

Vertical growth phase (VGP)

Definition Focal appearance either within an established radial growth (> 80%) phase or *ab initio* of a new population as an expanding spheroidal nodule which has a growth advantage over the cells of the radial phase.

Microscopy The cells appear different from those in the radial growth phase (e.g. may be amelanotic). The cell aggregates of the VGP are larger than those either in the epidermis or dermis of the RGP. The tumour cells extend into the lower half of the reticular dermis. The host lymphocytic response to the tumour is absent at the base of the tumour cells of the VGP.

Biological characteristics Cells cultured from the VGP rapidly form permanent cell lines in culture and these are tumorigenic in nude mice. Non-random abnormalities are found on chromosomes 1,6 and 7.

Natural history and prognosis The presence of a vertical growth phase correlates with the competence of the tumour cells to metastasize.

Classification

Superficial spreading melanoma

Epidemiology Commonest form and type with most rapidly increasing frequency.

Clinical features The appearances are variable but the commonest is bluish with admixed shades of dark brown. In some there may be depigmented patches (corresponding to areas of regression). The outine is frequently irregular. The surface is usually slightly raised above the surrounding normal skin. Dermal invasion (indicative of vertical growth phase) is usually associated with the appearance of a nodule on a previously flat lesion.

Microscopy The areas at the periphery of the lesion (where there is no dermal invasion) show atypical melanocytes at different levels of the epidermis either in clusters or as single cells (pagetoid spread). If a vertical growth phase has supervened the cells usually have abundant cytoplasm (epithelioid) and form one or more nodules significantly larger than the small nests associated with the radial phase.

Lentigo maligna (LM: Hutchinson's melanocytic freckle)

Epidemiology Usually occurs on sun-exposed skin in elderly whites. Commoner in males than females.

Site Common sites include malar and temple regions.

Clinical features Flat pigmented lesion.

Microscopy Melanocytes proliferate in a lentiginous pattern. In the pre-invasive period the atypical melanocytes are confined to the basal layer of the epidermis either singly or in small clusters. The epidermis tends to be atrophic. If an invasive lesion develops it is generally of the spindle-cell variety. Occasionally an aggressive invasive lesion will develop and these lesions are associated with marked reactive dermal fibrosis (desmoplastic melanoma).

Natural history and prognosis Best prognosis of the four types of melanoma. The proportion of these behaving in a malignant fashion is small (about 5%) and in those cases the benign phase ranges from 5–40 years.

Acral lentiginous melanoma

Epidemiology Rarest of the four types constituting approximately 4% of total. The commonest variety in dark-skinned races.

Site About 90% occur on the feet and 16% are beneath the nail (sub-ungual).

Microscopy There is an intraepidermal component (similar to lentigo maligna) but the cells have bizarre morphology. The epidermis is hyperplastic and the papillary dermis tends to be broadened and inflamed.

Natural history and prognosis Good if diagnosed early (90% 5-year survival) but very poor if the tumour has progressed to stage 2 (8% 5-year survival).

Nodular melanoma

Clinical features Presents as a red, grey or black nodule. There is no evidence of peripheral extension. The lesion may appear polypoid and ulceration is not infrequent.

Microscopy Little or no adjacent component (no more than three rete ridges involved at the periphery). There is a pure vertical growth phase *ab initio*.

Prognostic factors

1. Presence of a vertical growth phase.
2. Tumour thickness (Tables 43.11, 43.12). This is the single most important factor in superficial spreading and nodular melanomas. Measurement is vertically from the upper level of the granular epidermis to the deepest part of the tumour. At diagnosis nodular melanomas are much thicker than superficial spreading variety with only 25% of nodular melanomas < 1.69 mm deep compared with 77% of superficial spreading melanomas.

Level of invasion
First described by Clark.

Table 43.11 Association of tumour thickness and metastases

Thickness	Nodal metastases	Distant metastases
< 0.76 mm	2–3%	
0.76–1.50 mm	25%	8%
1.50–4.00 mm	57%	15%
> 4.00 mm	62%	72%

Table 43.12 Association of tumour thickness and survival

Thickness	7-year survival
≤ 1.69 mm	88%
1.70–3.99 mm	61%
> 4.00 mm	32%

Level 1   Tumour cells confined within the epidermis
Level 2   Tumour invades the papillary dermis
Level 3   Tumour cells have invaded through the papillary
           dermis and abut on the reticular dermis
Level 4   Tumour cells have invaded the reticular dermis
Level 5   Tumour cells are present in the subcutaneous
           tissues.

Within level 1 tumours the presence of ulceration and growth pattern are also prognostic indicators. In this level females have a significantly better prognosis than males and those tumours arising on the lower limb do better than those located elsewhere.

- **Anatomical site**   Those on the scalp, hands and feet have worse prognosis for equivalent thickness lesions.
- **Age**   Older patients do worse than younger patients.
- **Gender**   Females have a somewhat better prognosis than males.
- **Histological features**   Features suggesting a worse prognosis include a high mitotic rate, large tumour volume and the presence of satellite nodules.

....

CONNECTIVE TISSUE TUMOURS

Dermal connective tissue shows the same range of neoplasms as connective tissue in other sites.

Kaposi's sarcoma

Epidemiology   Formerly infrequent in most Western countries but found in relatively large numbers in sub-Saharan tropical Africa (endemic form) and in smaller numbers amoung Eastern Europeans and peoples of the Mediterranean basin (sporadic form). The incidence in the West has increased several hundred-fold which is confined for the most part to patients with AIDS. There is a difference in the prevalence of Kaposi's sarcoma in HIV+ homosexuals (36%) compared to haemophiliacs who have seroconverted as a result of receiving HIV-infected Factor VIII (1.6%).

Clinical features In the classic type the lesion presents as multiple bluish plaques or nodules on the lower extremities. Where the tumour is endemic in HIV+ and immuno-compromised patients the lesions are more variably distributed and behave aggressively. In these groups the finding of regional node and visceral involvement is by no means uncommon.

Microscopy The most characteristic appearance is of slits within the dermis which are lined by abnormal endothelial cells or spindle-shaped cells and contain red blood cells. The spaces appear to cleave the dermal collagen. There is an infiltrate of lymphocytes, iron-laden macrophages and other inflammatory cells. The precise nature of the lining cells remains controversial.

Fibrous histiocytoma (dermatofibroma, sclerosing haemangioma)

Site Most frequently on the lower leg.

Clinical features Presents as a papule or nodule which moves freely within the skin. Often deeply pigmented.

Microscopy The characteristic lesion is sited in the mid-dermis with a border of normal dermis between the lesion and the epidermis. The spindle-shaped cells are often arranged in a whorled (storiform) pattern and between these are macrophages which are often foamy (containing lipid).

Multi-nucleated giant cells may be seen. Mitoses are rare.

Natural history and prognosis Benign.

Dermatofibrosarcoma protuberans

Epidemiology Usually middle-aged individuals.

Site Commonest on the trunk.

Clinical features A plaque-like thickening which in time protrudes and shows a bluish or red colouration.

Microscopy Predominantly spindle cells in a storiform pattern. The tumour arises within the dermis but may spread downwards into the subcutaneous tissue. Mitoses are moderately frequent.

Natural history and prognosis   Local recurrences are not uncommon if surgical removal has been incomplete. Metastases are rare.

....

TUMOURS AND TUMOUR-LIKE LESIONS OF DERMAL BLOOD VESSELS

Pyogenic granuloma

Definition   A highly vascular nodule developing rapidly usually (but not always) at the site of injury to the skin.

Clinical features   Usually 5–10 mm diameter, polypoid and dusky red in colour.

Microscopy   Many small capillaries similar to those seen in granulation tissue set in an oedematous stroma rich in connective tissue mucins. Frequently ulcerated in which case there is an acute inflammatory infiltrate. The adjacent epidermis shows an appearance of a collarette.

Juvenile haemangioma (strawberry naevus)

Epidemiology   Occurs in about 1/200 infants.

Clinical features   Usually presents in first few weeks of life as a red macule that becomes elevated and reaches maximum size at about 6 months. Most regress with focal areas of greyish-white colour and by 7 years involution has occurred in 75% of cases.

Microscopy   This is a capillary haemangioma but in the early stages the proliferated blood vessels may be inconspicuous. At this time the lesion contains closely packed spindle cells with moderate numbers of mitoses.

Natural history and prognosis   Benign. No treatment required in most cases.

Cherry angiomas (Campbell de Morgan spots)

Epidemiology   Appear in adult life.

Clinical features   Multiple small lesions (few mm in greatest dimension). Well-demarcated with cherry red colour.

Microscopy Focal aggregates of dilated thin-walled blood vessels in the upper dermis. The overlying epidermis is often flattened.

Cavernous haemangioma

Epidemiology Most occur in infancy and may grow to considerable size. If very large there may be an associated thrombocytopenia due to sequestration of platelets within the lesion (Kasabach–Merritt syndrome). Cavernous hae-mangiomas are seen in the skin gut and other organs in the rare autosomal dominant condition known as **blue rubber bleb syndrome**.

Microscopy Aggregates of large dilated vessels lined by flattened endothelium and usually found in the deep dermis.

Glomus tumour

Definition Tumour derived from the neuromyoarterial glomus (consists of a complex system of anastamosing channels between digital arterioles and digital venules).

Site Mostly extremities with the nail-bed a particularly common site.

Clinical features Most are single and sporadic although some are multiple and familial (with autosomal dominant inheritance). Solitary tumours are pink nodules 1–20 mm diameter which are associated with pain either spona-neously or associated with pressure or temperature changes.

Microscopy The typical lesion shows dilated vascular channels in the dermis surrounded by rows of cuboidal glomus.

44 The skeletal system

BONE

ANATOMY

There are two bone types:

- cortical – dense and compact, predominates in shaft of long bones
- cancellous – appears spongy due to trabecular arrangement.

Organization

Epiphysis The area between the growth plate and the articular cartilage of long bones.

Metaphysis Includes the part of the growth plate furthest from the joint and the area joining the epiphysis to the shaft (area of most cell proliferation).

Diaphysis Shaft.

HISTOLOGY

Two types on the basis of organization: woven (occurs normally in embryonic life and childhood, characteristic of rapid bone formation and seen in osteogenesis imperfecta, scurvy, rickets, fracture callus, bone-forming tumours and Paget's disease of bone) with a random meshwork of birefringent collagen fibres and lamellae (characteristic of adult bone) showing parallel bundles/sheets of collagen fibres.

DEVELOPMENT IN EMBRYO

Bone formed in fetus from undifferentiated mesenchyme by either intramembranous ossification (bone formed directly from mesenchyme) or by endochondral ossification (initial cartilage-forming step).

Intramembranous ossification is the process of direct formation of bone from mesenchyme. Endochondral ossification has an intervening step of cartilage formation.

Most of the fetal skeleton is derived from cartilage growing through an interaction of growth and erosion of cartilage and deposition of bone. Bone formation starts in the mid-shaft in primary ossification centres.

These form cartilagenous models of adult bone which although smaller vary little in shape from their adult counterparts. The models grow by proliferation of chondrocytes and an increase in matrix. In long bones the primary ossification centres are mid-shaft. In the periochondrium of the cartilage, woven bone is deposited in a sleeve-like fashion while the proliferating chondrocytes eventually die and the matrix is calcified – under the influence of osteoblasts. Blood vessels grow into the centre. Some mesenchymal cells differentiate into osteoclasts which resorb the cartilagenous centres to leave hollow spaces.

Similar events occur at the secondary ossification centres at the ends of the long bones. Most pre-pubertal lengthening occurs at the bone ends as a result of the growth of the cartilagenous cylinder called the epiphyseal growth plate.

Bone remodelling

Removal and replacement of bone is an orderly occurrence with a turnover of 5–10% of the skeleton per year. This is achieved by a group of cells called the basic multi-cellular unit (BMU) consisting of osteoclasts, osteoblasts and other poorly characterized mononuclear cells. Around 1–10 million BMUs are present in the normal skeleton. Osteoclasts are formed from fusion of precursor cells at the bone surface and are derived from granulocyte-macrophage colony-forming units in the bone marrow. More bone will be reabsorbed if differentiation to osteoclasts increases or protease secretion of differentiated osteoclasts increases. Osteoclast differentiation is upregulated by interleukins 1, 3, 6 and 11, tumour necrosis factor and granulocyte-macrophage stimulating factor and downregulated by calcitonin, prostaglandins (except the E series) and tissue inhibitors of metalloproteinases. Osteoclast activity is upregulated by interleukins 1 and 6, tumour necrosis factor, α and β parathyroid hormone and gammainterferon. Osteoblasts are responsible for matrix mineralization. They do not divide and are derived from the same stem cell as chondroblasts, fibroblasts and adipocytes. Once mineralization has occurred some are incorporated into the bone as osteocytes.

In early life resorption and bone formation is in balance but after age 30–35 each cycle results in a small net loss of bone.

Processes of remodelling

Resorption Osteoclasts attach to bone surface and mobilize and digest mineral. Resorption in cortical bone occurs as tunnels originating in Haversian canals. In trabecular bone the resorption forms depressions (Howship's lacunae).

Reversal phase Macrophage-like cells modify the resorbed surface and lay down a collagen-poor 'cement line'.

Matrix formation Osteoblasts differentiate at resorption sites to deposit matrix (osteoid).

Mineralization Calcium in the form of hydroxyapatite is deposited in the new matrix.

....

FUNCTION

- structural framework
- reservoir for minerals: almost all body calcium and much of phosphorus and magnesium
- site of haemopoiesis.

DISORDERS OF BONE DEVELOPMENT

Disorders of epiphyseal plate

Achondroplasia

Genetics   May be autosomal dominant congenital disorder or sporadic.

Clinical   One of the commonest causes of dwarfism.

Pathogenesis   There is thinning of the growth plate with cartilage cells proliferating at a slower than normal rate.

Macroscopy   Bone thickness is normal. The head is disproportionately large. Spine is normal length. The limbs are shortened.

Morquio's syndrome

Genetics   Autosomal recessive inherited disorder.

Pathogenesis   Defective catabolism of intracellular carbohydrates resulting in the accumulation of keratan sulphates in many cells including chondrocytes. Spine and limb bones affected.

Clinical   Growth retardation, dental defects, mental retardation and corneal opacities.

Disorders of structure or quantity of collagenous matrix

Osteogenesis imperfecta

Epidemiology   Reported incidence of 1:20 000–1:60 000 live births.

Genetics   Heterogenous. Many genetic abnormalities resulting in similar clinical phenotypes.

Pathogenesis   Abnormal type I collagen structure and biosynthesis which is found in bones, tendons, ligaments, skin, dentine and sclerae. Genetic abnormalities resulting in the substitution of glycine by any other amino acid results in disruption of highly ordered triple helix consisting of three α chains (two α-1 and one α-2).

Clinical Dominant clinical expression is fragile bones. Also osteoporosis, hyperextensible joints, blue sclerae, abnormalities of tooth formation and onset of deafness (sensory) in adult life.

Classification

1. **Mild non-deforming**. 60%. Mildest, fractures unusual before walking, risk decreases after puberty. Blue sclerae (100%), some deafness (70%), dental abnormalities (25%). Autosomal dominant.

2. **Neonatal lethal**. 10%. Most severe and lethal in most cases. Multiple fractures in fetal life, neonates severely deformed, short limbs. Lack collagen type I in extracellular matrix. Autosomal recessive.

3. **Severe non-lethal**. 20%. Fractures present at birth, deformities of long bones, growth retardation. Scholiosis may cause respiratory problems including cor pulmonale. In familial cases autosomal recessive.

4. **Moderate and deforming**. 10%. Blue sclerae in infancy become white, moderate growth retardation, limb deformities may be severe. Most autosomal dominant.

....

DISORDERS OF BONE REMODELLING

Osteoporosis

Definition Decrease in bone mass leading to fractures following minimal trauma.

Epidemiology 1 in 3 women over 56 years will have had vertebral fracture and by extreme old age one in six men and one in three women will have had a hip fracture. Senile osteoporosis usually affects individuals over 70 years with M:F 1:2.

Aetiology Related to increasing age and female menopause.

Pathogenesis

1. **Menopause-related bone loss (type I osteoporosis)**: There is an accelerated phase of bone loss for 8–10 years after menopause involving loss of extra 2–3% above the loss associated with age. Oestrogen loss causes decrease

in secretion of TGF-beta, an increased IL-6 mediated osteoclast differentiation and increased secretion of lysosomal enzymes by osteoclasts.

2. **Age-related bone loss**: Trabecular bone loss begins at age 30 years and cortical loss at 40 years. In females 50% trabecular and 35% cortical bone is lost during lifetime while men loss two-thirds of this amount. Mechanism is due to the impaired filling of resorption cavities by new bone. This is thought to be related to impaired ability of bone marrow to produce osteoblast precursors.

3. **Secondary osteoporosis**: Associated with early oophorectomy, male hypogonadism, hyperthyroidism, Cushing's syndrome, chronic obstructive airways disease, disuse and treatments with glucocorticoids and some anti-convulsants.

Clinical features

Patients present with fractures most frequently of the vertebrae (44.8%) but also of the hip, wrist and other limbs. The occurrence and severity of osteoporosis is related to initial bone density, osteoblast function, calcium absorption, calcitonin levels (inhibits osteoclastic bone resorption: females have lower levels than males), obesity (protects against bone loss), exercise (stimulates osteoblastic activity), and cigarette smoking and heavy alcohol consumption (both risk factors for osteoporosis).

Osteomalacia

Definition   Characterized by defective mineralization of the osteoid matrix. The homologue of oteomalacia in children is rickets.

Pathogenesis   Reduction of mineralization of newly formed osteoid matrix and slowing down of the deposition of osteoid by osteoblasts. Mineralization normally occurs at the interface between the osteoid seam and the bone (the mineralization front) and mineralization lags behind osteoid formation by about 10 days. In osteomalacia the coupling between osteoid deposition and mineralization is lost, leading to an increase in the width of the osteoid seam.

Role of vitamin D

Synthesis in skin More than 90% of circulating vitamin D is derived from the action on 7-dehydrocholesterol of sunlight, forming pre-vitamin D3 which isomerizes to vitamin D3 at body temperature.

Dietary vitamin D Secondary role with relatively little derived from normal adult diet. However rickets/osteomalacia can occur in people with adequate sun exposure and in whom diet plays an important part. A high-risk diet for this is one rich in high extraction cereals and poor in meat, fish and dietary products. An explanation for this is that there may be an enterohepatic circulation in which vitamin D is excreted in bile and reabsorbed from gut lumen. Certain foods may interfere with the reabsorption resulting in increased faecal loss.

Absorption and/or loss of vitamin D from small gut Any disorder associated with malabsorption and steatorrhoca (e.g. coeliac disease) interferes with absorption of vitamin D (fat soluble).

Hydroxylation of vitamin D in the liver Vitamin D synthesized in the skin is transported to the liver associated with specific vitamin D-binding protein while vitamin D absorbed from the gut is transported in chylomicrons. In the liver cells there is hydroxylation at the 25 position (to form 25-hydroxycholecalcifcrol). Chronic liver disease (e.g. alcoholic liver disease and primary biliary cirrhosis) interferes with this hydroxylation. Biliary excretion of vitamin D metabolites may be increased following induction of enzymes by drugs such as phenytoin and phenobarbitone.

Hydroxylation of 25-OH cholecalciferol in the kidney Hydroxylation occurs at the 1-α position in the mitochondria of the epithelial cells of the proximal renal tubule resulting in the most active form of vitamin D, calcitriol (1-25-dihydroxycholecalciferol). This reaction is modulated by parathyroid hormone and plasma phosphate. Hydroxylation can also occur at other sites e.g. placenta and in osteoblasts, keratinocytes, macrophages after activation by gamma-interferon and activated macrophages in granulomas (e.g. in sarcoid). The kidney is also the source of the alternative form of vitamin D, 24-25-dihydroxycholecalci-ferol. The activity of the 24 hydroxylase enzyme is promoted by higher plasma concentrations of calcium and inorganic phosphorus. Calcitriol is 8 times more effective in promoting calcium absorption from the gut than 24–25-dihydroxycholecalciferol. Renal diseases associated with nephron loss will therefore be associated with progressive bone disease. Osteomalacia may be seen in Fanconi syndrome, myeloma kidney and heavy metal poisoning.

Biological effects of vitamin D   Calcitriol from the kidney is transported associated with vitamin D-binding protein. Actions are to promote transport of calcium from the gut lumen and to promote bone growth and mineralization. In bone this requires the successful binding to a receptor. Inherited vitamin D resistance (vitamin D-dependent rickets type II) is due to end-organ resistance.

Hypophosphataemic osteomalacia

Features   Second commonest cause of osteomalacia/rickets but much less common than vitamin D deficiency. Associated with sustained low levels of serum phosphate and resistance to treatment with vitamin D.

X-linked hypophosphataemic rickets
Genetics   X-linked dominant inheritance.

Clinical features   Children are well-nourished and healthy looking. Growth rate is initially normal but slows when weight-bearing starts.

Pathogenesis   Excessive loss of phosphate from the kidney due to abnormality of phosphate transport by tubular epithelium.

Tumour-associated osteomalacia
Epidemiology   Commonest in adults over 30 years. M:F 1:1.

Aetiology   Most associated with tumours of bone and soft tissue. Many are vascular tumours (haemangiopericytomas).

Pathogenesis   Secretion products from the tumour cause increased urinary loss of phosphate and also appear to inhibit hydroxylation of vitamin D at the 1-position.

Laboratory findings Serum phosphate and vitamin D are low.

Clinical features of osteomalacia syndrome

Severe bone deformities are now rarely seen in adults except in countries with endemic vitamin D deficiency from childhood to adult life.

Clinical features There is bone pain and bone tenderness. Muscle weakness is present in about 40%. Severe bone deformities (e.g. limb curvature, coxa vara and contracted pelvis) may occur. In rickets there is disturbance of endochondral ossification in addition to failure of mineralization. This affects mainly those bones growing rapidly in childhood (cranium, wrists and ribs) and leads to:

- widening of cranial sutures
- frontal bossing
- posterior flattening of the skull
- bulging of the costochondral junctions (known as a 'rickety rosary')
- enlargement of the wrist.

After the first year the bones most affected are those which both grow rapidly and weight-bear so abnormalities mostly affect the legs. If not treated there may be lifelong deformity. Muscle weakness may result in hypotonia in infants which is associated with a lax and protuberant abdomen.

Radiological features of osteomalacia

This is usually much less pronounced than in rickets. There is generalized osteopenia. The characteristic feature is Looser's zone or pseudofracture (mostly medial edge of long bones) which are linear areas of increased radiolucency roughly perpendicular to the long axis of long bones.

In rickets there is widening of the ends of the metaphysis with concavity of the usually straight transverse margin of the metaphysis.

Microscopy of osteomalacia

There is increased osteoid measured in terms of

1. Osteoid volume (expressed as percentage area of total trabecular bone).

2. Osteoid seam width (measured in relation to all trabeculae. Osteoid seam width of more than 3–4 collagen lamellae is abnormal).

3. Osteoid surface (expressed as fraction of the total perimeter length of all the trabecula in a section which is covered by osteoid).

Indices of mineralization are gained by examining biopsies from patients that have had time-spaced doses of tetracycline which is deposited in the mineralization fronts and can be seen under UV light. Partial or complete absence of tetracycline along the bone-osteoid interface indicates an abnormality of mineralization.

Secondary hyperparathyroidism due to low serum vitamin D and calcium leads to increased osteoclastic activity and increased unmineralized osteoid (particularly evident in renal osteodystrophy). This is not present in pure hypophosphataemic states as the serum calcium is normal and there is no secondary hyperparathyroidism.

In children with rickets the growth plate is widened due to disarray of the columns of cartilage cells. The normal progression of cartilage to primary spongiosa does not occur.

Hypophosphatasia

Genetics Believed to be autosomal dominant inheritance.

Pathogenesis Inability to mineralize bone or growth cartilage at the metaphysis.

Clinical features Usually presents in childhood with defective bone mineralization.

Laboratory findings Calcitriol levels are normal. Serum alkaline phosphatase levels are usually depressed. Often increase in urinary phosphoethanolamine levels.

Microscopy Identical to rickets but no histological features of secondary hyperparathyroidism.

Hyperparathyroidism

Definition Characterized by excessive osteoclastic resorption of bone.

Physiology of parathyroid hormone Most important regulator of blood or extracellular fluid calcium concentration.

Upregulated by low calcium. Effects mediated through resorption of calcium in the proximal and distal tubules of the kidney, increased bone resorption, increased calcium absorption from the small intestine. Hormone secretion is chiefly regulated by calcium levels. Phosphate levels can also cause increased secretion by lowering plasma-ionized calcium levels. Increased calcitriol levels lower hormone secretion probably acting at the mRNA level.

Primary hyperparathyroidism

Definition   Hypersecretion of parathyroid hormone outside the control of the normal negative feedback mechanism.

Aetiology   Either adenoma (about 80%; usually single but occasionally multiple), carcinoma (0.5–4%) or diffuse chief cell hyperplasia (about 15%). Both adenomas and hyperplasia may be associated with multiple endocrine neoplasia syndromes (most commonly type I).

Clinical features   Symptoms classically described as 'bones, stones, abdominal groans and psychic moans' but many (about 57%) are asymptomatic at diagnosis and picked up on screening biochemical investigations. Acute hypercalcaemia may be seen in about 14% with rapidly deteriorating renal function, nausea, vomiting, drowsiness and stupor.

Bone changes   Bone pain and occasionally pathological fracture. Bone shows increased osteoclastic resorption with trabecula showing indentations filled with well-vascularized connective tissue. In severe cases osteitis fibrosa cystica may develop (also known as brown tumours) where the bone trabeculum has been completely eroded and is replaced by vascular fibrous tissue with many osteoclasts.

Renal complications   Calcium-forming stones may develop (hyperparathyroidism accounts for about 5–10% of cases of calcium-containing renal stones). Nephrocalcinosis (precipitation of calcium and phosphate in the renal tubular epithelium) is rare and occurs in patients with long-standing disease. Functional changes in the renal tubules may be seen including metabolic renal acidosis (due to impairment of bicarbonate resorption caused by excess parathyroid hormone leading to hyperchloremic acidosis), phosphaturia, aminoaciduria, glycosuria and failure to concentrate urine.

Gastrointestinal complications Include development of peptic ulcer possibly in up to 10–20% of patients with hyperparathyroidism. Pancreatitis is a known association.

Neural and muscle complications Weakness associated with atrophy of proximal muscle groups (particularly lower limbs) associated with changes seen in denervated muscle groups.

Psychiatric changes Include depression, memory impairment and emotional lability. Due to hypercalcaemia.

Macroscopy Adenomas usually weigh 0.5–5.0g (normal gland 25–50 mg). Commonest in the inferior glands. Adenomas may be ectopically located in thymus, thyroid etc.

Secondary hyperparathyroidism

Aetiology Result of chronic hypocalcaemia. Associated with chronic renal failure, defective small bowel calcium absorbtion and inborn errors of vitamin D.

Pathogenesis Initially the feedback mechanism of low calcium concentrations leads to increased parathyroid hormone secretion. In time hyperplasia supervenes.

Laboratory findings Hypercalcaemia is not seen.

Clinical features Manifestations are associated with bone disease.

Microscopy Bone shows some histological evidence of osteomalacia and excess osteoclastic resorption with defective mineralization of osteoid.

Tertiary hyperparathyroidism

Definition Development of hypercalcaemia in patient with long-standing secondary hyperparathyroidism.

Hypercalcaemia associated with malignancy

Associations Commonest are lung cancer (35%), breast cancer (24%) and haematological malignancies (14%).

Pathogenesis

Mechanisms include the lytic resorption of bone in relation to secondary tumour deposits, generalized increase in bone resorption caused by circulating factors stimulating bone resorption and which may also increase tubular resorption of calcium by renal tubules (humoral hypercalcaemia of malignancy; most associated with squamous carcinoma of the lung and head and neck and carcinomas of the ovary and pancreas), bone resorption associated with inability to secrete calcium (associated with myelomatosis) and bone resorption due to increased absorption of calcium from the gut (seen in patients with leukaemia and lymphoma) and possibly associated with secretion of vitamin D by the malignant cells.

Paget's disease of bone

Epidemiology Affects 3–4% of the population aged over 40 years. Frequency increases with age. More common in the USA, Britain, France, Germany, Australia and New Zealand but rare in East Asia, Scandinavia and countries bordering the Mediterranean. Positive family history is common (up to 25% of cases).

Aetiology Obscure.

Pathogenesis The disease is characterized by excessive resorption of bone by osteoclasts, increase in bone mass and loss of normal lamellar architecture.

Clinical features May affect one or many bones. The commonest are the spine (76%) and the skull (65%) followed by the pelvis (43%), femur (35%), tibia (30%), clavicle (11%), sternum (7%) and humerus (2%). Deformities of the skull may be associated with narrowing of the forearm of the cranial nerves resulting in neuropathies. Deafness (sensory, conductive or both) is common – found in 30–50% of cases.

Laboratory findings There is a high level of bone-derived alkaline phosphatase. There is an increased level of plasma and urinary hydroxyproline.

Macroscopy Bones are enlarged and thickened (e.g. the calvarium of the skull may measure 2–3 cm thick) but the bone is softer. There is a considerable degree of deformity including protuberance of the frontal bones of the skull and bowing of the long bones (commonly anteriorly or lateral).

Microscopy The bone trabeculae are markedly enlarged and irregular. Evidence of excessive remodelling is prominent with resorption involving over 20% of the surface (normal about 3%). Osteoclasts are more numerous ($3/mm^2$ compared to $0.2/mm^2$ in normal people). The osteoclasts are abnormal containing many more nuclei than normal. Osteoblastic activity is florid and osteoid covers about 50% of the bone trabecula (normal 16%). The large trabeculae consist predominantly of lamellar bone but areas of woven bone are also present. The trabeculae have a mosaic appearance due to numerous bluish 'cement-lines'.

Natural history and prognosis Up to 60% of patients develop joint problems mostly in those associated with weight bearing. Fractures and fissure occur due to the weakness of the bones. Neurological disorders in relation to the skull occur. Neoplastic transformation into a sarcoma is 30 times more frequent occurring in 1–2% of Paget's disease patients. Osteogenic sarcoma is the most frequent followed by fibrosarcoma and chondrosarcoma. The prognosis for these sarcomas arising in the context of Paget's disease is poor.

Osteopetrosis

Definition Set of disorders characterized by an increase in bone mass and increased risk in developing pathological fractures.

Aetiology May be inherited or acquired.

Genetics Inherited cases may present in adult life or childhood. In the latter there is usually autosomal recessive inheritance. The adult form may be dominant or recessive.

Pathogenesis In most cases there is decreased bone resorption although an abnormal increase in bone formation would have the same effect.

Clinical fractures In most inherited cases presenting in childhood the disease is severe and usually fatal. Inherited cases presenting in adults tends to be less severe. The X-ray shows generalised increase in bone density. There is absent or delayed eruption of teeth.

Microscopy The bone trabeculae are large with normal or decreased numbers of osteoblasts.

PRIMARY BONE TUMOURS

When haematological tumours have been excluded:

- 21% show cartilage differentiation

  - 60% benign (osteochondroma, chondroma, chondro-blastoma, chondromyxoid fibroma)
  - 40% malignant (chondrosarcoma)

- approximately 19% are bone forming (show osteoid)

  - 13% benign (osteoid osteoma, osteoblastoma)
  - 87% malignant (osteosarcoma).

Benign cartilage-forming tumours

Osteochondroma (exostosis)

Definition Bone lesions with a cartilage cap projecting from the metaphysis of long bones. Usually solitary. Believed to be **hamartomas** rather than true neoplasms. Multiple osteochondromas may occur in childhood in **osteochondromatosis** (autosomal dominant).

Epidemiology Solitary lesions most common in adolescence. M:F 3:1

Site Long bones most commonly femur, tibia and humerus. Uncommon in small bones of hands or feet.

Clinical features Pain, localized swelling or deformity.

Macroscopy About 3–4 cm along longest axis. Project from bone either as sessile or pedunculated forms. Cartilaginous cap up to 1 cm thick.

Microscopy Superficial zone in the cap with haphazard arrangement of chondrocytes deep to which they are arranged in columns with ossification deep to this.

Natural history and prognosis Malignant change in less than 1% rising to 10% in cases with multiple lesions.

Chondroma (enchondroma)

Definition Benign neoplasm of mature hyaline cartilage.

Epidemiology Common. Any age but more in children, adolescents and young adults. M:F 1:1.

Site Solitary lesions most common in medullary cavity of small bones of hands and feet. Multiple lesions may occur in one or several bones:

- Ollier's syndrome = multiple unilateral enchondromas
- Mafucci's syndrome = multiple enchondromas and multiple soft tissue haemangiomas.

Clinical features Asymptomatic or painful, local swelling, tenderness or pathological fracture.

Macroscopy Well-circumscribed lobulated masses of bluish firm cartilage. Overlying bone is thinned/eroded.

Microscopy Lobules of mature hyaline cartilage surrounded by vascularized fibrous stroma. Chondrocytes irregularly distributed. Occasional dark nuclei and binuclear forms may be seen (not indicative of malignancy in children but more sinister in adults).

Natural history and prognosis Malignant transformation rare in hands/feet but may occur in flat bones and proximal limb chondromas. More likely in multiple chondroma syndromes (30–50%).

Chondroblastoma

Epidemiology Rare – less than 1% primary bone tumours. Most aged 10–20 years. M:F 2:1.

Site Typically in epiphyseal regions of long bones. Around knee and upper end of humerus is commonest.

Clinical features Pain and local tenderness is common.

Radiology Typically a central zone of bone destruction in epiphysis surrounded by narrow zone of increased bone density.

Macroscopy Usually 1–7 cm. Pinkish-grey cut surface with occasional areas of haemorrhage or necrosis. Involvement of articular cartilage is uncommon.

Microscopy Characterized by benign-appearing multinucleate cells (5–40 nuclei), islands of cartilaginous matrix and small mononuclear cartilage cells with mitoses. Other than in the areas of cartilaginous matrix, stoma is scanty.

Natural history and prognosis Most are cured by local removal (e.g. curettage) but some recur and occasional spread usually to lung can be seen.

Chondromyxoid fibroma

Epidemiology Rare (less than 1% primary bone tumours). Any age 3–70 years but most in 2nd and 3rd decade. Males more than females.

Site Most in metaphysis of long bones (tibia, femur, fibula) followed by flat bones (mostly ileum) and small bones of hands/feet.

Clinical features Pain is commonest presentation.

Radiology Eccentric, sharply circumscribed zone of rarefaction with its long axis parallel to that of the long bone.

Macroscopy Average diameter 5 cm. Cut surface is lobulated and cartilagenous or glistening white fibrous tissue.

Microscopy Varies from area to area. Some are frankly cartilaginous; others have myxoid matrix and areas of fibrous tissue are present. Lobular growth pattern with nuclei at the periphery of lobules.

Natural history and prognosis Benign. Curettage may be followed by local recurrence so wide excision may be indicated.

Malignant cartilage-forming tumours

Chondrosarcoma

Definition Malignant tumour which is differentiated for the most part into abnormal cartilage.

Epidemiology Second commonest primary malignant neoplasm of bone. About 25% are secondary developing within benign tumours (mostly osteochondromas). Primary chondrosarcomas tend to occur in middle age or later. M:F 3:2.

Site More than 75% occur in trunk (ribs and pelvis), and upper ends of femur and humerus. Few arise in hands/feet.

Clinical features Most present with either local swelling, pain or both.

Radiology Typically bony destruction associated with mottled densities representing focal calcification and ossification.

Macroscopy Characteristically lobulated. Size varies from a few millimeters to several centimetres.

Microscopy Low-grade chondrosarcomas can be difficult to differentiate from benign tumours. Features suggesting malignancy include many cartilage cells with plump nuclei, more than occasional binucleate cells and giant cartilage cells with single large or multiple nuclei. In **dedifferentiated chondrosarcoma** a low grade/well-differentiated area is seen in continuity with a highly malignant anaplastic sarcoma.

Natural history and prognosis Well-differentiated tumours grow slowly and seldom metastasize.

Dedifferentiated chondrosarcoma has a poor prognosis (80% dead in 2 years). Metastases are common (usually to lung) and are composed of the anaplastic component. Chondrosarcomas are resistant to radiotherapy.

Mesenchymal chondrosarcoma

Epidemiology Rare variant. Occurs in young (mean age 25 years).

Site Commonest is femur, humerus, ileum and os calcis.

Microscopy Mixture of cartilaginous tissue in various stages of differentiation and highly cellular areas with small darkly staining cells often spindle shaped and grouped around blood vessels.

Natural history and prognosis Local lymph node metastasis is common.

Clear cell chondrosarcoma

Epidemiology Peak incidence 20–40 years. M:F 2.6:1.

Site Most common in ends of long bones (60% in proximal end of femur).

Macroscopy Soft and lack hyaline appearance.

Microscopy Cells with central nucleus and clear cytoplasm arranged in indistinct lobules separated by fine connective tissue strands. Most contain a few benign-appearing giant cells.

Natural history and prognosis Most slowly growing with 18% patients having symptoms for more than 5 years.

Benign bone-forming tumours

Osteoma

Definition A set of lesions characterised by normally arranged mature bone.

Site Most common in the skull and facial bones.

Clinical features Usually asymtomatic. Some grow into paranasal sinuses or orbit and cause mechanical problems. Usually single but can be multiple as part of Gardner's syndrome.

Radiology Well-demarcated radio-opaque lesions.

Microscopy Dense mature lamellar bone with well-formed Haversian systems.

Osteoid osteoma

Definition Benign osteoblastic lesion consisting of a small round central area (nidus) surrounded by dense sclerotic bone.

Epidemiology About 12% of all benign bone tumours. Affects young (80% are 5–24 years). Marked male predominance.

Site End of shaft of femur or tibia in 50%. Vertebrae (especially arches) may be affected.

Clinical features Classically presents with pain. Localized swelling may occur.

Radiology Nidus appears as small radiolucent area surrounded by dense radio-opaque area.

Macroscopy Well-defined and fleshy. Usually 1–1.5 cm diameter. Nidus is redder.

Microscopy Nidus consists of interlacing, delicate bands of osteoid with haphazard arrangement surrounded by plump osteoblasts. The intervening spaces contain vascular fibrous tissue with variable numbers of benign looking giant cells. Cartilaginous differentiation is never seen. Surrounding sclerotic area is reactive bone.

Benign osteoblastoma (giant osteoid osteoma)

Definition Morphologically related to osteoid osteoma but larger, has different site and different reaction of surrounding bone.

Epidemiology Rare. Age similar to osteoid osteoma.

Site Tendancy to occur in vertebral column. Also in bones of hands/feet.

Macroscopy Usually larger than 1.5 cm. Well demarcated from surrounding bone. Granular friable cut surface with focal haemorrhage. Conspicuous surround of bone sclerosis is generally absent.

Microscopy Similar to osteoid osteoma with osteoid seams surrounded by plump osteoblasts. Mitoses may be present. In some cases dilated vascular channels may be present. Cases with atypical osteoblasts and poorly demarcated edge are termed **aggressive osteoblastomas** and may recur.

Malignant bone-forming tumours

Osteosarcoma

Definition Tumour with frankly sarcomatous stroma and evidence of formation of neoplastic osteoid and bone by malignant cells. May have predominant osteoid formation (**osteoblastic**), prominent neoplastic cartilage (**chondroblastic**) or cells resembling fibrosarcoma with abundant collagen (**fibroblastic**).

Epidemiology Commonest primary maligant tumour of bone. Rare before 10 years, peak 10–25 years. Cases occuring in middle-aged/elderly are associated with Paget's disease of bone. Males more than females.

Aetiology and pathogenesis Most are primary. Some are associated with pre-existing bone disease (particularly Paget's disease of bone) or irradiation (latent period 10–15 years). Osteosarcomas are seen in some children who have survived hereditary retinoblastoma.

Site Metaphyseal region of long bone (80%). About 50% around the knee. Commonest sites (descending frequency) are lower femur, upper tibia, upper humerus and ileum. Multi-centric osteosarcomas occur occasionally in childhood. Most arise from the medullary cavity, a small minority (usually occurring in diaphysis) arise within the cortex. Cases associated with Paget's disease of bone commonly occur in the pelvis, humerus, femur, tibia and skull.

Radiology   The cortex is almost always penetrated by tumour causing elevation of the periosteum leading to the radiological sign of **Codman's triangle** (bounded by periosteum with the base of cortical bone and containing reactive new bone with spicules perpendicular to the original cortex).

Macroscopy   Depends on degree of bone destruction, differentiation pattern of the tumour and pattern of local spread – extension down medullary cavity, penetration of cortex and elevation of periosteum, extension into epiphysis/joint space/adjacent soft tissue or appearance of separate nodules (skip metastases).

Microscopy   Frankly malignant connective tissue stroma in which the malignant cells are forming new bone or osteoid. Typically the osteoid is eosinophilic, has irregular outlines and is surrounded by a rim of malignant osteoblasts. Osteoblast-like giant cells are present in about 25%. The tumour cells contain large amounts of **alkaline phosphatase**. The stroma shows considerable variations from case to case.

Natural history and prognosis   In general highly malignant. Tendency to blood-borne metastasis to lung (98%), other bones (37%), pleura (33%) and heart (20%). Prognosis is adversely affected by the presence of Paget's disease of bone, site (skull and vertebral location is poor; osteosarcomas of the jaw and limb extremities better than proximal), multi-focality, differentiation pattern (e.g. telangiectatic variant has worse prognosis). Overall 5-year survival is 20% but improved to about 50% with combined chemotherapy followed by surgery.

Parosteal (juxtacortical) osteosarcoma

Epidemiology   Occur in slightly older people.

Site   Arise in the juxtacortical position in the mataphyseal region.

Macroscopy   May be large lobulated mass which encircles the shaft.

Microscopy Well-formed bone and osteoid in a spindle-cell stroma with scanty evidence of malignancy. The differential diagnosis is from myositis ossificans (which has orderly maturation of new bone at the periphery).

Natural history and prognosis Not all osteosarcomas in a juxtacortical position have a good prognosis: some (high-grade surface osteosarcomas) behave as aggressively as any other osteosarcomas.

Periosteal osteosarcoma

Site Superficial. Commonly the upper shaft of tibia or femur.

Radiology Areas of radiolucency on bone surface associated with spicules of new bone perpendicular to the shaft just below the periosteum.

Macroscopy Usually confined to the cortex.

Microscopy Frankly malignant stroma with conspicuous islands of cartilage.

Natural history and prognosis Prognosis is better than for usual osteosarcoma.

Osteosarcoma arising in the jaw

Epidemiology Older patient (mean 34 years).

Site Mandible and alveolar ridge of maxilla.

Microscopy Areas of cartilaginous differentiation are common.

Prognosis Relatively good.

Other tumours of bone

Giant cell tumour of bone

Epidemiology Account for just under 5% of primary bone tumours and 21% of benign neoplasms. Usually more than 80%) over 19 years with peak in 3rd decade. Slight female preponderance.

Site Commonly in long bone metaphyses – in descending order of frequency – around the knee (> 50%), lower end of radius and sacrum. May extend into metaphysis and break through cortex to the joint space. About 1% are multiple.

Radiology Lytic and radiolucent lesion expanding the bone.

Macroscopy Size varies from case to case. Cut surface is heterogenous with grey and red areas. There may be small blood-filled cysts. Overlying cortical bone is thinned.

Microscopy Two main elements are seen:

- **Stromal cells** with round/oval nuclei and ill-defined cytoplasm. Mitoses may be present but are not atypical.
- **Giant cells** which are large and have on average 20–30 nuclei with no mitoses or atypia. Natural history and prognosis. Considered benign but may be aggressive and some undergo malignant change (about 10%) with uncontrollable local recurrence or metastatic spread.

Ewing's tumour of bone

Definition A tumour belonging to the group of small round-cell tumours of childhood (with neuroblastoma, poorly-differentiated rhabdomyosarcoma and malignant small round cell tumour of the thoraco-pulmonary area [Askin tumour]) and believed to be related to primitive neuroectodermal tumours (PNET).

Epidemiology Accounts for 4.7% of all bone tumours and 6.1% of malignant tumours of bone. Peak incidence 5–20 years, rare over 30 years. Male preponderance.

Genetics About 85% show t(11;22).

Site Almost any bone. Long bones of the lower limbs and the pelvic girdle account for 60% with ribs the next most common site. In long bones the tumour arises in the medullary cavity.

Clinical features Pain and swelling are the commonest symptoms. There may be fever and raised erythrocyte sedimentation rate.

Radiology Lytic destruction and widening of the medullary cavity. Cortical infiltration may develop with elevation of the periosteum and new bone formation either perpendicular to the cortex or parallel with an onion-skin appearance.

Macroscopy Glistening greyish-white cut surface. Focal necrosis and haemorrhage is common.

Microscopy Sheets of small uniform round cells divided into islands by fibrous septae. Glycogen is present in the cytoplasm.

Natural history and prognosis An aggressive tumour with metastatic spread to lungs, pleura, other bones (especially the skull) and the central nervous system. With high dose irradiation followed by chemotherapy the 5-year survival has improved from 5–8% to about 75%.

FIBROBLASTIC TUMOURS

Malignant fibrous histiocytoma

Epidemiology Accounts for less than 1% of primary malignant bone tumours. Mean age is 40 years.

Aetiology About 30% are associated with foreign bodies, bone infarcts, Paget's disease of bone or previous irradiation.

Site 60% occur in long bones.

Clinical features Pain and swelling.

Radiology Lytic lesion.

Macroscopy Variable. Some are soft. Cut surface may be yellow (if lipid rich) or brownish-grey.

Microscopy Cartwheel pattern of pleomorphic cells. Plump fibroblastic spindle cells, multi-nucleate giant cells and macrophages containing lipid may be seen. Large atypical cells may be prominent. Mitoses are common.

Natural history and prognosis Highly aggressive tumours.

Fibrosarcoma

Definition Malignant spindle cell neoplasm which may or may not produce collagen but does not produce cartilage or osteoid.

Epidemiology Constitutes about 3% malignant primary bone tumours. Evenly distributed from 2nd to 7th decade. M:F 1:1.

Site More than 50% occur in long bones, principally metaphyseal, with 30% in the region of the knee.

Clinical features Pain and localized swelling.

Radiology Lytic due to destruction of medullary and cortical bone 'soap-bubble' appearance.

Macroscopy If collagen rich the tumour is firm and greyish-white; if not the tumours are soft friable and fleshy.

Microscopy In highly differentiated tumours the cells show a 'herring-bone' appearance with abundant collagen in whorls and bands. In others there is a high degree of cellular and nuclear pleomorphism with numerous mitoses.

Natural history and prognosis Metastases are common. five-year survival of about 25%.

Chordoma

Definition Tumour derived from the remains of the notochord.

Epidemiology Rare below 30 years. Males more than females.

Site Most in the sacrum but some occur in the spheno-occipital region.

Clinical features Sacral tumours present with symptoms/ signs of pressure on cauda equina and nerve roots. Intracranial tumours present with symptoms/signs of an intracranial mass.

Macroscopy Lobulated and well encapsulated. Gelatinous bluish-grey cut surface with focal haemorrhage or cystic change.

Microscopy Tumour cells are round or polyhedral growing in clumps or cords. The cytoplasm is vacuolated (physali-phorous cells). There is abundant mucin-rich stroma.

....

TUMOUR-LIKE LESIONS
Fibrous dysplasia of bone (Table 44.1)

Definition Non-neoplastic lesion in which bone is replaced by fibrous tissue containing spicules of woven bone. Occurs in three main forms.

Table 44.1 Types of fibrous dysplasia of bone

Type	Frequency	Age/Sex	Sites
Monostotic	70%	Older children/adolescents	Ribs, femur, tibia, maxilla, mandible, humerus
Polyostotic	25%	Younger children M:F 1:1	Femur, skull, tibia and humerus. Facial involvement in 50%
McCune–Albright syndrome (polyostotic with endocrine abnormality and patchy skin pigmentation)	3–5%	F > M	Skin and bone lesions on same side. Most commonly associated with precocious puberty. Skin lesions are large irregular areas.

Clinical features   Many of the monostotic cases are asymptomatic. Large lesions may present as pathological fractures. With cranial involvement presentation may be with facial deformity

Radiology   Cystic appearance.

Microscopy   Sheets of mature cellular fibrous tissue containing trabeculae of woven bone with sickle or fish-hook appearance which never mature into woven bone and lack a rim of osteoblasts.

••

MISCELLANEOUS BONE DISORDERS
Ischaemic necrosis of bone

Epidemiology   Accounts for 10% of joint replacements in USA. May be an isolated event, associated with local irradiation or the result of steroid therapy. May occur in adults or in children. In children it may effect the epiphysis of several different bones (**osteochondritis jeuvenilis**).

Pathogenesis   Bones have two blood supplies. The **nutrient artery** enters bone through a foramen, penetrates the cortex to reach medulla and divides into a plexus supplying medulla and inner half of cortex. **Periosteal vessels** perforate cortex perpendicular to surface and anastomose with nutrient arteries. In the cortex vessels run either parallel (haversian canals) or perpendicular (Volkmann's canals) to the long axis.

Interruption of the blood supply occurs under four circumstances:

1. Mechanical interruption (e.g. fracture or dislocation)
2. Thrombosis/embolism
3. Non-traumatic damage to vessel (vasculitis, post irradiation, chemically induced spasm)
4. Venous occlusion.

Mechanism   Ischaemia results in infarction of medullary bone (often clinically silent) or infarction of both medullary and cortical bone (most frequent in femur just below articular cartilage in hip and knee joints and in upper portion of humerus). Infarction elicits an inflammatory response, demolition of dead bone and replacement by new woven bone. The late stages may be associated with stress fractures with collapse and distortion.

Sites In children osteochondritis jeuvenilis occurs as:
- **Legg-Calvé-Perthes disease:** femoral head. Often a family history. Males more than females. Peak incidence 5–11 years
- **Kienboeck's disease:** lunate bone in hand
- **Kohler's disease:** navicular bone in foot
- **Frieberg's disease:** head of a metatarsal bone.

Acute osteomyelitis

Epidemiology Most in first two decades M:F 3:1.

Pathogenesis Pus-forming inflammation. Organisms may reach bone either by direct spread (e.g. with compound fracture, penetrating wound, surgical intervention) or via the bloodstream (often Staphylococcal from a trivial primary focus such as a boil). Patients with sickle cell disease are at risk of haematogenous osteomyelitis (most frequently salmonellae). The main target of haematogenous osteomyelitis is the metaphysis of the long bone. In rigid bones inflammation and oedema causes rise in interstitial pressure compromising blood supply and causing local bone necrosis. Bone necrosis is also due to the results of lysosomal enzymes from inflammatory cells.

If inflammation is not controlled the inflammation can extend through vessels a long haversian and Volkmann canals to involve the full length and thickness of the bone and into the periosteal tissue. Involvement of periosteal tissue results in lifting of the periosteum and may result in bone necrosis due to rupture of vessels or to spread within the periosteal space to involve joints.

Site In descending order of frequency – femur, tibia, humerus, radius. **Vertebral osteomyelitis** occurs mainly in adults with 50% due to *Staphylococcus aureus* and about 20% associated with enteric infections. Complications here include extension into dura, vertebral collapse and spinal cord compression.

Pathology Portions of dead bone separate from adjacent viable tissue (**sequestrum**). In some instances new bone may surround a central abscess (**Brodie's abscess**). New bone may also develop from the periosteum and surround the sequestrum giving a sheath of new bone (**involucrum**).

Complications Systemic complications include spread of infection into the bloodstream which may be associated with proliferation of organisms (septicaemia) and deposition of amyloid (usually AA-type). Local complications include acute bacterial arthritis, pathological fractures and onset of chronicity. Squamous carcinoma may develop after many years if sinuses to the skin have remained present. Sarcoma has occasionally developed in scar tissue in bone.

Tuberculous osteitis

Pathogenesis Usually due to blood bone infection.

Sites Mostly vertebrae and bones of hip, knee, ankle, elbow and wrist. In long bones the epiphysis and synovium is often involved. In the spine (**Pott's disease**) disease starts in vertebral body and extend into the disc space causing collapse.

Pathology Area of bone destruction associated with granulomatous inflammation with caseation. Little bone formation in seen.

DISORDERS OF THE JOINTS

NORMAL STRUCTURE AND FUNCTION

Definition Joints are connections between different bones.
- **diarthroses** move freely in relation to one another e.g. knee
- **synarthroses** are fixed and rigid e.g. sutures of the skull
- **amphiarthroses** have a slight degree of movement e.g. intervertebral joints.

Synovial joints

Structure These have a wide range of movement with adjacent bones reasonably widely separated by a joint cavity. This cavity is defined partly by articular cartilage covering the bone ends and parly by a tough fibrous capsule fused to the periosteum at or near the margins of the bone's articular surface.

Capsule Inner surface is lined by vascularized connective tissue and covered by cells in two functional groups which are usually not more than 1–2 layers thick.

- Type A cells: in macrophage family. Produce hyaluronic acid (important component of synovial fluid).
- Type B cells: Basically fibroblastic. Also produce some non-collagen proteins.

Articular cartilage Composed of chondrocytes embedded in an abundant extracellular matrix. Cartilage is avascular and is nourished by diffusion. The matrix consists of collagen (principally type II with some type IX and little type XI), large amounts of hydrophobic proteoglycans (mostly aggrecan) and a small amount of other proteins.

....

OSTEOARTHRITIS (OA)

Epidemiology Commonest joint disease affecting 14% of the adult population. Prevalence increases with increasing age with the slope of increase becoming steeper after 50 years. At its peak the prevalence may be as high as 75%.

Aetiology OA may result from either recurrent or increased load-bearing on normal articular cartilage, normal load-bearing on weakened articular cartilage, or both. Associations include obesity, female gender, mechanical factors (trauma, occupation and sport-induced stresses). There is a negative association with osteoporosis and cigarette smoking. Genetic factors play a part in polyarticular OA.

Pathogenesis Regarded as a disorder where the primary process is breakdown of the articular cartilage and exposure of the underlying bone.

Classification
- primary: no known aetiological association
- secondary: associated with known event or disease causally related to OA, e.g.

  - post trauma
  - congenital or developmental abnormalities which may be **localised** e.g. hip disease (Legg–Calvé–Perthes disease, congenital hip dislocation, shallow acetabulum, slipped femoral epiphysis) or **general-**

ized e.g. dysplasias or metabolic disorders such as haemochromatosis, Gaucher's disease and haemo-globinopathies.
— calcium pyrophosphate deposition (pseudogout)
— others diseases of bone e.g. avascular necrosis of the femoral head, rheumatoid arthritis, gout, septic arthritis, Paget's disease of bone and osteochondritis.
— other diseases not primarily of bone e.g. endocrine diseases, neuropathic joints, caisson disease, Kashin–Beck disease (due to eating bread containing toxin-producing fungi causing epiphyseal and metaphyseal dysplasia. Found in Siberia, northern China and Korea).

Clinical features The principal symptom is pain due to stimulation of pain fibres in the joint capsule and the periosteum, sub-chondrial microfractures and bursitis occurring as a result of muscle weakness. In addition there is reduction in the range and degree of movement. Signs of OA include joint deformity, crepitus and limitation of movement.

Macroscopy There are erosive changes in the cartilage (**fibrillation**) resulting in flaking off of small portions of cartilage. Exposed bone develops an ivory-like surface (**eburnation**). There is thickening of the sub-chondrial bone plate. Sub-chondrial bone pseudo-cysts may form due to entrance of synovial fluid under pressure through small fractures through the subchondrial plate. At the margins of the articular cartilage bony outgrowths (**osteophytes**) develop.

Microscopy Some chondrocytes undergo necrosis. More commonly there is proliferation of chondrocytes forming aggregates with large amounts of matrix.

Variants of OA

Nodal generalized osteoarthritis

Epidemiology Female preponderance. Peak onset in middle age.

Pathogenesis Possible autoimmune mechanism as there is a positive association with HLA A1 and B8, immune complexes are present in the cartilage and synovium of affected joints and IgG rheumatoid factor may be found.

Clinical features Polyarticular involvement of the inter-phalangeal joints of the fingers, good functional outcome as far as the fingers are concerned, predisposition for subsequent development of osteoarthritis of the knee, hip or spine and the presence of Heberden's (bony swellings associated with the distal interphalangeal joints) or Bouchard's (similar swellings at proximal interphalangeal joints) nodes which are initially and transiently red and tender.

Neuropathic joints (Charcot's joints)

Definition Severe disorganization of the joint following loss of normal nerve supply.

Aetiology first described by Charcot in relation to a patient with tabes dorsalis. Can be associated with severe diabetic neuropathy and, in the upper limb, syringomyelia.

Site The knee is commonest in tabes dorsalis.

Clinical features Recurrent swelling. Degenerative changes occur in the ligaments and tendons resulting in subluxation of the joint.

....

RHEUMATOID ARTHRITIS (RA)

Epidemiology Common. Affects 1–2% of the population.

Aetiology Unknown. Thought to be an interplay between genetic factors, sex hormones (more common in pre-menopausal females than males) and a putative infectious agent (possibly Epstein–Barr virus) triggering an autoimmune mechanism.

Pathogenesis Synthesis of rheumatoid factors is characteristic but not specific to the disease (also found in SLE, dermatomyositis, progressive systemic sclerosis and a number of non-rheumatic diseases such as liver cirrhosis, infective granulomatous diseases and pulmonary fibrosis). Rheumatoid factors are auto-antibodies principally of IgM type reacting preferentially with determinants on the Fc portion of IgG and are found in the serum of 80% of patients with rheumatoid arthritis (termed sero-positive). The production of rheumatoid factor may reflect local release of interleukin-6, a macrophage-derived cytokine that stimulates antibody production. Much evidence supports the suggestion that

T cells play a key role in rheumatoid arthritis. This includes the finding that CD4 (T_H) cells are the principal T-cell type and that these show numerous activation markers. Decline in the T-cell numbers lessens the severity of the disease. Animal experiments blocking IL-2 receptors produced an improvement while injection of T cell reacting with collagen II produced a severe arthritis.

Clinical features   Principal joints affected by arthritis are the small joints of the hands and feet, knees and hips. Distribution is often symmetrical. Sero-positivity is associated with severe and aggressive disease, increased likelihood of systemic manifestations and poorer prognosis.

Macroscopy   The articular surface is primarily unaffected. The initial abnormalities are of the synovium and its secretions. The synovial fluid volume is increased with increased cell content (primarily neutrophils), increased protein and possibly the presence of polymerized fibrin.

Microscopy   There is considerable thickening of the synovial cell lining (both A and B cells). The synovium is more vascular than normal. The deeper layers of the synovium contain more cells, initially in a perivascular distribution. Reactive lymphoid follicles may be present. Between the follicles there are numerous plasma cells. HLA class II molecules are expressed on nearly all cell types and endothelial cells show a marked upregulation of adhesion molecules such as ICAM-1 and E-selectin. The junction between the synovium, the articular cartilage and the bone becomes covered by vascular tissue continuous with the inflamed synovium (**pannus**). This is associated with degradation of the underlying cartilage and demineralization of the adjacent bone which becomes porotic.

Extra-articular manifestations of rheumatoid arthritis

Rheumatoid nodules

Epidemiology   Occur in about 30% of patients. Mostly in patients with aggressive disease and those with rheumatoid factors.

Site   Predilection for pressure areas such as the extensor areas of the forearm.

Microscopy Central area of eosinophilic coagulative necrosis surrounded by palisaded macrophages and fibroblasts. The overlying skin occasionally ulcerates usually associated with a necrotizing vasculitis.

Rheumatoid vasculitis

Pathogenesis Thought to be due to deposition of immune complexes within blood vessel walls.

Clinical features Depend on size of vessel affected.
* capillaries: 'glove and stocking' peripheral neuropathy
* arterioles: cutaneous ulceration with or without associated rheumatoid nodules
* small/medium arteries: severe compromise of affected organ
* veins: palpable purpura and recurrent episodes of wheals in the skin.

Laboratory findings Associated with high titres of IgG and IgM rheumatoid factors, cryoglobulinaemia, hypocomplementaemia and circulating immune complexes.

Microscopy Fibrinoid necrosis in the vessels associated with neutrophil infiltrate. Thrombosis may or may not be present. With time the affected segment of the vessel becomes occluded by vascular granulation tissue.

Lung changes

Clinical features Pleurisy is common. Intrapulmonary rheumatoid nodules may occur. Rarely there is diffuse interstitial fibrosis or fibrosing alveolitis (particularly associated with HLA DR3 and patients with the PiZ gene).

Cardiac abnormalities

Clinical features Asymptomatic pericarditis is common. Rheumatoid nodules may cause conduction disturbances. Vasculitis of coronary vessels may cause ischaemia and occasionally aortic root dilation leading to aortic valve incompetence.

Lymph node changes

Slight enlargement is common. Widespread palpable nodes are present in a few cases.

Bone abnormalities

Localized osteoporosis in relation to affected joints may be accompanied by generalized osteoporosis which may be due to decreased activity.

Eye involvement

Vasculitis may cause severe inflammation of the sclera (scleritis) causing a painful eye with blurred vision. Rheumatoid nodules may be present in the sclera and occasionally cause secondary glaucoma or scleral perforation.

Complications of rheumatoid arthritis

Amyloidosis

Rheumatoid arthritis is the commonest cause of reactive amyloidosis in Europe occurring in 2–5% of cases. May occur after many years. More likely in chronic active disease in which plasma concentrations of serum amyloid A have been raised. Deposited in many tissues but renal amyloidosis with renal dysfunction until recently carried a very poor prognosis.

Felty's syndrome

Definition Triad of rheumatoid arthritis, splenomegaly and neutropenia. Occurs in adult and juvenile forms. Defining criteria are the presence of splenomegaly and a white cell count of less than $2 \times 10^9/l$.

Epidemiology Rare. Present in about 1% hospital patients with rheumatoid arthritis.

Clinical features Joint disease is usually active with much cartilage destruction. Systemic manifestations are common. More than 50% of patients develop Sjögren's syndrome. Other signs are liver enlargement, lymphadenopathy and skin pigmentation.

Laboratory findings There is a high titre of IgG rheumatoid factor in more than 90%. Granulocyte-specific complement fixing anti-nuclear antibodies are present in many patients.

Juvenile rheumatoid arthritis (JRA)

Definition Although by definition this is a disease that occurs in individuals less than 16 years old it is not merely rheumatoid arthritis that affects juveniles.

Clinical features Some of the features, such as disturbances of skeletal growth, are related to the patient's age; others are intrinsic to the disease. These include a high spiking fever, high white cell count, macular rash chiefly on the trunk and limbs in which the macules are 2–5 mm diameter, salmon pink and surrounded by a zone of pallor; characteristically, they appear in the afternoon accompanied by fever and may have disappeared by the next morning. There is prediction for involvement of the temporomandibular joint, cervical spine and wrists. There is radial rather than ulnar deviation of the fingers, involvement of the distal interphalangeal joints, a high prevalence of iridocylitis, rare seropositivity and rarely rheumatoid nodules. Three main presentations have been described:

1. **Systemic onset juvenile rheumatoid arthritis (Still's disease)** presents in 20% patients with JRA. Systemic manifestations from time of onset include enlargement of liver, spleen and lymph nodes and a typical rheumatoid rash.
2. **Polyarticular onset** is present in 40%. Numerous joints involved. Most closely resembles adult RA. Many are seropositive.
3. **Pauciarticular** accounts for 40%. No more than four joints are affected at presentation. Early onset pauciarticular JRA affects girls more commonly than boys while the reverse is true for late onset pauciarticular JRA. In the early onset type there are often anti-nuclear antibodies in the serum and 50% have chronic iridocyclitis while in late onset disease sacroiliac joint involvement is common and some go on to develop ankylosing spondylitis.

....

THE SPONDYLOARTHROPATHIES

Definition A set of disorders that may present purely as arthropathies or as arthropathies in association with disease in other systems.

Pathogenesis There is a strong association with HLA-B27 but the role of this in the pathogenesis is unknown. It has been suggested that it may be a receptor for a micro-organism or peptide produced by an infective organism or that there is molecular mimicry between part of HLA-B27 and a peptide antigen derived from the processing of a micro-organism by an antigen-presenting cell.

Clinical features   There is a great deal of overlap between the spondyloarthropathies which all share some common features.

- strong association with HLA-B27 (seen in 50% cases associated with psoriasis and chronic inflammatory bowel disease and more than 95% of cases associated with ankylosing spondylitis)
- arthritis tends to affect sacrum and intervertebral joints
- rheumatoid factors are negative (hence the term seronegative arthropathies)
- pathological changes especially seen in the insertions of ligaments or tendons into bone (entheses)
- other organs involved include the eye, aortic valve and ascending aorta, skin and lung
- may be complicating reactive amyloidosis
- there is a tendency for aggregation in family groups.

Ankylosing spondylitis (AS)

Definition   The defining criteria are:
- limitation of movement of the lumbar spine in three planes
- pain in lumbar spine or in dorsolumbar junction
- limitation of chest expansion to < 2.5 cm
- radiological evidence of severe sacroiliitis.

Epidemiology   Prevalence is about 0.25–1% of population. Most whites with AS are HLA-B27 positive and 5–10% people with HLA-B27 develop AS. M:F is 2.5:1. Disease usually starts in early adult life.

Clinical features   About 20–30% develop arthritis in peripheral joints (commonly the hip and shoulder). This is more common in people developing the disease early. Extra-articular manifestations include constitutional symptoms (e.g. low grade fever, weight loss, raised ESR and either hypochromic or normochromic anaemia), iritis, infiltrative and fibrotic lung disease (upper lobes), cardio-vascular complications (aortic incompetence, cardiomegaly and persistent conduction defects).

Macroscopy There is ossification of the discs, sacroiliac joints and epiphyseal joints. The site of the pathological changes is the area in which the ligaments, tendons and capsules are inserted into the bone (enthesis).

....

REACTIVE ARTHROPATHIES

Reiter's syndrome

Clinical features Three syndromes related to joints can occur:

- A peripheral arthritis syndrome affecting 2–4 joints (chiefly ankles and knees). Sausage-like swelling of the digits due to involvement of the tendon sheath is characteristic.
- An enthesopathic syndrome in which the entheses of various bones become painful (particularly the heel).
- A pelviaxial syndrome in which dorsal low back or buttock pain occurs.

Various extra-articular manifestations can occur including urethritis, cervicitis, diarrhoea and mucocutaneous problems such as balanitis and keratoderma blenorrhagium. Conjunctivitis is common in the early stages. The first episode usually subsides within three to six months but small joint disease, heel pain, balanitis and psoriatic lesions may be stubborn. About 75% of patients will be in remission within two years but relapses generally begin three to four years after the initial episode.

Enteropathic arthropathy

Associations Clinically overt inflammatory bowel disease (e.g. ulcerative colitis and Crohn's disease), Whipple's disease, jejunocolic bypass, collagenous colitis, mild gut symptoms or with asymptomatic mild histological gut inflammation.

Psoriatic arthropathy

Epidemiology   Occurs in 7% of patients with psoriasis. M:F about 1:1. Peak incidence in 3rd and 4th decade.

Clinical features   Usually peripheral joints as well as axial skeleton and sacroiliac joints. Patients complain of morning pain and stiffness. Joints are affected asymmetrically; there is erythema over the joints and rheumatoid factors are rare (about 10%).

Infective arthropathies

Definition   Presence of multiplying organisms within the joints.

Pathogenesis   Infection may occur by blood-borne spread from a distant site (commonest), by direct penetration or by direct spread from a contiguous infected site. Septic arthritis following blood-borne spread occurs more frequently in individuals with pre-existing structural abnormalities of the joint, when the infective organism (e.g. *Staphylococcus aureus* or *Neisseria gonorrhoae*) is better adapted to colonization of the joint either by adhesion to the synovial tissue or by toxin production that facilitates colonization or when the host is in an immunocompromised state. The acute inflammatory reaction can result in severe and rapid effect on the underlying cartilage due to bacterial products and lysosomal enzymes.

Gonococcal arthritis

Epidemiology   Commonest form of infective arthritis in adults. Peak incidence 15–30 years (75% of cases). More common in females. Patients are usually healthy and sexually active and have no pre-existing joint disease.

Aetiology   *Neisseria gonorrhoeae.*

Clinical features   Migratory involvement of several joints is common (effusions may not be purulent) but some have monoarthritis with purulent effusion. Hip involvement is uncommon. Fever, rash and tenosynovitis are common in those with polyarthritis.

Laboratory findings Organisms are identifiable on Gram stain of effusion in 25% and cultures of synovial fluid are positive in 50%. No increase in synovial fluid lactate.

Natural history and prognosis Rapid response to antibiotics with full recovery in most cases.

Non-gonococcal bacterial arthritis

Epidemiology Most common in very young and very old. Pre-existing joint disease is common (10% of cases occur in patients with rheumatoid arthritis). Male more commonly affected.

Aetiology *Staphylococcus aureus* (40–50%), *Staphylococcus epidermidis* (10–15%), *Streptococcus pneumoniae* (2%), other streptococcal species (20%), Gram-negative bacilli (15%), *Haemophilus influenzae* (2%) and various anaerobic species (5%).

Clinical features Usually monoarticular (80%) with knee involvement in 50% and hip in 20%. May be evidence of associated infections e.g. skin, lung or urinary tract.

Laboratory findings Gram stain of synovial fluid shows organisms in 50–65% of cases (75% in staphylococcal infection; 50% in Gram-negative bacterial infections) and cultures of synovial fluid are positive in 90%. Marked elevation of synovial fluid lactate.

Natural history and prognosis Response to antibiotics is often slow and open drainage may be required. Mortality rate is about 10% and up to 30% have residual joint damage after resolution of inflammation.

Tuberculosis and joint disease

Pathogenesis Either haematogenous dissemination of organisms or direct spread from a focus of tuberculous osteitis in adjacent bone.

Clinical features Several clinical syndromes occur including tuberculous spondylitis (Pott's disease of the spine), peripheral arthritis, tuberculous osteomyelitis, dactylitis (affecting long bones of the hands/feet), tenosynovitis and bursitis and Poncet's disease (aseptic arthritis associated with tuberculous lesion elsewhere).

Microscopy   In the peripheral arthritis there is an effusion that is rich in neutrophils. Synovial biopsy shows typical granulomatous lesions in more than 90% of cases but acid-fast bacilli are seldom identified in either the synovial fluid or tissue. However culture gives positive results in 80%.

Lyme disease

Epidemiology   Lyme disease is endemic in mammals, particularly rodents in North America and Europe. It is the leading vector-borne disease in North America with 9600 cases reported in 1992. The early stages of the disease are most commonly seen between June and October when the nymph stage of the ticks and the outdoor activities of the human are at their height. Later manifestations are seen throughout the year.

Aetiology   Caused by the spirochaete *Borrelia burgdorferi*.

Transmission   By the bite of various ticks.

Clinical features   Lyme disease may affect the skin, nervous system, heart and the joints. Three clinical stages occur but these may not appear in an orderly pattern and they show considerable overlap. The first two stages occur early in the disease manifesting within a few weeks of infection. The third stage makes its appearance after 6–12 months or even some years.

Stage 1   Macular rash known as erythema migrans in 60–80% usually accompanied by low grade fever, headache, shifting arthralgia, muscle pain and lymphadenopathy. The skin lesion can occur between 3 days and 6 weeks after initial infection (mean 10 days). The macule is large (mean diameter 15 cm), round/oval with a well-demarcated edge. The initial erythematous lesion expands and may reach a 30-cm diameter while the centre clears at least in part. Erythema migrans usually resolves after 3–4 weeks although it may recur.

Stage 2   This is the early disseminated stage. Multiple ring-like lesions occur in the skin which are smaller than the primary lesion. Fever and associated constitutional symptoms are still present. Some patients develop bluish-red nodules most commonly in the nipples and the ear lobes (**borrelial lymphocytoma**). There may be cranial neuritis most commonly manifest by facial palsy (may be bilateral). Peripheral neuropathies and/or lymphocytic meningitis or meningo-encephalitis may occur. In Europe the commonest neurological manifestation is Bannwarth's syndrome (severe root pain commonly experienced at night and lymphocytosis in the CSF but without overt signs of meningitis). A small proportion of patients (about 8%) develop various degrees of atrial-ventricular heart block.

Stage 3 Clinical features of chronic disease may occur months to years after initial infection. Chronic arthritis is fairly uncommon: it usually affects joints asymetrically and especially the large joints, particularly the knee. Examination of the synovium shows villous hypertrophy, fibrin deposits and increased vascularity. There is a plasma cell and macrophage infiltrate and lymphoid follicles may be seen. Involvement of the nervous system includes a sub-acute encephalopathy with cognitive disturbance and disturbance of mood and sleep. The skin shows acrodermatitis chronica atrophicans. These are bluish-red areas with a doughy consistency that become atrophic with wrinkling of the skin.

Natural history and prognosis Antibiotics including doxycycline, tetracycline, cefuroxime, erythromycin, ceftazidime, azithromycin and imipenem appear effective in humans.

....

CRYSTAL ARTHROPATHY

Monosodium urate deposition: gout

Definition Set of disorders associated with deposition of monosodium urate deposition in tissues and abnormally high concentrations of uric acid in body fluids.

Aetiology Body-fluid uric acid concentration depends on the balance between purine ingestion and synthesis and uric acid elimination. There may be polygenic control of uric acid levels but environmental factors such as dietary intake of purine, high alcohol consumption and high body weight/bulk are also important. Excretion of uric acid involves glomerular ultrafiltration with reabsorption of urate in the proximal tubule via and active transport system linked to reabsorption of sodium. Active secretion of urate occurs more distally with some post-secretory reabsorption. In 75–90% of patients the hyperuricaemia is associated with decreased fraction excretion (due to decreased urate excretion, increased absorption or a combination of these), 10–15% have increased uric acid production and excretion and in about 10% gout is due to increased cell turnover or increased purine catabolism. Secondary hyperuricaemia may be associated with chronic renal disease and drugs (e.g. thiazide diuretics, salicylates in low doses, ethambutol and pyrazinamide).

Three single-gene defects are associated with severe gout due to increased purine synthesis

Lesch–Nyhan syndrome

Genetics X-linked recessive.

Enzyme defect Hypoxanthine guanine phosphoribosyl transferase.

Clinical manifestations Choreoathetosis, mental deficiency, spasticity and a strange behavioural disturbance characterized by self-mutilation.

Phosphoribosyl pyrophosphate synthetase deficiency

Genetics X-linked recessive.

Clinical manifestations Gout and renal stones in childhood/early adult life. Deafness may be seen both in the male children and the heterozygous mothers.

Glucose-6-phosphatase deficiency

Clinical manifestations Gouty arthritis before the end of the first decade with chronic tophaceous gout with kidney involvement in those surviving to adulthood.

Pathogenesis Gouty arthritis occurs when monosodium urate crystals are deposited from supersaturated solutions. There is usually a long period of 'silent' hyperuricaemia and deposition may be triggered by alcohol, dietary indiscretions, trauma, surgery and infection. Once the crystals have been deposited they absorb immunoglobulin, fibrinogen, fibronectin and some complement components which act as opsonins promoting phagocytosis. In macrophages the crystals cause rupture of phagolysosome membranes, spillage of lysosomal contents and complement activation together with release of acute inflammatory mediators.

Clinical features

There are four stages:

1. Hyperuricaemia with no symptoms.

2. Acute gouty arthritis.

Epidemiology M:F 8:1. Rare in males before puberty and rare in females before the menopause. Peak incidence in males is 30–60 years.

Clinical features Metatarsophalangeal joint of the big toe is commonest site (70%). Usually sudden onset of pain with signs of acute inflammation (red, hot, swollen, painful and tender). Attacks often start at night.

Microscopy Clusters of crystals in the synovium and individual crystals are seen in neutrophils.

Natural history and prognosis Untreated attacks will resolve spontaneously in hours, days or weeks.

3. Intercritical phase

Definition Asymptomatic phase between episodes of acute arthritis. May last months or years.

4. Chronic tophaceous gouty arthritis

Clinical features Asymmetrical swelling of joints. Development of large yellowish-white masses of urate crystals visible to the naked eye (tophus) typically in periarticular tissues, bursae, tendon sheaths and cartilage of the outer ear but may also be found in the eye, skin, larynx, tongue and heart.

Gout may affect the kidney giving acute uric acid nephropathy and acute renal failure (due to sudden precipitation of urate crystals in the renal-collecting ducts and ureters), chronic renal disease or uric acid stones.

Calcium pyrophosphate dihydrate deposition: pseudogout and chondrocalcinosis

Calcium pyrophosphate dihydrate crystals (CPPD) may be deposited in synovium giving arthritis (pseudogout) or in articular or meniscus cartilage (chondrocalcinosis).

Aetiology CPPD deposition may occur as a sporadic disease associated with ageing, as a familial disease, associated with some metabolic diseases (e.g. hyperparathyroidism, haemochromatosis, hypophosphatasia, hypomagnesaemia, alkaptonuria and hypothyroidism) and following surgery or trauma to a joint.

....

TUMOURS AND TUMOUR-LIKE LESIONS
Pigmented villonodular synovitis and giant-cell tumour of tendon sheath

Definition Almost certainly a benign neoplasm rather than a reactive or inflammatory condition. Although the two conditions are more or less identical morphologically pigmented villonodular synovitis (PVNS) usually involves the synovium of the joint diffusely while the giant cell tumour of tendon sheath (GCTTS) is usually a discrete nodule.

Epidemiology Peak incidence of PVNS is the 3rd to 5th decade. M:F 1:1.

Site PVNS occurs most frequently in the knee (80%) but may involve the hip, toes, ankle, wrist, elbow and small joints of the hand. GCTTS is most frequently found in the tendon sheaths of the hand.

Microscopy
- **PVNS**: numerous macrophages with finely vaculated cytoplasm. Synovial lining cells, macrophages and spindle-shaped stromal cells contain haemosiderin.

Moderate numbers of lymphocytes and multi-nucleate giant cells are present.

- **GCTTS**: well-defined lobulated masses. Dual cell population consisting of spindle cells and 'foamy' macrophages (due to intracellular lipid accumulation). Multi-nucleate cells are often abundant and haemosiderin is usually present.

Synovial chondromatosis

Definition Islands of cartilage present within the synovial tissues.

Site Hip and knee most frequently.

Clinical features Some of the deposits become detached causing pain, stiffness and swelling.

Microscopy Cartilaginous islands within the synovium which appear disorganized with clustering of chondrocytes and some cytological atypia. Some may undergo ossification (synovial osteochondromatosis).

Ganglion

Definition A thin-walled cyst containing mucoid fluid associated with a joint.

Site Most commonly extensor surface of the hand or foot. Particular predilection for the wrist.

Pathogenesis May arise from areas of myxoid degeneration in the connective tissue of the tendon sheath.

TUMOUR AND TUMOUR-LIKE LESIONS OF SOFT TISSUE

Epidemiology Account for less than 1% of all invasive neoplasms but at least 2% of deaths from malignant disease.

Classification According to the mature tissue the tumour most resembles. The commonest are:

- liposarcomas (17%)
- leiomyosarcomas (smooth muscle; 14%)
- rhabdomyosarcomas (skeletal muscle; 12%)

- malignant fibrous histiocytoma (11%)
- malignant nerve sheath tumour (9.5%)
- synovial sarcoma (6%)
- No other group amounts to more than 4% and 10–15% are unclassified

Aetiology Mostly unknown (see Table 44.2).

Cytogenetics Certain cytogenetic translocations are associated with specific entities (see Table 44.3).

Morphological correlates to behaviour

- size: the larger the tumour the more likely to be aggressive

Table 44.2 Aetiology of soft-tissue lesions

Genetic associations	• Type 1 neurofibromatosis (von Recklinghausen's disease) associated with multiple neurofibromata. May be complicated by malignant schwannoma • Hereditary haemorrhagic telangiectasia (Osler–Weber–Rendu syndrome) • Gardner's syndrome in which intestinal polyps are associated with fibromatosis.
Radiation	• Mainly malignant fibrous histiocytoma and extraosseous osteosarcoma. Latent period is about 10 years after exposure. Outlook is often poor.
Foreign bodies	• Some cases have been reported associated with foreign bodies (e.g. bullets, shrapnel, surgically implanted material). Latent period is 2–50 years. Most frequently malignant fibrous histiocytoma and angiosarcoma.

Table 44.3 Cytogenetic translocations and specific entities

• synovial sarcoma	translocation	t(X;18)
• Ewing's sarcoma	translocation	t(11;22)
• alveolar rhabdomyosarcoma	translocation	t(2;13)
• myxoid liposarcoma	translocation	t(12;16)
• neuroblastoma with poor prognosis	deletion	1p
• malignant mesothelioma (pleura)	deletion	1p and/or 3p and/or 22

- position: superficial lesions likely to be less aggressive. Deep lesions are more likely to metastasize
- growth rate: tumours that grow rapidly (e.g. have many mitoses) and show necrosis are likely to be aggressive.

....

TUMOURS WITH ADIPOSE TISSUE DIFFERENTIATION

Benign tumours (lipoma)

Epidemiology Commonest soft tissue tumour of adulthood. Mostly middle-aged or elderly.

Clinical features Slow growing masses of subcutaneous tissue of trunk or limbs. Measure 1–20 cm and are usually painless. The angiolipoma variant is painful in 50% of cases.

Prognosis Local recurrence after excision is uncommon. Almost never undergo malignant change. Of those that occur within or between muscles (about 2%), about 15% recur unless widely excised as they have a more infiltrative edge.

Microscopy Composed of well-defined lobules of mature adipose tissue. Variants exist. (see Table 44.4).

Malignant tumours (liposarcoma)

Epidemiology Commonest malignant connective tissue tumour. Rare in children but can occur at any time in adult life. Peak incidence 40–60 years. Slight male predominance.

Site Most occur on lower limb or retroperitoneal space.

Clinical features Symptoms relate to the presence of a mass at the particular site.

Microscopy Hallmark for diagnosis is the lipoblast which contains two or more lipid-filled cytoplasmic droplets that indent the nucleus. Four sub-types:

- **well-differentiated**: four sub-types of which the commonest is 'lipoma-like' containing cells resembling mature adiposities. Occasional lipoblasts. Few stellate or spindle cells.
- **myxoid**: commonest. Small undifferentiated mesenchymal cells with variable number of lipoblasts in

Table 44.4 Variants of benign tumours of adipose tissue

Angiolipoma	• up to 10% of lipomas • predominantly in young/middle-aged adults • most frequent in upper limb • 50% are painful • associated with network of thin-walled blood vessels occupying a significant portion of the lesion
Angiomyolipoma	• essentially hamartomas • most frequent in kidney but may be extrarenal
Spindle-cell lipoma	• less than 2% of lipomas • predominantly middle/old age; most commonly males aged 50–80 years • commonest on back of neck or upper back • microscopically contain mature adiposities, short collagen bundles and small basophilic spindle cells
Pleomorphic lipoma	• similar to spindle cell lipoma clinically and microscopically but histologically is associated with bizarre multi-nucleate giant cells. Occasionally a few lipoblasts with small intracytoplasmic vacuoles can be seen
Lipoblastoma	• rare • almost exclusively in infants • most frequent on limbs • may be encapsulated or diffuse • benign, recurrence is very uncommon • microscopically they have lobules of adiposities with variable differentiation ranging from primitive pre-lipoblasts to mature adiposities. A complex network of thin-walled blood vessels is often present
Hibernoma	• cells show differentiation into 'brown fat' • occur in middle-aged adults • most common between shoulder, in the neck or axilla • microscopically they are well encapsulated. Cells are multi-vacuolated or granular

a myxoid stroma. Characteristically has a complex anastamosing vasculature giving a 'chicken-wire' appearance.
• **round cell**: uncommon variant. Mostly uniform small to medium, round, basophilic cells with little cytoplasm. Few lipoblasts.

- **pleomorphic**: Mixed population of spindle cells, numerous tumour giant cells and small number of lipoblasts. Numerous mitoses.

Prognosis   Two main prognostic factors – histological sub-type and location.

Sub-type	well-differentiated	excellent
	myxoid	good, metastasis rare
	round cell	commonly metastasize. 5-year survival is about 20%
	pleomorphic	metastasis common
Site	retroperitoneal	5-year survival only 35%
	limbs	easier to excise completely so better prognosis

....

SMOOTH MUSCLE TUMOURS

Benign tumours (leiomyoma)

Site   Many locations including uterus, gut, dermis/sub-cutis and deep soft tissue (rarest). Angioleiomyomas arise from smooth muscle of blood vessels.

Microscopy   those arising in the uterus and gut have been discussed in the relevant sections. The tumours arising in the skin/subcutis are of two types. Table 44.5 shows the microscopic and clinical features of each type. Note that the clinical features are different for each type.

Malignant smooth muscle tumours (leiomyosarcoma)

Site   May occur in a hollow viscus (e.g. uterus or stomach). Non-visceral leiomyomas occur in specific sites (Table 44.6).

Microscopy   Spindle-cell tumour. Identification of smooth muscle differentiation may be difficult and can be aided by electron microscopy (thin myofilaments, dense bodies and a basal lamina) and/or immunohistochemistry (stain for desmin and smooth muscle actin). Malignant potential assessed by size (e.g. > 7.5 cm in retroperitoneal smooth muscle tumour implies malignancy), mitotic rate (in skin/subcutis 2 mitoses per 10 high power fields is indicator of

Table 44.5 Microscopic and clinical features of leiomyoma

	Angioleiomyoma	Pilar leiomyoma
Microscopic features	• Well circumscribed • Composed of bundles of smooth muscle cells with eosinophilic cytoplasm, distinct cell borders and blunt-ended nuclei orientated around thick-walled blood vessels which may have compressed lumens	• Infiltrative edge • Interlacing bundles of smooth muscle cells
Clinical features	• Usually single nodule on a limb • Peak incidence in middle age • Females more often than males • Painful in 50% of cases	• Less common than angioleiomyoma • Usually multiple • Often limbs or trunk of young adult • About 15% of cases appear to be inherited (autosomal dominant)

malignancy but in retroperitoneum 5 mitoses per 10 high power fields denotes malignancy), areas of necrosis and cellular pleomorphism.

Table 44.6 Sites of non-visceral leiomyomas

Abdominal cavity	• usually mesenteric or retroperitoneal • relatively common • usually late adult. Slight female predominance • difficult to remove and may recur
Dermis	• originate in arrector pili muscle • usually < 3 mm diameter • tend to occur on limbs of middle-aged males • painful • recurs if incompletely excised. Low metastatic potential.
Subcutaneous tissue/ intramuscular	• similar age to dermal tumours • tend to be larger • 40% metastasize
Blood vessels	• usually large vessels • females more often than males; peak 40–60 years • often metastasize early

TUMOURS WITH SKELETAL MUSCLE DIFFERENTIATION

Benign tumours (rhabdomyoma)

Epidemiology   Very rare (2% of primary muscle tumours). Three types are shown in Table 44.7.

Cardiac rhabdomyoma

Epidemiology   Rare. Occurs in infancy. Around 50% are associated with tuberous sclerosis. Congenital abnormalities present in 14%.

Site   Usually multiple. Left and right ventricle affected with equal frequency. Atria affected in 30% of cases. Usually intramural but may protrude into the chambers.

Macroscopy   Well-defined rounded nodules usually < 1 cm diameter.

Microscopy   Polygonal cells with central mass of eosinophilic cytoplasm. From this narrow striated processes extend to the periphery of the cell where there is a zone of striated cytoplasm. Intracytoplasmic glycogen gives a clear appearance to the cytoplasm.

Prognosis   Most fatal by 5 years.

MALIGNANT TUMOURS (RHABDOMYOSARCOMA)

Epidemiology   Commonest malignant soft tissue tumour of infants and young children. Less common in adults.

Site   In children most occur outside muscle. In adults most are intramuscular.

Prognosis   Two-year survival rate has risen from 20% to > 70% with combination of surgery, radiotherapy and chemotherapy. Prognosis depends on the stage as shown in Table 44.8.

Classification   Different types of rhabdomyosarcoma are recognized with different sites of origin, epidemiological features and microscopic appearances.

Table 44.7 Types of benign rhabdomyoma

Type	Occurrence	Site	Microscopic features
Adult	• Mean age > 50 years • M:F 4:1	Most in head and neck. May present as a solitary polypoid lesion in larynx, pharynx, palate or mouth. Sometimes arises within muscle of tongue	• Well-circumscribed mass • Large round or polygonal cells with abundant eosinophilic cytoplasm • Cells contain intracytoplasmic glycogen • Cross striations are rare
Fetal	• Rarest form • Exclusively in boys less than 3 years	Most frequently head and neck (commonly post-auricular region)	Immature skeletal muscle cells in a loose myxoid stroma
Genital	• Affects middle-aged females	Cervix, vagina and vulva	Large rhabdomyoblasts with cross striations and intracytoplasmic bodies

Table 44.8 Clinical staging and prognostic factors for rhabdomyosarcoma

	Findings
1. Stage	
I	• Localized disease completely excised
II	• Localized disease with microscopic evidence of residual tumour. Spread to lymph nodes with complete excision or microscopic evidence of residual disease
III	• Incomplete excision. Macroscopically obvious residual disease
IV	• Distant metastases at presentation
2. Anatomical site	• Best for orbit, head and neck and some genitourinary • Less favourable for lesions in limbs • Tumours located close to meninges (e.g. paranasal or middle ear) have 35% chance of spread to CNS which is usually fatal in 1 year
3. Histological sub-type	• Alveolar rhabdomyosarcoma have shorter survival than other sub-types (difference mainly seen in patients with localized disease)

Embryonal rhabdomyosarcoma

Epidemiology Accounts for two-thirds of rhabdomyosarcomas. Most occur aged < 6 years. Males more than females.

Site Commonest in orbit and paratesticular regions. Other sites include nasopharynx, middle ear, prostate, urinary bladder, limbs and retroperitoneum.

Classification **Botryoid** rhabdomyosarcoma is a variant of embryonal but the tumour has a polypoid configuration and myxoid stroma; they frequently occur in mucosa-lined organs.

Microscopy Variable. Some principally have small rounded or spindle cells with dark-staining nuclei and basophilic cytoplasm in a myxoid stroma. Others have bundles of spindle cells. A third variant has stellate cells in a reticular pattern. All have rhabdomyoblasts (large round, elongated or oval cells with eosinophilic fibrillated cytoplasm, 50–60% have cross striations) but in variable numbers.

Alveolar rhabdomyosarcoma

Epidemiology About 25% of rhabdomyosarcomas. Most aged 10–20 years.

Site Almost always intramuscular in limbs (especially arms) or trunk.

Microscopy Pattern of honeycomb spaces bounded by fibrous tissue and lined by small round or oval cells. Mitoses are frequent. In the centre of these alveolar spaces there is loss of cellular cohesion and large multinucleate giant cells are seen. Occasional rhabdomyoblasts are seen.

Pleomorphic rhabdomyosarcoma

Epidemiology Rarest sub-type. Most adult rhabdomyosarcomas are of this type.

Microscopy Principally large cells with eosinophilic cytoplasm and single or multiple atypical nuclei. Cross striations are rarely seen.

....

TUMOUR OF UNCERTAIN ORIGIN/ DIFFERENTIATION

Synovial sarcoma

Definition Unrelated to synovium.

Epidemiology Wide age range. Peak 15–35 years.

Site Origin within a joint is rare. About 90% occur in soft tissue, often near a joint capsule, tendon or tendon sheath. Lower limb most frequently affected (60–70%) with thigh and knee points of predilection.

Microscopy Biphasic histology in two-thirds of cases with an epithelial element (nests or glands) and spindle-cell component. Spindle cells are most commonly arranged in sheets. May be grouping around blood vessels. Variable mitotic rate but mostly in spindle cell component. Mast cells are prominent. Calcification or ossification may be seen. One third are monophasic composed of spindle cells only. Immunohistochemistry show the presence of epithelial markers – cytokeratin and epithelial membrane antigen

(EMA) – with epithelial cells strongly positive and occasional spindle cells positive.

Ultrastructure Epithelial cells component indistinguishable from other malignant epithelial cells (e.g. in adenocarcinoma). Microvilli may be seen in relation to slit-like intercellular spaces in monophasic tumours.

Cytogenetics Both biphasic and monophasic tumours show t(X; 18)(p11.2;q11.2).

Prognosis Ten-year survival is about 30%. Local recurrence occurs in 50% often within two years of primary excision but sometimes later. May spread to lung (commonest) regional nodes or bone.

Alveolar soft part sarcoma

Epidemiology Rare (less than 1% of sarcomas). M:F 1:1. Peak incidence 20–29 years.

Site Usually deep in soft tissue of buttock/thigh (39%), popliteal region (17%), chest wall/trunk (13%) or forearm (10%).

Macroscopy Often quite large. Firm. Often variegated colours due to areas of haemorrhage and necrosis.

Microscopy Tumour cells are large and rounded or polygonal with granular eosinophilic cytoplasm. The cytoplasm contains PAS positive diastase resistant material (i.e. not glycogen). In 20% this material is in the form of crystalline structures. The cells are arranged in a ball-like structure with a centre that is often necrotic (alveolar pattern). In some cases the nests bulge into vascular spaces (glomeruloid pattern).

Prognosis Little data available. If no evidence of metastatic disease at diagnosis the mean survival can be 11 years. If metastases are present this falls to three years.

Epithelioid sarcoma

Epidemiology Peak incidence 15–35 years. Males more commonly affected than females.

Site Most present as multi-nodular masses in the dermis or subcutaneous tissue of limbs; wrist and hand are sites of predilection.

Microscopy   Cellular nodules often with central necrosis. The cells are plump, polygonal and epithelial-like. In the periphery of the nodules the cells become eosinophilic and more spindled. Immunohistochemistry shows positive staining for epithelial markers (cytokeratin and/or epithelial membrane antigen: [EMA]).

Prognosis   Local recurrence in 75%. Distant metastases in 40% via lymphatic and blood vessels. The course of the disease may, however, be prolonged.

....

FIBROHISTIOCYTIC TUMOURS
Malignant fibrous histiocytoma (MFH)

Definition   There is debate as to whether this is a specific entity, a non-specific morphological pattern or both. Tumours that have a pattern recognized as that of malignant fibrous histiocytoma account for a substantial number of soft tissue sarcomas. Several different sub-types.

Pleomorphic/storiform malignant fibrous histiocytoma

Epidemiology   Commonest variant (60–70% of cases of MFH). Tumour of late adult life, peak incidence in 7th decade.

Site   Limb skeletal muscle (especially thigh) with retroperitoneum as second most common site.

Clinical features   Presents as a slow-growing painless mass, often present for months.

Macroscopy   Usually multinodular and infiltrating. Grey-white with areas of haemorrhage and necrosis.

Microscopy   Irregularly arranged plump, eosinophilic spindle cells with dark staining, often bizarre nuclei. Frequent mitoses. In some areas the cells have a whorled pattern.

Myxoid malignant fibrous histiocytoma

Epidemiology   Accounts for 10–20% of cases of MFH.
Site   Most in limbs. Often subcutaneous.

Macroscopy   Mucoid/myxoid cut surface.

Microscopy   Different from pleomorphic MFH in respect of the stroma that is rich in extracellular stromal mucin much of which appears to be hyaluronic acid.

Prognosis   Local recurrence is common (66% of cases). Metastasis less frequent (23%).

Giant cell malignant fibrous histiocytoma

Epidemiology   Accounts for 5–15% of cases of MFH.

Site   Commonest on the limbs (especially leg). Up to one-third occur in subcutaneous tissue.

Macroscopy   Multi-nodular with prominent haemorrhage.

Microscopy   Overall similar to pleomorphic MFH but also have osteoclast-like giant cells. In about half there are foci of osteoid or mature bone at the periphery of the tumour nodules.

Prognosis   Recurrence in 30–50%. Metatstasis less common in subcutaneous (20%) compared to deeper sites (75%).

Inflammatory malignant fibrous histiocytoma

Epidemiology   Accounts for 5–10% of cases of MFH.

Site   Predilection for retroperitoneal space but may occur on limbs.

Macroscopy   Cut surface often appears yellow.

Microscopy   Many xanthoma cells. Typically there are sheets of xanthoma cells mixed with inflammatory cells (mostly neutrophils). Background featureless hyaline matrix. In some instances areas merge with more typical pleomorphic MFH areas.

Prognosis   Tendency to recur in retroperitoneum as they are difficult to resect. Metastases in about 30%. Five-year survival about 30%.

Angiomatoid malignant fibrous histiocytoma

Epidemiology   Accounts for 1–3% of cases of MFH. Peak incidence in 1st and 2nd decades.

Site Most commonly in dermis and subcutis of limbs, especially upper limb.

Macroscopy Often well defined with cystic change and haemorrhage.

Microscopy Characteristically has sheets of histiocytes intimately related to large blood-filled spaces, intense inflammation and extensive scarring. The blood-filled spaces lack endothelial linings (i.e. not true vascular spaces).

Prognosis Recurrence in 60% of cases. Metastasis rare.

....

NON-NEOPLASTIC AND NEOPLASTIC FIBROBLASTIC LESIONS

Benign fibroblastic lesions

Keloid scars

Epidemiology Commonest in adolescents and young adults. Predilection for blacks. Females more than males.

Pathogenesis Excessive connective tissue reaction to minor trauma.

Site Face, neck, sternum, forearms and ear-lobes commonest.

Clinical features Present as smooth plaques that are itchy or tender. Often extend beyond margins of antecedent trauma.

Microscopy In early stages consist of cellular fibrous tissue arranged in nodules and interlacing bundles. Normal mitoses may be present. In later stages there is hyalinized eosinophilic and relatively acellular collagen.

Prognosis Tend to recur after excision.

Hyperplastic scar

Epidemiology No predilection for blacks. No sex difference.

Pathogenesis Excessive connective tissue reaction to minor trauma.

Site Any.

Clinical features Does not extend beyond area of antecedent trauma.

Microscopy Persists as nodules of relatively cellular fibrous tissue. Collagen does not hyalinize.

Prognosis Recurs only occasionally.

Nodular fasciitis

Epidemiology Most common in adolescents and young adults.

Site Usually in subcutaneous fat. Volar surface of arm is commonest site but other sites include trunk and lower limbs.

Clinical features Presents as a rapidly growing nodule reaching maximal size of a few centimetres' diameter in about 3 months.

Macroscopy Well circumscribed.

Microscopy In the early stages lesions are composed of plump immature fibroblasts in short bundles and whorls. Lesions are cellular. Normal mitoses are frequent. No cellular pleomorphism. With maturation pools of myxoid material accumulate forming microcysts. May contain lymphocytes, red blood cells and multi-nucleate giant cells. In late lesions there is hyalinization and the blood vessels atrophy.

Prognosis Excision is usually curative. Around 1% recur after surgery.

Elastofibroma

Epidemiology Usually present in late adult life.

Site Frequently just below scapula.

Clinical features Long history of slow growing, ill-defined mass. May be bilateral.

Microscopy Irregular fascicles of collagen in subcutaneous fat with short thick elastic fibres which have a beaded or globular appearance.

Fibromatoses

Classification
- palmar fibromatosis: Dupuytren's contracture
- plantar fibromatosis

- Peyronie's disease: fibromatosis involving the penis
- fibromatosis colli: affects sternocleidomastoid muscle of neonates. About 10% proceed to permanent torticollis.

Clinical features   In later stages patients develop contracture. Palmar fibromatosis occurs with increased frequency in alcoholics, diabetics and epileptics.

Microscopy   All characterized by nodules of fibroblasts arranged in long sweeping bundles. Nuclear pleomorphism and mitotic rate are trivial in degree.

Prognosis   Local recurrence is common.

Deep fibromatoses (desmoid fibromatoses)

Site   Usually deep intramuscular location.

Macroscopy   Generally large (up to 10–15 cm). Infiltrative margin.

Prognosis   High rate of recurrence.

Desmoid fibromatosis of anterior abdominal wall

Epidemiology   Less common than extra-abdominal counterpart. Usually young adults, particularly women who have borne children.

Site   Usually deep in rectus muscle. May occur in surgical scars.

Intra-abdominal desmoid fibromatoses

Epidemiology   Rare. Usually young adults. Association with Gardner's syndrome.

Site   Most in mesentery. May involve retroperitoneum. May be history of previous surgery with lesion within the surgical field.

Extra-abdominal desmoid fibromatoses

Epidemiology   Principally 3rd and 4th decades. M:F 1:1. No relationship to previous trauma.

Site   Pectoral and pelvic girdles most frequently.

Clinical features   Lesions grow slowly to form large masses.

Prognosis   Most aggressive of the fibromatoses. Recurrence rate is 60–70%.

Fibrosarcoma

Classification   Classified into two broad categories:

Adult
- usually painless masses
- deep in soft tissue of lower limb or trunk
- usually middle-age adult
- M:F 1:1
- local recurrences in 50%
- 5-year survival is 40%; 10-year survival 30%.

Infantile
- typically < 2 years, may be present at birth
- males more than females
- either in subcutaneous tissue or muscle
- mostly in limbs with distal portions more often affected
- more benign behaviour than adult. Local recurrence in 20%
- metastases in 10–15%.

Microscopy   Bundles of spindle cells arranged at angle to each other (herring-bone appearance). Variable amount of stromal collagen (the more there is the better the prognosis). Mitoses are frequent and a proportion will be abnormal. Little pleomorphism and no multi-nucleate cells (differing from MFH).

ALTERATIONS OF INTRACRANIAL PRESSURE

After fusion of the skull sutures, the brain in enclosed within a rigid container. The cranium itself is further divided into compartments by unyielding folds of dura mater constituting the tentorium cerebri and the falx cerebri.

Cerebro-spinal fluid (CSF) is produced by the choroid plexus and the rate of production equals the rate of resorption by the arachnoid villi. Normal volume of CSF is about 140 ml. Rate of production/resorption is about 20 ml/h. A rise in the volume of the intracranial contents therefore causes a greater rise in pressure than would be seen in other organs. A rise in intracranial pressure causes displacement of CSF followed by compression of the ventricles. Eventually there is displacement of the brain, most commonly towards the foramen magnum. Portions of the brain may herniate under the tentorium or falx.

Increased CSF volume due to disturbance of the CSF production/resorption equilibrium (usually defective absorption) leads to hydrocephalus with dilation of the cerebral ventricles.

Obstructive hydrocephalus

Divided into two classes on the basis of site of obstruction.

- **non-communicating**: obstruction within the ventricular system (commonly in narrow areas such as the foramen of Munro, the aqueduct of Sylvius, and the exit foramina from the 4th ventricle). There is no

communication between fluid in the ventricles and the lumber CSF
- **communicating**: obstruction located in sub-arachnoid space

Obstruction may be congenital or acquired.

Congenital or infantile hydrocephalus
Usually due to developmental malformation such as variants of Chiari malformation, isolated stenosis of aqueduct of Sylvius, Dandy–Walker malformation or to obstruction of foramina of Magendie or Luschka by fibrous organization of cerebellar haemorrhage.

In young infants (before fusion of sutures) this results in cranial enlargement. This may be drained by insertion of a shunt into ventricles. If not drained there may be irreparable brain damage and severe mental retardation.

Very young infants (< 2 months) have relatively little myelin and tolerate ventricular dilation better than older infants.

Acquired hydrocephalus
May result from a focal lesion (e.g. tumour, abscess, haematoma) or of a diffuse process (e.g. meningitis, sub-arachnoid haemorrhage). Clinical effects depend upon whether there is associated raised intracranial pressure (ICP).

Raised ICP associated with mental dullness, nausea, vomiting and papilloedema. In some instances the hydrocephalus stabilizes through changes in production/resorption of CSF with normalization of ICP (normal pressure hydrocephalus) and is associated with dementia, gait disorder and urinary incontinence. **Hydrocephalus ex vacuo** refers to dilation of the ventricles due to loss of brain tissue (e.g. atrophy, ischaemia). ICP is normal.

Raised intracranial pressure

Different pressure levels are associated with different effects:

- 0–1.3 kPa: normal
- 2–3 kPa: mild. No treatment

- 4kPa: moderate. Treatment required
- > 5 kPa: severe. Associated with some cerebral ischaemia and decline in electrical activity.

Rate of rise is the important factor. Faster increases are associated with worse clinical effects.

Causes
- obstructive hydrocephalus
- local space-occupying lesions (neoplasm, infection, infarction)
- cerebral oedema (vasogenic, cytotoxic, associated with infection, post-traumatic, associated with hypercapnia).

Effects
Mainly associated with location of lesion.

1. Supra-tentorial

   - haemorrhage due to rupture of vessels from basilar artery to brain stem (Duret's haemorrhages)
   - uncinate process of temporal lobe may herniate through the tentorium stretching the 3rd cranial nerve leading to ptosis, lateral displacement of the eye and dilation of the pupil
   - compression of the pyramidal tract in the crus cerebri of the opposite side against the tentorium leads to motor paralysis on the same side as the expanding lesion.

2. Infra-tentorial

   - herniation of cerebellar tonsils through the foramen magnum. This affects the respiratory centres leading to apnoea and death.

Clinical features
- headache: worse in morning, often described as bursting. Due to tension in dura and distortion in cerebral vessels which are both pain sensitive
- vomiting: due to distortion or ischaemia of lower brain stem
- papilloedema: swelling of optic disc seen on fundoscopy. Due to accumulation of axoplasm in optic disc associated with block of normal axoplasm flow from retinal ganglion along optic nerve.

CONGENITAL AND GENETIC DISORDERS

Neural tube defects

Spina bifida

A set of disorders in which the posterior arches of the lower lumbar vertebrae are not fused.

Spina bifida occulta

- mildest form
- only vertebral arches affected
- overlying skin may show dimple, patch of hair or nodule of adipose tissue.

Meningocele

- more severe
- CSF-filled sac of meningeal tissue protrudes through vertebral defect.

Meningomyelocele

- still more severe
- sac contains part of spinal cord
- associated with major neurological defects affecting lower limbs, bladder and rectum.

Spina bifida aperta

- very rare
- most severe form
- complete failure of fusion of caudal end of neural plate
- unfused plate lies exposed on skin surface
- severe neurological defects affecting lower limbs, bladder and rectum.

Anencephaly

Complete failure of development of cranial end of neural tube. Incompatible with life.

Encephalocele

Homologue of menigomyelocele but containing brain tissue.

Arnold–Chiari malformation

There are four types.

1. *Ectopia of cerebellar tonsils*

   - tonsils may herniate through foramen magnum and be associated with arachnoiditis and thickening of meninges
   - may be associated with syringomyelia (development of fluid-filled spaces in spinal cord).

2. *Elongation of medulla*

   - seen with or without S-shaped deformity and prolongation and herniation of vermis of the cerebellum into foramen magnum
   - may be associated with meningomyelocele
   - hydrocephalus develops, especially if meningomyelocele is repaired.

3. *Cervical spina bifida with herniation of cerebellum through foramen magnum forming myelocerebello-meningocele*

4. *Cerebellar hypoplasia*

Dandy–Walker malformation

Rare cause of hydrocephalus in early life. Typically there are three abnormalities present:

- malformed cerebellar vermis
- obstruction of 4th ventricle foramina with cystic dilation of 4th ventricle
- elevated tentorium.

....

INFECTIONS

Infections of the meninges (meningitis)

These may be acute or chronic.

Acute meningitis

Usually involves leptomeninges (pia mater and arachnoid). These are bathed in CSF making dissemination within cranial cavity almost inevitable.

Infections of the dura (**pachymeningitis**) occur rarely and may be secondary to cranial or cervical osteomyelitis or an epidural abscess. Tertiary syphilis gives pachymeningitis. In meningitis:

- bacterial infections are associated with purulent exudate
- viral infections are associated with a lymphocytic cellular reaction.

Acute bacterial meningitis

Organisms involved depend on patient's age and the route of infection.

- *Streptococcus pneumoniae*
  - commonest cause of acute meningitis
  - especially affected are very young and very old
  - source is likely to be pneumonia, endocarditis or sinusitis
  - increased risk associated with alcoholic and splenectomized patients.

- *Neisseria meningitidis* (meningococcus)
  - may be sporadic (group B) or epidemic (group A or C)
  - commonest in children under 5 but has increasing prevalence in children in 2nd decade of life.

- *Haemophilus influenzae*
  - commonest in children up to age of 6 years but can occur at other ages
  - results from spread from pharyngeal or middle ear infections
  - associated with risk of mental defect in children who survive infection.

- *Escherichia coli*
  - causes meningitis in neonatal period
  - increased risk associated with low birth weight, prematurity and congenital malformations.

- *Listeria monocytogenes*
  - can cause meningitis in healthy adults
  - more important cause of disease in neonates following infection from maternal genital tract.

Routes of infection
- via bloodstream
- direct from infections of middle ear or sinuses
- direct implantation following trauma or surgical/therapeutic manoeuvres.

Clinical features
- headache
- neck stiffness
- photophobia
- fever
- clouding of consciouness in some.

Diagnostic test
- examination of CSF following lumbar puncture
- cloudy with numerous acute inflammatory cells
- Gram stain may show organisms
- increased protein (> 5 g/l)
- low glucose to less than 50% blood level (normal is about 66% blood level).

Macroscopy
- loss of normal transparency of leptomeninges
- changes most obvious over hemispheres in pneumococcal meningitis
- changes most obvious over base of brain in haemophilus meningitis.

Microscopy
- vasodilation
- large number of inflammatory cells in sub-arachnoid space extending into sulci
- in early stages neutrophils are most numerous but later macrophages predominate
- some inflammatory reaction extends into parenchyma. Perivascular inflammatory cells may be present.

Complications
- cerebral oedema – usually generalized
- thrombosis associated with small vessel involvement in sub-arachnoid space leading to small ischaemic lesions in underlying brain
- cranial nerve palsies associated with involvement of certain nerves (e.g. 6th) as they pass through sub-arachnoid space

- scarring which may occlude some foramina leading to hydrocephalus
- ependymitis – usually fatal. Lining of ventricle appears roughened. Ventricle may fill with pus.

Chronic bacterial meningitis

Tuberculous meningitis

Clinical features Most often affects infants and children. Insidious onset with non-specific prodrome including anorexia, malaise and episodes of vomiting lasting 2–3 weeks.

This is followed by signs of meningeal irritation which are less severe than in acute bacterial meningitis.

Diagnostic test CSF examination:

- CSF usually clear
- protein content may be raised
- delicate clot may be present
- glucose and chloride concentrations are lowered
- increased cell population including polymorphs and lymphocytes.

Macroscopy Base of brain most severely affected. Subarachnoid space may be filled by grey-green gelatinous material.

Microscopy Well-formed granulomas may be infrequent. Inflammatory reaction may be non-specific with many macrophages and plasma cells arranged haphazardly.

Viral meningitis

Organisms

- enteroviruses (Coxsackie virus, Echo virus)
- mumps virus
- herpes simplex type 2
- varicella zoster
- arenavirus causing lymphocytic choriomeningitis.

Clinical features

- fever
- drowsiness
- headache
- neck stiffness
- nausea and vomiting.

Diagnostic test CSF examination
- increased cellular content. Mainly lymphocytes
- slightly raised protein concentration
- normal glucose concentration.

Infections of the brain parenchyma (encephalitis)

Bacterial infections

1. Cerebral abscess

Route of infection Spread from infective lesions in middle ear, mastoid air cells or sinuses. May also be blood-borne e.g. from suppurative bronchiectasis, lung abscess or empyema.

Clinical features Abscess acts as a space-occupying lesion causing increased intracranial pressure. May be associated with diffuse suppurative encephalitis. Rupture of abscess may give suppurative ventriculitis or meningitis.

Macroscopy Commonest sites are frontal, temporal and parietal lobes and cerebellum.
- often oval
- frequently multi-locular
- in early lesions there are small foci of suppurative encephalitis or microabscesses in surrounding white matter. The capsule is poorly defined
- later lesions have thicker firmer capsules.

Microscopy Well-established abscesses have five zones:
- central necrotic area with debris, pus and macrophages
- granulation tissue with new capillaries and proliferating fibroblasts
- granulation tissue with lymphocytes and plasma cells
- dense collagenous fibrous tissue
- oedematous white matter with gliosis.

2. Tuberculoma
- localized mass of caseation necrosis
- may be single or multiple
- cerebral hemispheres commonly affected in adults
- cerebellum involved more commonly in children.

3. Parenchymous neurosyphilis

4. Tabes dorsalis

Clinical features
- severe loss of function, especially loss of deep pressure, vibration and positional sensations and co-ordination
- characteristic stamping gait
- loss of deep tendon reflexes
- shooting pains (lightning pains) in limbs
- lack of pain sensation may lead to post-traumatic disorganization of joints such as knee and ankle (Charcot's joints).

Macroscopy
- atrophy of of posterior columns of spinal cord which appear shrunken and grey
- overlying leptomeninges are thick
- posterior nerve roots are atrophic.

Microscopy
- posterior columns show fibre loss and demyelination
- similar changes may be seen in proximal parts of the nervous system e.g. optic discs, third cranial nerve
- organisms very difficult to find in lesions.

5. General paresis of the insane

Clinical features
- in early stages there is deterioration of personality and changes in mental function. May be delusions which may be bizarre and grandiose
- changes progress to complete dementia
- may be tremors of lips and tongue, general weakness, minor seizures and disturbances of finer movements.

Macroscopy Brain is shrunken and cerebral cortices are disorganized.

Microscopy
- degeneration of nerve cells and fibres
- proliferation of astrocytes and glial fibres
- small intracerebral vessels show cuffing by lymphocytes and plasma cells with endothelial cell swelling
- organisms can be quite easily identified in lesions.

Viral encephalitis

Routes of infection
- via bloodstream
- via nerves (e.g. rabies)
- large areas of necrosis.

Microscopy Perivascular cuffing of small vessels by lymphocytes and plasma cells. In severe cases the basement membrane around the perivascular space ruptures and inflammatory cells spread into surrounding tissue.

Neuronal changes include loss and shrinkage of neurones with darkly staining nuclei and eosinophilic cytoplasm. Inclusion bodies:

- herpes simplex: Cowdray type A inclusions (intranuclear)
- rabies: Negri bodies (round/oval, cytoplasmic. Stains red with eosin)
- tissue necrosis: phagocytosis of necrotic neurones (neuronophagia) by microglia is seen.

Neuropathology of AIDS

Sub-acute encephalitis (AIDS encephalopathy)
Clinical features Associated with AIDS-related dementia.

Diagnostic test Virus can be detected as budding retroviral particles under EM or by the use of immunocytochemistry or in-situ hybridization.

Microscopy Characterized by presence of one or both of:

- microglial nodules: small clusters of lymphocytes and macrophages in white-matter, basal ganglia, pons, cerebellum and more rarely cortex
- multi-nucleated macrophage cells.

Vacuolar myopathy
Microscopy Characterized by vacuolation of the spinal cord predominantly involving the lateral and posterior columns of the thoracic portion. Lesion starts as swelling in myelin sheath progressing to vacuolation and secondary degeneration of axons.

Opportunistic infections
- *Bacterial* These occur seldom in AIDS with the exception of atypical mycobacterial infections (e.g. *Mycobacterium avium intracellulare*) which are usually associated with systemic disease.

- *Viral* Cytomegalovirus is most common (seen in up to 26% cases of AIDS). No consistent clinical/pathological effects; may be asymptomatic.

Microscopy Ranges from single cells with intranuclear inclusions to areas of necrosis either in perventricular regions of the brain or the spinal cord and nerve roots.

1. Fungal

Cryptococcus neoformans is commonest (found in 2.6% of brains from AIDS patients at post-mortem). This usually produces basal meningitis and the organism can be identified in CSF. Initially may be associated with little inflammatory response but later produces either a mixed inflammatory cell infiltrate or a granulomatous response.

Other fungal infections include candidiasis, aspergillosis, coccidiomycosis and histoplasmosis.

2. Parasitic

Toxoplasma gondii is seen in 10% of AIDS patients. It is the most ubiquitous intracellular parasite. Most cases are sub-clinical infections, but encysted forms of the parasite persist and may be reactivated when immune system is depressed.

Brain lesions may be widespread and involve white and grey matter.

CNS neoplasms associated with AIDS

1. Lymphomas

Usually-high grade B cell lymphomas of large cell or Burkitt type often associated with Epstein–Barr virus in the tumour cells (especially Burkitt lymphoma).

2. Kaposi's sarcoma

Rarely seen in CNS.
If present, it is associated with disseminated disease involving multiple organs.

Fungal infections of brain parenchyma

Usually secondary to fungal disease elsewhere (e.g. lung) and reaching brain via blood. Some have characteristic geographic distribution:

Coccidiodes (south-western United States, Mexico, South America)
Blastomyces (USA, Canada, Mexico)
Histoplasma (USA, southern Africa, South America).

Many produce granuiomatous meningitis and/or granulomas in brain (e.g. *Coccidiodes*, *Blastomyces*, *Histoplasma*). Some produce abscesses (e.g. *Candida*, *Aspergillus*).

Mucor is especially seen in uncontrolled diabetics and produces acute necrotizing meningitis and abscesses.

Protozoal infections of the brain

Cerebral malaria

Aetiology Malaria is caused by various *Plasmodium* species:

- *Plasmodium falciparum* (responsible for most malaria deaths)
- *Plasmodium vivax*
- *Plasmodium malariae*
- *Plasmodium ovale*.

They are usually transmitted by bite of infected *Anopheles* mosquitoes. Cerebral malaria is the most frequent and most dangerous manifestation of falciparum malaria.

Clinical features Strictly it is defined as unrouseable coma in association with malaria but in practice diagnosed if *impaired* consciousness in patient with malaria.

- patient is usually febrile
- no evidence of meningeal irritation or papilloedema
- retinal haemorrhages in about 15%
- focal neurological deficits uncommon
- may be phasic increases in tone with extensor posturing of decorticate or decerebrate types. Opisthotonos may occur.

Mortality of untreated cases is about 100%. Following appropriate treatment 15% of children and 20% of adults still die. In adults risk of death is increased to about 50% in pregnancy. About 3% of adults and 10% children who survive have residual neurological impairment.

Macroscopy The brain is slightly swollen. Petecheal haemorrhages in white matter demonstrated on cut surface.

Microscopy most micro-vessels are packed with red blood cells containing mature *P. falciparum*. Haemozoin pigment is seen within and outside red blood cells.

Accumulation of glial cells may be seen in relation to haemorrhagic foci which follow rupture of vessels blocked by parasitized red cells.

Toxoplasmosis

This is common in AIDS patients and may be passed on to fetus by pregnant mother (congenital toxoplasmosis).

- 1–2 per 1000 live births

Clinical features
- intellectual impairment
- hydrocephalus
- megaloencephaly
- chorioretinitis
- calcification within the brain.

Amoebiasis

1. Meningoencephalitis

- usually caused by *Naegleria fowleri* which is acquired by swimming in warm lakes or pools contaminated by amoebi
- spread via nasal passages
- olfactory bulbs most often involved by the resulting purulent meningitis
- inflammation spreads into cortex where necrotizing vasculitis may occur.

2. Amoebic brain abscess

- caused by *Entamoeba histolytica*
- rare. Only found following haematogenous spread from liver abscess.

Trypanosomiasis

1. African trypanosomiasis

- caused by *T. gambiense* (causes sleeping sickness) and *T. rhodesiense*
- transmitted by bite of tsetse fly

- both varieties cause a combination of pancarditis (more conspicuous with *T. rhodesiense*) and encephalitis (more characteristic of *T. gambiense*)

Microscopic features
- meningoecephalitis with striking cellular cuffs around small intracerebral vessels consisting of lymphocytes and plasma cells
- usually involves deep white matter, basal ganglia, brainstem and cerebellum
- in severe cases aggregates of lymphocytes and plasma cells are seen not in relation to blood vessels
- parasites are not seen in the brain tissue. Diagnosis depends on their identification in blood.

2. **South American trypanosomiasis** (Chagas' disease)

- caused by *T. cruzi*
- transmitted by house bugs
- infection usually occurs in children but may be dormant for many years
- in acute cases there may be encephalitis characterized by focal inflammation of white matter associated with small aggregates of lymphocytes, plasma cells and microglia.

....

NUTRITIONAL DISORDERS

Vitamin deficiencies

Vitamin B₁ deficiency

1. Wernicke's Encephalopathy

In the developed world most often associated with malnutrition resulting from chronic alcoholism. May also be associated with excessive vomiting and malabsorption associated with small intestinal disease.

The deficiency causes pyruvate deficiency.

Clinical features

In the acute phase:
- disturbance of consciousness
- paralysis of extraocular muscles
- nystagmus.

Macroscopy
- in acute phases, congestion of the mamillary bodies with petechial haemorrhages
- in chronic cases, atrophy of mamillary bodies

Other areas affected are the anterior nucleus of the thalamus, walls of the 3rd ventricle, periaqueductal tissue and floor of fourth ventricle.

Microscopy
- in acute stages, neurone and axons are preserved but haemorrhages are prominent
- in chronic stages, there is loss of mamillary body myelin, reactive gliosis and haemosiderin deposition.

2. Korsakoff's psychosis

Clinical features
- short-term memory loss and confabulation
- commonly associated with Wernicke's encephalopathy but may be associated with other disorders of the diencephalon
- may be irreversible.

Vitamin B_2 deficiency

Pellagra   Caused by deficiency of nicotinic acid or its precursor tryptophan.

In developed world associated with antibiotic related abnormalities of normal gut flora, massive resection of small intestine and some chronic diarrhoeal illnesses.

Clinical features
- dermatitis
- diarrhoea
- dementia.

Vitamin B_6 deficiency

In developed world most often associated with drugs.

Vitamin B_{12} deficiency

Commonest cause of megaloblastic anaemia.

Vitamin E deficiency

Associated with chronic malabsorption, bile salt deficiency, abetalipoproteinaemia.

Results in dying-back type of neuropathy affecting central and peripheral axons of sensory ganglion cells.

....

DEMYELINATING DISORDERS

Characterized by loss of myelin ensheathing the axons without damage to axons themselves. May be caused by:

- damage to myelin-forming oligodendrocytes
- direct injury to myelin sheaths.

Multiple sclerosis

Epidemiology   The commonest demyelinating disease, with a peak incidence in 20–40 year age group. Rare after 60 years of age. There is a distinct geographical distribution, with frequency increasing with distance from Equator (more marked in Northern Hemisphere). Emigration to low risk area before age of 15 years is associated with decreased risk. Older emigrants maintain risk of area of origin.

Genetic factors   Associated with HLA DW2 and DR2 in Europeans and with DR6 and BW22 in Japanese.

Clinical features   Mode of onset and rate of progression is variable. Most patients start with single, focal neurological deficit such as visual disturbance (30%) or limb weakness (50%). Others have tremor, vertigo or sensory symptoms.

These initial deficits frequently remit. The remissions may be quite longlasting. Occasional severe cases starting in adult life show relentless progression with no remissions.

Macroscopy   Sharply defined plaques of demyelination in brain and spinal cord appearing as grey/translucent areas of variable size (few millimetres to several centimetres).

Any area may be affected but common sites are areas bordering the ventricles, the optic nerves, chiasm and optic tracts, cerebellum, cerebral white matter, brain stem and spinal cord.

Microscopic features   Sharply defined areas of loss of myelin (seen best in sections stained for myelin e.g. by luxol fast blue).

In acute lesions there is cuffing of small venules by lymphocytes, plasma cells and macrophages. Most lymphocytes are T cells. T-suppressor cells are seen in perivenular space; T-helper cells are seen at edge of plaques.

Blood vessels are surrounded by reactive astrocytes. In chronic lesions there is a decrease in oligodendrocytes.

CSF changes   Increase in IgG with oligoclonal bands (not specific – also seen in sub-acute sclerosing panencephalitis, syphilis and Guillain–Barré disease).

Acute perivenular encephalomyelitis (acute disseminated post-viral encephalomyelitis)

Progressive illness characterised by extensive, acute, irreversible demyelination. It may:

* follow a variety of viral infections (e.g. mumps, measles, varicella) with an interval of a few days to 3 weeks
* occur after immunization against smallpox, rabies or whooping cough.

. . . .

BASAL GANGLIA AND BRAIN STEM DEGENERATIONS

Parkinson's disease

Clinical features
* tremor
* rigidity
* inhibition of movement (bradykinesia)
* dementia (some cases).

Disease of the dopaminergic system in the substantia nigra and corpus striatum.

Types
* idiopathic (possibly related to free radical-induced oxidative damage)
* post-encephalitic
* drug related (including phenothiazines, haloperidol, reserpine, α-methyl-dopa, procaine and heroin)
* toxic damage (e.g. carbon monoxide, cycad, chronic manganese poisoning)

- post-traumatic (e.g. in boxers following chronic cerebral injury)
- ischaemia
- striatonigral degeneration
- Shy–Drager syndrome (Parkinson-type features associated with autonomic dysfunction such as postural hypotension, inability to sweat, urinary incontinence and impotence).

Macroscopy Pallor of the substantia nigra.

Microscopy
- decrease in number of pigmented neurones
- other neurones in the same region show shrinkage and vacuolation
- loss of neurones elicits macrophage response with macrophages containing dark pigment (neuromelanin)
- marked degree of astrocyte gliosis.

Lewy bodies

A characteristic feature of the microscopic picture of Parkinsonism.

- concentrically ringed hyaline bodies
- 20 μm or more in diameter
- dark eosinophilic core surrounded by rings of structureless material
- found in some affected cells, usually only one within a single cell
- present in 90% of cases of idiopathic Parkinson's
- rare in post-encephalitic Parkinson's, striatonigral degeneration and Shy–Drager syndrome
- not confined to substantia nigra. May be found in cortex or peripheral ganglia.

....

PRIMARY DEGENERATIVE DISORDERS AFFECTING CEREBELLAR FUNCTION

1. Congenital ataxias of unknown cause
2. Ataxias with recognized metabolic causes

- ataxia telangiectasia
- xeroderma pigmentosum
- Hartnup disease

- abetalipoproteinaemia
- urea cycle enzyme deficiencies.

3. Early onset ataxia appearing to be inherited as autosomal recessive

- Friedreich's ataxia

Clinical features
- unsteadiness
- dysarthria
- starts in childhood and progresses
- most patients wheelchair bound by 20s.

4. Late onset ataxias (olivoponto-atrophies)

- chiefly (but exclusively) autosomal dominant inheritance
- may be associated with mitochondrial function defect.

Clinical features Cerebellar ataxia. Many other neurological features with marked heterogeneity between cases.

Macroscopic features Shrinkage of pons and cerebral peduncles. Cerebellar cortical atrophy may be present. Atrophy of the inferior olives and olivocerebellar fibres is seen.

....

DEGENERATIVE DISORDERS OF THE PYRAMIDAL SYSTEM: MOTOR NEURONE DISEASE

Amylotrophic lateral sclerosis

- familial cases make up 5–10%
- linkage analysis suggests role for long arm of chromosome 21
- affects cortico-spinal tracts whch are laterally placed in spinal cord
- loss of both upper and lower motor neurones
- upper motor neurone defect leads to spasticity, hyperreflexia and abnormal plantar reflexes
- lower motor neurone defect gives atrophy of muscles and fasciculation
- some cases are associated with motor cortex loss.

Macroscopy Shrunken, greyish atrophic anterior nerve roots with normal-sized white posterior nerve roots.

Microscopy Loss of myelinated fibres originating from motor neurones in anterior horn of the spinal cord. Lateral columns appear chalky with extensive myelin loss accompanying the axonal loss. Muscles supplied by the affected neurones are shrunken and pale.

Progressive muscular atrophy

- preferential degeneration of anterior horn motor neurones
- lower motor neurone (flaccid) paralysis
- muscle fasciculation is prominent.

Progressive bulbar palsy

- degeneration affects medullary motor nuclei
- lower motor neurone paralysis of the jaw, tongue and pharyngeal muscles.

DEMENTIA

An acquired global impairment of intellect, memory and personality without impairment of consciousness. Risk increases with age: about 1/20 over the age of 65 have severe dementia and about 2/20 will have mild or moderate dementia.

Many causes:

- Alzheimer's disease (> 50%)
- vascular disease (15%)
- combined Alzheimer's disease and vascular disease (10%)
- Pick's disease
- cerebral neoplasia
- alcoholism
- drugs
- hypothyroidism.

Alzheimer's disease

Epidemiology
- affects about 5% people in their 60s and about 15% older than 80 years
- M:F 2:1 (increases with age over 70 years).

Macroscopy
- may be normal
- atrophy
- reduction in weight of brain (often < 1 kg [normal 1.2–1.3 kg])
- affects whole brain but most pronounced in frontal and temporal lobes
- dilation of ventricles
- widening of sulci (particularly in relation to Sylvian fissure).

Microscopy
- loss of neurones particularly in the hippocampus, noradrenergic locus ceruleus in the brain stem and in the cholinergic basal nucleus of Meynert in the basal forebrain
- disorganization of cerebral cortex
- neuritic plaques

    - occasionally found in brains of non-demented elderly patients but there is correlation between number of plaques and degree of cognitive impairment
    - rounded areas in cortex up to 150 μm in diameter
    - best demonstrated using silver salt-based stain
    - central dense core of amyloid fibrils surrounded by cuff of abnormally distended degenerating nerve cell processes intermingled with glial processes
    - amount of amyloid increases with age of plaque
    - found in all areas of cerebral cortex although the main sensory and motor areas tend to be spared. Hippocampus, basal nucleus of Meynert and amygdala tend to most severely affected
- neurofibrillary tangles

    - not specific for Alzheimer's disease
    - bundles of filaments within cytoplasm of affected neurone
    - stain positive with silver salts

- contain amyloid
- consist of a mixture of antigens including tau protein

- amyloid

  - found in cores of senile plaques and in the wall of vessel in meninges and cerebral cortex
  - small molecule known as β-protein (or A4 protein)

- granulo-vacuolar degeneration

  - mainly found in the hippocampus in the cytoplasm of pyramidal neurones
  - single cell may contain many vacuoles
  - centre of vacuole contains a tiny dot (stains positive with silver stains). containing abnormal phosphory-lated proteins

- Hirano bodies

  - not specific to Alzheimer's (may be found in elderly patients of normal intellect but markedly increased in brains of demented patients)
  - present in neurones – mainly of hippocampus
  - rod shaped/pyramidal eosinophilic bodies
  - consist of cytosceletal elements.

Binswanger's disease

- dementia associated with hypertension
- ischaemic lesions are present in deep white matter of cortex
- deep white matter is reduced in amount and cysts may be present.

Huntington's chorea

Epidemiology and genetics
- autosomal dominant with high penetrance (almost 100%)
- abnormality located near end of short arm of chromosome 4
- prevalence rate in Northern Europe is 4–7/100 000
- much rarer in North American blacks and Japanese.

Clinical features
- average age of onset is mid-40s
- survival of 5–30 years (average 15 years)
- severe mental deterioration.

Microscopy
- most severe changes are in putamen and caudate nucleus
- severe degree of atrophy due to neurone loss accompanied by gliosis
- appears to be selective loss of small neurones (normally most numerous in corpus striatum).

Biochemical examination of brain Marked decrease in GABA (and its synthesizing enzyme glutamic acid decarboxylase) within the corpus striatum and substantia nigra.

Pick's disease

Epidemiology
- rare
- mostly in 6th decade
- survival 1–10 years from onset
- women are slightly more often affected than men
- occasional familial cases have been described.

Clinical features Indistinguishable from Alzheimer's disease.

Macroscopic features
- severe localized atrophy of the brain mostly affecting frontal and temporal lobes
- sulci are very much widened
- gyri, particularly near the tips, show severe atrophic change giving appearance likened to a walnut.

Microscopic features
- severe neuronal loss mainly in outer parts of the cortex associated with gliosis
- some of the surviving neurones show a characteristic swelling, becoming round or pear-shaped with the nucleus pushed to one end and uniformly eosinophilic cytoplasm
- some of the swollen cells contain intracytoplasmic inclusions (Pick bodies) which stain positively with silver stains and contain neurofilaments and neurofibrillary tangles.

....

TRANSMISSILE SPONGIFORM ENCEPHALOPATHIES

Creutzfeldt–Jakob disease (CJD)

Clinical features
- rapidly progressive global dementia
- myoclonus
- progressive motor dysfunction
- usually fatal within 1 year.

Transmissibility   Infective agents have no nucleic acid 1 and are called prions (proteinaceous infectious particle).

Microscopic features
- loss of neurones
- spongy appearance of affected parts of brain caused by formation of small cystic cavities in cortex
- brisk astrocytic response
- amyloid plaques and in some cases deposition of amyloid in blood vessels.

Biochemical features   Modification of prion protein into amyloid. This protein is coded for by a normal cellular gene.

Gerstmann–Sträussler–Scheinker syndrome

Epidemiology and genetics   Often familial with autosomal dominant pattern.

Clinical features   Dementing illness often associated with ataxia.

Microscopic features   Similar to those of Creutzfeldt–Jakob disease.
- amyloid plaques
- amyloid in blood vessels is not present in all cases.

Kuru

Epidemiology   A disease confined to Fore tribe in New Guinea; it was common in children and adult females but rare in males. Kuru has been disappearing in the last 25 years; its demise is associated with the disappearance of ritual cannibalism as a mark of respect to dead kinsmen. Removal of the brain was carried out by females and the brain was then scooped by hand into bamboo cylinders with a high risk of inoculation by infected material.

Clinical features
- cerebellar ataxia
- severe tremor
- progressive motor dysfunction associated with dysarthria
- progresses to death within a year of onset of symptoms.

VASCULAR DISORDERS OF THE CENTRAL NERVOUS SYSTEM

NORMAL VASCULATURE

The major part of the cerebral hemispheres is supplied by the internal carotid arteries. The vertebral arteries supply the base of the brain and the cerebellum. The two systems are connected at the base of the brain in the circle of Willis. There is therefore an efficient collateral circulation if the circle of Willis is anatomically normal and free from significant degrees of atheroclerosis. The small cerebral vessels have no collateral circulation and stenosis or occlusion of these vessels inevitably leads to ischaemia.

STROKE

Definition   Sudden onset of focal loss of neurological function lasting longer than 24 hours with a vascular origin (ischaemia or haemorrhage).

Epidemiology   Third commonest cause of death in the UK (about 10% of all deaths). There are half a million new cases per year in the USA of which 50% die. Only 10% of the remainder regain full function. The elderly are most frequently involved but 30% of cases occur in the 35–65 age group.

Aetiology   Up to 84% are due to ischaemia which may be associated with thrombosis (53%) or embolus (31%; derived from the heart or the neck arteries). Rare causes of ischaemia are vasospasm, venous occlusion and inflammatory vasculitides such as polyarteritis nodosa. The remaining 16% are caused by haemorrhage which may be intracerebral (10%) or sub-arachnoid (6%). The commonest association is with hypertension but some are associated with vascular malformations, vascular neoplasms and abnormal bleeding tendencies.

Risk factors for stroke (Table 45.1)

Cerebral infarction

Aetiology Embolic stroke accounts for about 30% cases. In addition to thromboembolism the emboli may be gaseous.

- air: complicating cardiac, brain or pulmonary surgery and catheterization procedures
- nitrogen: either associated with hyperbaric decompression – when there is a reduction from an abnormally high atmospheric pressure to normal the nitrogen comes out of solution and forms bubbles obstructing flow in small vessels – or hypobaric decompression, when there is reduction from normal atmospheric pressure to an abnormally low one.

In fat embolism white matter is studded with petechial haemorrhages. Grey matter shows fat globules but no damage due to short capillaries and many anastamoses. Small infarcts may occur in the deeper cortex, especially frontal lobes, the brain stem and pons. Other causes include aggregates of tumour cells, parasitic larvae or clumps of meconium and keratinocytes (e.g. amniotic fluid embolism).

Site/clinical features The effects of occlusion of arteries depends on the vessel occluded.

Table 45.1 Risk factors for stroke

Factor	Relative risk
Existence of ischaemic heart disease	2–5
Hypertension	6
Diabetes mellitus	2–4

Internal carotid artery occlusion

Due to thrombosis in 80%. Emboli do occur, most frequently impacting at the upper end of the internal carotid. Flow is only significantly reduced with 80–90% occlusion. Five patterns of ischaemic damage may follow occlusion of the internal carotid artery.

1. Massive infarction involving the whole territory of the middle cerebral artery.
2. Infarction of the cortex round the Sylvian fissure with or without involvement of the internal capsule and basal ganglia.
3. Infarction restricted to the internal capsule.
4. Small infarcts within the white matter supplied by the middle cerbral artery.
5. Infarction in the boundary between zones supplied by the middle cerebral artery and the anterior cerebral arteries or more rarely boundary between middle and posterior cerebral arteries (watershed areas).

Subclavian artery occlusion

Obstruction of the subclavian or inominate artery proximal to the origin of the vertebral artery may lead to retrograde flow of blood down the vertebral artery to supply blood to the arm. Blood is therefore stolen from the circle of Willis (subclavian steal syndrome). Exercise of the arm may precipitate cerebral ischaemia.

Occlusion of the vertebrobasilar system

Aetiology Cervical osteoarthritis, sudden hyperextension of the atlanto-occipital joint in rheumatoid arthritis and damage sustained as a result of twisting and traction of the neck in infants in the course of delivery. In the basilar artery itself the commonest cause is atherothrombosis.

Clinical features Vertebrobasilar insufficiency leads to vertigo and nystagmus which may be associated with nerve palsies, dysarthria and problems with swallowing. Basilar artery occlusion leads to flaccid quadriplegia, coma or bulbar palsy.

Middle cerebral artery occlusion

Epidemiology Commonest site of intracranial arterial occlusion.

Pathogenesis Embolism is the commonest (two-thirds of cases).

Clinical features Contralateral hemiparesis and contralateral cortical-type sensory loss. If occlusion occurs on the left side there is usually expressive aphasia. If the optic radiation is involved there may be hemianopia.

Macroscopy Size varies from a few mm to massive lesions affecting the whole territory of the artery. The infarct might be anaemic (pale) or haemorrhagic. The latter is characteristically associated with embolic occlusion where the embolus may fragment and the vessel dilate with the result that there is distal movement of the embolus and reperfusion takes place behind it. Haemorrhagic infarcts may also be seen with venous thrombosis.

The appearances are dependent on time from the onset of ischaemic damage (see Table 45.2).

Transient ischaemic attacks

Definition Focal neurological deficit that is fully reversible usually lasting no more than a few minutes but may be prolonged up to 24 hours.

Pathogenesis Either breaking off of small portions of mural thrombus from the surface of an atherosclerotic plaque or heart valve which impact in small cerebral vessels or sudden decline in cardiac output. Hypercoagulable and high blood viscosity states (e.g. polycythaemia).

Natural history and prognosis Constitutes an advance warning of future cerebral infarction (occurs in about 13–50%).

Intracerebral haemorrhage

Classification Two main types:
- primary: usually associated with hypertension; accounts for about 80% of cases
- secondary: due to local or systemic disease e.g. aneurysm, vascular malformation, amyloid or bleeding disorders.

Primary intracerebral haemorrhage
Epidemiology Most common in late middle age.

Table 45.2 Appearances dependent on time from onset of ischaemic damage

Time from onset	Macroscopy	Microscopy
0–6 hours	No gross changes	From 4–6 hours there is evidence of neuronal death. Cells show intense eosinophils with vacuolation of the cytoplasm and poor nuclear staining
24 hours	May be some loss of demarcation between grey and white matter. Affected area is softer than normal	Evidence of later stages of neuronal necrosis with ghost-like appearance. The neuropil looks spongy. Demyelination occurs within the infarct and by 18–24 hours it is possible to see a sharp demarcation between abnormal myelin within the lesion and normal myelin at the periphery. Large numbers of neutrophils are seen at the periphery
4 days	Softening of the infarct is more marked and there may be breakdown of the centre	Macrophages are present in the lesion in large numbers and are foamy and in haemorrhagic infarcts contain red cells
Weeks–months	In most cases there is cyst formation. In haemorrhagic infarcts the wall shows reddish-yellow colour	At the edge there is proliferation of astrocytes and abundant new glial fibres that wall off the lesion from the surrounding tissues. The fibres in gliosis are confined within the membranes of the astrocyte and its process

Site   Most common sites are the lentiform nucleus (capsular haemorrhage; 80%) and the pons or white matter of the cerebellum (20%).

Pathogenesis   Most favoured suggestion is that they occur as a result of rupture of tiny microaneurysms (Charcot–Bouchard aneurysms, miliary aneurysms) measuring up to 1–2 mm diameter. These are present in 50% hypertensives compared with 5% non-hypertensives and are seen in 90% of individuals dying of hypertensive cerebral haemorrhage. Aneurysm number is related to duration and severity and duration of the hypertension. Aneurysmal rupture is likely to result from sudden rises in blood pressure in an already hypertensive individual.

Clinical features   Rapid evolution with a complex array of different neurological deficits appearing over a period of minutes or hours.

Macroscopy   Large haematomas cause deformation and destruction of brain tissue tracking along planes of least resistance, splitting and separating white matter. Not infrequently the haematoma bursts into the lateral ventricles or sub-arachnoid space. Functionally there is increased intracranial pressure which may lead to herniation through the tentorium and secondary brainstem haemorrhage. If the patient survives, the haematoma becomes absorbed, leaving a cavity with an orange-brown coloured rim.

Sub-arachnoid haemorrhage

Epidemiology
Accounts for about 6% of cerebrovascular disease. Peak incidence 55–60 years. Incidence in USA is 11–12/100 000 per year.

Pathogenesis
Spontaneous sub-arachnoid haemorrhage arises from the following causes:
- rupture of a sacular aneurysm of one of the major cerebral arteries (65%)
- bleeding from an arteriovenous malformation (5%)
- bleeding secondary to a blood dyscrasia (2.5%)
- extension of an intracerebral bleed (2.5%)

- rupture of a mycotic aneurysm or no obvious cause (25%).

Macroscopy In those that die there is usually massive bleeding with rupture into the ventricular system. Other possible findings include sub-arachnoid blood clot, cerebral infarction and intracerebral haematoma.

Natural history and prognosis About 27% die in the first week. A third of patients will have another bleed within a month with a mortality of 42% at that time. Risk of recurrence is greatest between 5th and 9th day. Risk of recurrence falls so that 10% of those surviving 6 weeks rebleed within a year while in those surviving over a year there is a 5% risk of recurrence for each year that passes and about 50% of those will die as a consequence.

Vascular abnormalities: saccular aneurysm (Berry aneurysm)

Definition Rounded focal defects involving only part of the circumference of the vessel wall.

Epidemiology Found in about 1–2% of the population. Females more than males.

Site
- seen at the junction between internal carotid–posterior communicating arteries (40%)
- anterior cerebral–anterior communicating arteries (30%)
- bifurcation of the middle cerebral artery in the Sylvian fissure (20%)
- the point where the basilar artery divides into the posterior cerebral arteries (4%).

Pathogenesis Arise on the basis of focal defects in the tunica media of cerebral arteries at their junction points. Not present at birth. May be associated with coarctation of the aorta, autosomal dominant form of polycystic kidney or some forms of connective tissue disease (Ehlers–Danlos syndrome). Rupture may be associated with transiently raised blood pressure (this explains the association with physical exertion and heightened emotional tone).

Microscopy Aneurysm wall consists of fibrous tissue lined by a single layer of endothelial cells. There is no muscle or connective tissue. Some larger aneuryms contain layered thrombus.

Natural history and prognosis A critical diameter of 8–10 mm has been suggested at which time the wall measures approximately 40 µm. Early consequences of rupture depends on whether the blood is localized to the site of rupture or spreads diffusely through the sub-arachnoid space. If the aneurym is embedded in the underlying brain bleeding is mostly intracerebral. Late complications include cerebral infarction (as a result of arterial compression by haematoma, vasospasm or the effects of raised intracranial pressure) or hydrocephalus because of block of CSF circulation due to clot.

Mycotic aneurysm

Definition Aneurysm caused by infection or artery wall.

Aetiology Most are associated with impaction of infected embolus in cases of infective endocarditis (3–10% patients with endocarditis develop these). Most commonly *Streptococcus pyogenes* and *Staphylococcus aureus*. Fungal aneurysms are occasionally seen (most commonly *Aspergillus.*)

Clinical features About 65% rupture within 5 weeks of the endocarditis (mortality about 80%).

Fusiform aneurysm

Definition Whole circumference of the affected segment of artery is involved.

Site Most commonly in the basilar artery.

Aetiology Associated with atheroma.

Clinical features Abnormalities of flow predispose to thrombus formation which may lead to transient ischaemic attacks. Occasionally there is thrombotic occlusion and rarely the aneurysms rupture.

Arteriovenous malformations

Epidemiology Usually present some time in 2nd to 4th decades. Cavernous haemangiomas present in the 3rd to 5th decades.

Site Most common in relation to the cerebral hemispheres and may lie on the surface of the brain or penetrate into the substance. Cavernous haemangiomas are found in the white matter.

Clinical features Recurrent sub-arachnoid haemorrhages. Cavernous haemangiomas are associated with epilepsy (38%), intracranial bleeding (23%), headache (28%) and focal neurological deficits (12%).

Microscopy Meshwork of poorly formed vessels (arteries and veins) surrounded by brain tissue showing gliosis and haemosiderin-laden macrophages.

....

HYPOXIC INJURY TO THE BRAIN

Normal regulation of blood flow

Degree of oxygenation of tissues relies on the amount of blood flow and the oxygen content of the blood. Autoregulation of cerebral blood flow is mediated via changes in the resistance of the cerebral arterioles. The limits of autoregulation are in the region of 50 mm Hg systolic and 160 mm HG systolic. Hypoxia and hypercapnia also lead to vasodilation and increased blood flow.

Categories of hypoxia

1. **Stagnant hypoxia**: inadequate blood flow e.g. following cardiac arrest or dysrrhythmias.
2. **Anoxic/hypoxic hypoxia**: Oxygen levels are inadequate to meet metabolic demand.
3. **Histotoxic hypoxia**: Both cerebral bloodflow and oxygen content are normal but there is a failure to use the oxygen due to poisoning of the respiratory enzymes (e.g. cyanide poisoning).
4. **Anaemic hypoxia**: Inadequate amounts of haemoglobin cause low oxygen content. Mimicked by carbon monoxide poisoning.
5. **Hypoxic damage resulting from hypoglycaemia**: leads to inability to use oxygen.

Brain damage secondary to cardiac arrest

Aetiology Irreversible damage is likely if the period of 'shut-down' exceeds 5–7 min at normal body temperature.

Macroscopy Indistinct patchy or laminar necrosis in the depths of the sulci and the CA1 region of the hippocampus. In survivors there is marked atrophy: decreased brain weight and enlargement of the ventricles. The cortex of the parietal and occipital lobes appear to be particularly severely affected.

Microscopy There is diffuse neuronal necrosis with some areas more affected than others. The Purkinje cells in the cerebellum are severely and diffusely affected. Damage to brainstem nuclei can also occur. This is more severe in infants and young children than in adults.

Natural history and prognosis Severe brain damage associated with cardiac arrest is usually fatal within a few days but some survive with severe neurological deficits.

Brain damage due to hypotension

Site Tends to be concentrated in the arterial boundary zones between the main cerebral and cerebellar artery territories. Infarcts of varying size develop most likely to occur in the parietal and occipital lobes (boundary zone of the anterior, middle and posterior cerebral arteries). There is variable involvement of the basal ganglia. The hippocampus and brainstem is usually spared.

Aetiology Seen during neurosurgical procedures undertaken in the sitting position, sudden decreases in arterial pressures, after occlusion of the carotid artery, dental anaesthesia in a semi-recumbent position, in severe non-missile head injury and over-enthusiastic treatment of hypertension.

Brain damage due to carbon monoxide poisoning

Clinical features Severe headache, fatigue and impaired judgement. A concentration of 60–70% carboxyhaemoglobin leads to loss of consciousness and more than 70% is rapidly fatal.

Macroscopy If death occurs within a few hours the brain is bright pink in colour. If the patient survives more than

36–48 hours the brain shows congestion and there are often petechiae in the corpus callosum and in other parts of the white matter.

'Respirator brain'

Definition Synonymous with brain death.

Aetiology Arrest of cerebral circulation due to severe brain swelling.

EEG findings Iso-electric and the brainstem reflexes are abolished. Spinal reflexes may persist.

Macroscopy There is increased weight due to oedema. The brain is soft and diffluent and may pour out of the opened cranium like porridge. Herniation of the cerebellar tonsils through the foramen magnum is common. On sectioning there is blurring of the boundary between grey and white matter.

Microscopy There is severe and extensive neuronal necrosis. The dying cells show marked cytoplasmic eosinophilia. The necrosis elicits no tissue reaction.

....

HEAD INJURY

Epidemiology Accounts for about 1% of all deaths in the UK. Responsible for 25% of deaths from trauma and 50% of those resulting from road traffic accidents.

Classification Two main types: missile and non-missile (blunt) injury. Damage may result from primary (occurring at the moment of injury e.g. scalp injury, skull fracture, cerebral contusion, intracranial haemorrhage and diffuse axonal injury) or secondary (comprising complications of the primary injury e.g. associated with raised intracranial pressure, hypoxia, brain swelling and infection).

Non-missile injury

Pathogenesis Two main mechanisms are thought to be involved.

1. **Contact effects** – usually focal. Resulting from an object striking the head (essentially local effects such as scalp injury, skull fracture, extradural haematoma, intracerebral haemorrhage and some varieties of brain contusion).

2. **Acceleration effects** – usually diffuse. Produced by rapid movement of the head at the instant of the injury. Acceleration leads to shear, tensile and compressive strains and to changes in intracranial and intracerebral pressure. There are two serious types of damage:

   • acute subdural haemorrhage resulting from tearing of subdural bridging veins
   • diffuse axon damage due to shear strains generated within the brain as a result of modulations in the acceleration/deceleration conditions.

....

FOCAL INJURIES

Haemorrhage

Extradural haematoma
Epidemiology   Occurs in about 2% of cases of head injury.

Aetiology   Most often associated with skull fracture especially if the groove in the which the middle meningeal artery runs is involved. This artery is involved in 70–80% of cases.

Clinical features   In children extradural haematoma occurs not uncommonly without skull fracture. The initial injury may seem trivial and there is often a lucid interval before the effects of the haemorrhage become apparent often in the form of declining consciousness and ultimately coma.

Macroscopy   As the blood clot enlarges it peels away the dura from the underlying skull forming an ovoid mass which compresses the underlying brain.

Subdural haemorrhage
Epidemiology   Occurs in 26–63% of cases of non-missile head injury.

Aetiology   Most commonly the result of a fall or blow to the head.

Pathogenesis Tearing of bridging veins in the sub-dural space. The result of rapid acceleration or deceleration.

Clinical features The neurosurgical classification depends on the haematoma.
- Acute: dark red semi-liquid blood.
- Subacute: mixture of clotted and fluid blood.
- Chronic: dark turbid fluid and some fresh blood.

Intracerebral haemorrhage
Epidemiology Occurs in about one-sixth of fatal head injuries.

Site Principal sites are the temporal lobes and the sub-frontal region.

Pathogenesis Thought to be rupture of small intracerebral blood vessels at the time of injury.

Cerebral contusion
Definition Post-traumatic haemorrhagic lesions in the brain substance occuring in the presence of an intact pia-arachnoid.

Site Affects the crests of the gyri but may extend into the sulci and gyral white matter. Chief targets are the frontal lobe poles, the orbital gyri, the cortex above the Sylvian fissure, the temporal lobe poles and the lateral and inferior aspects of the temporal lobes.

Classification Based on the site of the contusion and the site of injury to the head.
- **Coup**: at the site of impact in the absence of a fracture.
- **Contrecoup**: at a site diametrically opposite the site of impact.
- **Herniation**: contusions occuring where the medial parts of the temporal lobe are pushed up against the edge of the tentorium or where the cerebellar tonsils are forced down into the foramen magnum at the moment of injury.

Diffuse injury

Definition Pathological correlate of immediated pro-longed unconsciousness not associated with a mass lesion.

Epidemiology Occurs in about 50% patients with severe head injury. Responsible for over a third of deaths from head injury.

Pathogenesis Results from severe shearing strains on nerve fibres within the substance of the brain at the moment of injury.

Macroscopy There are focal haemorrhagic lesions in the region of the corpus callosum (often involve the interventricular septum) and focal lesions of different sizes in the dorsolateral quadrant of the rostal brainstem adjacent to the superior cerebellar peduncles.

Microscopy If survival has been a matter of days numerous eosinophilic swellings on nerve fibres are seen. If the patient has survived for a few weeks there are many clusters of microglial cells scattered throughout the white matter. Fat laden macrophages and reactive astrocytes are seen.

TUMOURS OF THE NERVOUS SYSTEM

Any tumour that arises at an intracranial site has the potential to exert an effect solely by its presence within a rigid cranium causing:

- compression of adjacent structures the effects of which may be reversible
- destruction of surrounding tissue due to infiltration – this is irreversible
- obstruction to flow of CSF
- oedema
- irritative effects on neural function which may cause epileptiform seizures.

The combination of a space-occupying lesion, surrounding oedema and hydrocephalus (if present) often leads to raised intracranial pressure.

....

NEUROECTODERMAL TUMOURS
Astrocytomas

Site Well-differentiated astrocytomas of the cerebellum and brainstem account for 45% of primary neuroectodermal tumours of children and 10% in adults. Most adult astrocytomas occur in the cerebral hemispheres of individuals under 30 years.

Clinical features The presentation depends on the location, e.g. brainstem asstrocytomas may present with quadriplegia while cerebellar tumours cause ataxia.

Classification A commonly used system divides astrocytomas into three groups: well-differentiated astrocytoma, anaplastic astrocytoma and glioblastoma multiforme. Another system classifies astrocytomas into four grades on the basis of nuclear atypia, mitoses, endothelial cell proliferation and necrosis.

Natural history and prognosis Site is important as this determines whether a tumour can be sucessfully excised without damage to vital surrounding brain tisuue. The grade of the tumour is also prognostic with a 4-year median survival for grade 2 lesions compared with 1.6 years for grade 3 and 0.7 years for grade 4 tumours.

Well-differentiated astrocytoma

Macroscopy Usually white ill defined masses. Pilocytic variants are usually firm while protoplasmic astrocytomas are soft and gelatinous. Cerebellar astrocytomas are often cystic.

Microscopy
* Protoplasmic astrocytomas: stellate cells with fine processes containing glial fibrils. There may be small cystic spaces.
* Fibrillary astrocytomas: these have rather more glial fibres, and pilocytic astrocytomas (found most commonly in the cerebellum of children and adolescents) are composed of elongated cells with long thin processes containing glial fibrils. Some of these contain long eosinophilic club-like structures (**Rosenthal fibres**).

Gemistocytic change may occur in which the cells of the astrocytoma become large and plump with abundant cytoplasm.

In patients with tuberous sclerosis (autosomal dominant inheritance) the astrocytomas are characteristically in the region of the thalamus and composed of large astrocytes with eccentrically placed nuclei (sub-ependymal giant-celled astrocytoma).

Natural history and prognosis Approximately 50% 2-year survival.

Anaplastic astrocytoma

Site   Usually in cerebral hemispheres. Uncommon in brainstem and cerebellum.

Aetiology   Thought to arise from previously well-differentiated astrocytomas.

Microscopy   There is usually a well-differentiated area and an area with increased cellularity, increased pleomorphism, a substantial mitotic rate and prominent blood vessels.

Natural history and prognosis   Worse survival than well-differentiated astrocytomas but better than glioblastoma mutliforme.

Glioblastoma multiforme

Epidemiology   Commonest neuroectodermal tumour affecting principally middle-aged and elderly patients. Peak incidence in the 6th decade.

Site   About 75% occur in the frontal and temporal lobes. Another 20% occur in the parietal lobes.

Macroscopy   Large greyish-white tumour with better defined edges than other astrocytomas. Obvious central necrosis may be present. May be confined to one hemisphere or spread across the midline as a butterfly-shaped mass.

Microscopy   There is cellular pleomorphism with giant cells and bizarre mitoses, necrosis (with or without haemorrhage), capillary endothelial proliferation (some of which terminate in a tangle of capillaries – glomeruloid areas), pseudopallisading of rod-shaped astrocytes around areas of necrosis, and small rod-shaped anaplastic cells.

Natural history and prognosis   Poor; majority dead within 1 year.

Oligodendroglioma

Epidemiology   Account for 3–6% glial tumours. Occur at any age but more common in adults.

Site   Most commonly cerebral hemispheres.

Clinical features   Most common presentation is with focal neurological deficit or adult onset epilepsy. Radiologically there may be spotty calcification.

Macroscopy   Often plum-coloured and well demarcated. May involve the surface.

Microscopy Cells are uniform and have small round nuclei, clear cytoplasm and well-defined cytoplasmic membrane. There is a fine network of capillaries.

Natural history and prognosis Tumours with low cellularity have a moderate prognosis (median survival 91 months); those with high cellularity, particularly if associated with necrosis, have median survival of 18 months and 5-year survival of 9%.

Ependymoma

Epidemiology About 4% of glial tumours. Bimodal age distribution with sharp peak at 5 years and broader peak in adults.

Site In children 60% arise above the tentorium and the majority are intracranial. In adults tumours are equally distributed between cranium and spinal cord. Overall about 38% arise in the floor of the 4th ventricle, 20% in the cerebral ventricles, 14% in the spinal cord and 28% in the corda equina.

Clinical features Depends on tumour site. Blockage of the 4th ventricle leads to hydrocephalus. Invasion of the floor of the 4th ventricle is associated with brainstem-related neurological deficit. Tumours of the spinal cord and corda equina result in backache and invasion of the spinal cord give long tract signs.

Macroscopy Pink or cream tumours within the ventricles or coating the spinal cord or corda equina.

Microscopy Variable between tumours. Rarely the tumours are very well differentiated with well-formed rosettes lined by ependymal cells that are ciliated or show basal bodies (blepharoblasts). More commonly there are pseudorosettes with aggregates of ependymal cells around blood vessels with fine processes abutting on the blood vessel wall. Occasionally there is a papillary pattern.

Natural history and prognosis Most are benign. A few are anaplastic, grow rapidly and have a poor prognosis.

Myxopapillary ependymoma
Definition Distinctive variant of ependymoma.
Epidemiology Usually 20–40 years but some in children.

Site Almost exclusively the cauda equina. Originates from the conus medullaris of the filum terminale.

Macroscopy Symptomatic tumours are large, sausage-shaped masses often with a nodular surface. Compress or envelope the roots of the cauda equina.

Microscopy Well differentiated cuboidal or low columnar cells surround central cores of acellular hyaline connective tissue containing small blood vessels and often mucin. Solid masses of polygonal cells are also found away from the papillae and rarely there may be tubule formation.

Natural history and prognosis Behave benignly unless complete removal is impossible when recurrences are likely.

Choroid plexus tumours

Epidemiology Papillomas are rare. Less than 1% of intracranial tumours. Half are less than 20 years.

Definition Most are papillomas but some show malignant characteristics (carcinoma).

Site Usually cerebral ventricles.

Clinical features Most present with hydrocephalus due to either obstruction of CSF flow or over-production of CSF by the tumour.

Macroscopy Pink papillary mass growing in the ventricular cavity. The stroma may be calcified giving a gritty feel.

Microscopy Papillae of well-vascularized connective tissue covered by columnar or less often cuboidal epithelium. Immunocytochemistry shows presence of carbonic anhydrase C, S100 protein and focally cytokeratin and GFAP.

Primitive neuroectodermal tumours (PNET)

Definition Small round cell tumours of the nervous system which include neuroblastoma, aesthesioneuroblastoma, retinoblastoma, medulloblastoma, cerebral neuroblastoma and pinealoblastoma.

Microscopy The cells have a high nuclear to cytoplasmic ratio and fine fibrillary processes. The nuclei are small, oval and deeply staining; mitoses are common. Many show neuronal, glial or ependymal differentiation.

Medullablastoma

Epidemiology Commonest primary brain tumour in childhood. About 43% occur before 15 years with two peaks at 3–4 years and 8–9 years.

Site In children almost exclusively in the vermis in the midline of the cerebellum. In young adults they arise more laterally in the cerebellar hemispheres.

Clinical features Depends on site. Cerebellar damage causes ataxia. Blockage of CSF flow causes hydrocephalus. If the floor of the 4th ventricle is involved there may be brainstem signs.

Microscopy These are very cellular. The cells are small with little cytoplasm. The nuclei are round and stain deeply. Mitoses are frequent. Mostly there is no architecture but some may show rosette formation with the nuclei at the periphery and the centre occupied by tapering cytoplasmic processes (Homer Wright rosettes). If the tumour abuts on the meninges there is a marked connective tissue response mimicking sarcoma (desmoplastic medulloblastoma).

....

TUMOURS OF THE MENINGES

Meningioma

Definition Tumour arising from the arachnoid.

Epidemiology Account for 15% of primary intracranial tumours in Western Europe and North America but more common in Africa. For cranial meningiomas M:F 1:2.5 but for spinal menigiomas M:F 1:9. Most common in middle age with peak incidence in Britain in 6th decade.

Clinical features Depends on speed of growth and site. Tumours at the base of the brain cause focal neurological deficits, those over the convexity of the cerebral hemispheres and in the falx cerebri may present late and be of considerable size before causing signs. Menigiomas of the vertebral column cause compression of the long tracts.

Macroscopy Typically firm, rounded well-encapsulated lesions with cream or pink cut surface. Usually adherent to dura and easily separated from the brain. Some are gritty to cut.

Microscopy For the most part there is a uniform cell population with pale open nuclei and 1–2 nucleoli. The cytoplasm has a delicate fibrillary pattern. Common histological variants are:

- Meningothelial: sheets of tumour cells with or without whorls. Cell borders are rather indistinct. Little or no reticulin between tumour cell bundles.
- Fibroblastic: sheets of cells that are elongated with no evidence of whorls.
- Transitional: features of both meningothelial and fibroblastic types.
- Psammomatous: large numbers of calcified laminated spheres (psammoma bodies).

Natural history and prognosis Tend to be slow growing and the majority are benign.

NERVE SHEATH TUMOURS

Schwannoma (neurilemmoma, neuroma)

Epidemiology Account for about 8% of intracranial tumours and about 25% of intraspinal. Most frequent in middle age.

Clinical features Depends on site. About 80% of intracranial schwannomas arise from the 8th nerve and present with deafness and tinnitus.

Macroscopy Smooth lobulated lesions with soft rubbery consistency. Usually attached to nerve or nerve root.

Microscopy Two major patterns:
- **Antoni A**: compact areas with regular interlacing bundles of fusiform cells. Often foci of pallisading which may be arranged in regular repetetive array (Verocay bodies).
- **Antoni B**: Looser, more open areas in which cells are small with rounded nuclei and fine cytoplasmic processes. Mast cells are common.

Neurofibroma

Epidemiology Frequently multiple as part of von Reckinghausen's disease (peripheral neurofibromatosis occurs in 1/3000 live births with autosomal dominant inheritance; central neurofibromatosis occurs in 0.1/100,000 live births).

Genetics In peripheral neurofibromatosis there is a deletion on the long arm of chromosome 17 (gene NF1). In central neurofibromatosis the deletion is on chromosome 22).

Microscopy In the skin the tumours are usually poorly delineated and composed of loosely packed bundles of spindle cells. Nerve fascicles are frequently expanded by the lesion.

Natural history and prognosis For those treated by resection and radiotherapy the 5-year survival is 40–55% and 10-year survival 30–40%.

THE PERIPHERAL NERVES

FUNCTION

1. To carry commands from the anterior horn cells to the muscles.
2. To carry signals to the effector organs controlled by the autonomic nervous system.
3. To carry afferent signals from sensory transducers in the skin, muscle, joint and other organs to the central nervous system.

STRUCTURE

The nerves consist of bundles of axons (fascicles) connecting the periphery to the central nervous system. In each fascicle there are nerve fibres the functional elements of which are the axons and associated Schwann cells. The nerve fibres are embedded in specialized connective tissue (the endoneurium) and are surrounded by a sheath of cells (the perineurium) that are arranged in layers and connected by tight junctions.

The perineurium

Continuous with the pia-arachnoid. Functions as a protective layer and a diffusion barrier.

The endoneurium

Specialized extracellular space consisting of longitudinally orientated collagen fibres in mucopolysaccharide rich matrix. Also contains capillaries supplying the nerve fibres. Tight junctions between the endothelial cells provide a blood–brain barrier but this is less effective in the sensory ganglia where there are fenestrations in the capillary endothelium.

The epineurium

The outermost sheath surrounding peripheral nerves. Rich in collagen and containing fibroblasts and occasional mast cells with a vascular bed of small arteries, veins and lymphatics.

Myelinated nerve fibres

Based on size there are two populations of myelinated fibres. Small axons (mean diameter 4 μm) and larger ones (mean diameter 11 μm) with a ratio small:large of 2:1. Large fibres conduct impulses at high speed (about 100 m/sec) and are particularly concerned with motor functions and light touch. The smaller fibres conduct impulses more slowly (12–30 m/sec) and are associated with pain and temperature.

Unmyelinated nerve fibres

More numerous than myelinated. Range in size 0.2–3 μm. Each fibre is enveloped in the cytoplasm of a single Schwann cell which separates unmyelinated fibres from each other. They conduct slowly (0.3–1.6 m/sec) and conduct pain sensations and also constitute post-ganglionic autonomic axons.

Myelination and the Schwann cell

Myelin consists of lipid bilayers in which transmembrane proteins are embedded. The axon segment myelinated by a single Schwann cell is the internode. The sheath is interrupted at regular intervals where one Schwann cell abuts another (node of Renvier). In the smallest diameter fibres an internode may be as short as 100 μm while in a large fibre it may be as long as 1 mm. All internodes along a single fibre are the same length. In the peripheral nervous system each Schwann cell myelinates only one segment of the axon. Myelination starts in the 17th week of gestation. As the axon enlarges it becomes enveloped by a chain of Schwann cells lying at intervals along the axon. These Schwann cells spin out spirals of plasma membrane which wrap around the axon. As the process goes on the cytoplasm is extruded from the spirals and the compacted Schwann cell plasma membranes form the myelin sheath.

....

INJURY TO PERIPHERAL NERVES

Axonal degeneration

Aetiology   Results from damage either to the neurone (e.g. poliomyelitis, motor neurone disease) or the axon itself (e.g. trauma, toxic damage, metabolic disorders).

Microscopy

1. **Wallerian degeneration**: Axonal fragmentation is seen initially in the portion distal to the injury. The myelin sheath retracts from the underlying degenerating segment. The axon tends to break at the nodes of Ranvier. The axonal debris and myelin start to accumulate in the Schwann cells but later macrophages take over this role. Myelin lipid breaks down over 6–7 days forming cholesterol esters that can be detected by Sudan III/IV dyes. During the first few days axonal transport continues in the proximal segment. The distal part of the proximal portion becomes swollen (diameter 50–100 μm) due to many mitochondria and vesicles. Within about 36 hours of nerve injury the Schwann cells

proliferate to form a continuous column ensheathed by their basement membrane (**bands of Büngner**). These act as a guide for newly formed regenerating axons and provide myelin sheaths for these axons. If no regenerating axons penetrate the axons then they undergo atrophy.

2. **Regeneration of axons**: Starts about a week after injury. The neural cell body swells with displacement of the nucleus away from the axon hillock. Nissl substance fades away. Regenerating axons arise either at the site of interruption or from the pre-terminal nodes of Ranvier. They grow along the bands of Büngner with a growth rate of about 2–5 mm/day. If they reach the appropriate end organ they may grow to normal size although the new internodes are shorter than normal. Effectiveness of regeneration is dependent on the size of the nerve and degree of injury (large nerve and severe injury means chances of restoration are slim).

In some cases scar tissue forms between proximal and distal ends making connection with the distal end by sprouting axons impossible. These will then spread out randomly to form a tangle of small fibres: **stump** or **amputation neuroma**.

Segmental demyelination

Definition   Loss of one or more segments of myelin from a nerve in the absence of damage to the axon.

Pathogenesis   In primary demyelinating disease the myelin is first ingested by the Schwann cells but later this role is taken over by macrophages. In autoimmune demyelination (e.g. Guillain–Barré syndrome) macrophages appear to play a more active role and insert their processes through the Schwann cell membrane and attack the myelin sheath exposing the underlying axon. The loss of myelin from axonal segments stimulates remyelination which is preceded by proliferation of Schwann cells which move along the denuded segment and line up along it. New nodes of Ranvier form where these cells abut. New internodes are defined before the process of remyelination has really got under way. New internodes are shorter than normal and the remyelinated segments are variable in length. If there are repeated episodes of demyelination and remyelination excess Schwann cells are produced. These arrange themselves in a whorled pattern round the axon (onion bulbs). These structures are seen in several hereditary neuropathies associated with demyelination such as Charcot–Marie–Tooth disease and in sporadic relapsing segmental demyelinating neuropathies.

....

PERIPHERAL NEUROPATHIES

Classification

1. **Clinical** classification includes two factors:
   a) Distribution

   - mononeuropathy – single nerve only involved
   - mononeuritis multiplex – asymetric involvement of several nerves
   - polyneuropathy – usually diffuse symmetrical process starting distally and extending proximally.

   b) Fibre affected

   - sensory neuropathy
   - motor neuropathy
   - mixed sensory–motor neuropathy
   - autonomic neuropathy.

2. **Pathological classification**
   a) Neuronopathies

   - Affecting the spinal cord, such as loss of anterior horn cells (e.g. poliomyelitis), motor neurone disease, spinal muscular atrophy, spinal cord tumours, paraneoplastic encephalomyelitis, syringomyelia and menigomyelocele.
   - Affecting the dorsal root ganglia, such as virus infections, hereditary sensory neuropathies and ataxia telangiectasia.
   - Affecting the autonomic nervous system, such as diabetes mellitus and amyloidosis.

b) Axonopathies

- Affecting spinal or cranial nerve roots, such as prolapsed intervertebral disc, spinal osteoarthritis, spinal trauma, vertebral collapse, neoplasms, bacterial meningitis and arachnoid adhesions.
- Affecting peripheral nerve trunks, such as direct trauma, compression and vascular disorders (especially the vasculitides).
- Affecting distal axons, such as toxins (e.g. organophospates), nutritional disturbances, drugs and infections (e.g. leprosy).

....

MECHANICAL INJURY

Nerve injury may be classified in ascending order of severity.

Neuropraxia

Mildest degree of peripheral nerve dysfunction expressed in the form of focal conduction block associated with some degree of disorganization of the paranodal structure. Demyelination and axon degeneration are not seen.

Aetiology   Most due to mild compression injury.

Microscopy   Believed to be associated with retraction of myelin in the nodal region. If more severe there may be segmental demyelination of the affected internode.

Natural history and prognosis   Recovery may take weeks but is usually complete.

Axonotmesis

Definition   Injury in which there is axonal as well as myelin damage. The basal lamina of the Schwann cell remains intact.

Aetiology   Likely to occur with persistent nerve compression (e.g. carpal tunnel syndrome).

Pathogenesis   Wallerian degeneration takes place distal to the lesion with associated signs of degeneration such as muscle atrophy. Regeneration starts rapidly, aided by the preservation of the nerve framework.

Microscopy A zone of narrowing is seen in the nerve with expansion of the endoneurium on both sides of the compression but particularly on the proximal side. Compression leads to impaired axonal transport and bulbous swelling on the proximal side, while the distal side starts to atrophy. Demyelination and axon degeneration may be seen at the compression site. At a later stage the nerve fascicle becomes scarred with proliferation of Schwann cells and fibroblasts. Deposits of mucopolysaccharide may be seen and ovoid hyalin bodies (**Renaut bodies**) appear in the endoneurium.

Carpal tunnel syndrome

Definition Commonest entrapment neuropathy. Median nerve compressed within the anatomical compartment defined by the transverse carpal ligament.

Associations Pregnancy, hypothyroidism, rheumatoid disease, diabetes mellitus, acromegaly and amyloidosis.

Clinical features May be bilateral. There is tingling and pain in the hands followed by weakness and later atrophy of the thenar muscles. There is sensory loss in the palm and the three and a half fingers on the radial side of the hand.

Neurotmesis

Aetiology Occurs when nerve continuity including connective tissue sheath is interrupted.

Pathogenesis The absence of intact basal lamina sheaths removes the tubes which guide the regenerating nerve fibres.

....

TOXIC NEUROPATHIES

Most are sensorimotor neuropathies associated with distal axonopathy.

Acrylamide (in monomeric form)

Clinical features   Distal sensorimotor neuropathy associated with limb ataxia. Tendon areflexia is present even in the mildest form. Patients complain of excessive sweating.

Microscopy   Selective loss of myelinated fibres. Myelinated fibres affected only in severest cases.

Hexacarbons

These include n-Hexane, used as a solvent in glues, and n-butyl-ketone, used in the manufacture of PVC.

Pathogenesis   Possibly via the common metabolite 2,5-heaxanedione.

Clinical features   Distal sensorimotor neuropathy developing slowly and progessing for about 4 months after exposure has ceased.

Microscopy   Focal axonal enlargement (some neuro-filamants up to 10 nm diameter) with thinning of the myelin sheath.

Organophosphorus compounds

Pathogenesis   Most cases have resulted from exposure to one single large oral dose. The axonopathy has a lag phase occuring 7–21 days after exposure.

Clinical features   Abrupt onset of distal limb paraesthesiae followed by development of predominantly motor neuropathy. Not infrequently there is atrophy of leg muscles and interosseus muscles of the hand. Signs of corticospinal tract dysfunction are common.

Microscopy   Distal axonal degeneration associated with axon loss in the corticospinal tract and in the gracile fasciculi.

Drugs

Aetiology   Associated with several drugs including isoniazid, vincristine, nitrofurantoin, chloraquine, amiodarone, metronidazole and gold.

Clinical features   Most produce a chronic and progressive sensorimotor polyneuropathy.

Microscopy   Variable. With vinca alkaloids there is accumulation of neurofilaments and paracrystalline material in neuronal cell bodies and in axons.

....

INFECTIVE AXONOPATHY

Leprosy

Pathogenesis   Depends on the immune reaction to *Mycobacterium leprae* with the two extremes, lepromatous and tuberculoid leprosy, having counterparts in the nerves.

Lepromatous leprosy

Clinical features   The neuropathy is diffuse with a distribution that reflects the requirement of the bacilli for low temperature for proliferation. Thus the distal extremities of the limbs, the nose, ears, supra-orbital regions and the skin of the zygomatic arch may be affected. Sensory loss affects pain and temperature. The peripheral nerves may become thickened, producing a superimposed entrapment neuropathy.

Microscopy   In the early stages the nerve shows inflammatory reaction in the perineurium and epineurium. Numerous bacilli are present within fibroblasts in the perineurium and epineurium, within macrophages and within Schwann cells. Loss of myelinated and unmyelinated axons is present and there is evidence of demyelination.

Tuberculoid leprosy

Clinical features   There are localized areas of skin anaesthesia with sharply demarcated edges and associated anhydrosis. Cutaneous nerves are often thickened and there are lesions within the nerves resembling cold abscesses.

Microscopy   Epithelioid granulomas are present. Few bacilli are seen. In late stages there is extensive and severe endoneurial scarring associated with disorganization of the nerve architecture.

PERIPHERAL NEUROPATHIES CHARACTERIZED BY DEMYELINATION

Acquired

Acute inflammatory demyelinating polyradiculopathy (Guillain–Barré syndrome)

Epidemiology Now the commonest acute neuropathy and the commonest cause of paralysis in Europe and the USA. Males more than females. Peak incidence 20–50 years.

Aetiology About two-thirds give a history of infection 1–4 weeks before appearance of the neuropathy including trivial upper respiratory tract or gastrointestinal infections, infections with cytomegalovirus, Epstein–Barr virus or mycoplasma.

Pathogenesis Thought to be an autoimmune process involving both cellular and humoral mechanisms.

Clinical symptoms Mostly a symmetrical motor weakness associated with early loss of tendon reflexes. Distal muscle groups are affected initially but this is associated with ascending paralysis which may involve respiratory muscles. Distal sensory loss and autonomic abnormalities may occur.

Laboratory findings CSF protein is raised but the cell count is normal. Anti-neural antibodies may be detected.

Electrodiagnostic findings Significant reduction in nerve conduction velocity, conduction block and signs of denervation are present.

Microscopy The nerves show an inflammatory reaction which is initially perivascular but migrates into the endoneurium. Macrophages dominate the cell population. These insert their processes into the myelin sheath and strip away the lamellae of myelin from the axons. The segmental demyelination is accompanied by Schwann cell proliferation and remyelination. Usually the axons remain intact, but there may be secondary loss.

Natural history and prognosis Recovery may take up to 3–6 months or longer. The high mortality previously seen has fallen but deaths do occur mostly due to respiratory paralysis and its complications.

Chronic inflammatory demyelinating polyradiculoneuropathy (CIDP)

Clinical features Similar to Guillain–Barré syndrome but follows a chronic relapsing course.

Microscopy Widespread demyelination in peripheral nerves and spinal roots associated with variable degrees of inflammation. Oedema may be present in the myelin sheath. 'Onion bulbs', denoting episodes of demyelination and remyelination, may be seen.

Diabetic neuropathy

Symmetrical polyneuropathy

Pathogenesis Loss of axons most prominent distally but may affect dorsal nerve roots. In some cases there is segmental demyelination and occasional small 'onion bulbs'. May be due to diabetic microvascular disease affecting endoneurial capillary networks.

Clinical features Earliest features are the loss of vibration sense, deep pain sensation and temperature sense. This is commonest in the feet but may involve the hands ('glove and stocking' distribution). Motor neuropathy leads to atrophy of interosseus muscles and results in failure to counter long flexor muscles giving a high arch and clawing of the toes. Some develop painful neuropathy with burning pain in the feet, shins and anterior surfaces of the thigh, which is worse at night. An autonomic neuropathy gives a variety of features including cardiovascular abnormalities (tachycardia, loss of sinus rhythm, postural hypotension), urinary bladder abnormalities (loss of tone and stasis), gastrointestinal tract abnormalities (gastroparesis, vomiting, diarrhoea) and impotence.

Focal or multifocal neuropathy

Clinical features May occur in acute or chronic form. The acute form affects particularly nerves supplying the lower limb and cranial nerves most notably the 3rd nerve. In chronic neuropathies more than 50% show involvement of the radial or ulna nerve.

Microscopy Focal demyelinating lesions are seen in the affected cranial nerves and a variable degree of fibre loss is seen in the focal and multifocal neuropathies. Endoneurial blood vessels show basement membrane thickening.

··

HEREDITARY DEMYELINATING PERIPHERAL NEUROPATHIES

Hereditory sensorimotor neuropathies

Type I: Charcot–Marie–Tooth disease, Roussy–Lévy syndrome.

Genetics Autosomal dominant inheritance in most cases, recessive in a few.

Clinical features Presents in childhood with foot deformities (pes cavus). Distal weakness, muscle wasting and sensory impairment follow and this may spread to upper limb. Roussy-Lévy syndrome additionally has ataxia and upper limb postural tremor.

Microscopy Segmental demyelination, loss of myelinated fibres and 'onion bulbs'. Nerve trunks may be enlarged and thickened.

Type II: neuronal Charcot–Marie–Tooth disease

Definition Progressive axonal disorder presenting later in life and is less severe than type I disorder.

Genetics Both autosomal dominant and recessive (more severe) inheritance has been reported.

Microscopy Axonal loss and relatively little demyelination. Clusters of regenerating axons may be present. Loss of anterior horn cells and dorsal root ganglion cells.

Type III: Déjérine–Sottas Disease

Genetics Autosomal recessive inheritance.

Clinical features Presents in childhood with delayed motor development, limb weakness, skeletal deformities and ataxia. Peripheral nerves are thickened and may be palpable.

Microscopy Extensive development of 'onion bulbs'. Central axons have either a thin myelin sheath or no myelin. There is extensive axonal loss.

Hereditary sensory and autonomic neuropathy (HSAN)

Type I

Genetics Autosomal dominant inheritance.

Clinical features Usually presents in the 2nd decade or later. There is loss of pain and temperature sensation, especially in the feet.

Pathogenesis Degeneration of cells in the dorsal root ganglia initially of the lumbo-sacral region but later affecting the ganglia of the upper limbs.

Microscopy Nerve biopsy shows loss of small myelinated and unmyelinated axons. Large myelinated fibres less severely affected.

Type II

Genetics Autosomal recessive inheritance.

Clinical features Presents usually in infancy with severe and widespread sensory loss affecting all types of sensation. Autonomic disturbance restricted to anhydrosis and gustational facial sweating.

Microscopy Severe loss of myelinated fibres with relative preservation of unmyelinated axons.

Type III (Riley–Day syndrome)

Genetics Autosomal recessive inheritance most often affecting Ashkenazi Jews.

Clinical features Affected infants have difficulty feeding associated with frequent vomiting and risk of developing lung infections. Autonomic disturbances include defective tear formation, postural hypotension, episodic hypertension and defective temperature control. Tendon areflexia and loss of pain sensation are present from birth.

Pathogenesis Aplasia of small sensory and autonomic neurones (sympathetic more affected than parasympathetic).

Microscopy   Sensory nerves show loss of small myelinated axons. Sensory and autonomic ganglia show decreased numbers of neurones.

Other inherited neuropathies
Friedreich's ataxia

Definition   Degenerative spinocerebellar disorder.

Clinical features   In the early stages there is loss of sense of joint position and vibration together with tendon areflexia.

Microsocpy   **No** abnormality in the motor fibres. There is degeneration of sensory fibres, dorsal nerve roots and cells of the lower lumbo-sacral ganglia. Thick myelinated fibres suffer badly. Fine unmyelinated axons tend to be preserved.

Hereditary liability to pressure palsies

Genetics   Autosomal dominant inheritance.

Clinical features   Recurrent nerve palsies associated with mild mechanical compression.

Microscopy   Focal sausage-shaped areas of hypermyelination. Paranodal and segmental demyelination may occur.

Familial amyloid polyneuropathies

Genetics   All autosomal dominant inheritance.

Pathogenesis   Seven varieties. In five types the amyloid is derived from abnormal transthyretin. In type III (van Allen type) amyloid is derived from variant apolipoprotein A1 and in type IV (Finnish type) amyloid is derived from gelsolin.

HEREDITARY METABOLIC NEUROPATHIES
Metachromatic leucodystrophy

Genetics   Autosomal recessive inheritance.

Biochemistry   Set of conditions associated with accumulation of sulphatides due to deficiency of aryl sulphatase A.

Pathogenesis Demyelination in central and peripheral nervous system.

Microscopy Metachromatic membrane-bound inclusions are seen in Schwann cells.

Krabbe's globoid cell leucodystrophy

Genetics Autosomal recessive inheritance.

Biochemistry Lack of galacto-cerebroside-β-galactosidase.

Pathogenesis Accumulation of galacto-cerebroside in macrophage-like cells (globoid cells).

Microscopy Peripheral nerves show demyelination and endoneurial scarring. Globoid cells are seen in the central but not peripheral nervous systems.

Refsum's disease

Genetics Autosomal recessive inheritance.

Biochemistry Accumulation of phytanic acid.

Clinical features Chronic, distal, symmetrical sensorimotor neuropathy. Associated with pigmentary degeneration of the retina and ataxia.

Microscopy Nerves are enlarged due to accumulation of mucoid material in the endoneurium and to Schwann cell hyperplasia and 'onion bulb' formation. The number of myelinated fibres is decreased.

Fabry's disease (angiokeratoma corporis diffusum)

Genetics X-linked recessive inheritance.

Biochemistry Deficiency of ceramide-trihexoside-α-galactosidase A.

Clinical features Affects the skin (dark red telangiectatic lesions), cornea, heart, nervous system and kidney. Peripheral nerve involvement gives mild sensory and autonomic neuropathy with episodes of severe pain in limbs (Fabry crises).

Microscopy Affected nerves show loss of small axons (myelinated and unmyelinated). Inclusions are present in endothelial and perineurial cells showing alternating dark and light lines.

Tangier disease (hereditary deficiency of high density lipoprotein)

Genetics   Autosomal recessive inheritance.

Biochemistry   Absence of apolipoprotein A1 giving low plasma levels of high density lipoprotein. There is no increase in plasma cholesterol but large amounts of cholesterol esters are deposited in tonsil (large and yellow in colour), spleen, lymph nodes, bone marrow, skin and the submucosa of the gastrointestinal tract.

Clinical features   About 50% have neuropathy of varying patterns.

Microscopy   There is severe depletion of small myelinated and unmyelinated axons. Schwann cells contain droplets of neural lipid and cholesterol ester.

Abetalipoproteinaemia (Bassan–Kornzweig disease)

Genetics   Autosomal recessive inheritance.

Biochemistry   Failure of synthesis of apolipoprotein B48 in intestinal lining cells with failure of chylomicron formation. Neuropathy appears to be the result of secondary deficiency of vitamin E.

Clinical features   Malabsorption, abnormal red blood cells (acanthocytes), pigmentary retinal degeneration and symmetrical distal neuropathy.

Microscopy   Demyelination and loss of axons.

The porphyrias

Peripheral nerve involvement may occur in the hepatic porphyrias (acute intermittent porphyria, variegate porphyria, hereditary coproporphyria and porphyria cutania tarda).

Genetics   All hepatic porphyrias (except amino-levulinic acid dehydratase deficiency) show autosomal dominant inheritance.

Acute intermittant porphyria

Epidemiology   Presents in early adult life. Females more than males.

Aetiology May be triggered by alcohol, barbiturates and oral contraceptives.

Clinical features Abdominal pain and vomiting (90%), sensorimotor peripheral neuropathy (70%), tachycardia and hypertension (70%) and neuropsychiatric disorders.

Microscopy Distal axonopathy of dying-back type.

Variegate porphyria

Clinical features Combination of features of acute inter-mittent porphyria and porphyria cutania tarda. There are bullous skin lesions associated with UV light.

....

MISCELLANEOUS NEUROPATHIES
Neoplasm-associated neuropathies

Pathogenesis Neuropathies may develop as a result of direct invasion of the nerve by tumour. Non-metastatic complications of neoplastic disease include a sensorimotor neuropathy (principally lower limbs; associated with carcinoma of lung particularly small cell carcinoma) and a sub-acute sensory neuropathy (associated with small cell carcinoma of the lung) in which there is loss of fibres in the peripheral nerves and sensory roots. In the latter type the loss of ganglion cells in the dorsal roots is associated with a perivascular infiltration of lymphocytes in the ganglia sug-gesting an immune mechanism.

Uraemic neuropathy

Epidemiology Seen in about two-thirds of patients with chronic renal failure.

Clinical features Symmetrical, distal sensorimotor neu-ropathy.

Microscopy Axonal degeneration which is most severe distally.

NORMAL MICROANATOMY AND PHYSIOLOGY

Size Diameter 50–100 mm. Length is variable with an average of about 3 cm although lengths of 4 cm are not uncommon.

Embryology Each fibre develops from fusion of several fetal cells (myoblasts). The nuclei of these cells persist and lie just below the plasma membrane.

Organization Muscle fibres are grouped into bundles (fascicles). Each fibre is enclosed in a delicate endomysium containing capillaries. Each fascicle is bound by a delicate perimysium. Groups of fascicles lie in fibro-adipose tissue in which the larger blood vessels and lymphatics run (epimysium).

HISTOLOGY

The most striking histological feature is the presence of striations. Each myofibril consists of several functional units (sarcomeres) about 2–3 μm long. Electron microscopy shows each sarcomere to have dark and light bands made up of the contractile filaments arranged parallel to the long axis of the sarcomere.

- dark (A) bands: thick filaments (predominantly myosin)
- light (I) bands: thin filaments (actin) attached to the Z disc marking the end of the sarcomere.

Sliding of the actin and myosin filaments past each other is responsible for contraction. This contraction occurs when a signal passes from the motor nerve to the muscle cell generating a potential in the plasma membrane leading to alterations in calcium ion levels within the cytosol of the muscle cell.

Muscle fibres within a single muscle show physiological differences in respect to their twitch speed and fatiguability:

- Type 1: slow twitch. Fatigue resistant.
- Type 2A: fast twitch. Intermediate fatiguability.
- Type 2B: fast twitch. Fatigue rapidly.

Table 45.3 ATPase reactions at different pH

Fibre type	pH 9.4	pH 4.6	pH 4.3
Type 1	pale	dark	dark
Type 2A	dark	pale	pale
Type 2B	dark	intermediate	pale

These can be distinguished by myosin ATPase reactions at different pHs (Table 45.3).

Muscle cells within a single unit are of the same type but fibres consist of several units, and a normal fibre therefore shows a mosaic pattern. Terms used in muscle pathology are given in Table 45.4.

Table 45.4 Terms used in muscle pathology

Hypertrophy	Increase in calibre of the fibre.
Atrophy	Decrease in the size of a fibre.
Fibre splitting	Clefts in the individual muscle fibres.
Malposition of nuclei	Normally nuclei in muscle cells are situated peripherally. Only about 3% lie internally.
Ring fibres	A muscle cell in which the peripheral myofilaments have become reorientated so that they run circumferentially.
Cytoplasmic bodies	Composed of actin filaments packed together to form a central mass from which less densely packed filaments radiate.
Nemaline bodies	Rod-shaped or thread-like bodies 2 μm in length occurring between the muscle in congenital (nemaline) myopathy.
Cores	Well-demarcated areas in type 1 fibres that have been stained to show oxidative enzymes.
`Moth-eaten' fibre	A muscle cell in which there are areas of pallor in fibres stained to show oxidative enzymes. The presence of irregular edges distinguishes them from cores.
Target fibres	Variants of cores with a central granular mass within the muscle surrounded by a halo and then by normal myofibrils.
Vacuoles	Spaces within muscles. Variable in size and content.
Contraction bands	Segments where the muscle fibres stain intensely with eosin. Due to an influx of calcium ions which activate myosin ATPase leading to segmental hypercontraction.

DISORDERS OF SKELETAL MUSCLE

Myopathies

Classification of myopathies (Table 45.5).

Definition Disorder in which the muscle is the primary target.

THE MUSCULAR DYSTROPHIES

The defining characteristics of this disease group is that the conditions are genetically determined, destructive and progressive.

Table 45.5 Classification of myopathies

Destructive myopathies	
Dystrophies	Duchenne type muscular dustrophy Becker type muscular dystrophy Limb girdle dystrophy Fascioscapulohumeral dystrophy Oculopharyngeal dystrophy Scapuloperoneal dystrophy
Inflammatory myopathies	Dermatomyositis associated with polymyositis
Infections	Bacterial or viral infections (e.g. Coxsackie) or infestations
Toxic/drug related	Alcohol Emetine Penicillamine
Non-destructive myelopathies/myotonic syndromes	
Congenital/genetically determined	Myotonic dystrophy Congenital myotonia Centronuclear myopathy Central core disease Minicore disease Nemaline myopathy Mitochondrial myopathy
Associated with type 2 fibre atrophy	Polymyalgia rheumatica Steroid myopathy Endocrine myopathies
Metabolic	Glycogenosis (McArdle's disease) Periodic paralysis Malignant hyperthermia

Duchenne type muscular dystrophy (DMD)

Epidemiology Incidence of 1/3500 live male births and prevalence of about 1 in 1000. Occasionally occurs in females.

Genetics X-linked recessive inheritance. Sporadic mutations account for a substantial proportion of cases. The gene is located on the short arm of the X chromosome (Xp21). In females with the disease there is usually a translocation involving the short arm of the X chromosome. Gives flexibility to the cell membrane thus protecting it during contraction.

Pathogenesis Lack of production of the protein dystrophin which is usually situated on the inner surface of the sarcolemma. It may act as a transmembrane connector between the contractile fibrils within the muscle cells and elements of the extracellular basement membrane. Dystrophin is thought to impart flexibility to the cell membrane and thus to protect it during contraction and relaxation. If flexibility is absent small membrane defects occur allowing excess calcium ions into the cells triggering hypercontraction and ultimately coagulative necrosis.

Clinical features Presents early in childhood, usually by 4 years. Pelvi-femoral muscles appear earliest affected causing clumsiness of gait, frequent falls and difficulty rising. Characteristically the calf muscles are hypertrophied but this disappears with disease progression. The proximal muscle weakness first seen in the lower limbs spreads to the shoulder girdle, arm, neck and trunk. The patients frequently become wheelchair bound between 10–12 years and death usually occurs before the age of 20 years due to either cardiac arrythmia or respiratory difficulties and eventually pneumonia.

Laboratory findings In the early stages there is gross increase in plasma creatinine phosphokinase (10 000 IU/L – normal 60 IU/L). As the muscle mass becomes depleted during the course of the disease these levels gradually decrease.

Microscopy There is segmental necrosis of the muscle fibres followed by invasion of the affected cells by phagocytic macrophages. Small clusters of muscle cells are generally affected. Regeneration follows but fails to compensate for muscle fibre loss. The endomysium and perimysium show fibrosis in the early stages and later there is replacement of muscle by fibro-adipose tissue. In addition to the necrotic fibres there are occasional enlarged and rounded fibres showing deeply eosinophilic cytoplasm (hyaline fibres) representing the hypercontracted fibres.

Becker type muscular dystrophy (BMD)

Genetics   X-linked recessive inheritance.

Pathogenesis   The mutation in the dystrophin gene differs from DMD. Dystrophin is synthesized but is abnormal.

Clinical features   Similar to DMD but milder. The onset of weakness is delayed in some cases to the 2nd decade, the course is more benign and some patients may survive up to 50 years.

Laboratory findings   In some the plasma creatinine phosphokinase levels may be as high as DMD but in others the level is only 10 x normal.

Microscopy   Necrosis and phagocytosis are much less prominent than in DMD though there is still variation in fibre size. An additional feature is fibre splitting which increases in amount with disease progress. Extensive fibrosis and replacement of the muscle by fibro-adipose tissue tends to occur only in the end stages of the disease.

....

GENETICALLY DETERMINED MYOTONIC SYNDROMES

Myotonic dystrophy

Genetics   Autosomal dominant inheritance. The gene (*MyD*) is on the long arm of chromosome 19 (19q13.3). Congenital myotonic dystrophy is occasionally seen. It occurs only in children born to mothers with the disease (even though the expression in the mother may be mild).

Clinical features   Usually presents after the age of 20 years. The clinical hallmarks are myotonia (prolongation of muscle contraction after voluntary effort has ceased) and muscle weakness which in the early stages affects the facial and anterior neck muscles as well as the distal muscle groups of the limbs. There is involvement of multiple organs which results in frontal baldness, cataract (90%), diabetes mellitus and other endocrine abnormalities, cardiomyopathy (leading to cardiac dysrhythmias), mitral valve prolapse, multiple pilomatrixomas of the skin, gonadal atrophy, dementia and smooth muscle dysfunction. In the congenital form hypotonia rather than myotonia is often seen in the neonatal period and the infants may show severe respiratory difficulties. Motor development may be delayed and mental retardation is often present.

Microscopy One of the earliest findings is selective atrophy of type 1 fibres which is accompanied by hypertrophy of type 2 fibres. Central nuclei are seen at an early stage of the disease. Staining for myosin ATPase reaction shows ring fibres. Blebs appear on the sarcolemma which contain eosinophilic cytoplasm staining positively with PAS but not containing myofibrils. Necrosis of the muscle cells is rare. The clinical appearance of wasting is due to muscle atrophy.

Histological examination of biopsies from children with the congenital form shows immaturity of muscle rather than the features described above.

··

CONGENITAL MYOPATHIES

This is a group of often familial diseases presenting with hypotonia, delayed motor development, proximal muscle weakness, facial weaknes in many instances. Death occurs in infancy frequently due to respiratory failure.

Centronuclear myopathies

Genetics The more severe form has an X-linked recessive inheritance (also known as myotubular myopathy) but a milder form shows an autosomal dominant inheritance.

Clinical features In the X-linked form the infants show striking hypotonia and are at risk of dying from repiratory failure early in life. In the autosomal form there tends to be later onset and slow progression giving a picture similar to limb-girdle dystrophies.

Microscopy In the X-linked form there are centrally placed nuclei and sections stained for myosin ATPase show an unstained perinuclear halo. Type 1 fibres predominate. In the autosomal form there are also central nuclei but the muscle cells are much larger and appear more mature.

Nemaline myopathy

Genetics Evidence of autosomal dominant and autosomal recessive inheritance patterns.

Clinical features Affected infants tend to present with hypotonia and muscle weakness. Respiratory failure may cause death in infancy. Skeletal abnormalities such as kyphoscoliosis and high arched palate may be seen and the muscles of the face may be particularly affected.

Microscopy There is predominance of type 1 fibres and very large numbers of small rod-shaped bodies within the sarcoplasm.

Electron microscopy The rod-shaped bodies show the same periodicity and lattice structure as Z discs.

Central core disease

Genetics May be sporadic or show autosomal recessive or dominant inheritance.

Clinical features Onset of muscle weakness is usually delayed until the child has started to walk or later.

Microscopy Great preponderance of type 1 fibres. There are well-demarcated, centrally located zones of pallor (cores). The myofibrils within these cores may be disrupted or normal but there is a lack of mitochondria and/or the junctions between T-tubules and the sarcoplasmic reticulum.

Mitochondrial encephalomyopathies

Classification Some clearly defined syndromes associated with mutations of the mitochondrial genome include:

- **C**hronic **p**rogressive **e**xternal **o**phthalmoplegia (**CPEO**). Characterized by ptosis and ophthalmoplegia which is followed by weakness in the muscles of the shoulder girdle and upper limbs. Associated with large deletions on certain mitochondrial genes. Sporadic.
- **M**yopathy, **e**ncephalopathy, **l**actic **a**cidosis, **s**troke (**MELAS**). Associated with point mutations on mitochondrial certain genes. Inherited through the maternal line.
- **M**yoclonic **e**pilepsy and **r**agged **r**ed **f**ibres (**MERRF**). Associated with point mutations on certain mitochondrial genes. Inherited through the maternal line.

Pathogenesis Mitochondrial proteins are derived from two sources. DNA from the cell's nucleus with the proteins transported across the mitochondrial membrane from the cytosol or from mitochondrial DNA which shows a strictly maternal rather than Mendelian pattern of inheritance. Cells most severely and commonly affected are the 'permanent' cells such as neurones, cardiac muscle and skeletal muscle.

Microscopy The defining morphological criterion of mitochondrial myopathies is the ragged red fibre – a muscle fibre containing large aggregates of peripheral and interfibrillar mitochondria appearing as red granules in frozen section stained with a modified Gomori trichrome stain. The abnormal fibres show more fine droplets of neutral lipid than normal.

....

METABOLIC MYOPATHIES

Definition This term is applied to specific enzyme defects interfering with normal energy production of the muscle cell (principally derived from glycogen, glucose and free fatty acids).

Clinical features Disorders are expressed in two main forms, either with progressive weakness or muscle cramps induced by exercise (may or may not be associated with muscle necrosis and myoglobinuria).

Microscopy Vacuoles are present within the muscle cells. These contain either accumulations or carbohydrate or lipid.

The gycogenoses

Type II (infantile form = Pompe's disease)

Biochemistry Acid maltase deficiency.

Clinical features Pompe's disease (infantile form) is generalized and usually fatal. Infants are floppy with massive cardiomegaly and less pronounced hepatomegaly. Death due to cardiac or respiratory failure usually occurs before 2 years. The childhood/adult forms present with myopathy without cardiac involvement. In childhood there is calf hypertrophy similar to Duchenne muscular dystrophy. Death may occur in the second or third decade; in the childhood form usually due to respiratory failure.

Microscopy In the infantile form the vacuoles in the muscle are very numerous but this is less marked in the childhood and adult forms. The accumulated glycogen is stored in lysosomes and in the cytoplasm where it may form large pools.

Type III (Cori–Forbes disease)

Biochemistry Debrancher deficiency.

Clinical features Childhood disease with hepatomegaly, failure of normal growth and fasting hypoglycaemia. Significant myopathy is uncommon but some affected individuals develop wasting of the leg muscles and intrinsic muscles of the hand in the third or forth decade.

Microscopy Severe vacuolar myopathy.

Type IV (Andersen's disease)

Biochemistry Branching enzyme deficiency.

Clinical features Liver disease is prominent leading to cirrhosis. Death usually occurs by 4 years due to liver failure or from bleeding associated with portal hypertension.

Microscopy Basophilic deposits are present which are stained with periodic acid Schiff stain.

Electron microscopy Granules are an abnormal polysaccharide with a filamentous and/or granular structure.

Type V (McArdle's disease)

Biochemistry Deficiency of muscle phosphorylases.

Genetics Autosomal recessive inheritance. Gene is located on the long arm of chromosome 11.

Clinical features There is exercise intolerance characterized by muscle pain, early fatigue and muscle cramps caused by brief intense exercise or sustained less intense exercise. Some will develop muscle necrosis and myoglobinuria associated with the exercise. Permanent muscle weakness is seen in some patients, particularly the elderly.

Microscopy Glycogen vacuoles are present in both subsarcolemmal and interfibrillary locations.

Type VII (Tarui's disease)

Biochemistry Muscle phosphofructokinase deficiency.

Genetics Autosomal recessive inheritance.

Clinical features Similar to McArdle's disease although muscle necrosis and myoglobinuria is less common. Differentiation between the two requires biochemical studies of muscle.

Microscopy Resembles McArdle's disease.

Type IX

Biochemistry Phosphoglycerate kinase deficiency.

Clinical features May be silent or present in one of two forms either with mental retardation, seizures and haemolytic anaemia in infancy/early childhood or with exercise intolerance and recurrent episodes of myoglobinuria in childhood/early adult life.

Type X

Biochemistry Phosphoglycerate mutase deficiency.

Clinical features Extremely rare. There is intolerance to extreme exercise associated with muscle pain, cramps and myoglobinuria.

Type XI

Biochemistry Lactic acid dehydrogenase deficiency.

Clinical features Extremely rare. Presents with exercise intolerance and recurrent myoglobinuria.

....

INFLAMMATORY MYOPATHIES

Clinical features All share the same clinical features. There is gradual and insidious onset of muscle weakness with the precise manifestation depending on the muscle groups involved.

Laboratory findings There are increased plasma concentrations of creatine phosphokinase.

Dermatomyositis

Epidemiology Affects both genders. May occur at any age.

Pathogenesis Possible that the muscle necrosis is secondary to ischaemia due to an antibody mediated attack on capillaries.

Clinical features In adults about 15% are associated with malignancy (most commonly adenocarcinoma of the stomach, breast, ovary, lung and colon). In some resection of the neoplasm is followed by regression of symptoms.

Microscopy There is all stages of segmental necrosis and regeneration of fibres. The inflammatory infiltrate is predominantly B lymphocytes and is concentrated in the perimysial connective tissue. T lymphocytes (mainly CD4 positive, helper) are seen in the endomysial region. Areas of necrosis involve small groups of fibres suggesting ischaemic damage and there is a relative decrease in capillaries in the affected areas. The skin changes seen in this disease are either those of non-specific dermatitis or similar to those seen in systemic lupus erythematosus.

Polymyositis

Pathogenesis Thought that the muscle injury is due to attack by cytotoxic T cells.

Microscopy T cells are accompanied by macrophages. The necrotic muscle cells are surrounded by CD8 positive T cells. The inflammatory infiltrate is focal and predominantly endomysial.

Inclusion body myositis

Epidemiology Predominantly affects the elderly.

Clinical features Insidious onset. Unresponsive to steroids (in contrast to dermatomyositis and polymyositis).

Microscopy The inflammatory infiltrate is chiefly endomysial and is mainly composed of cytotoxic T cells. The defining criteria are the presence of vacuoles bordered by basophilic material within the muscle fibres (believed to be lysosomal) and the presence of eosinophilic inclusions within muscle cells.

....

RHABDOMYOLYSIS

Aetiology Sometimes associated with influenza. Many drugs and toxins have been implicated.

Clinical features In the acute form there is sudden onset of severe pain, flaccid paralysis of the affected muscles and myoglobinuria which may be severe enough to cause acute renal failure.

Laboratory findings Greatly inceased plasma levels of creatine phosphokinase.

Microscopy There is coagulative necrosis of muscle fibres which elicits a mild interstitial inflammatory response.

....

THE EFFECTS OF DENERVATION

Aetiology Results from damage to lower motor neurones.

Microscopy There is a combination of atrophy of muscle fibres and cytoplasmic changes. A single anterior horn cell innervates many muscle cells that are close to each other but admixed with cells innervated by other motor units. Interruption of the nerve supply results in atrophy of the group of fibres innervated by the affected nerve. As the myofibrils and myofilaments of an individual fibre atrophy that fibre become compressed by adjacent fibres and assumes an angular shape. Eventually the fibre becomes completely atrophic and the nuclei condense to form aggregates. The cytoplasmic changes include darker staining of sections stained for oxidative enzymes. Target fibres occur in up to 20% of cases.

THE EFFECTS OR REINNERVATION

Pathogenesis Denervated fibres act as the stimulus for the sprouting of new nerve fibres from the pre-terminl regions of adjacent normal axons. This sprouting is associated with branching of the terminal axon so that a single axon may supply a number of muscle fibres. The physiological and enzyme pattern of the individual muscle cells depends on the electrical stimuli received from the nerve thus leading to a change in the muscle fibre type.

Microscopy There may be quite large groups of muscle fibres of the same type (type grouping). Rapidly progressive disease is reflected by type 1 fibre predominance while slowly progressive denervation is usually associated with type 2 fibre grouping.

DEFECTS IN NEUROMUSCULAR TRANSMISSION

Myasthenia gravis and other myesthenic syndromes

Definition A set of autoimmune disorders in which antibodies bind either to the acetylcholine receptor on the motor end plate (myasthenia gravis and neonatal myasthenia) or to the presynaptic membrane (Lambert–Eaton syndrome associated with malignancy).

Pathogenesis In myasthenia gravis and neonatal myasthenia IgG autoantibodies that bind to epitopes of the acetylcholine receptor are present in the serum. Binding of these antibodies to the receptor blocks the action of acetylcholine and binds complement leading to the destruction of the receptor. Neonatal myasthenia occurs in 10–15% of infants born to mothers with myasthenia gravis due to anti-acetylcholine receptor IgG antibodies crossing the placenta. The Lambert–Eaton syndrome is associated with muscle wasting in the proximal limbs and trunk and is due to an autoantibody that binds to the pre-synaptic membrane inhibiting the release of acetylcholine.

Associations Myasthenia gravis shows strong associations with abnormalities of the thymus. Up to 40% patients with myasthenia gravis have a thymoma (symptoms relieved by thymectomy) and up to 75% of the remainder have thymic hyperplasia (symptoms also relieved by thymectomy). Lambert–Eaton syndrome is most often associated with small cell carcinoma of the lung.

Clinical features There is abnormal muscle fatiguability and muscle weakness.

Special senses

DISORDERS OF THE EYELIDS

Developmental abnormalities

Dermoid cysts

Site Often affect the upper lid. Rest on or attached to periostium of orbital ridges.

Clinical features Rounded lesions not greater than 1 cm diameter, soft and non-tender.

Microscopy Cyst lined by well-differentiated epidermis and containing keratinous debris.

Inflammatory disorders

STY (hodeolum)

Definition Acute suppurative inflammation involving the hair follicles or the ducts of the sebaceous or apocrine glands.

Aetiology *Staphylococcus aureus* is frequently implicated.

Clinical features Red and tender lesion which may discharge pus through the eyelash follicle.

Chalazion

Definition Chronic inflammatory lesion involving the meibomian glands.

Pathogenesis Blockage of the gland causes increased intraductal pressure and rupture releasing lipid-rich material.

Microscopy Florid inflammatory reaction with lipid-laden macrophages lymphocytes and plasma cells.

Cysts of Moll's glands

Clinical features Thin-walled transparent blister-like lesions.

Site Free margin of lid.

Microscopy Unilocular cysts usually lined by atrophic cuboidal epithelium.

Xanthelasma

Site Medial aspect of both lids.

Clinical features Yellow plaque-like lesions. In young people they are associated with hyperlipidaemic states but in the middle aged and elderly there is no association with lipid metabolism.

Microscopy Aggregates of lipid-laden macrophages.

....

TUMOURS OF THE EYELID

In general these are tumours that may occur at other skin sites.

Naevus of ota

Definition A pigmented melanocytic naevus which is thought to be an extrasacral form of Mongolian blue spot.

Epidemiology Most common in orientals and Afro-Caribbeans.

Site Region supplied by the first and second branches of the trigeminal nerve.

....

DISEASES OF THE CONJUNCTIVA

Degenerative disorders

Pinguecula

Site Bulbar conjunctiva in the inter-palpebral area.

Clinical features Small yellowish area of thickening.

Microscopy Elastosis of the subepithelial tissues with hyalinization of the interfibrillar ground substance. In some the epithelium is atrophic while in others it is thickened.

Pterygium

Site Junction between the sclera and cornea and spreads to involve the corneal conjunctiva.

Clinical features As the lesion spreads over the cornea it causes opacification and visual impairment.

Microscopy There is elastosis, new blood vessel formation and chronic inflammation.

Squamous metaplasia

Definition Replacement of the thin non-keratinizing epithelium by thick opaque keratinized squamous epithelium.

Aetiology Several conditions predispose to squamous metaplasia including dry eyes (lack of tears), vitamin A deficiency, severe exophthalmos, paralysis of the muscles or the eyelids and graft-versus-host disease.

Inflammatory diseases: infective

Definition May involve the conjunctiva alone (conjunctivitis), the cornea alone (keratitis) or both (keratoconjunctivitis).

Bacterial

Epidemiology Common, especially in childhood.

Aetiology *Haemophilus aegyptius*, staphylococci and *Streptococcus pneumoniae*. Infection with *Neisseria gonorrhoeae* may occur in the newborn following transmission from the birth canal during delivery. Congenital syphilis affects the cornea causing interstitial inflammation for 2–3 months followed by new blood vessel formation.

Viral

Aetiology Most common are caused by herpes viruses and adenoviruses. Measles may cause a mild to moderate conjunctivitis.

Clinical features   Herpes infection may cause ulceration. In sub-Saharan Africa measles is frequently associated with corneal ulceration followed by scarring and blindness.

Chlamydial

Trachoma

Epidemiology   Single most important cause of blindness in developing countries.

Aetiology   *Chlamydia trachomatis* mainly serotypes A, B and C. Spread by eye–eye contact through flies.

Microscopy   There are large lymphoid follicles with germinal centres which may undergo necrosis. Inclusions can be found in the epithelial cells. The cellular infiltrate is replaced by granulation tissue and then scar tissue.

Chlamydial ophthalmitis in neonates

Aetiology   Generally serotypes D–I. Infection during delivery.

Protozoal

Aetiology   *Acanthamoeba castellani* and *A. polyphaga*. Found in brackish or sea water but can contaminate contact lens cleaning solutions (saline).

Pathogenesis   Repeated minor trauma associated with contact lens use may promote infection.

Helminthic

Aetiology   Onchocerciasis (Loa Loa) caused by *Onchocerca volvulus*. Transmitted by blackflies which inject lava into host dermis. Microfilaria migrate from skin of face.

Clinical features   Conjunctiva and cornea show fluffy opacities which in the cornea lead to scarring and blindness.

Non-Infective causes

Immune

Aetiology   Allergic conjunctivitis may occur when there is contamination of the atmosphere by pollens (vernal conjunctivitis).

Site Bilateral.

Clinical features Flat-topped papillae on oedematous conjunctiva.

Microscopy The infiltrate is rich in eosinophils.

Tumours of the conjunctiva

Papilloma

Epidemiology Relatively common.

Aetiology Possibly related to human papilloma virus infection.

Clinical features In children it is frequently bilateral. Tends to recur.

Microscopy Typical appearances of a papilloma with varying degrees of keratinization and acanthosis.

Intraepithelial carcinoma (carcinoma in situ)

Clinical features Area of leukoplakia or papillary lesion. May complicate pterygium.

Microscopy Identical to those of carcinoma in situ at other mucous membranes.

Invasive squamous carcinoma

Microscopy Similar to that of squamous carcinomas elsewhere but some deeply infiltrative tumours may have an adenosquamous pattern similar to mucoepidermoid carcinoma.

Melanocytic naevi and malignant melanoma

Epidemiology Melanocytic naevi are not uncommon but melanoma is very rare.

Microscopy Naevi tend to be either junctional or compound and often show cystic epithelial inclusions.

....

DISORDERS OF THE CORNEA

Keratoconus

Definition Congenital ectasia of the central part of the cornea.

Epidemiology Usually within first decade. Associated with atopy and Down's syndrome.

Microscopy Breaks in Bowman's membrane (below epithelium) with thinning of stroma.

Fuchs' endothelial dystrophy

Epidemiology Age-related disorder.

Pathogenesis Affects endothelium and Descemet's membrane (posterior surface of the corneal stroma; covered by a layer of endothelial cells which controls fluid content of corneal stroma). Loss of endothelium results in failure to control fluid content and results in corneal oedema. May be precipitated by cataract surgery.

Inherited corneal dystrophies

Lattice dystrophy

Genetics Autosomal dominant inheritance.

Microscopy Amyloid deposition within the stroma and scarring of Bowman's membrane.

Granular dystrophy

Genetics Autosomal dominant inheritance.

Microscopy Protein crystals deep to Bowman's membrane in central part of cornea.

Macular dystrophy

Genetics Autosomal recessive inheritance.

Clinical features Usually severe visual impairment by 30 years of age.

Microscopy Deposition of glycosoaminoglycan in the cornea.

Herpes infection of the cornea

Dendritic ulceration

Clinical features Ulcers have a branched appearance which can be seen by fluorescein staining (stains expose

Bowman's membrane). If Bowman's membrane is intact healing is without scarring.

Microscopy Damage largely confined to the epithelium.

Stromal keratitis

Microscopy Stromal and epithelial oedema frequently with damage to Bowman's membrane. Patchy infiltrate of neutrophils and lymphocytes is seen. Characteristic nuclear inclusions are present and giant cells can be seen in Descemet's membrane.

....

THE LENS
Cataract

Definition Opacification of the lens.

Aetiology Many different aetiologies:

- genetic with cataract alone (autosomal dominant)
- genetic with systemic syndrome (Alport's and Marfan's syndromes)
- congenital (associated with trisomy 13, consequence of rubella infection)
- galactosaemia
- diabetes
- drugs (long-term steroids, dinitophenol)
- long-term exposure to UV light or irradiation
- trauma
- age related.

....

THE UVEAL TRACT (IRIS, CILIARY BODY AND CHOROID)
Uveitis

Definition Inflammation may principally involve one of the areas e.g. the iris (iritis), ciliary body (cyclitis) or the choroid (choroiditis).

Clinical features There is a red painful eye with sensitivity to bright light, blurring of vision, slight pupillary constriction and in some cases pus in the anterior chamber of the eye.

Aetiology May be an isolated phenomenon or associated with some other disease such as Reiter's syndrome, ankylosing spondylitis, ulcerative colitis, juvenile rheumatoid arthritis and Behçet's disease.

Sympathetic ophthalmitis

Definition Penetrating injury resulting in protrusion of uveal tract is followed by uveal tract inflammation in the contralateral eye.

Pathogenesis Thought to be an autoimmune disease.

Clinical features The lag phase is usually 4–6 weeks but may be up to several years. Removal of the injured eye prevents damage in the other eye if performed before such damage begins.

Microscopy Granulomatous inflammation affecting the choroid.

Glaucoma

Definition Disorders resulting in raised intraocular pressure.

Open-angle glaucoma

Definition Increased resistance to outflow in trabecular meshwork.

Epidemiology The primary form is usually seen in the elderly and may be familial.

Aetiology May be primary or secondary due to blockage of the meshwork by red cells, macrophages (following rupture of hypermature cataract) or exfoliated flakes of glycoprotein from basement membrane.

Closed-angle glaucoma

Aetiology Obstruction to the meshwork at the root of the iris. May be primary or secondary due to adhesions between peripheral part of the cornea and iris.

Natural history and prognosis High pressure may cause damage to the cornea, retina or optic nerve.

THE RETINA

Inherited disorders of the retina

Retinitis pigmentosa

Genetics Mostly autosomal recessive inheritance but occasionally autosomal dominant or X-linked recessive.

Pathogenesis There is degeneration of photoreceptor cells and accumulation of pigment within the retina.

Clinical features Visual fields become limited with disease progression. Fundoscopy reveals pale optic nerve and attenuation of retinal blood vessels.

Vascular diseases

Occlusion of the central retinal artery

Aetiology Usually impaction of embolus from the left side of the heart (e.g. infective endocarditis, atrial myxoma) or from an atherosclerotic plaque in the carotid vessels.

Pathogenesis Irreversible ischaemic damage is due to this being an anatomical end-artery.

Clinical features There is often sudden onset of blindness. The retina is pale and the arterial branches are thread-like. The choroid lying deep to the macula is seen as a central red spot (cherry red spot; also seen in Tay–Sachs' disease).

Occlusion of the central retinal vein

Epidemiology Mostly elderly.

Aetiology Associated with glaucoma, hypertension and atherosclerotic disease.

Pathogenesis Occlusion is associated with marked engorgement of retinal veins draining into the central vein which can lead to haemorrhages and there is also severe retinal oedema.

Clinical features In 20% of patients new vessels form which may affect the anterior surface of the iris and lead to adhesions and to closed-angle glaucoma.

Retrolental fibroplasia

Epidemiology Virtually restricted to premature infants.

Aetiology   Exposure to high concentrations of oxygen.

Pathogenesis   High oxygen concentration leads to obliteration of developing blood vessels resulting in lack of normal vascularization of the peripheral part of the retina. From this ishaemic part there is secretion of vascular growth factor leading to overgrowth of new vessels, traction on the retina, retinal detachment and blindness.

Senile macular degeneration

Epidemiology   Cause of visual impairment in the elderly.

Aetiology   Unknown.

Clinical features   Loss of central vision with preservation of peripheral vision for long periods.

Microscopy   Accumulation of lipid-rich material in the pigmented epithelial cells and within Bruch's membrane (limiting zone between the pigmented epithelium and the retina proper).

....

INTRAOCULAR TUMOURS

Malignant melanoma

Epidemiology   Commonest malignant intraocular tumour in adults.

Site   Derived from the pigment-producing cells of the uveal tract. Choroid (85%) or ciliary body (10%) most frequently.

Microscopy   Three varieties are described which may occur alone or, more frequently, in combination.

- Spindle cell A – slender cells with small fusifiom nuclei and no nucleoli.
- Spindle cell B – larger and more pleomorphic. Large oval nuclei with prominant nucleoli. Higher number of mitoses.
- Epithelioid – largest cells of all with irregular appearance. Abundant cytoplasm and often multiple and bizarre nuclei.

Natural history and prognosis   Death due to metastases may occur in 46% following enucleation of affected eye.

Important prognostic factors include cell type (epithelioid the worst, while spindle-cell A can almost be regarded as benign tumours), size, site (tumours in iris have best prognosis), extra-scleral invasion, necrosis and prominence of nucleoli.

Retinoblastoma

Epidemiology Commonest intraocular tumour in childhood.

Clinical features Most commonly presents with a white pupillary reflex and less commonly with a squint.

Microscopy Dense masses of small round cells with dark staining nuclei and little cytoplasm. If better differentiated there may be rosettes. Patchy necrosis is common. Darkly staining debris is seen in the walls of small blood vessels.

Natural history and prognosis Tumours may invade the optic nerve and then spead to brain or metastasize via cerebrospinal fluid. Uveal invasion is common. Metastases may be extracranial (mostly skeletal). If treatment is adequate survival for unilateral retinoblastima is more than 90%. Bilateral tumours have lower survival.

Aetiology May arise on the basis of pre-existing naevus.

THE EAR

NORMAL STRUCTURE

The external ear

Consists of a pinna, the external auditory meatus and a canal from the pinna to the tympanic membrane. The pinna is largely cartilage covered by skin. Glands open on to the meatal surface that secretes a waxy substance (cerumen).

The middle ear

Cavity separating the tympanic membrane from the semicircular canals and cochlea. Communicates anteriorly with the pharynx via the eustachian tube and posteriorly with the mastoid air cells.

The inner ear

Consists of the semi-circular canals and cochlea. The vestibular and auditory nerves arise from the inner ear and travel to the brain via the internal auditory meatus.

....

DISORDERS OF THE EXTERNAL EAR

Developmental abnormalities

Pre-auricular sinus

Pathogenesis Abnormal fusion of the facial folds producing a blind-ending epithelial track.

Site Anterior to the external auditory meatus.

Natural history and prognosis May become blocked to form a keratin-filled cyst or may become infected.

Diagonal ear lobe crease

Site Crease runs downward and backward from external auditory meatus.

Natural history and prognosis Thought to be associated with an increased risk of death from cardivascular disease.

Inflammatory disorders

Relapsing polychondritis

Definition Disorder affecting cartilage, eye and heart.

Pathogenesis Thought to be an autoimmune disorder.

Clinical features In the ear there is reddening, swelling and pain of the pinna associated with atrophy and distortion as the cartilage is destroyed.

Cauliflower ear

Definition Thickening and distortion of the pinna.

Pathogenesis Partial organization of repeated haematomas secondary to trauma.

Chondrodermatitis nodularis chronica

Pathogenesis Possibly secondary to trauma or cold.

Clinical features Painful nodule on the superior portion of the helix. There is often ulceration of the skin.

Microscopy The cartilage under the ulceration is degenerate and there is inflammation of the perichondrium.

....

DISORDERS OF THE MIDDLE EAR

Inflammatory disorders

Otitis media

Epidemiology Common in children.

Aetiology Usually bacterial and often follows an upper respiratory tract infection.

Pathogenesis Impaired drainage of the middle ear due to blockage of eustachian tube predisposes to infection.

Clinical features Earache. Otoscopic examination shows reddened and tense tympanic membrane.

Natural history and prognosis Complications include spread to the mastoid air spaces and thus to the meninges and brain. Chronic otitis media may develop (but may also develop in the absence of an acute presentation) causing persistent earache, conduction deafness and chronic discharge from the external auditory meatus. There may be granulation tissue which protrudes through a tympanic membrane perforation (aural polyp). Cholesterol granuloma (yellow nodules in the tympanic cavity and mastoid) are granulomatous inflammation around cholesterol crystals usually as a consequence of previous haemorrhage. Tympanosclerosis may develop with dense hyalinized collagen within the middle ear especially affecting the tympanic membrane and crura of the stapes, with or without spotty dystrophic calcification. Otitis media with effusion (glue ear) is a common complication and causes impaired hearing in children; it is characterized by an effusion in the middle ear which does not drain due to blockage of the eustachian tube.

Cholesteatoma

Definition A mass of actively growing keratinizing stratified squamous epithelium within the middle ear.

Classification
- congenital – believed to arise from an epithelial rest in the developing middle ear
- acquired – usually occurs in the upper and posterior portion of the middle ear. Can expand and erode the adjacent bony structures including the ossicles.

Disorders of the ossicles

Otosclerosis

Site Affects mainly the cochlea and the footplate of the stapes with fixation of the stapes.

Clinical features A major cause of conduction deafness.

Microscopy The footplate of the stapes resembles the appearances of Paget's disease of bone with foci of woven bone and numerous 'cement lines'.

Neoplasms of the middle ear

Paraganglioma (Glomus jugulare)

Site Most paragangliomas arise from paraganglionic tissue in the wall of the jugular bulb. A few arise from paraganglia sited near the middle ear surface of the promontory.

Clinical features Present as red masses behind the tympanic membrane or within the external auditory canal.

Microscopy There are well-defined nests of catecholamine containing cells separated from each other by vascular connective tissue. The nests are surrounded by an attenuated layer of sustentacular cells which do not contain catecholamine but mark for S100 protein.

Natural history and prognosis Usually slow growing but may invade deeply into the petrous bone. Metastases occur only rarely but recurrences are common.

....

DISORDERS OF THE INNER EAR

Presbyacusis

Definition Degenerative condition involving various parts of the cochlea.

Pathogenesis   There is loss of hair cells.

Ménière's disease

Epidemiology   More common in males than females.

Site   Bilateral in 20% cases.

Clinical features   Affects hearing and balance and causes episodic deafness, tinnitus and vertigo.

Pathogenesis   Excess fluid accumulates in the endolymphatic spaces of the cochlea leading to their distention. The elastic Reissner's membrane bulges into the vestibular cavity.

Acoustic neuroma

Site   From the Schwann cells of the VIIIth cranial nerve. Most are unilateral but 10% are bilateral and associated with neurofibromatosis type 2.

Index

Abetalipoproteinaemia, 374, 923
Abscess, 46–7
  breast, 599
  cerebral/brain, 871, 876
  crypt, in ulcerative colitis, 393
  lung, 311–12
Acanthamoebiasis, 942
Acanthosis nigricans, 188
Acathanolytic dermatosis, 760
Accessory spleen, 738
2-Acetyl-aminofluorine, 207–8
Achalasia, 350
Achondroplasia, 804–5
Acid phosphatase, 188
Acid secretion, gastric, 354
Acidosis, renal tubular, 488
Acinar emphysema, 296–7, 297
Acinic cell carcinoma, 346–7
Acinus
  hepatic, 410
    fibrosis, 424
  pulmonary, 291
Acne vulgaris, 768–9
Acoustic neuroma, 953
Acral lentiginous melanoma, 795–6
Acromegaly, 614–15
Acrylamide neurotoxicity, 915
Actinomycosis, 332
Activated partial thromboplastin
    time, 686
Addison's disease, 622–3
Adenocarcinoma
  cervix, 566
  fallopian tubes, 590–1
  kidney, 508–10
  large bowel, 382, 402
  lung, 314, 317
  small bowel, 377
  stomach, 367
  vaginal, 587
Adenochondroma, 318–19
Adenoid cystic carcinoma, 345–6
Adenolymphoma, 344–5
Adenoma, 165
  adrenocortical, 627

breast, 602
gallbladder, 458
large bowel, 402
oxyphilic/oncocytic, see
    Oncocytoma
pancreas, 464
parathyroid, 811
pituitary, 617–19
renal cortical, 507
salivary, 344, 345
small bowel, 377
thyroid, 644–5
Adenomatoid tumour
  myometrium, 568
  testis, 536
Adenomatous polyposis coli,
    familial, 200, 204, 403
Adenomyosis, 559
Adenosine deaminase deficiency,
    84–5, 706
Adenosis
  breast, 601
  vaginal, 586
Adenosquamous carcinoma,
    endometrial, 561
Adenoviruses, 135–6, 288
Adhesion
  platelet, 141, 679
  tumour cell, 176
Adhesion molecules and
    inflammation, 30–2
Adipose tissue tumours, 848–50
Adnexal tumours, skin, 789
Adrenal glands, 620–9
  hyperplasia, congenital, 169, 624
  metastases, 183
Adrenocorticotrophic hormone
    (ACTH), tumours producing,
    619, 625
Adrenoleukodystrophy, 624–5
Adult respiratory distress syndrome,
    307–8
Adynamic bowel syndrome, 398
Aesthesioneuroblastoma, 285–6
Aflatoxin, 208

Agammaglobulinaemia, Bruton's, 86
Age
 aortic valve changes, 247
 atherosclerosis and, 234
 immune deficiency and, 87
 macular degeneration and, 948
 testicular changes, 525
 wound healing and, 58
Agenesis, renal, 469–70
AIDS, *see* HIV disease
Air embolism, 149, 889
Airways, *see also* Respiratory system
 anatomy, 291–2
 chronic obstructive disease,
  294–300
Alagille's syndrome, 444–5
Alcoholic liver disease, 425–9
Aldosterone, excess secretion, 624–5,
  627
Alkaline phosphatase,
  carcinoplacental, 189
Alkylating agents, 208
Allergic alveolitis, extrinsic, 303–4
Allergic angiitis and granulomatosis,
  277–8
Allergic conjunctivitis, 942–3
Allergic rhinitis, 283
Allergy, 90–1
Alloimmune haemolytic anaemia,
  672–3
α-1-antitrypsin deficiency, 295,
  436–7
α-cell tumour, 635–6
α-chain disease, 379
Alphafetoprotein, 189
α-granule deficiency, 683
Alveolar rhabdomyosarcoma, 855
Alveolar soft part sarcoma, 858
Alveolitis, 302–4
Alveolus, 291–2
 clearance (macrophage function),
  294
 diffuse damage, 307–8
Alzheimer's disease, 884–5
Amoebiasis, *see also*
  Acanthamoebiasis
 CNS, 876
 GI tract, 390
cAMP, 38
Amyloid/amyloidosis, 123–8, 745
 cardiovascular, 127, 256
 CNS, 128, 885
 peripheral, familial, 921
 in rheumatoid arthritis, 835
Amyotrophic lateral sclerosis, 882–3

Anaemia, 651–77
 Fanconi's, 204, 676
 haemolytic, *see also* Haemolysis
 iron-deficiency, 360, 656–7
 in neoplasia, 186
 refractory, 699, 700
Anal disorders, 406–9
Analgesic nephropathy, 492
Anaphylatoxins, 34
Anaphylaxis, 90–1
Anaplastic/undifferentiated
  tumours
 astrocytoma, 903
 seminoma, 532
 thyroid carcinoma, 647
Andersen's disease, 933–4
Androblastoma, 579
Androgen(s)
 deficiency/resistance, 527–8
 oversecretion, 626, 627
Androgenital syndrome, 626
Anencephaly, 866
Aneuploidy, 216–19
 sex chromosome, 218–19, 552
Aneurysms, 267–71
 cerebral, 894–5
 mycotic, 251, 895
 ventricular, 242
Angiitis, *see* Vasculitis
Angina (pectoris), 152, 239–40
Angiodysplasia, 400
Angiofibroma, juvenile, 284
Angiofollicular lymph node
  hyperplasia, 717–18
Angiogenesis, tumours, 175
Angioimmunoblastic lymphoma,
  733
Angiokeratoma, diffuse, 922
Angioleiomyoma, 851
Angiolipoma, 849
Angioma, *see* Haemangioma
Angiomatoid malignant fibrous
  histiocytoma, 858–9
Angiomyolipoma, 508, 849
Angioneurotic oedema, 288
Angiosarcomas
 breast, 611
 liver, 442–3
 spleen, 748
Ankylosing spondylitis, 106, 837–8
Ann Arbor staging system, 722
Annular pancreas, 461
Antibody (antibodies), 68, 71–3
 anti-idiotypic, 97–8
 factor VIII, 689

Antibody (antibodies) (contd)
  graft rejection and, 102–3
  in immune haemolytic anaemia,
    672–3, 673–4
  in infection, 81–2, 82
  in syphilis, 119–20
  to self-antigens (autoantibodies)
    in glomerulonephritis, 479
    in systemic lupus
      erythematosus, 498, 499
    in systemic sclerosis, 502
    in vasculitis, 272
  tumours and, 191
  in type II hypersensitivity, 91
  in type V hypersensitivity, 93
Antibody-mediated inflammation,
    62
Anticardiolipin antibodies, 119
Antidiuretic hormone, see
    Vasopressin
Antigen(s), 67–8
  processing/recognition, 77–8
  self-, tolerance vs autoimmunity,
    94–5, 96–7
  transplantation, 99–103
  tumour-associated, 190–1
Antigen-presenting cells, 75, 78, 711
Antigenic drift and shift, viral, 138
Antiglomerular basement membrane
    disease, 479–80
Anti-idiotypic antibodies, 97–8
Antineutrophil cytoplasmic
    autoantibodies, 272
Antithrombin III, 686
  abnormalities, 144, 690
α_1-Antitrypsin deficiency, 295, 436–7
Antrum, pyloric, 354
Anus, 406–9
Aorta
  aneurysms, 268–80
  coarctation, 263
  dissection, 270
Aortic valve disease, 246–8
  rheumatic, 246
Aphthous ulcers, 335
Aplasia, renal, 470
Aplastic anaemia, 675–7
Apocrine metaplasia, 601
Apoptosis, 23–4
Appendix, 380–2
Arachidonic acid metabolism, 36
Arenaviruses, 139, 421
Arnold–Chiari malformation, 867
Aromatic amines, 207
Arrhenoblastoma, 579

Arteries, see also Vasculature
  graft rejection and, 103
  kidney, 466–7
  in pulmonary hypertension,
    lesions, 326–7
Arterioles in pulmonary
    hypertension, 327
Arteriovenous malformation, 895–6
Arteritis, 273–4
Arthritis, 830–6
  gouty, 844, 844–5
  rheumatoid, see Rheumatoid
    disease
Arthropathies, 830–45
Articular cartilage, 830
Asbestos, 319–21
Ascites, 450
Aspirin, antiplatelet effects, 684
Asthma, 299–300
Astrocytoma, 901–3
Astrovirus, 388
Ataxia, 881–2
  Freidreich's, 921
Ataxia telangiectasia, 85, 204, 727
Atherosclerosis (and atheromatous
    plaque), 142–3, 232–4
  aortic aneurysm in, 269
  embolism from plaque, 150
Athlete's foot, 780
Atopic eczema, 761–4
Atrial natriuretic peptides and heart
    failure, 265
Atrium
  left, in rheumatic valve disease,
    245
  septal defect, 261
Atrophic candidiasis, 334
Atrophic gastritis, 359
Atrophy, 170
  muscle, see Muscle
  olivopontocerebellar, 882
  testicular, 528
Autoantibodies, see Antibody
Autocrine motility factor, 178
Autoimmune disorders/disease, 63,
    94–107
  adrenal, 622–3
  splenomegaly, 744–5
  thyroid, 640, 641–2
Autoimmune haemolytic anaemia,
    673–5
Autoimmune hepatitis, chronic, 423
Autonomic neuropathy, hereditary
    sensory and, 920–1
Autopsy, 7–9

Autosomal disorders, 221–3
Axon regeneration, 911
Axonopathies, 911
Axonotmesis, 913–14
Azathioprine, 104
Azo dyes, 207

B cell (B lymphocyte), 69, 80, 710–11
  deficiencies, 86
  in lymph nodes, 74, 710–11
B-cell acute lymphoblastic
    leukaemia, 695
Bacteraemia, infective endocarditis
    and, 250
Bacterial infection
  in aortic aneurysm, 269
  bladder, 516
  CNS, 623, 868–70, 871–2, 873
  conjunctival, 941
  cutaneous, 771–5
  genitalia, male, 541–4
  immune response, 81–2
  intestinal, 383–7
  joints, 839–42
  oral, 332
  pericardial, 258–9
  thyroid, 643
Bacterial killing, 39–40, 108–9
  disorders, 41–2
Bacterial overgrowth, 373–4
Bacterial toxins, 14–16
  septic shock and, 266–7
Balan(oposth)itis, 540
Bare lymphocyte syndrome, 706
Barrett's oesophagus, 351–2
Bartholin's cysts, 582–3
Bartonella henselae, 714
Basal cell carcinoma, 788–9
Basal cell papilloma, 787–8
Basal ganglia degeneration, 880–1
Basement membrane, 633
  diabetes and, 633, 633–4
  glomerular, 467
    disorders, 479–80, 484, 633–4
  tumour spread and, 176–8
Bassan–Kornzweig disease
    (abetalipoproteinaemia), 374,
    923
Bazin's disease, 775
Becker-type muscular dystrophy, 929
Behçet's syndrome, 541
Berger's disease, 484–5
Bernard–Soulier syndrome, 141,
    683–4

Berry aneurysm, 894–5
β-cell tumour, 635–6
Bicuspid aortic valve, 247
Bile, 412, see also Cholestasis
Bile duct, drug damage, 454
Biliary cirrhosis, 429–31
  primary, 426, 429–31
  secondary, 432, 443–6
Biliary disorders, 412–14, 455–60
  childhood, 443–4
Bilirubin, 412
  disorders (incl.
      hyperbilirubinaemia),
      412–13
Binswanger's disease, 884
Bladder, urinary, 514–19
  hypertrophy, 168
Blasts
  in myelodysplastic syndromes,
      699, 700
  transformation (crisis), 697
Bleeding, see Haemorrhage
Bleeding disorders, 678–9, 680–4,
    687–9
Bleeding time, 686
Blistering disorders, 755–61
Blood disorders, see Haematological
    disorders
Blood flow
  disorders, 141–50
  myocardial, 237
  pulmonary, in congenital heart
      disease, 261–3
Blood vessels, see Vasculature
'Blue bloater', 298
Blue naevus, 791
Bombesin and neoplasia, 172
Bone, 801–29
  in cancer
    metastases, 182–3
    non-metastatic changes, 187
  necrosis, see Necrosis
  remodelling, 802–3
    disorders, 805–14
  repair, 59–60
Bone marrow
  embolism, 150
  transplantation, graft-vs-host
      disease, see Graft-vs-host
      disease
Borrelia burgdorferi, 841–2
Botryoid sarcoma, 588, 854
Botulinum toxin, 16
Bowel, 369–409
Bowen's disease, 544, 788

Bowenoid papulosis, 544–5
Brain, *see also* Central nervous
        system *and entries under*
        Encephal-
    injury, 896–901
    metastases, 183
Brainstem degenerations, 880–1
BRCA-1/-2, 202, 605
Breast, 596–612
    cancer, *see* Malignant disease
    hyperplasia, 169
Brenner tumour, 573–4
Bronchi, 291
Bronchiectasis, 300–1
Bronchioles, 291
Bronchitis, chronic, 294–6
Bronchoalveolar carcinoma, 317
Bronchopneumonia, 309
Brunner's gland hamartoma, 376–7
Brunn's nests, 515
Bruton's agammaglobulinaemia, 86
Budd—Chiari syndrome, 448
Buerger's disease, 275
Bulbar palsy, progressive, 883
Bullous disorders, 755–61
Burkitt's lymphoma, 379, 726, 731

CA125, 570
Cachexia, cancer, 185
Cadherins, 176
Calcification, heterotopic, 162–3
Calcium oxalate/phosphate stones,
        505–6
Calcium pyrophosphate dihydrate
        deposition, 845
Calculi (stones)
    biliary, 455–6
    renal, 505–7
    salivary, 341–2
Calymmatobacterium granulomatis,
        542
Campbell de Morgan spots, 799–800
Campylobacter jejuni, 384
Cancer, *see* Malignant disease
Candidiasis, 334–5, 780–2
    oral, 334–5, 781
Caplan's syndrome, 323
Carbon monoxide poisoning, 897–8
Carbuncles, 771
Carcinoembryonic antigen, 189
Carcinogenesis, *see* Oncogenesis
Carcinoids
    gastric, 366–7
    large bowel, 381

    pulmonary, 318
    small bowel, 377–8
Carcinoma, 165, *see also specific
        tissues and types*
Carcinoma in situ, *see* Intraepithelial
        neoplasia
Carcinoplacental alkaline
        phosphatase, 189
Cardia, 354
Cardiac disorders, *see* Heart *and
        entries below*
Cardiogenic shock, 266
Cardiolipin, antibodies to, 119
Cardiomyopathies, 252–9
Cardiovascular system, 231–80
    amyloidosis, 127, 256
    liver failure and, 451
Carotid disease, 890
Carpal tunnel syndrome, 914
Cartilage, articular, 830
Cartilage-forming tumours, 815–19
Caruncle, urethral, 522
Caseation necrosis, 24
Castleman's disease, 717–18
Cat-scratch disease, 714
Cataracts, 945
Cauliflower ear, 950
Cavernous haemangioma, 400, 442,
        800
CD3 complex, 78
CD4+ T cells, 78–9
    HIV disease and, 89
CD8+ T cells, 79
Cell(s)
    death, *see* Death
    differentiation, disturbances, 164,
        173
    growth and proliferation, *see*
        Growth and proliferation
    host, in viral infection, 129–32,
        133–4
    in inflammation, 26, 30–42
        in regeneration phase, 51–2
    injury, *see* Injury
Cell cycle, 167
    oncogenesis and, 194
Cell-mediated hypersensitivity, 93
Cell-mediated immunity, 68, 82, 82–3
Cellulitis, 771
Central core disease, 931
Central nervous system, 863–908
    amyloidosis, 128, 885
    granulomatous angiitis, 275
    radiation damage, 18
    repair, 61

Central nervous system (*contd*)
  syphilis effects, 121–2, 871–2
Centriacinar emphysema, 296–7
Centrocytic and centroblastic
      lymphomas, 726, 729–30
Centronuclear myopathies, 930–1
Cerebellum
  congenital anomalies, 867
  degenerative disease, 881–2
Cerebral artery occlusion, middle,
      890–1
Cerebral haemorrhage, *see*
      Intracerebral haemorrhage
Cerebrovascular disorders, 888–901
Cervix, 562–6
  intraepithelial neoplasia, 166, 564
Chagas' disease, 877
Chalazion, 939
Chancre, tuberculous, 772
Chancroid, 542
Charcot joint, 832
Charcot–Marie–Tooth disease, 919
Chediak–Higashi syndrome, 41
Cheilitis, candidal, 335
Chemical carcinogens, 206–7
  skin cancer and, 785–6
Chemical injury
  endothelium, 143
  kidney, 488
Chemokines, 36–7
Chemotaxis, 33, 42
  defects, 41
Cherry angioma, 799–800
Chickenpox, 777
Children, *see also* Infants; Newborn
  haemolytic uraemia syndrome,
      504
  liver disorders, 443–7
  respiratory infections, 295
  tuberculosis, 115–16
Chlamydia spp.
  intestinal infection, 387
  trachomatis, 542–3, 942
Cholangiocarcinoma, 441
Cholangitis
  ascending, 457
  sclerosing, 431–2
Cholecystitis, 457–8
Choledochal cyst, 445–6
Cholelithiasis, 455–6
Cholera (*V. cholerae*), 383
  toxin, 15
Cholestasis, 414
Cholesteatoma, 951–2
Cholesterol and plaque genesis, 233

Cholesterol stones, 455
Cholesterolosis, 458
Chondroblastoma, 816–17
Chondrocalcinosis, 845
Chondrodermatitis nodularis
      chronica, 950–1
Chondroid hamartoma, 318–19
Chondroma, 815–16
Chondromatosis, synovial, 846
Chondromyxoid fibroma, 817
Chondrosarcoma, 817–19
Chordoma, 825
Choriocarcinoma
  ovary, 575
  stomach, 367
  uterus, 595–6
Choroid plexus tumour, 905
Christmas disease, 688
Chromosome abnormalities, 215–19,
      see also Genetics
  analysis, 215
  cancer and, 203
    colorectal, 404
    haematological, 692–3
    lung, 313
    oral, 337
    soft tissue, 847
  translocations, *see* Translocations
Chromosome structure, 214
  abnormalities, 215–16
Chronic disease, anaemia of, 658–9
Chronic obstructive airway disease,
      294–300
Churg–Strauss syndrome, 277–8
Ciliary (Moll's) gland, cysts, 940
Cirrhosis, 423–37
  Indian childhood, 446
Clear cell carcinoma
  endometrial, 561
  ovarian, 573
  vaginal, 587
Clear cell chondrosarcoma, 818–19
Clear cell sarcoma, renal, 512
Cleft lip/palate, 330
Clostridium botulinum toxin, 16
Clostridium difficile, 384–5
Clostridium tetani toxin, 16
Clotting (and clotting system), 141,
      685–9, *see also*
      Hypercoagulability
  co-factors, 142, 680, 684–7
    deficiencies/abnormalities,
      687–8, 689
  inflammation and, 35
  liver disease affecting, 452–3, 689

Clotting (and clotting system) (contd)
neoplasms affecting, 186
wound healing and, 53
Clubbing, cancer, 187
Coagulation, see Clotting
Coagulative necrosis, 24
Coal miners' pneumoconioses,
296–7, 322–3
Codon
deletion, 225
stop, mutations, 226
Coeliac disease, 106, 371–2
Cold, common, 282
Cold antibodies, 674
Colitis, 392–5, see also
Enterocolitis
pseudomembranous, 384–5
Collagenous colitis, 394
Colloid tumours, see Mucinous
tumours
Colon, 395–406
Colony stimulating factors, 66,
70–1
haemopoiesis, 650
Comedo carcinoma, 604
Common variable
immunodeficiency, 87
Complement system, 33–4, 80–1
membrane injury and, 11
Complex sclerosing lesion, 600
Compound naevi, 791
Condyloma acuminata, 543
Congenital and developmental
disorders, see also specific
disorders
bladder, 515–16
bone, 804–5
CNS, 864, 866–7
ear (external), 950
eyelid, 939–40
genital tract
female, 551–4
male, 525–8, 538–9
heart, 247, 259–63
intestine, 370–1, 397–8, 407
kidney, 469–73
larynx, 287
oesophagus, 349
oral cavity, 330–1
pancreas, 461
penis, 538–9
pituitary, 614
stomach, 356
thyroid, 639
urethra, 520, 538–9

Congestion, 157–8, 310
venous, 157–8, 447
Congestive splenomegaly, 741
Conjunctival disorders, 940–3
Connective tissue disorders
hereditary, bleeding disorders, 678
oesophageal dysfunction, 350
Connective tissue tumours
skin, 797–9
small bowel, 378–9
stomach, 367–8
Conn's syndrome, 624–5
Contact dermatitis, 764
Contact urticaria, 764
Cori–Forbes disease, 923
Corneal disorders, 943–5
Coronary (ischaemic) heart disease,
236–42
Coronaviruses, 139
Cortex
adrenal, 620, 621–2
disorders, 622–7
renal
adenoma, 507
necrosis, 503
Coxsackie virus type A, 333
Cranial arteritis, 274
Craniopharyngioma, 617
Creutzfeldt–Jakob disease, 887
Cri du chat syndrome, 215
Crigler–Najkar syndrome, 413
Crohn's disease, 390–2, 408
Cronkhite–Canada syndrome, 376
Cryoglobulinaemia, essential mixed,
279
Cryptogenic fibrosing alveolitis,
302–3
Cryptorchidism, 525
Cryptosporidiosis, 389
Crystal arthropathy, 842–5
Cushing's, 625
Cutaneous disorders, see Skin
Cyanosis, shunt, 261–2
Cyclins and cyclin-dependent
kinases, 194, 201
Cyclo-oxygenase pathway, 36
Cyclosporin A, 104
Cyst(s)
breast, 600
choledochal, 445–6
cutaneous, 786–7
eyelid, 939, 940
fallopian tubes, 590
renal, 470–4
splenic, 747–8

Cyst(s) (contd)
  vulval, 582
Cystadenocarcinoma, ovary, 572
Cystadenoma, 165
  ovary, 572
  pancreas, 464
Cystic fibrosis, 426, 463–4
Cystic teratoma, mature, 576
Cystic tumour, pancreas, 464
Cystine stones, 507
Cystitis, 516–18
Cystitis cystica and glandularis, 515
Cytokines (incl. lymphokines)
  lymphocyte-derived, 68, 69–71
  macrophage activity and, 42
  in septic shock, 267
  in wound healing, 57–8
Cytomegalovirus, 420, 874
Cytopathology, 7
Cytoplasm in cell death, 22
Cytoplasmic proteins as tumour
    suppressors, 200
Cytotoxicity, T cell-mediated, 79–80

Dandy–Walker malformation, 867
Darier's disease, 759–60
de Quervain's thyroiditis, 643
Death
  cell, 22–5
    viral infection and, 132
  person, myocardial infarction, 242
Decalcification, 4
Decidual reaction, cervical stroma,
    563–4
Defence mechanisms, respiratory
    tract
  lower, 293–4
  upper, 282, 293
Déjérine–Sottas disease, 919–20
Deletions
  chromosome, 215
    colorectal cancer and, 404
    lung cancer and, 313
  gene, 223–5
Dementia, 883–6
Demyelinating disorders
  CNS, 879–80
  peripheral, 911–12, 917–21
Dendritic corneal ulcer, 944–5
Denervation, 936–7
Dermatitis (eczema), 760–4
  seborrhoeic, 754
Dermatitis herpetiformis, 757–8
Dermatofibroma, 798

Dermatofibrosarcoma protuberans,
    798–9
Dermatology, see Skin
Dermatomyositis, 188, 935
Dermatopathic lymphadenopathy,
    713
Dermatophytes, 779–80
Dermis, 751
  tumours, 797–9, 851
  in wound healing, 54–5
Dermoid cyst, 939
Desmoid fibromatoses, 861
Developmental disorders, see
    Congenital and
    developmental disorders
Di George syndrome, 86, 705
Diabetes insipidus, 616
  nephrogenic, 487
Diabetes mellitus, 629–45, 918–19
  atherosclerosis in, 235
  juvenile, 107
  nephropathy, 492–3, 633–4
  neuropathy, 918–19
  skin lesions, 783
  wound healing in, 58–9
Diamond–Blackfan syndrome,
    677
Diarrhoea, traveller's, 383–4
Differentiation disorders, cell, 164,
    173
Diffuse brain injury, 900–1
Diffuse large B-cell lymphoma, 730
Diffuse lymphocyte-predominant
    Hodgkin's disease, 721
Diffuse small cleaved cell
    lymphoma, 729–30
Dilated cardiomyopathy, 254–5
Diphallus, 539
Diphtheria, 287
  toxin, 15–16
Discoid lupus erythematosus,
    766–7
Disseminated intravascular
    coagulation, 681–2
Diverticula
  colonic, and diverticular disease,
    398–9
  pharyngoesophageal, 351
  small bowel, 375
    Meckel's, 370–1
DNA
  repair defect, 785
  tumour cell, transformation using,
    196
DNA techniques, 6–7

DNA viruses, 134–7
  replication, 131
Dominant mutations, 219, 221, 222
Down's syndrome, 203, 216–17
Drug reactions/drug-induced
      disorders
  blood cells, 674–5, 676–7
  erythema multiforme, 759
  kidney, 104, 489, 492
  liver, 453–4
  peripheral nerves, 915–16
  systemic lupus erythematosus, 98
  type II hypersensitivity, 91–2, 489
Dubin–Johnson syndrome, 413
Duchenne muscular dystrophy,
      928–9
Ductal carcinoma, 606–7
Ductal carcinoma in situ, 603–4
Ductal papilloma, 602–3
Ductus arteriosus, patent, 260–1
Duodenum
  mucosal protection, 355–6
  ulcer, 361, see also Peptic ulcer
Duplications, gene, 225
Dysentery, 384
Dysgerminoma, 574–5
Dyslipidaemia, see Hyperlipidaemia
Dysphagia, 349–53
Dysplasia (developmental)
  fibrous, 825–7
  neuronal intestinal, 398
  renal, 470–1
Dysplasia (epithelial premalignant),
      166
  gastric, 364
Dysplastic naevus syndrome, 792
Dystrophic calcification, 162

Ear, 949–53
Eaton–Lambert syndrome, 938
Ebola virus, 421
Eclampsia, 592, 593
Ectopia
  cerebellar tonsils, 867
  pancreas, 461
  testis, 525
Ectopic hormone production, 187
Ectopic pregnancy, 591
Eczema, see Dermatitis
Edward's syndrome, 218
Elastofibroma, 860
Elderly, see Age
Electron microscopy, 6
Elliptocytosis, hereditary, 664

Embolism (and embolization)
  in aortic aneurysm, 269
  fat, 149–50, 889
  in infective endocarditis, 251
  pulmonary, 148, 323–4
  stroke due to, 889
  thrombus-derived, 147, 148
Embryonal carcinoma, 533–4
Embryonal rhabdomyosarcoma, 588,
      854
Emphysema, 294–7
Encephalitis, 871–6
Encephalocele, 866
Encephalomyelitis, acute
      disseminated/perivenular,
      880–1
Encephalomyopathy, mitochondrial,
      932
Encephalopathy, hepatic, 450–1
Enchondroma, 815–16
Endocarditis
  infective, 148, 249–52
  non-bacterial thrombotic, 252
Endocardium
  fibroelastosis, 257
  in rheumatic fever, 244–5
Endocrine system/organs, 613–48
  amyloidosis, 128
  disorders
    in candidiasis, 781–2
    in liver failure, 452
    in neoplasia, 186–7
Endocytosis, 108, see also
      Phagocytosis
Endoderm sinus tumour, see Yolk
      sac tumour
Endometrioid tumour/carcinoma,
      560, 573
Endometriosis, 558–9
Endometritis, 556–7
Endometrium, 554–62
  cancer, 210, 559–62
Endomyocardial fibrosis, 256
Endothelium
  in atherosclerosis, 231
  corneal, dystrophy, 944
  in inflammation, 30–2
  injury, 143
  platelets and, 141, 687
Endotoxins (lipopolysaccharide), 14
  and septic shock, 266–7
Enhancer sequences, oncogene
      activation, 197
Enterocolitis, 383–91, see also Colitis
  necrotizing, 400

Enteropathic arthropathy, 838
Enteroviruses, 137–8
Enzyme-mediated fat necrosis, 25
Enzymopathies
  crystal arthropathy, 843–4
  red cell, 664–6
Eosinophilic cystitis, 518
Eosinophilic granuloma, 305–6,
    735
Ependymoma, 904–5
Epidermal growth factor, 56–7
Epidermis, 750–1
  tumours, 786–90
  in wound healing, 53–4
Epidermodysplasia verruciformis,
    778–9
Epidermolysis bullosa, 760–1, 762
Epididymis, 523–37
Epiglottis, acute, 287
Epiphyseal plate disorders, 804
Epispadias, 539
Epithelia
  hyperplasia, breast, 600–1
  iron deficiency effects, 657
  in tissue regeneration, 51
Epithelioid cells, 109–10
Epithelioid sarcoma, 858–9
Epstein–Barr virus, 135, 212, 420,
    714, 726
Epulis, congenital, 331
Erysipelas, 771
Erythema gyratum repens, 188
Erythema induratum, 775
Erythema multiforme, 758, 759
Erythrocyte, see Red cell
Erythroplasia of Queyrat, 544
Erythropoiesis, compensatory,
    662
Escherichia coli
  enteritis, 383–4
  meningitis, 868
Ethnicity (race) and atherosclerosis,
    234
Ewing's tumour, 823–4
Exomphalos, 371
Exostoses, 815
Exotoxins, 14, 15–16
Exstrophy, bladder, 515–16
Extracellular matrix and tumour
    spread, 176–9
Extradural haematoma, 899
Exudate, 154
  inflammatory, 30–40
    malfunction due to, 47
    types, 45–6

Eye, 939–49
  in diabetes, 634–5
  in rheumatoid disease, 835
Eyelid, 939–40

Fabry's disease, 922
Factor VII$_c$, elevated, 691
Factor VIII
  antibodies, 689
  deficiency, 687–8
Factor IX deficiency, 688
Factor XI deficiency, 688
Factor XII, 34–5, 685
Falciparum malaria, 743
Fallopian tubes, 551, 588–91
Fallot's tetralogy, 261–2
Familial adenomatous polyposis
    coli, 200, 204, 403
Familial amyloid polyneuropathy,
    921
Familial Mediterranean fever, 127
Fanconi's anaemia, 204, 676
Fasciitis
  necrotizing, 543–4, 771–2
  nodular, 860
Fat, pigments associated with, 161
Fat embolism, 149–50, 889
Fat necrosis, 24–5, 598–9
Fatty change, 20–1
  liver, 21, 427
Fatty streak, 231–2
Felty's syndrome, 744–5, 835
Feminization, testicular, 527
Fertility disorders, males, 526–8
α-Fetoprotein, 189
Fever, cancer, 185
Fibrinogenaemia, 691
Fibrinoid necrosis, 44, 497
Fibrinolysis, 35, 687
  inherited disorders, 691
Fibroadenoma, 601–2
Fibroblastic lesions
  bone, 824–5
  soft tissue, 859–62
Fibrocystic change, 599–601
Fibroelastosis, endocardial, 257
Fibrolamellar carcinoma, 440–1
Fibrolipid plaque, 232
Fibroma, see also Elastofibroma
  chondromyxoid, 817
  ovary, 579
Fibromatoses, 860–1
Fibronectin and tumour spread, 179
Fibroplasia, retrolental, 947–8

Fibrosarcoma, 824–5, 862
Fibrosing alveolitis, cryptogenic,
302–3
Fibrosis
breast, 601
endomyocardial, 256
hepatic, 424
congenital, 447
pulmonary, progressive massive,
322
Fibrous dysplasia, 825–7
Fibrous histiocytoma
benign, skin, 798
malignant
bone, 824
soft tissue, 857–8
Filovirus, 421
Fish tank granuloma, 775
Fissure, anal, 407
Fistula, anal, 407–8
5q syndrome, 699–701
Fixation, 4
Fluid accumulations, 154–8, see also
Oedema
Focal nodular hyperplasia, 437
Focal segmental glomerulonephritis,
478–9
Folate deficiency, 655
Follicle-stimulating hormone, see
Gonadotrophins
Follicular adenoma, 644–5
Follicular carcinoma, 646
Follicular cystitis, 517
Follicular hyperplasia, lymphoid,
707, 712
Follicular keratosis, 759–60
Follicular lymphomas, 726
Folliculitis, 771
Fordyce's granules, 331
Foreign body
inflammatory response, 59
oesophagus, 349
soft-tissue lesions, 847
Fournier's gangrene, 543–4, 771
Fractures, healing, 59–60
Frameshift mutations, 226
Free radicals (incl. oxygen-derived
forms)
damage by, 12–13, 48
myocardial, 238
phagocyte-derived, 48
in bacterial killing, 38–9
Freidreich's ataxia, 921
Frozen sections, 5
Fructosaemia, 444

Fuch's endothelial dystrophy, 944
Fungal infections
CNS, 874–5
in AIDS, 874
oral, 334–5
skin, 779–82
spleen, 743
upper respiratory, 284, 288
Furuncles, 771
Fusiform aneurysm, 895
Fusion mutations, 225

Galactosaemia, 444
Gallbladder, 455–60
Gallstones, 455–6
Ganglion, 846
Gangrene, 25
Fournier's, 543–4, 771
Gardner's syndrome, 204, 403
Gas, diffusion in alveolus, 293
Gas embolism, 149, 889
Gas gangrene, 25
Gastric acid secretion, 354
Gastrin-releasing peptide, 172
Gastrinoma, 636
Gastritis, 356–63
Gastrointestinal tract (gut),
330–409
atrophy, 170
in hyperparathyroidism, 812
hypertrophy, 168
reactive arthropathy, 838
Gastrointestinal tract, radiation
injury, 18
Gastro-oesophageal reflux, 349, 351
Gaucher's disease, 742
Gender (sex) and atherosclerosis, 234
General paresis of insane, 122,
871–2
Genetic disorders, 214–27
amyloidosis in, 126–7
of blood, 660–71
haemoglobin, 223, 225, 655,
666–71
of blood vessels, 678
cardiomyopathy, 254
of immune system, 84–6, 87, 705–6
infertility (males), 526–8
of liver, 444–5
of muscle, 927, 928–35
of peripheral nerves, 919–24
thrombosis risk, 144–5, 690–1
tumours in, 203–5
soft tissue, 847

Genetics and genetic factors, *see also* Chromosome abnormalities
cancer, 203–6
  bladder, 519
  breast, 605
  colon, 403–4
  gastric, 363
  haematological, 692, 692–3, 696, 697, 698
  lymphoid, 725–6
  oral, 337
  renal, 508, 510
coeliac disease, 372
peptic ulcer, 361
refractory anaemias, 699
Genital tract, *see* Reproductive system
Germ cell(s), 523–4
Germ cell tumours, 530–2, 574–7
  mixed sex cord and, 535–6
  ovaries, 574–7
  testes, 530–2, 535–6
  thymus, 709
Gerstmann–Strässler–Scheinker syndrome, 887
Giant cell(s), multinucleated, 110
Giant cell arteritis, 274
Giant cell malignant fibrous histiocytoma, 858
Giant cell tumour
  bone, 822–3
  tendon sheath, 845–6
Giant lymph node hyperplasia, 717–18
Giant osteoid osteoma, 820
Giardiasis, 388–9
Gigantism, 614–15
Gilbert's syndrome, 412–13
Glanzmann's disease, 683
Glaucoma, 946
Glioblastoma multiforme, 903
Globin, 651
  disorders/defects, 655, 661, 666–71
Globoid cell leucodystrophy, 922
Glomerulonephritis, 156, 477–86
  mesangioproliferative, 252, 484
Glomerulus, 466, 474–86
  disease/changes, 474–86, 498–502
  in graft rejection, 103
Glomus jugulare, 952
Glomus tumour, 800
Glucagonoma, 636
Glucocorticoids, 621–2
  oversecretion, 625, 627
  wound healing and, 58

Glucose tolerance, impaired, 631
Glucose 6–phosphatase deficiency, 843–4
Glucose-6-phosphate dehydrogenase deficiency, 665–6
Glycogenoses, 933–5
Glycolysis, defects on, 664–5
Glycosylated proteins, 632
cGMP, 38
Goitre, 642–3
Gonadoblastoma, 580
Gonadotrophins (FSH and LH)
  inadequate, 526
  pituitary adenoma producing, 619
Gonads, defective development/dysgenesis, 203, 552–3
Gonorrhoea
  arthritis, 839–40
  urethritis, 521
Goodpasture's syndrome, 480
Gout, 842–5
Graft(s) (transplants), 99–107
  bone marrow, graft-vs-host disease, 105, 394
  MHC and, 99–107
  renal, 103, 512–13, 786
Graft-vs-host disease, 105, 394
Granular cell(s), mesangial, 468
Granular cell tumour, oral, 338–9
Granulocyte-monocyte CSFs, 66, 70
Granuloma
  eosinophilic, 305–6, 735
  fish tank/swimming pool, 775
  pyogenic, 288, 799
  sperm, 536–7
Granuloma annulare, 783
Granuloma inguinale, 542
Granulomatosis
  allergic angiitis and, 277–8
  Wegener's, 276–7
Granulomatous angiitis of CNS, 275
Granulomatous disease, chronic, 41–2
Granulomatous endometritis, chronic, 557
Granulomatous inflammation/disorders, 62, 108–22
  breast, 599
  larynx, 288
  skin, 783
  spleen, 743
Granulomatous orchitis, 530

Granulomatous prostatitis, 547
Granulomatous salpingitis, 589–90
Granulomatous thyroiditis, 643
Granulosa cell tumours, 577–8
Graves' disease, 641–2
Great vessels, transposition, 262
Grey platelet syndrome, 683
Grover's disease, 760
Growth and proliferation, cell
  neoplastic disturbances, 164, 171–3
  non-neoplastic disturbances,
    167–70
Growth factors
  neoplasia and, 172, 172–3
  wound healing and, 55–7
Growth hormone overproduction,
  615–16
  adenoma, 619
Guillain–Barré syndrome, 917
Gummatous necrosis, 121
Gut, see Gastrointestinal tract
Gut-associated lymphoid tissue,
  369–70
Gynaecological disorders, 551–612
Gynaecomastia, 611–12

Haemangioendothelioma, infantile,
  442
Haemangioma (angioma)
  colorectal, 400
  cutaneous, 798–9
  hepatic, 442
Haematological disorders, 649–703
  in liver failure, 452
  in neoplasia, 186
  splenomegaly in, 745
Haematuria, 375
  in glomerulopathy, 484–5
Haemochromatosis, 426, 433–4
Haemodynamic injury,
  endocardium, 250
Haemoglobin, 650–1
  disorders of, 655, 666–71
    inherited, 223, 225, 655, 666–71
  glycosylated, 632
  pigments derived from, 160–1
Haemoglobinuria, paroxysmal
  nocturnal, 671–2
Haemolysis/haemolytic anaemia,
  652, 659–79, 745
  immune, 91, 672–5
Haemolytic uraemia syndrome, 503–4
Haemophilias, 687–8
Haemophilus ducreyi, 542

Haemophilus influenzae, 868
Haemopoietic system, 649–703
  radiation injury, 18
Haemorrhage, see also Bleeding
    disorders
  brain, 891–6
    traumatic, 899–900
  tumour-associated, 185
Haemorrhagic cystitis, 518
Haemorrhagic disease of newborn,
  688–9
Haemorrhagic inflammation, 44
Haemorrhagic telangiectasia,
  hereditary, 678
Haemorrhoids, 408
Haemosiderosis, 161, 432–5
Haemostasis (and disorders), 141–8,
  678–84
Hageman factor, 34–5, 685
Hailey–Hailey disease, 760
Hairy cell leukaemia, 698–9
Hairy leukoplakia, 336
Halothane hepatitis, 453–4
Hamartoma, 166
  chondroid, 318–19
  large bowel, 401
  small bowel, 376–7
  splenic, 748
Hand–Schüller–Christian
  syndrome, 735
Hashimoto–Pritzker syndrome, 735
Hashimoto's thyroiditis, 640
Head injury, 898–901
Healing, wound, 48, 53–60
Heart
  amyloidosis, 127
  arrest, brain damage in, 896–7
  congenital disease, 247, 259–63
  hypertrophy, 168
  ischaemic disease, 236–42
  muscle, see Myocardium
  radiation injury, 18
  rhadomyoma, 852
  rheumatoid disease, 834
  rupture (external), 241
  valvar disease, 242–52
Heart failure, 263–5
  congestive, oedema in, 155, 306,
    306–7
  in infective endocarditis, 251
Heat in inflammation, 26, 27
Heat shock proteins, 13–14
Helicobacter pylori, 356–8
Helminths
  bladder, 517

Helminths (*contd*)
  conjunctiva, 942
  immune response, 83
Hemifacial hypertrophy, 330
Henoch–Schönlein purpura, 279
Hepadnaviruses, 137
Heparin cofactor II, 686
Hepatic artery, 411
  arterial underperfusion, 448
Hepatic venous drainage disorders,
    447–9
Hepatitis, 415–19, *see also*
    Steatohepatitis
  alcoholic, 427–8
  chronic, 421–2, 423–4
  halothane, 453–4
  peliosis, 449
  viral, 415–19
    HAV, 415
    HBV, 137, 212–13, 416, 417,
        418
    HCV, 417
    HDV, 417–18
    HEV, 419
Hepatoblastoma, 441–2
Hepatocellular carcinoma, 438–41
Hepatocytes (liver cell), 411
  drug-related injury, 454
Hepatoid adenocarcinoma, stomach,
    367
Heredity,, *see entries under* Genetic
Hermaphroditism, true, 552–3
Hernia, hiatus, 352
Herpes simplex virus, 775–6
  corneal lesions, 944–5
  hepatic lesions, 420
  mucocutaneous lesions, 775–6
    oral lesions, 333
    penile lesions, 543
  oesophagus, 352
Herpes viruses, 135, 212, 272, 420
Herpes zoster (shingles), 776
  oral, 333
Heterolysis, 23
Heteroplasia, 166
Hexacarbon neurotoxicity, 915
Hiatus hernia, 352
Hibernoma, 849
High density lipoprotein, hereditary
    deficiency, 923
Hirschsprung's disease, 397–8
Histiocytic necrotizing
    lymphadenitis, 717
Histiocytoma, fibrous, *see* Fibrous
    histiocytoma

Histiocytosis
  Langerhans cells (histiocytosis X),
    305–6, 735
  pulp, 712
  sinus, *see* Sinus histiocytosis
Histochemistry, 5
Histocompatibility antigens, *see*
    Major histocompatibility
    complex
HIV disease/AIDS, 88–90, 873–4
  lymphadenopathy, 715
  neuropathology, 873–4
  oral lesions, 334
  tumours, 728, 797–8, 874
HLA, *see* Major histocompatibility
    complex
Hodgkin's disease, 718–22
  non-Hodgkin's lymphoma and,
    728
  splenic, 746–7
  thymic, 709
Hordeolum, 939
Hormones, *see also* Endocrine system
    and specific hormones
  hyperplasia in target organs of,
    169
  in tumourigenesis, 210
  tumours producing, 186–7
    pancreas, 635–7
    pituitary, 618–19
Horseshoe kidney, 470
HPV, 211, 334, 543, 565, 776–8
HTLV-1, 213, 272, 727
Human immunodeficiency virus, *see*
    HIV
Human papilloma virus, 211, 334,
    543, 565, 776–8
Human T-cell leukaemia virus-1
    (HTLV-1), 213, 272, 726
Huntington's chorea, 885–6
Hydatidiform mole, 592–4
Hydrocephalus, 863–4
Hydrogen peroxide, detoxification
    of, 40
21-α-Hydroxylase deficiency, 624,
    626
Hyperaemia, 157–8
Hyperbilirubinaemia, *see* Bilirubin
Hypercalcaemia
  in malignancy, 812–13
  non-metastatic, 187
Hypercoagulability, 689–91
Hyperfibrinogenaemia, 691
Hyper-IgM syndrome, X-linked,
    87

Hyperlipidaemia
  atherosclerosis in, 235
  immunosuppressed patients, 105
Hypernephroma, 508–10
Hyperparathyroidism, 810, 810–12
Hyperpigmentation, 159–60
Hyperpituitarism, 615–16
Hyperplasia, 168–9
  adrenal
    bilateral nodular, 626–7
    congenital, 169, 624
  cervical microglandular, 563
  endometrial, 557–8
  epithelial, breast, 600–1
  hepatic, 437
  islet cell, 635–7
  lymphoid/lymph node, 712
    follicular, 707, 712
    giant, 717–18
  prostatic, 169, 547–8
  thyroid, 169, 641–2
  vulval squamous, 581–2
Hyperplastic polyps, 401
Hyperplastic scar, 859–60
Hypersensitivity, 90–3
  drug-induced, 91–2, 489
  in tuberculosis, 115
Hypersensitivity vasculitis, 278–9
Hypersplenism, 740
Hypertension, 495–8
  atherosclerosis in, 235
  essential, 495–6
  malignant, 497
  portal, 427, 449–50
  pulmonary, 325–8
  secondary, 495
    immunosuppressed patients, 105
Hyperthyroidism, 640–3
Hypertrophic cardiomyopathy, 253–4
Hypertrophic pyloric stenosis, 356
Hypertrophy, 168
  benign prostatic (nodular hyperplasia), 169, 547–8
  hemifacial, 330
Hypocalcaemic osteomalacia, 807–8
Hypochromic anaemia, 653
Hypocomplementaemic vasculitis, 279
Hypogammaglobulinaemia of infancy, transient, 87
Hypogonadotrophic hypogonadism, 526, 553–4
Hypophosphataemic rickets, 808

Hypopituitarism, 614–15
Hypoplasia, congenital adrenal, 623
Hypoplastic anaemia, congenital, 677
Hypospadias, 538
Hyposplenism, 740–1
Hypotensive brain damage, 897
Hypothyroidism, 639–40
Hypovolaemic shock, 265–6
Hypoxaemia, pulmonary circulatory effects, 298
Hypoxia, 19–20, 896
Hypoxic brain damage, 896–8
Hypoxic pulmonary vascular disease, 327

Idiotypic bypass, 97
Immune complexes, 48
  in infective endocarditis, 251–2
  and type III hypersensitivity, 92–3
Immune haemolysis, 91, 672–5
Immune response, 76–83
  tumours, 190, 191–2
  viral infection, 82–3, 133–4
Immune system, 67–107, *see also* Defence mechanisms
  anatomy, 73–6
  blistering diseases and, 755–9
  coeliac disease and, 372
  disorders, 84–93
    in neoplastic disease, 185–6
  granulomatous reactions and, 111
  splenectomy and, 741
  upper respiratory tract, 282
  urticaria and, 765
Immune thrombocytopenia, 681
Immunoblastic lymphoma, 633, 730–1, 734–5
Immunocompromised patients, infections, *see* Infections
Immunocytoma, 728–9
Immunodeficiency, 84–90, 705–7, 727
  in iron deficiency, 657
  tumours and, 105, 190, 727
Immunoglobulin(s), 71–3, *see also* Antibody
  light chains, amyloidosis and, 124–5
Immunoglobulin A, 72–3
  deficiency, 86
Immunoglobulin A nephropathy, 484–5
Immunoglobulin D, 73
Immunoglobulin E, 73

Immunoglobulin G, 72
  antibodies, 672–3
Immunoglobulin gene superfamily,
  30–1
Immunoglobulin M, 73, *see also*
  Hyper-IgM syndrome
  antibodies, 672
Immunoglobulin(s)
Immunohistochemistry, 5–6
Immunophenotyping, lymphoma,
  724, 728–33
Immunoproliferative small intestinal
  disease, 379
Immunosuppressive drugs, 104–5
Impetigo, 770
In-situ hybridization, 6
Inclusion bodies (in viral infection),
  132
Inclusion body myositis, 936
Indian childhood cirrhosis, 446
Infants, *see also* Newborn
  hydrocephalus, 864
  liver disorders, 442, 443–7
  premature, retinopathy, 947–8
  renal papillary necrosis, 493
Infarction, 153
  cerebral, 889–90
  myocardial, 240–2, 266
  renal, 502–5
Infections, 112–18, 119–22, 129–40,
  see also Infestations *and specific
  (types of) pathogen*
  CNS, 867–77
  conjunctival, 941–2
  corneal, 944–5
  erythema multiforme, 759
  glomerulonephritis following,
    481–2
  granuloma formation, 112–18,
    119–22
  hepatic, 414–21
  immune response, 81–3
  immunocompromised patients,
    104, 308–9
    AIDS, 873–4
  inflammatory response, 59
  joint, 839–42
  large bowel, 383–91
  lymph node, 713–15
  oesophageal, 352
  oral, 332–5, 781
  penile, 541–4
  pericardial, 258–9
  peripheral nerve, 917
  respiratory

    childhood, 295
    lower, 136, 308–11
    upper, 282–3, 283–4, 287–8
  skin, 770–82
  splenic, 742–3
  testicular, 528–30
  thyroid, 643
  tumour-associated, 185
  urinary tract
    diabetes, 634
    lower, 516–17
    upper, 492–3
  vaginal, 585–6
  vasculitis in, 272
Infective endocarditis, 148, 249–52
Infertility, males, 526–8
Infestations, 782
Inflammation, 26–66
  acute, 30–42
    natural history, 48–66
  cells in, 26, 30–42
  chronic, 62–6
  factors modifying inflammatory
    reaction, 43–8
  granulomatous, *see*
    Granulomatous
    inflammation
Inflammatory bowel disease, 391–5,
  408
Inflammatory carcinoma, 608
Inflammatory disorders
  anus, 407–8
  biliary system, 457–8
  breast, 598
  cervix, 563–4
  conjunctiva, 941–3
  ear, 950–1, 951–2
  endometrium, 556–8
  fallopian tubes, 589–90
  oral cavity, 332, 341–3
  pancreas, 462–4
  penis, 540–3
  prostate, 546–7
  respiratory tract, 282–4, 287–8
  spleen, 743–5
  testis, 528–30
  urinary tract (lower), 516–17, 521–2
  vagina, 585–6
Inflammatory malignant fibrous
  histiocytoma, 858
Inflammatory myopathies, 935–6
Inflammatory polyneuropathies,
  917–18
Influenza, 138
Inheritance, *see entries under* Genetic

Inhibin, 570
Injury, see also Traumatic injury
  brain, 896–901
  cell, 10–21
    red, 675
  endothelial, 143
  inflammation in, see Inflammation
  kidney
    glomerulus, mechanisms, 475
    medulla, 488
  peripheral nerve, 910–24
Insertions, gene, 225
Insulin-dependent diabetes mellitus,
      629–30
Insulinoma, 635–6
Integrins
  in inflammation, 30–1
  in tumour spread, 176
Interferons
  T cell-derived, 70
  viral infection and, 133–4
Interleukin(s), 69–71
  haemopoiesis and, 650
  IL-1, 37, 57, 69, 650
    in inflammation, 37, 65
    in wound healing, 57
  IL-8, 36–7, 65, 69, 650
  lymphocyte-derived, 69–70
Interstitial cystitis, 518
Interstitial disease
  kidney, 487–93
  lungs, 302–6
Intestine, 369–409
Intima
  graft rejection and, 103
  thrombosis and, 142–3, 234
Intracerebral haemorrhage, 891–3
  traumatic, 900
Intracranial pressure, 863–5
Intradermal naevi, 791
Intraepithelial neoplasia (carcinoma
      in situ)
  breast, 603–5
  cervical, 166, 564
  conjunctival, 943
  laryngeal, 289
  penile, 544–5
  vaginal, 586–7
  vulval, 583
Intratubular germ cell neoplasia, 531
Inversions, chromosome, 216
Iodide-deficiency goitre, 642–3
Ionizing radiation
  cancer associated with, 210–11,
      786, 847

colitis due to, 394–5
  injury by, 17–19
    skin, 18, 786
Iron, 655–7
  deficiency, anaemia of, 360, 656–7
  storage disorders, 160–1, 257,
      432–5
Ischaemia, 151–3
  cerebral, damage due to, 891, 892
  intestinal
    large, 399–400
    small, 374–5
  myocardial, 236–9
  in sickle cell disease, 667
Ischaemic attacks, transient, 891
Ischaemic gangrene, 25
Ischaemic heart disease, 236–42
Ischaemic necrosis of bone, 827–8
Islet cell tumours/hyperplasia,
      635–7
Isochromosomes, 216
Isospora belli, 389

Jaundice, paediatric, 443–7
Jaw, osteosarcoma, 822
Joint disorders, 829–46
Junctional naevi, 790–1
Juxtacortical osteosarcoma, 821–2
Juxtaglomerular apparatus, 468–9

Kaposi's sarcoma, 797–8, 874
Karyotype, normal, 215–16
Karyotyping, 215
Kawasaki's disease, 278, 717
Keloid scar, 859
Keratoacanthoma, 789–90
Keratopathy, 943–5
Keratosis
  follicular, 759–60
  seborrhoeic, 787–8
Ketoacidosis, diabetic, 630
Kidney, 466–513
  diabetic disease, 492–3, 633–4
  drugs toxic/adversely affecting,
      104, 489, 492
  failure, 475, 493–5
    acute, 493–5
    chronic, 475, 486
  in hyperparathyroidism, 811
  in infective endocarditis, 252
  oedema, 156
  salt and water retention, 155
  transplantation, 103, 512–13, 786

Kiel classification, 723
Kikuchi's disease, 717
Kimmelstiel—Wilson lesion, 634
Kinin system, 35
Klebsiella pneumonia, 311
Klinefelter's syndrome, 203, 218–19, 526
Koch phenomenon, 114–15
Krabbe's disease, 922
Kuru, 887–8
Kwashiorkor, 21, 156

Lactating adenoma, 602
Lambert—Eaton syndrome, 938
Lamina propria
  bladder, 515
  cells of, 76
Langerhans cells histiocytosis
    (histiocytosis X), 305–6, 735
Large bowel, 395–406
Large cell lung carcinoma, 314, 318
Large cell lymphomas, 730, 733, 734–5
Laryngitis, 287, 288
Laryngotracheobronchitis, acute, 287
Larynx, 286–90
Lassa fever, 421
Lead poisoning, 659
Left-to-right shunts, 259–61
Legionella pneumonia, 310
Leiomyoma (and leiomyomatosis), 850
  uterine, 566–7
Leiomyosarcoma, 568–9, 850–1
Leishmaniasis, 744
Lennert's lymphoma, 733
Lens, 945
Lentigo maligna, 795
Leprosy, 117–18, 916
Lesch—Nyhan syndrome, 843
Letterer—Siwe disease, 734
Leucocytes (white cells)
  in inflammation, 26
  in liver failure, 452
  splenectomy and, 741
Leucodystrophy, 921–2
Leukaemia, 691–701, 747
Leukoplakia, 335–6
  candidal, 335
Lewy bodies, 881
Leydig cells, 524
  tumours, 524–5
Lice, 784
Lichen planus, 765–6

Lichen sclerosis (et atrophicus)
  penis, 540
  vulva, 581
Lip, congenital disorders, 330, 331,
    see also Cheilitis
Lipid cell tumours, 579–80
Lipoblastoma, 849
Lipofuscins, 161
Lipoma, 848
Lipopolysaccharide, *see* Endotoxins
Liposarcoma, 848–50
Lipoxygenase pathway, 36
Liquefaction necrosis, 24
Listeria monocytogenes, 868
Liver, 410–54
  coagulopathy due to, 452–3
  fatty change, 21, 427
  metastases, 182, 443
  radiation injury, 18
  venous congestion/oedema, 158,
    447
Loa loa, 942
Lobar pneumonia, 49–50, 309, 309–10
Lobular carcinoma, 608
Lobular carcinoma in situ, 604–5
Lobular hepatitis, chronic, 422
Low density lipoprotein,
    glycosylated, 632
Lung, 290–328
  anatomy/function, 290–3
  cancer, 312–19
    secondary (metastases), 182
    smoking and, 207, 312–13
  in liver failure, 452
  oedema, 158, 306–8
  radiation injury, 18
  rheumatoid disease, 323, 834
  tuberculosis, 115–16, 116
  vascular problems, *see entries
    under* Pulmonary
Lupoid hepatitis, chronic, 423
Lupus erythematosus, 766–7
  systemic, 98, 499–501
Lupus vulgaris, 772
Luteinizing hormone, *see*
    Gonadotrophins
Lyell—Ritter disease, 770
Lyme disease, 841–2
Lymph nodes, 73–5, 710–37, *see also*
    Mucocutaneous lymph node
    syndrome
  disorders (non-metastatic), 718–37,
    834
  lymphocyte traffic, 76
  tumour cells in (metastases), 189

Lymph nodes (*contd*)
    breast cancer, 608
    gastric cancer, 365–6
Lymphadenitis, 711, 714, 715
Lymphangiectasia, congenital, 374
Lymphangioleiomyomatosis, 306
Lymphatic system, 710
    large bowel, 396
    penis/scrotum, anomalies, 539
    tumour spread, 179–80
    breast cancer, 610
Lymphoblastic leukaemia, acute, 694–5
Lymphoblastic lymphoma, 731–2, 734
Lymphocyte-depleted Hodgkin's disease, 721–2
Lymphocyte-predominant Hodgkin's disease, 720–1
Lymphocyte traffic, 76, *see also* B cell; Bare lymphocyte syndrome; T cell
Lymphocytic leukaemia, chronic, 697–9
Lymphocytic lymphoma, 726, 727–9, 732
Lymphoedema, 157
Lymphogranuloma venereum, 542–3, 714
Lymphoid hyperplasia, *see* Hyperplasia
Lymphoid (lymphoreticular) system, 704–49
    radiation injury, 18
Lymphokines, *see* Cytokines
Lymphoma, 723–35, 746–7
    Hodgkin's, *see* Hodgkin's disease
    non-Hodgkin's/in general, 723–35, 746–7
    in AIDS, 728, 875
    breast, 611
    gastric, 368
    ovarian, 580
    small bowel, 379
    splenic, 746–7
    testicular, 536
    thymic, 709
Lymphoproliferative disorders, post-transplant, 105
Lymphoreticular system, *see* Lymphoid system
Lynch syndrome, 403–4
Lysosomes, 36

disorders, 13, 41
    storage disease, 13, 742–3
fusion, 39, 41

McArdle's disease, 934
Macrocytic anaemia, 653, 653–9
Macroglobulinaemia, Waldenström, 736–7
Macrophages, 65–8, 108–10
    alveolar, 294
    in atherosclerosis, 233
    in inflammation, 42, 44, 65–8, 108–10
    tumours and, 191
Maculopathy, 944, 948
Magnesium ammonium phosphate stones, 506
Major histocompatibility complex (MHC; HLA), 77–8
    associated disease, 105–7
    transplants and, 99–103
Malabsorption, 371
Malakoplakia, 518
Malaria, 743–4, 875–6
Malignant disease (cancer), 165, 175–83, 193–213, *see also* Tumours *and histological types*
    adrenal cortex, 627, 629
    bladder, 518–19
    bone, 817–19
    breast, 202, 603–10
        males, 612
    cell differentiation in, 174
    eye
        conjunctiva, 943
        intraocular, 948
    fallopian tubes, 590–1
    gallbladder, 458–9
    haematological, 691–9
    hypercalcaemia in, 812–13
    of immune system, 88
    ionizing radiation and, 210–11, 786, 847
    kidney, 508–12
    large bowel, 381, 382, 402, 403–6, 409
    liver, 438–42, 442–3
    lymph node, 718–35
    oesophagus, 352–3
    oral cavity, 336–9, 345–7
    ovary, 571, 572, 573, 574, 576–7
    pancreas, 465, 636
    penis, 545

Malignant disease (cancer) (*contd*)
  pituitary, 619
  pleura, 321
  prostate, 548–60
  respiratory tract
    lower, *see* Lung, cancer
    upper, 284–6, 289–90
  salivary gland, 285, 343–7
  skin, 732–3, 785–6, 788–90, 792–8
    sunlight and, 210, 785, 793
  small bowel, 377–8, 379
  soft tissue, 848–50, 850–1, 852–9, 862
  spleen, 746–7, 748–9
  spread, 175–83, *see also* Metastases
    breast cancer, 611
    gastric cancer, 365–6
    lung cancer, 315–16
    oesophageal cancer, 353
    oral cancer, 338
  stomach, 263–8, 360
  testis, 533–4, 535, 536
  thrombosis and, 145–6
  thyroid, 645–8
  urethra, 522
  uterus, 595–6
    cervix, 564–6
    endometrium, 210, 559–61
    myometrium, 568–9
  vagina, 587–8
  vasculitis in, 273
  vulva, 583–5
Malignant hypertension, 497
Malnutrition, *see* Nutritional status
MALT, *see* Mucosa-associated lymphoid tissue
Mantle cell lymphoma, 379, 726, 729–30
Marburg virus, 421
Marginal zone lymphoma, splenic, 747
Marjolin's ulcer, 786
Mast cells, 35–6
Meckel's diverticula, 370–1
Mediterranean fever, familial, 127
Mediterranean lymphoma, 379
Medulla
  adrenal, 620
  renal
    cystic disease, 472–3
    damage, 488
Medulla oblongata, elongation, 867
Medullary carcinoma
  breast, 607
  thyroid, 647–8

Medulloblastoma, 906
Megacolon
  acquired, 398
  congenital, 397–8
Megaloblastic anaemia, 653–5
Meibomian cyst (chalazion), 939
Melanin pigmentation, 159–60, 331
Melanocytic lesions, 791–7
  conjunctiva, 943
Melanoma, malignant, 792–7
  conjunctival, 943
  intraocular, 948–9
  vulval, 585
Membrane, cell
  injury, 11
    exotoxins, 16
  in myocardial ischaemia, 238
  neoplastic change and, 171–2
  viral infection and, 130, 132
Membranous glomerulonephritis, 477–8
Membranous inflammation, 43
Ménière's disease, 953
Meningioma, 906–7
Meningitis, 867–71
  meningococcal, 623, 868
Meningocele, 866
Meningococcal meningitis, 623, 868
Meningoencephalitis, 876
Meningomyelocele, 866
Meningovascular syphilis, 121
Menopause
  bone loss, 805–6
  breast at, 598
Menstrual cycle and disorders, 555–6
Merkel cell tumour, 790
Mesangiocapillary glomerulonephritis, 482–4
Mesangioproliferative glomerulonephritis, 252, 484
Mesangium, 468
Mesenchymal chondrosarcoma, 818
Mesoblastic nephroma, congenital, 511
Mesonephric duct, *see* Müllerian duct
Mesonephroid carcinoma, ovary, 573
Mesothelioma, malignant, 321
Metabolic disturbances
  diabetes, 630, 632–3
  leukaemia, 693–4
Metabolic myopathies, 932–5

Metabolic neuropathies, hereditary, 921–4
Metachromatic leucodystrophy, 921–2
Metaplasia, 174
  apocrine, 601
  endometrial, 557
  squamous, *see* Squamous metaplasia
Metastases
  distant, 165, 181–3
    in liver, 182, 443
    from lung, 315
    in ovaries, 580
    process of metastasis, 175, 181–3
    in spleen, 749
    from stomach, 366
  lymph node, *see* Lymph nodes
Metastasizing leiomyomatosis, benign, 567
Metastatic calcification, 162–3
MHC, *see* Major histocompatibility complex
Microcytic anaemia, 653, 655–9
Microvasculature/circulation (small blood vessels)
  in acute inflammation, 26
  inflammation of, 276–9
  syphilis affecting, 121
  type III hypersensitivity and, 92–3
Miliary tuberculosis, 115
Mineralocorticoids, 621
Missense mutations, 226
Mitochondrial disorders, 220, 227, 932
Mitral valve disease, 248–9
  rheumatic, 245–6
Mixed-cellularity Hodgkin's disease, 721
Mole (molar pregnancy), 592–4
Mole (skin), *see* Naevus
Molecular pathology, 6–7
Moll's gland, cyst, 940
Monoclonal gammopathy, benign, 737
Mononuclear phagocytes, 42
Mononucleosis, infectious, 714–15
Monosomy 21, 216
Morbid anatomy, 7–9
Morquio's syndrome, 804
Motor neurone disease, 882–3
Mucinous (colloid) tumours
  breast, 607
  ovary, 572
Mucocutaneous candidiasis, 781–2

Mucocutaneous lymph node syndrome, 278, 717
Mucoepidermoid carcinoma, 346–7
Mucoid adenocarcinoma, stomach, 367
Mucormycosis, 384
Mucosa
  gastroduodenal, 354, 355–6
  large bowel, 396–7
Mucosa-associated lymphoid tissue (MALT), 75–6
  lymphomas of, 368
Mucoviscidosis (cystic fibrosis), 426, 463–4
Müllerian (mesonephric) duct development, 551
  abnormal, 551–2
  remnants, 582
Müllerian tumours, mixed, 561–2
Multiple endocrine neoplasias, 637
  type I, 637
  type IIa/IIb, 205, 637, 647
Multiple lymphomatous polyposis, 379
Multiple myeloma, 735–6
Multiple sclerosis, 879–80
Mumps, 529–30
Muscle
  atrophy, 170
    progressive, 883
  heart, *see* Myocardium
  in hyperparathyroidism, 812
  in neoplastic disease, 187–8
  skeletal, *see* Skeletal muscle
  tumours of, 850–5
Muscular dystrophy, 927–9
Muscularis propria
  bladder, 515
  bowel, 397
Musculoskeletal system, *see* Bone; Joint; Muscle
Mutations, *see* Single gene defects
Mutator genes, 202
Myasthenia gravis (and myasthenic syndromes), 98, 107, 707, 937–8
Mycobacterium
  avium intracellulare, 387, 713
  leprae, 117–18, 916
  marinum, 775
  tuberculosis, *see* Tuberculosis
Mycoplasma spp., 272
Mycosis fungoides, 732–3
Mycotic aneurysms, 251, 891

Myelin, 910, *see also* Demyelinating
    disorders
  nerve fibres with/without, 909
Myelodysplastic syndromes,
    699–701
Myelofibrosis, idiopathic, 702–3
Myeloid leukaemia
  acute, 695–6
  chronic, 692–3, 696–7
Myeloma, multiple, 735–6
Myelomeningocele
    (meningomyelocele), 866
Myeloproliferative disorders, 701–3,
    746
Myocarditis, 257–8
Myocardium, *see also*
    Endomyocardial fibrosis
  infarction, 240–2, 266
  ischaemia, 236–9
  in rheumatic fever, 244
  structural/functional
    abnormalities, 252–9
Myoclonic epilepsy and ragged red
    fibres, 932
Myometrium, 566–9
Myopathies, 927–36
  vacuolar, 873
Myotonic dystrophy, 929–30
Myxoid malignant fibrous
    histiocytoma, 857–8
Myxopapillary ependymomoa,
    904–5

Naevus
  melanocytic, 790–2
  Ota's, 940
  strawberry, 799
  white sponge, 331
Nail, candidiasis, 781
2-Naphthylamine, 207
Nasopharynx, 282–6
Natural killer cells and tumours, 191
Necrobiosis lipoidica diabeticorum,
    783
Necrosis, 24–5, *see also* Infarction
  bone, 60
    ischaemic, 827–8
  fat, 24–5, 598–9
  fibrinoid, 44, 497
  gummatous, 121
  renal cortical, 503
  renal papillary, 492–3, 634
Necrotizing enterocolitis, 400
Necrotizing fasciitis, 543–4, 771–2

Necrotizing lymphadenitis,
    histiocytic, 717
Neisseria gonorrhoeae, *see* Gonorrhoea
Neisseria meningitidis
    (meningococcus), 623, 868
Nemaline myopathy, 931
Neonates, *see* Newborn
Neoplasms, *see* Tumours
Nephritic syndrome, 156, 252, 474
Nephritis, interstitial, 489
Nephroblastoma (Wilms' tumour),
    199, 510–12
Nephrology, *see* Kidney
Nephroma, congenital mesoblastic,
    511
Nephronophthisis, juvenile, 472–3
Nephrosclerosis, 496–7
Nephrotic syndrome, 146, 156, 474
  minimal change, 476–8
Nerve sheath tumours, 907
Nerve supply, *see also* Denervation;
    Reinnervation
  large bowel, 396
  oesophagus, 348
Nervous system, 863–931, *see also*
    Central nervous system;
    Peripheral nervous system
  in neoplastic disease, 187–8
  radiation damage, 18
  repair, 61
  toxins, 16
Neural tube defects, 866–7
Neurinoma, *see* Neuroma
Neuroblastoma, olfactory, 285–6
Neurodegeneration
  CNS, 880–8
  peripheral nerve, 910–11
Neuroectodermal tumours, 901–6
  primitive, 823, 905
Neuroendocrine tumours
  skin, 790
  stomach, 366–7
Neurofibroma, 908
Neurofibromatosis, 205–6
  type 1 (and NF-1 gene), 200
Neurohypophysis, 613, 614
  disorders, 616–17
Neuroma (neurinoma;
    schwannoma), 907, 953
  acoustic, 953
Neuromuscular disorders, 937–8
Neuronal Charcot–Marie–Tooth
    disease, 919
Neuronal intestinal dysplasia, 398
Neuronopathies, 910

Neuropathic joints, 832
Neuropathies, 910–24
    amyloid (hereditary/familial),
        126–7, 127
    oesophageal peristalsis, 350
Neuropraxia, 913
Neurosyphilis, 121–2, 871–2
Neurotmesis, 914
Neurotoxins, bacterial, 16
Neutropenia, 40–1
Neutrophils
    cytoplasmic autoantibodies, 272
    defective function, 40–2
    in inflammation, 30, 32–3
Newborns/neonates, see also Infants
    haemolytic disease, 673
    haemorrhagic disease, 688–9
    ophthalmitis, 942
Nezelof syndrome, 86, 705
Niemann–Pick, 742–3
Nipple
    adenoma, 602
    Paget's disease, 607
Nitric oxide, 109
    septic shock and, 267
Nitrogen embolism, 149, 889
Nitrosamines and nitrosamides, 208
Nodular fasciitis, 860
Nodular glomerulosclerosis, 634
Nodular goitre, toxic, 642
Nodular hyperplasia
    focal (liver), 437
    prostatic, 169, 547–8
Nodular lymphocyte-predominant
        Hodgkin's disease, 720
Nodular melanoma, 796
Nodular sclerosis Hodgkin's disease,
        721
Nodular transformation (liver),
        437–8
Nodular tuberculide, 774–5
Nodules, rheumatoid, 833–4
Nodulocystic acne, 769
Non-insulin-dependent diabetes
        mellitus, 630–1
Nonsense mutations, 226
Norwalk virus, 388
Nose, 282–6
    defence mechanisms, 282, 293
Nucleic acid, viral, uncoating, 130–1
Nucleus
    in cell death, 22
    injury, 11
    proteins in, as tumour
        suppressors, 200

Null-cell adenoma, 618
Nutritional status (incl.
        malnutrition)
    CNS and, 877–9
    immunity and, 88
    oedema and, 156
    wound healing and, 58

Obstruction
    bladder outflow, 516
    small bowel, 375–9
    tumours causing, 184
Obstructive airway disease, chronic,
        294–300
Occupation carcinogens, 208, 209
    lung cancer, 313
Ocular disorders, see Eye
Oedema (swelling), 154–8
    acute cellular, 18–19
    angioneurotic, 288
    cardiogenic, 155, 206–7, 306
    in inflammation, 26, 27–8, 47
    pulmonary, 158, 306–8
Oesophagus, 348–53
Oestrogens
    endometrial carcinoma and, 210
    menstrual disorders and, 555–6
Olfactory neuroblastoma, 285–6
Oligodendroglioma, 903–4
Olivopontocerebellar atrophy, 882
Onchocerciasis, 942
Oncocytoma (oncocytic/oxyphilic
        adenoma)
    pituitary, 618
    renal, 510
    salivary gland, 345
Oncogene(s), 193–7
Oncogenesis (carcinogenesis;
        tumourigenesis), 193–212
    lung cancer and, 313
    viruses in, see Viral infection
Ophthalmic disorders, see Eye
Ophthalmoplegia, chronic
        progressive external, 932
Opsonins/opsonisation, 33, 39, 108
Oral cavity, 330–9
    infections, 332–5, 781
Oral contraceptives, 145
Orchitis, 528–30
Organization (wound), 50
Organophosphate poisoning, 915
Orthomyxoviruses, 138
Osler–Rendu–Weber syndrome,
        678

Osteitis, tuberculous, 829
Osteoarthritis, 830-2
Osteoblastoma, benign, 820
Osteochondroma, 815
Osteogenesis imperfecta, 804-5
Osteoid osteoma, 819-20
Osteoma, 819-20
Osteomalacia, 806-10
Osteomyelitis, vertebral, 828
Osteopetrosis, 814
Osteoporosis, 170, 805-6
Osteosarcomas, 820-2
Ostium primum/secundum, 261
Ota's naevus, 940
Otitis media, 951
Otosclerosis, 952
Ovaries, 569-80
    development, 551
Oxygen radicals, see Free radicals
Oxyphilic adenoma, see Oncocytoma

p16, 202
p53, 201-2
Paget's disease (bone), 813-14
Paget's disease (skin)
    nipple, 607
    perianal, 409
    vulval, 583-5
Pain in inflammation, 29
Palate, cleft, 330
Panacinar emphysema, 297
Pancreas, 461-5, 629-37
Pancreatitis, 462-3
Papillary adenoma, 464
Papillary carcinoma
    renal cell, 509
    serous (endometrial), 560
    thyroid, 645-6
Papillary carcinoma in situ, 604
Papillary muscles, 249
    rupture, 241
Papillary necrosis, renal, 492-3, 634
Papilloma, 165
    basal cell, 787-8
    brain, 905
    conjunctiva, 943
    upper respiratory, 284, 289
Papilloma viruses, 211
    human, 211, 334, 543, 565, 776-8
Papovaviruses, 137
Papulonecrotic tuberculide, 774-5
Papulosis, bowenoid, 544-5
Papulosquamous disorders, 765-9
Paracortical hyperplasia, 712

Paraffin section, 4-5
Paraganglioma, 952
Paramyxoviruses, 138-9
Paranasal sinuses, 282-6
Paraneoplastic syndromes (systemic
        abnormalities), 185-8
    lung cancer, 316
Parasites, see Helminths; Protozoa
Parathyroid disorders, 810, 810-12
Parenteral nutrition, total, infant, 445
Parkinson's disease, 880-1
Parosteal osteosarcoma, 821-2
Parotid glands, 339
Parotitis, chronic recurrent, 342
Paroxysmal nocturnal
        haemoglobinuria, 671-2
Patau's syndrome, 217
Pediculosis, 784
Peliosis hepatitis, 449
Pellagra, 878
Pelvis, renal, urothelial tumours, 512
Pemphigoid, bullous, 757
Pemphigus, benign familial, 760
Pemphigus erythematosus, 756-7
Pemphigus foliaceus, 756
Pemphigus vegetans, 756
Pemphigus vulgaris, 755-6
Penis, 537-45
Pepsin secretion, 355
Peptic ulcer, 63, 298, 360-3
Perfusion
    pulmonary, 292
    wound healing and, 59
Pericardial effusions, 258
Pericarditis, 258-9
    rheumatic fever, 244
Periosteal osteosarcoma, 822
Peripheral nervous system, 908-24
    repair, 61
Peritoneal leiomyomatosis,
        disseminated, 567
Pernicious anaemia, 654
Peutz—Jeghers syndrome, 160,
        376-7, 401
Peyer's patches, 75
Peyronie's disease, 539
Phaeochromocytoma, 205, 628-9
Phagocytes
    harmful effects, 47-8
    mononuclear, 42
    movement/chemotaxis, 33
    respiratory burst, 39-40, 108-9
Phagocytosis, 39, 42, 108
    disorders, 41
    in splenic cords, 738-9

Pharyngitis, 136, *see also*
    Nasopharynx
Pharyngoesophageal diverticula,
    351
Philadelphia chromosome, 692–3,
    696
Phosphoribosyl pyrophosphate
    synthetase deficiency, 843
Phyllodes tumour, 610–11
Physical agents, carcinogenic,
    210–11
Pick's disease, 886
Picornaviruses, 137–8
Pigment stones, 455–6
Pigmentation, 159–62
    oral, 331
    in Peutz–Jeghers syndrome, 376
Pigmented villonodular synovitis,
    845–6
Pilar cyst, 787
Pilonidal sinus, 408
Pinguecula, 940–1
'Pink puffer', 298
Pituitary, 613–19
Pityriasis rosea, 767–8
Pityriasis rubra pilaris, 768
Pityriasis versicolor, 779
Placental site trophoblastic tumour,
    596
Plasma cells
    Castleman's disease, 718
    dyscrasias, 735–7
Plasminogen activators, 687
Platelet(s), 141–2, 679–84
    disorders, 144, 680–4
        in cancer, 186
    endothelium and, 141, 687
    in haemostasis, 141–2, 679–84
    splenectomy and, 741
Platelet-activating factor, 36
Platelet-derived growth factor
    atherosclerosis and, 233
    neoplasia and, 172
    wound healing and, 56
Pleural disease, 328–9
    asbestos-related, 321
Pneumococcus, *see Streptococcus
    pneumoniae*
Pneumoconioses, 296–7, 319–23
Pneumonia, 136, 308–11
    lobar, 49–50, 309, 309–10
Point mutations, 225
Polyarteritis nodosa, 276
Polychondritis, relapsing, 950
Polycyclic hydrocarbons, 206–7

Polycystic ovary syndrome, 570
Polycystic renal disease, 471–2
Polycythaemias, 701–2
Polymerase chain reaction, 6–7
Polymyositis, 188, 936
Polyneuropathies, 917–18, 921
Polyoma virus, 211–12
Polyps (and polyposis)
    cervical, 563
    endometrial, 559
    large bowel, 200, 204, 382, 401, 403
    nasal, 283
    small bowel, 376, 379–80
    vocal cord, 288–9
Pompe's disease, 933
Porphyrias, 923–4
Portal fibrosis, 424
Portal hypertension, 429, 449–50
Portal vein, 411
Posterior urethral valves, 520
Post-mortem, 7–9
Poxviruses, 134–5
Preauricular sinus, 950
Precancer, *see also* Intraepithelial
        neoplasia
    gastric, 364
    skin, 788
Pre-eclampsia, 592, 593
Pregnancy, 591–6
    breast cancer risk and parity,
        605
    breast in, 598
Prematurity, retinopathy of, 947–8
Presbyacusis, 952
Pressure palsy, hereditary liability,
    921
Primitive neuroectodermal tumours,
    823, 905
Progesterone and menstrual
        disorders, 556
Prolactinoma, 618–19
Proliferation, *see* Growth and
        proliferation
Prostate, 545–50
    hyperplasia, 169, 547–8
Protein C, 686–7
    deficiency, 144–5, 690–1
    resistance, 145, 691
Protein S, 686
    deficiency, 145, 691
Protein undernutrition, wound
        healing, 58
Proteinuria, 375
Proteolytic enzymes and tumour
        spread, 177

Prothrombin time, 686
Proto-oncogenes, *see* Oncogenes
Protozoal infection
    brain, 875–7
        in AIDS, 874
    conjunctiva, 942
    immune response, 83
    intestinal, 388–90
    splenic, 743–4
Pseudogout, 845
Pseudohermaphroditism
    female, 553
    male, 527
Pseudomembranous colitis, 384–5
Psoriasis, 752–4
    arthropathy, 839
Pterygium, 941
Ptyalism, 341
Pubic lice, 784
Pulmonary atresia, 262
Pulmonary circulation, 292–3, 323–8
    in congenital heart disease, 261–3
    embolism, 148, 323–4
    hypoxaemia effects, 298
Pulmonary non-vascular problems,
        see Lung
Pulmonary valve disease, 249
Pulp histiocytosis, 712
Pulseless disease, 273–4
Purine nucleoside dephosphorylase
        deficiency, 706
Purulent (suppurative) inflammation,
        43
Purpura
    Henoch–Schönlein, 279
    thrombocytopenic, *see*
        Thrombocytopenic purpura
Pyelonephritis, 489–91
Pyloric antrum, 354
Pyloric stenosis, hypertrophic, 356
Pyogenic granuloma, 288, 799
Pyramidal system, degenerative
        disorders, 882–3
Pyruvate kinase deficiency, 664–5

Race and atherosclerosis, 234
Radial scar, 600
Radiation, *see* Ionizing radiation;
        Ultraviolet
Rapamycin, 104
Ras
    colorectal cancer and, 404
    leukaemias and, 693
    lung cancer and, 313

Reactive arthropathies, 838–42
Reactive epithelial hyperplasia, 170
Reactive systemic amyloidosis,
        125–6
REAL classification, 724
Recessive mutations, 219, 221–2
Rectum, 395–406
    ulcer, solitary, 395
Red cells (erythrocytes), 650–77
    disorders of/affecting, 651–77
        in liver failure, 452
        in neoplasia, 186
Red pulp, 740
Reed–Sternberg cells, 719
Refsum's disease, 922
Regeneration
    axon, 911
    tissue, 50–1
Reifensteins's syndrome, 527–8
Reinnervation, 937
Reiter's syndrome, 521–2, 838
Renal arteries, 466
    stenosis, 497–8
Renal cell carcinoma, 508–10
Renal tissue, *see* Kidney
Renal vein thrombosis, 503
Rendu–Osler–Weber syndrome,
        678
Renin-angiotensin system and heart
        failure, 265
Reoviruses, 140
Reproductive system, 523–612
    female, 551–612
    male, 523–50
Resolution, 49–50
    pneumonia, 310
'Respirator brain', 898
Respiratory burst, 39–40, 108–9
Respiratory distress syndrome,
        adult, 307–8
Respiratory system, 282–329
    infections, *see* Infection
Restrictive cardiomyopathy, 255–7
Restrictive ventilatory impairment,
        302–8
Retention polyp, juvenile, 401
Retinoblastoma (and RB gene),
        198–9, 200–1, 605, 949
Retinoic acid receptor, 693
Retinopathy, 947–9
    diabetic, 634–5
Retrolental fibroplasia, 947–8
Retroviruses, 140
    oncogenic, 194
    replication, 131

Reye's syndrome, 446
Rhabdoid tumour of kidney, 511–12
Rhabdomyolysis, 936
Rhabdomyoma, 852, 853
Rhabdomyosarcoma, 852–5
    embryonal, 588, 854
Rhabdoviruses, 139
Rheumatic fever/heart disease,
        242–6
Rheumatoid disease/arthritis, 106,
        744–5, 832–6
    coalminers with, 323
Rhinitis, allergic, 283
Rhinoscleroma, 283
Rickets, 808
Rickettsial infections, 272
Riedel's thyroiditis, 644
Right-to-left shunts, 261–3
Riley—Day syndrome, 920–1
Ringworm (tinea), 779–80
RNA splice mutations, 226
RNA viruses, 137–40
    oncogenic, 195
    replication, 131
Rosacea, 769–70
Rosai—Dorfman disease, 716
Rotavirus, 387–8
Rotor syndrome, 413
Roussy—Lévy syndrome, 919

Saccular aneurysm, 894–5
Salivary glands, 339–47
    tumours, 285, 343–7
Salmonella spp., 385–6
Salpingitis, 589–90
Salt retention, 155
Sarcoidosis, 118–19, 304–5, 716
Sarcoma(s), 165
    bone, 817–19, 820–2, 824–5
    breast, 611
    endometrial stromal, 561
    hepatic, 442–3
    Kaposi's, 797–8, 874
    myometrial, 568–9
    renal, 512
    soft tissue, 848–50, 850–1, 852–7
    splenic, 748
Sarcoma botryoides, 588, 854
Sarcomatoid renal cell carcinoma,
        509
Sarcoptes scabei, 782
Scabies, 782
Scar
    hyperplastic, 859–60

keloid, 859
    radial, 600
Scar tissue, granulomas, 111
Scatter factor, 178
Schistosomiasis, 517
Schwann cells, 910
Schwannoma, see Neuroma
Sclerosing adenosis, breast, 601
Sclerosing cholangitis, 431–2
Sclerosing haemangioma, 798
Scrotum, 537–45
Seborrhoeic dermatitis, 754
Seborrhoeic keratosis, 787–8
Selectins, 30
Seminoma, 531–2
Senear—Usher syndrome, 756–7
Sensorimotor neuropathy,
        hereditary, 919–20
Sensory and autonomic neuropathy,
        hereditary, 920–1
Septic shock, 266–7
Serous tumours
    endometrium, 560
    ovary, 571–2
    pancreas, 464
Sertoli cells, 523
Severe combined immune
        deficiency, 84–5, 705–6
Sex and atherosclerosis, 234
Sex chromosomes
    anomalies/aneuploidy, 218–19,
        552–3
    single gene defects, see X-linked
        disorders
Sex cord-stromal tumours
    ovary, 577–80
    testis, 535–6
Sexual development
    females, 551–2, 597–8
        abnormalities, 551–4
    males, 524–5
        abnormalities, 525–8, 538–9
Sézary syndrome, 733
Shigella dysentery, 384
Shingles, see Herpes zoster
Shock, 265–7
Shock lung, 307–8
Shunts, cardiac, 259–63
Sialadenitis, 342
Sialorrhoea, 341
Sickle cell disease, 666–8
    renal problems, 493
Sideroblastic anaemia, 655, 658, 659
Signal transduction, 38
Silicosis, 323

Simian vacuolating virus, 212
Sinus histiocytosis, 712
    with massive lymphadenopathy,
        716
Sinuses, paranasal, 282–6
Sinusoid (liver), 411
    portal hypertension and, 450
Sjögren's syndrome, 342–3
Skeletal muscle, 925–38
    tumours, 852–5
Skeletal system, see Bone; Joint;
        Muscle
Skin, 750–800
    cancer-associated disorders, 188
    in liver failure, 453
    radiation effects, 18, 786
    tumours, 785–800, 850
        malignant, see Malignant
            disease
Small cell carcinoma
    lung, 314, 317
    stomach, 367
Small intestine, 369–79
Small lymphocytic lymphoma,
        727–9, 732
Smoking
    atherosclerosis and, 234–5
    cancer and, 207
        lung, 207, 312–13
    chronic bronchitis/emphysema
        and, 295
Smooth muscle cells and plaque
        genesis, 233
Smooth muscle tumours, 850–1
Soft tissue changes in cancer, 187
Spasm, oesophageal, 350
Sperm granuloma, 536–7
Spermatic cord, torsion, 537
Spermatocytic seminoma, 532
Spherocytosis, hereditary, 663–4
Sphingolipidoses, 742–3
Spina bifida, 866
Spindle-cell lipoma, 849
Spirochaetosis, intestinal, 387
Spitz naevus, 792
Spleen, 75, 737–49
    venous congestion/oedema,
        158
Splenectomy, effects, 740–1
Splenomegaly, 741–7
Spondylitis, ankylosing, 106, 837–8
Spondyloarthropathies, 836–8
Spongiform encephalopathies,
        transmissible, 887–8
Sprue, tropical, 373

Squamous cell carcinoma
    anal, 409
    cervical, 564–6
    conjunctival, 943
    cutaneous, 788
    laryngeal, 289, 290
    oral, 337–8
    penile, 545
    vaginal, 587
    vulval, 585
Squamous hyperplasia, vulval,
        581–2
Squamous metaplasia, 174
    conjunctiva, 941
Staining, section, 5
Staphylococcal scaled skin
        syndrome, 770
Steatocystoma multiplex, 787
Steatohepatitis, 424, 427–8
Stem cell deficiency, 84
Steroid cell tumours, 579–80
Stevens – Johnson syndrome, 758
Still's disease, 836
Stomach, 353–68
    ulcer, 360, see also Peptic ulcer
Stones, see Calculi
Stop codon mutations, 226
Storage diseases
    glycogen, 933–5
    lysosomal, 13, 742–3
Storage pool disease, 683
Strawberry naevus, 799
Streptococcal sore throat, 243
Streptococcus pneumoniae
        (pneumococcus)
    meningitis, 868
    pneumonia, 309–10
Stress proteins, 13–14
Stroke, 888–96
Stroma
    cervical, decidual reaction,
        563–4
    neoplasia and the, 164
    spread of, 177–8
Stromal keratitis, 945
Stromal tumours
    breast, 610–12
    endometrial, 561–2
    sex cord, see Sex cord-stromal
        tumours
Sty, 939
Subarachnoid haemorrhage, 893–4
Subclavian artery occlusion, 890
Subcutaneous tissue, 751
Subdural haematoma, 899–900

Subendocardial myocardial
   infarction, 240
Sublingual glands, 339
Submandibular glands, 339
Submucosa, large bowel, 397
Sunlight and skin cancer, 210, 785,
   793
Suppurative inflammation, 43
Surgical pathology, 3–6
SV40, 212
Swallowing, 348–9
   problems (dysphagia), 349–53
Swelling, see Oedema
Swimming pool granuloma, 775
Sympathetic ophthalmitis, 946
Synovial chondromatosis, 846
Synovial joints, 829–30
Synovial sarcoma, 857–8
Synovitis, pigmented villonodular,
   845–6
Syphilis, 119–22
   aortic aneurysms, 268, 270
   CNS effects, 121–2, 871–2
   male genitalia, 529, 541–2
   oral lesions, 332
Systemic lupus erythematosus, 98,
   499–501
Systemic sclerosis, 501–2

T cell (T lymphocyte), 69, 69–71, 76,
   78–80, 80, see also Human
   T-cell leukaemia virus
   activation, 78–80
   antigen recognition, 78
   autoimmunity and, 97
   deficiencies, 86, 705
   graft rejection and, 102
   in HIV infection, 89
   in lymph nodes, 75, 711
   tumours and, 191
T-cell acute lymphoblastic
   leukaemia, 695
T-cell lymphomas, 733–5
   enteropathy-associated, 379
Tabes dorsalis, 121–2
Tacrolismus, 104
Takayasu's arteritis, 273–4
Tamponade, cardiac, 258
Tangier disease, 923
Tarui's disease, 934
Telangiectasia
   ataxia, 85, 204, 727
   hereditary haemorrhagic, 678
Temporal arteritis, 274

Tendon sheath, giant cell tumour,
   845–6
Teratoma
   ovary, 576–7
   testis, 532–4
Testis, 523–37
Testosterone, inadequate, 526
Tetanus toxin, 16
Tetralogy of Fallot, 261–2
Thalassaemias, 668–71
   α-, 223, 668–9
Thecoma, 578
Thrombasthenia, 683
Thrombin time, 686
Thrombocythemia, essential, 703
Thrombocytopenia, 680–1
Thrombocytopenic purpura
   idiopathic, 745–6
   thrombotic, 504–5, 681
Thrombophlebitis obliterans, 275
Thrombosis, 141–8, 690–1, see also
   Embolism
   atheromatous plaque and, 142–3,
      233–4
   intraventricular, 241–2
   risk factors, 144–6, 690–1
   venous, see Veins
Thrombotic endocarditis,
   non-bacterial, 252
Thrombotic thrombocytopenic
   purpura, 504–5, 681
Thrush, 334
Thymus, 704–9
Thyroid, 637–48
   hyperplasia, 169, 641–2
Thyroiditis, 640, 643–4
Thyrotrope adenoma, 619
Tinea (ringworm), 779–80
Togaviruses, 139–40
Tolerance (immune), 94–5
Tophaceous gout, 844–5
Total parenteral nutrition, infant,
   445
Toxic neuropathies, 914–16
Toxic nodular goitre, 642
Toxins, bacterial, see Bacterial toxins
Toxoplasma gondii
   encephalitis, 874, 876
   lymphadenitis, 715
Trachoma, 942
Transcoelomic tumour spread, 181
Transcription
   mutations affecting, 226
   promoters, in oncogene activation,
      196–7

Transforming growth factors (TGF), 56-7
TGF-α, 56-7, 172
TGF-β, 57, 66, 71, 172-3
Transfusion reactions, 673
Transient ischaemic attacks, 891
Transitional carcinoma, urinary, 512, 518-19
Translocations, chromosomal, 197, 215-16, 847
lymphoma, 726
Transmural myocardial infarction, 240-1, 241-2
Transplantation, see Graft
Transposition of great vessels, 262
Transudate, 154
Traumatic injury
head, 898-901
nerve, 913-14
spleen, 746
Treponema pallidum, see Syphilis
Trichilemmal cyst, 787
Triglyceride, intracellular accumulation, 20-1
Trisomies, 216-18
chromosome 21 (Down's syndrome), 203, 216-17
Trophoblastic disease, 592-6
Tropical splenomegaly, 744
Tropical sprue, 373
Truncus arteriosus, persistent, 262-3
Trypanosomiasis, 876-7
Tuberculoid leprosy, 118, 916
Tuberculosis, 112-17, 772-5
bone, 829
CNS, 870, 871
cutaneous, 772-5
intestinal, 386-7
joints, 840-1
laryngeal, 287-8
lymph node, 713
oral, 332
pericardial, 258-9
testicular, 529
Tubular adenoma, 602
Tubular carcinoma, 606-7
Tubules, renal, 487-93
salt/water retention, 155
Tumour(s) (neoplasms), 164-6, 171-212
adrenal, 627-9
bladder, 518-22
bone, 815-25
breast, 202, 601-10, 612
cervix, 564-6

classification, 165
ear, 952, 953
endometrium, 210, 559-62
eye
conjunctiva, 943
intraocular, 948-9
eyelid, 940
fallopian tubes, 590-1
gallbladder, 458-60
haematological, 691-9
heart, 852
in HIV disease/AIDS, 728, 797-8, 874
host effects of, 184-9
host effects on, 190-2
of immune system, 88
immunodeficiency/immunosuppression-related, 105, 190, 727
initiation and promotion, 208-9
joints, 845-6
kidney, 507-12
large bowel, 381-2, 402-6, 409
liver, 438-43
lymph node, 718-37
malignant, see Malignant disease
myometrium, 566-9
nervous system, 901-8, 924
oesophagus, 352-3
oral cavity, 336-9
osteomalacia and, 808-9
ovary, 570-80
pancreas, 464-5, 635-7
parathyroid, 811
penis, 544-5
pituitary, 617-20
prostate, 548-60
respiratory tract
lower, 312-19
upper, 284-6, 289-90
salivary gland, 285, 343-7
skin, 785-800, 850
small bowel, 377-9
soft tissue, 846-59
spleen, 746-7, 748-9
spread, see Malignant disease
stomach, 363-8
testis, 530-6
thymus, 707-9
thyroid, 644-8
urethra, 522
vagina, 586-8
vulva, 583-5
Tumour-like conditions
bone, 825-7
breast, 601-3

Tumour-like conditions (*contd*)
  joints, 845–6
  liver, 437–8
  penis, 543–4
  skin, 786–8, 799–800
  soft tissue, 859–62
Tumour necrosis factors (TNF), 66, 70
  TNF-α, 37–8, 57–8, 66, 70
Tumour suppressor genes, 197–202
Tumourigenesis, *see* Oncogenesis
Turcot syndrome, 205, 403
Turner syndrome, 218, 552

Ulcer(s), 47
  aphthous, 335
  dendritic corneal, 944–5
  Marjolin's, 786
  peptic, 63, 298
  rectal, solitary, 395
  venous, 281
  vulval, 582
Ulcerative colitis, 392–4
Ultraviolet light and skin cancer, 210, 785, 793
Undifferentiated tumours, *see* Anaplastic tumours
Urachus, congenital anomalies, 516
Uraemic neuropathy, 924
Urate arthropathy, 842–5
Ureter, urothelial tumours, 512
Urethra, 519–22
  developmental disorders, 520, 538–9
Uric acid stones, 506–7
Urinary bladder, *see* Bladder
Urinary tract, 466–522
  infections, *see* Infections
  radiation injury, 19
  upper, 466–513
Urothelium, 514–15
  tumours, upper urinary, 512
Urticaria, contact, 764
Urticarial vasculitis, 279
Uterus, 554–69
  developmental abnormalities, 551–2
Uveitis, 945–6

Vacuolar myopathy, 873
Vagina, 551, 585–8
Valsalva's sinus, aneurysm, 269

Valves, heart, disorders, 242–52
Varicella-zoster virus, *see* Chickenpox; Herpes zoster
Varicocele, 537
Varicose veins, 280–1
Vasculature (blood vessels)
  bleeding disorders due to, 678–9
  cerebral, disorders, 888–901
  dermal, tumours/tumour-like lesions, 799–800
  graft rejection and, 103
  hepatic, 411
    disorders, 447–9
  intestinal, 369, 395–6
    disorders, 399–400
  intima, *see* Intima
  new, in tumours, 175
  pituitary, 613
  in pulmonary hypertension, lesions, 325–7
  radiation injury, 17
  renal, 466–7
    disorders, 502–5
  retinal, disorders, 947–8
  small, *see* Microvasculature
  testicular, disorders, 537
  tumour spread in, 180
Vasculitis (angiitis), 271–9
  rheumatoid, 834
Vasoactive compounds and inflammation, 35–6
Vasoactive intestinal peptide-secreting tumour, 636–7
Vasopressin (ADH), 614
  abnormal production, 616–17
Vegetations, infective endocarditis, 251
Veins, 279–81, *see also* Vasculature
  congestion, 157–8, 447
  kidney, 467
  leiomyomatosis, 567
  occlusion, ischaemia in, 151
  thrombosis, 146–8
    renal, 503
Veno-occlusive disease
  hepatic, 448
  pulmonary, 327
Venous hypertension, pulmonary, 327
Ventilation, 292
  restrictive ventilatory impairment, 302–8
Ventricular aneurysm, 242
Ventricular dilatation, 264

Ventricular infarction, right, 241
Ventricular septum
  congenital defect, 260, 262
  rupture, 241
Ventricular thrombosis, 241–2
Verruca, *see* Wart
Verrucous carcinoma
  oral, 338
  penile, 545
  vulval, 584
Vertebra, 836–8
  infections, 828, 829
Vertebrobasilar disease, 890
Vibrio cholerae, *see* Cholera
VIPoma, 636–7
Viral infection, 129–40
  bladder, 516
  CNS, 870–1, 872–3, 874
  conjunctival, 941–2
  cutaneous, 775–9
  hepatic, 414–21, *see also* Hepatitis
  intestinal, 387–8
  oral, 333–4
  pericardial, 258
  protective response, 82–3, 133–4
  respiratory, 282–3
  tumourigenesis and, 132, 133,
      194–6, 211–13
    lymphoma, 726
Vitamin(s), wound healing and, 58
Vitamin B complex deficiencies,
    877–8
Vitamin D and osteomalacia, 807–8
Vitamin E deficiency, 878–9
Vitamin K, 685
  coagulopathies and, 688–9
Vocal cord polyps, 288–9
  penis, 543
von Recklinghausen's disease
    (NF-1), 200
von Willebrand's disease, 141, 684
Vulva, 581–5

Waldenström macroglobulinaemia,
    736–7
Wallerian degeneration, 910
Warm antibodies, 673–4

Wart (verruca), viral, 776–8
  genital (condyloma acuminata),
      543
Warthin's tumour, 344–5
Wassermann antibodies, 119
Water retention, 155
Waterhouse—Friderichsen
      syndrome, 623
Wegener's granulomatosis, 276–7
Wernicke's encephalopathy, 877–8
Whipple's disease, 373
White cells, *see* Leucocytes
White pulp, 739
White sponge naevus, 331
WHO classification, lymphoma, 724
Wilms' tumour, 199
Wilson's disease, 435–6
Wiskott—Aldrich syndrome, 85–6,
    727
Working Formulation (lymphomas),
    723–4
Wound healing, 48, 53–60

X-linked disorders, 223, *see also* Sex
      chromosomes
  immune deficiency, 86, 87
Xanthelasma, 940
Xanthogranulomatous
      pyelonephritis, 491
Xeroderma pigmentosum, 203–4, 785
Xerostomia, 340–1
XO (Turner) syndrome, 218, 552
XXX superfemale, 219
XXY (Klinefelter's) syndrome, 203,
      218–19, 526
XYY syndrome, 219

Yellow fever, 419
Yersinia enterocolitis, 385
Yersinial lymphadenitis, 714
Yolk sac (endodermal sinus) tumour
    ovary, 575
    testis, 534

Zinc and wound healing, 58